M000287441

Ganong's
Medical Physiology
Examination &
Board Review

Kim E. Barrett, PhD

Distinguished Professor, Department of Medicine
University of California, San Diego
La Jolla, California

Susan M. Barman, PhD

Professor, Department of Pharmacology/Toxicology
Michigan State University
East Lansing, Michigan

Scott Boitano, PhD

Professor, Physiology and Cellular and Molecular Medicine
Arizona Respiratory Center
Bio5 Collaborative Research Institute
University of Arizona
Tucson, Arizona

Jane F. Reckelhoff, PhD

Billy S. Guyton Distinguished Professor
Chair, Department of Biochemistry
Director, Women's Health Research Center
University of Mississippi Medical Center
Jackson, Mississippi

McGraw Hill Education

New York   Chicago   San Francisco   Athens   London   Madrid   Mexico City
Milan   New Delhi   Singapore   Sydney   Toronto

This book was set in Adobe Garamond Pro by Cenveo® Publisher Services.
The editors were Michael Weitz, Brian Kearns, and Peter J. Boyle.
The production supervisor was Catherine H. Saggese.
Art management was by Armen Ovsepyan.
Project management was provided by Anubhav Singh, Cenveo Publisher Services.

This book was printed on acid-free paper.

Dedication

This volume is dedicated to William Francis ("Fran") Ganong, renowned physiologist and neuroendocrinologist. From the first edition in 1963, until the 22nd, he was the sole author of *Review of Medical Physiology*. At the time of his death in 2007, it was one of the most widely used physiology textbook in the world, and it retains an intensely loyal following. His dedication to the volume was legendary, and he was well known for always carrying index cards at his long-term institution, the University of California, San Francisco, where he was a faculty member for almost 50 years and chaired the Department of Physiology from 1970 to 1987. The cards would be used to gather facts from colleagues and visiting speakers, and the facts would be accumulated to inform the next edition of his text—remarkably, completed without fail every 2 years. It is fitting that this new derivative of his life-long work will serve to educate new generations of medical and other health professional students.

Contents

Preface

We have been gratified by the response we have received since taking over the helm of *Ganong's Review of Medical Physiology* with the 23rd edition, and now with two additional editions under our belt. It has been our goal to reorganize and update this venerable resource, while maintaining the features of the book that gave it such an important place in the worldwide marketplace for physiology texts for the 22 editions produced by the extraordinary Professor Fran Ganong. We have paid particular attention to overhauling the graphical aspects of the volume to aid in consistency among chapters and to take advantage of its new full-color format and have added new pedagogical features, such as clinical correlations and therapeutic highlights. Throughout our endeavors to uphold Professor Ganong's unique perspective we have noticed that the book's comprehensive nature reduces its utility as a tool to review physiology content in preparation for Step 1 of the United States Medical Licensing Exam (USMLE). We also felt that the current edition could be improved with supplemental resources with which students can assess their own mastery of the content.

With these limitations in mind, we are pleased to present this companion title, *Ganong's Medical Physiology Examination & Board Review*. Our primary goal has been to streamline the text of the "parent" volume for ease of review, retaining only the most high-yield concepts and illustrations. We have specifically reworked the self-study questions from the original book so that they are consistent with the "clinical vignette" format found in the USMLE and have added many additional questions. In fact, this new book has more than 350 questions to test basic physiology knowledge in an applied context. Finally, every question carries a comprehensive explanation of why the right answer is in fact correct and why the distractors are wrong, further enhancing conceptual understanding of physiology rather than simply reinforcing rote memorization. With these new features, this companion volume represents a robust resource for USMLE preparation.

This new volume also introduces a change in the authorship team. While Professor Heddwen Brooks will continue to contribute to the parent volume, other commitments precluded her involvement in the current project. We are very fortunate to have been able to recruit Professor Jane Reckelhoff to the author group. Janie is an acclaimed teacher of medical and graduate students at the University of Mississippi Medical Center and brings a wealth of experience in the areas of renal, cardiovascular, and gender-related physiology research to our group. Janie's involvement, furthermore, means that three past presidents of the American Physiological Society are now included among the book's authors—perhaps a record for a physiology text.

We hope that a new generation of students will benefit from *Ganong's Medical Physiology Examination & Board Review*—either in conjunction with *Ganong's Review of Medical Physiology*, or as a standalone resource. We also hope that the late Professor Ganong would have been pleased with this evolution of the text that became his life's work.

SECTION I CELLULAR & MOLECULAR BASIS FOR MEDICAL PHYSIOLOGY

The detailed study of physiologic system structure and function has its foundations in physical and chemical laws and the molecular and cellular makeup of each tissue and organ system. This first section provides an overview of the basic building blocks that provide the important framework for human physiology. It is important to note here that these initial sections are not meant to provide an exhaustive understanding of biophysics, biochemistry, or cellular and molecular physiology, rather they are to serve as a reminder of how the basic principles from these disciplines contribute to medical physiology discussed in later sections.

In the first part of this section, the following basic building blocks are introduced and discussed: electrolytes; carbohydrates, lipids, and fatty acids; amino acids and proteins; and nucleic acids. Students are reminded of some of the basic principles and building blocks of biophysics and biochemistry and how they fit into the physiologic environment. Examples of direct clinical applications are provided in the Clinical Boxes to help bridge the gap between building blocks, basic principles, and human physiology. These basic principles are followed up with a discussion of the generic cell and its components.

In the second part of this introductory section, we take a cellular approach to lay groundwork for understanding groups of cells that interact with many of the systems discussed in future chapters. The first group of cells presented contribute to inflammatory reactions in the body. These individual players, their coordinated behavior, and the net effects of the "open system" of inflammation in the body are discussed in detail. The second group of cells discussed are responsible for the excitatory responses in human physiology and include both neuronal and muscle cells. A fundamental understanding of the inner workings of these cells and how they are controlled by their neighboring cells helps the student to understand their eventual integration into individual systems discussed in later sections.

This first section serves as an introduction, refresher, and quick source of material to best understand systems physiology presented in the later sections. For detailed understanding of any of the chapters within this section, several excellent and current textbooks that provide more in-depth reviews of principles of biochemistry, biophysics, cell physiology, and muscle and neuronal physiology are available. Students who are intrigued by the overview provided in this first section are encouraged to visit such texts for a more thorough understanding of these basic principles.

General Principles & Energy Production in Medical Physiology

OBJECTIVES

After studying this chapter, you should be able to:

- Define units used in measuring physiologic properties.
- Define pH and buffering.
- Understand electrolytes and define diffusion, osmosis, and tonicity.
- Define and explain the significance of resting membrane potential.
- Understand in general terms the basic building blocks of the cell: nucleotides, amino acids, carbohydrates, and fatty acids.
- Understand higher-order structures of the basic building blocks: DNA, RNA, proteins, and lipids.
- Understand the basic contributions of the basic building blocks to cell structure, function, and energy balance.

INTRODUCTION

In humans and other vertebrate animals, specialized cell groups form into organs and include a gastrointestinal system to digest and absorb food; a respiratory system to take up O_2 and eliminate CO_2; a urinary system to remove wastes; a cardiovascular system to distribute nutrients, O_2, and the products of metabolism; a reproductive system to perpetuate the species; and nervous and endocrine systems to coordinate and integrate the functions of the other systems. While this book is concerned with the way these systems function and the way each contributes to the functions of the body as a whole, this first chapter focuses on a review of basic biophysical and biochemical principles and the introduction of the molecular building blocks that contribute to cellular physiology.

■ GENERAL PRINCIPLES

THE BODY AS ORGANIZED "SOLUTIONS"

The cells that make up the bodies of all, but the simplest multicellular animals are exposed to **extracellular fluid (ECF)** enclosed within the integument of the animal. Cells take up O_2 and nutrients from this fluid, and they discharge metabolic waste products into it. The composition of ECF closely resembles that of the primordial oceans in which, presumably, all life originated.

In animals with a closed vascular system, the ECF is divided into the **interstitial fluid,** the circulating **blood plasma,** and **the lymph fluid that bridges these two domains.** The plasma and the cellular elements of the blood fill the vascular system, and together they constitute the **total blood volume.** The interstitial fluid is that part of the ECF that is outside the vascular and lymph systems, bathing the cells. About one-third of the **total body water** is extracellular; the remaining two-thirds is intracellular **(intracellular fluid).** In the average young adult male, 18% of the body weight is protein and related substances, 7% is mineral, and 15% is fat. The remaining 60% is water. The distribution of this water is shown in **Figure 1–1A.** Flow between these compartments is tightly regulated.

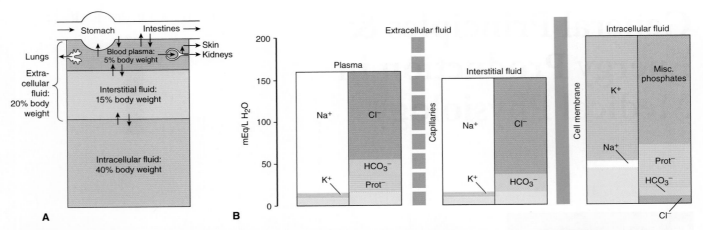

FIGURE 1–1 Organization of body fluids and electrolytes into compartments. (A) Body fluids can be divided into intracellular and extracellular fluid compartments (ICF and ECF, respectively). Their contribution to percentage body weight (based on a healthy young adult male; slight variations exist with age and gender) emphasizes the dominance of fluid makeup of the body. Transcellular fluids, which constitute a very small percentage of total body fluids, are not shown. Arrows represent fluid movement between compartments. **(B)** Electrolytes and proteins are unequally distributed among the body fluids. This uneven distribution is crucial to physiology. Prot⁻, protein, which tends to have a negative charge at physiologic pH.

WATER, ELECTROLYTES, & ACID/BASE

The water molecule (H_2O) is an ideal solvent for physiologic reactions. H_2O has a **dipole moment** where oxygen slightly pulls away electrons from the hydrogen atoms and creates a charge separation that makes the molecule **polar**. This allows water to dissolve a variety of charged atoms and molecules. It also allows the H_2O molecule to interact with other H_2O molecules via hydrogen bonding. The resulting hydrogen bond network in water allows for several key properties relevant to physiology: (1) water has a high surface tension, (2) water has a high heat of vaporization and heat capacity, and (3) water has a high dielectric constant. In layperson's terms, H_2O is an excellent biologic fluid that serves as a solute; it provides optimal heat transfer and conduction of current.

Electrolytes (eg, NaCl) are molecules that dissociate in water to their cation (Na^+) and anion (Cl^-) equivalents. Because of the net charge on water molecules, these electrolytes tend not to reassociate in water. There are many important electrolytes in physiology, notably Na^+, K^+, Ca^{2+}, Mg^{2+}, Cl^-, and HCO_3^-. It is important to note that electrolytes and other charged compounds (eg, proteins) are unevenly distributed in the body fluids (**Figure 1–1B**).

The maintenance of a stable hydrogen ion concentration ($[H^+]$) in body fluids is essential to life. The **pH** of a solution is defined as the logarithm to the base 10 of the reciprocal of the H^+, that is, the negative logarithm of the $[H^+]$. The pH of water at 25°C, in which H^+ and OH^- ions are present in equal numbers, is 7.0. For each pH unit less than 7.0, the $[H^+]$ is increased 10-fold; for each pH unit above 7.0, it is decreased 10-fold. In the plasma of healthy individuals, pH is slightly alkaline, maintained in the narrow range of 7.35–7.45 (**Clinical Box 1–1**). Conversely, gastric fluid pH can be quite acidic (on the order of 3.0) and pancreatic secretions can be quite alkaline (on the order of 8.0). Enzymatic activity and protein structure are frequently sensitive to pH; in any given body or cellular compartment, pH is maintained to allow for maximal enzyme/protein efficiency.

Molecules that act as H^+ donors in solution are considered acids, while those that tend to remove H^+ from solutions are considered bases. Strong acids (eg, HCl) or bases (eg, NaOH) dissociate completely in water and thus can most change the $[H^+]$ in solution. In physiologic compounds, most acids or bases are considered "weak"; that is, they contribute or remove relatively few H^+ from solution. Body pH is stabilized by the **buffering capacity** of the body fluids. A **buffer** is a substance that has the ability to bind or release H^+ in solution, thus keeping the pH of the solution relatively constant despite the addition of considerable quantities of acid or base. Of course, there are a number of buffers at work in biologic fluids at any given time. All buffer pairs in a homogenous solution are in equilibrium with the same $[H^+]$; this is known as the **isohydric principle.** One outcome of this principle is that by assaying a single buffer system, we can understand a great deal about all of the biologic buffers in that system.

When acids are placed into solution, there is dissociation of some of the component acid (HA) into its proton (H^+) and free acid (A^-). This is frequently written as an equation: $HA \rightleftharpoons H^+ + A^-$. According to the laws of mass action, a relationship for the dissociation can be defined mathematically as: $K_a = [H^+][A^-]/[HA]$, where K_a is a constant, and the brackets represent concentrations of the individual species. With some mathematical rearrangement, this can be written in a more conventional form known as the **Henderson-Hasselbalch equation:** $pH = pK_a + \log [A^-]/[HA]$, where pH is the $-\log$ of $[H^+]$ and pK_a is the $-\log$ of the above defined constant. This relatively simple equation is quite powerful. One thing that can be discerned right away is that the buffering capacity of a particular weak acid is best when the pK_a of that acid is equal to the pH of the solution (eg, $[A^-] = [HA]$, $pH = pK_a$). Similar equations can be set up for weak bases. Important biologic buffers include carbonic acid, phosphates, and proteins.

DIFFUSION & OSMOSIS

Diffusion is the process by which a gas or a substance in a solution expands, because of the motion of its particles, to fill all the available volume. The particles (molecules or atoms) of a substance dissolved in a solvent are in continuous random movement. A given particle is equally likely to move into or out of an area in which it is present in high concentration. However, because there are more particles in the area of high concentration, there is a **net flux** of solute particles from areas of high concentration to areas of low concentration. The time required for equilibrium by diffusion is proportional to the square of the diffusion distance. The magnitude of the diffusing tendency from one region to another is directly proportional to the cross-sectional area across which diffusion is taking place and the **concentration or chemical gradient,** and can be represented as **Fick's law of diffusion.** Thus

$$J = DA\frac{\Delta c}{\Delta x},$$

where J is the net rate of diffusion, D is the diffusion coefficient, A is the area, and $\Delta c/\Delta x$ is the concentration gradient. The minus sign indicates the direction of diffusion. When considering movement of molecules from a higher to a lower concentration, $\Delta c/\Delta x$ is negative, so multiplying by $-DA$ gives a positive value. Diffusion is a major force affecting the distribution of water and solutes in the body.

When a substance is dissolved in water, the concentration of water molecules in the solution is less than that in pure water, because the addition of solute to water results in a solution that occupies a greater volume than does the water alone. If the solution is placed on one side of a membrane that is permeable to water but not to the solute, and an equal volume of water is placed on the other, water molecules diffuse down their concentration (chemical) gradient into the solution (**Figure 1–2**). The diffusion of **solvent** molecules into a region in which there is a higher concentration of a **solute** to which the membrane is impermeable is called **osmosis.** The tendency for movement of solvent molecules to a region of greater solute concentration can be prevented by applying pressure to the more concentrated solution. The pressure necessary to prevent solvent migration is the **osmotic pressure** of the solution.

Osmotic pressure depends on the number rather than the type of particles in a solution. In an **ideal solution,** osmotic pressure (P) is related to temperature and volume in the same way as the pressure of a gas:

$$P = \frac{nRT}{V},$$

where n is the number of particles, R is the gas constant, T is the absolute temperature, and V is the volume. If T is held constant, it is clear that the osmotic pressure is proportional to the number of particles in solution per unit volume of solution. For this reason, the concentration of osmotically active particles is usually expressed in **osmoles.** One osmole (Osm) equals the gram-molecular weight of a substance divided by the number of freely moving particles that each molecule liberates in solution. For

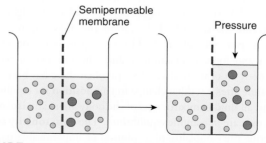

FIGURE 1–2 Diagrammatic representation of osmosis. Water molecules are represented by small open circles, and solute molecules by large solid circles. In the diagram on the left, water is placed on one side of a membrane permeable to water but not to solute, and an equal volume of a solution of the solute is placed on the other. Water molecules move down their concentration (chemical) gradient into the solution, and, as shown in the diagram on the right, the volume of the solution increases. As indicated by the arrow on the right, the osmotic pressure is the pressure that would have to be applied to prevent the movement of the water molecules.

biologic solutions, the milliosmole (mOsm; 1/1000 of 1 Osm) is most commonly used.

If a solute is a nonionizing compound such as glucose, the osmotic pressure is a function of the number of glucose molecules present. If the solute ionizes and forms an ideal solution, each ion is an osmotically active particle. For example, NaCl would dissociate into Na^+ and Cl^- ions, so that each mole in solution would supply 2 Osm. However, body fluids are not ideal solutions, and although the dissociation of strong electrolytes is complete, the number of particles free to exert an osmotic effect is reduced owing to interactions between the ions. Thus, it is actually the effective concentration (**activity**) in the body fluids rather than the number of equivalents of an electrolyte in solution that determines its osmotic capacity. The more concentrated the solution, the greater the deviation from an ideal solution.

The osmolal concentration of a substance in a fluid is measured by the degree to which it depresses the freezing point, with 1 mol of an ideal solution depressing the freezing point by 1.86°C. The number of milliosmoles per liter in a solution equals the freezing point depression divided by 0.00186. The **osmolarity** is the number of osmoles per liter of solution (eg, plasma), whereas the **osmolality** is the number of osmoles per kilogram of solvent. Therefore, osmolarity is affected by the volume of the various solutes in the solution and the temperature, while the osmolality is not. Osmotically active substances in the body are dissolved in water, and the density of water is 1, so osmolal concentrations can be expressed as osmoles per liter (Osm/L) of water. In this book osmolality is expressed in milliosmoles per liter (of water). Note that although a homogeneous solution contains osmotically active particles that can exert an osmotic pressure only when it is in contact with another solution across a membrane permeable to the solvent but not to the solute.

OSMOLAL CONCENTRATION OF PLASMA: TONICITY

The freezing point of normal human plasma averages −0.54°C, which corresponds to an osmolal concentration in plasma of 290 mOsm/L. The osmolality might be expected to be higher than this, because the sum of all the cation and anion equivalents in plasma is over 300 mOsm/L. However, plasma is not an ideal solution and ionic interactions reduce the number of particles free to exert an osmotic effect. Except when there has been insufficient time after a sudden change in composition for equilibrium to occur, all fluid compartments of the body are nearly **isosmotic;** that is, they are in osmotic equilibrium. The term **tonicity** is used to describe the osmolality of a solution of impermeable particles relative to plasma. Solutions that have the same tonicity as plasma are said to be **isotonic; hypertonic** and **hypotonic** refer to higher or lower tonicities as plasma, respectively. All solutions that are initially isosmotic with plasma (ie, that have the same actual osmotic pressure or freezing-point depression as plasma) would remain isotonic if it were not for the fact that some solutes diffuse across cell membranes and others are metabolized. Thus, a 0.9% saline solution remains isotonic because there is no net movement

of the osmotically active particles in the solution into cells and the particles are not metabolized. On the other hand, a 5% glucose solution is isotonic when initially infused intravenously, but glucose can move across the plasma membrane, and can be metabolized, so the net effect is that of infusing a hypotonic solution.

All but about 20 of the 290 mOsm in each liter of normal plasma are contributed by Na^+ and its accompanying anions, principally Cl^- and HCO_3^-. Other cations and anions make a relatively small contribution. Although the concentration of the plasma proteins is large when expressed in grams per liter, they normally contribute less than 2 mOsm/L because of their very high molecular weights. The major nonelectrolytes of plasma are glucose and urea, which in the steady state are in equilibrium with cells. Their contributions to osmolality are normally about 5 mOsm/L each but can become quite large in hyperglycemia or uremia. The total plasma osmolality is important in assessing dehydration, overhydration, and other fluid and electrolyte abnormalities (**Clinical Box 1–2**).

NONIONIC DIFFUSION, DONNAN EFFECT & NERNST POTENTIAL

Some weak acids and bases are quite soluble in cell membranes in the undissociated form, whereas they cannot cross membranes in the dissociated form. Consequently, if molecules of the undissociated substance diffuse from one side of the membrane to the other and then dissociate, there is appreciable net movement of the undissociated substance from one side of the membrane to the other. This phenomenon is called **nonionic diffusion.**

When an ion on one side of a membrane cannot diffuse through the membrane, the distribution of other ions to which the membrane is permeable is affected in a predictable way. For example, the negative charge of a nondiffusible anion hinders diffusion of the diffusible cations and favors diffusion of the diffusible anions. The **Gibbs–Donnan equilibrium states** that in the presence of a nondiffusible ion, the diffusible ions distribute themselves so that at equilibrium their concentration ratios are equal. This holds for any pair of cations and anions of the same valence.

The Donnan effect on the distribution of ions has three effects in the body introduced here and discussed below. First, because of charged proteins ($Prot^-$) in cells, there are more osmotically active particles in cells than in interstitial fluid, and because animal cells have flexible walls, osmosis would make them swell and eventually rupture if it were not for **Na, K ATPase** pumping ions back out of cells. Thus, normal cell volume and pressure depend on Na, K ATPase. Second, because at equilibrium the distribution of permeant ions across the membrane is asymmetric, an electrical difference exists across the membrane whose magnitude can be determined by the **Nernst equation** (see further). Third, because there are more proteins in plasma than in interstitial fluid, there is a Donnan effect on ion movement across the capillary wall.

The forces acting across the cell membrane on each ion can be analyzed mathematically. Chloride ions (Cl^-) are present in higher concentration in the ECF than in the cell interior, and they tend to diffuse along this **concentration gradient** into the cell. The interior of the cell is negative relative to the exterior, and chloride ions are pushed out of the cell along this **electrical gradient.** An equilibrium is reached between Cl^- influx and Cl^- efflux. The membrane potential at which this equilibrium exists is the **equilibrium potential.** Its magnitude can be calculated from the Nernst equation, as follows:

$$E_{Cl} = \frac{RT}{FZ_{Cl}} \ln \frac{[Cl_o^-]}{[Cl_i^-]}$$

where E_{Cl} = equilibrium potential for Cl^-
  R = gas constant
  T = absolute temperature
  F = the Faraday number (number of coulombs per mole of charge)
  Z_{Cl} = valence of Cl^- (–1)
  $[Cl_o^-]$ = Cl^- concentration outside the cell
  $[Cl_i^-]$ = Cl^- concentration inside the cell

Converting from the natural log to the base 10 log and replacing some of the constants with numeric values holding temperature at 37°C, the equation becomes

$$E_{Cl} = 61.5 \log \frac{[Cl_i^-]}{[Cl_o^-]} \text{ at } 37°C$$

TABLE 1–1 Concentration of some ions inside and outside mammalian spinal motor neurons.

Ion	Concentration (mmol/L of H_2O)		Equilibrium Potential (mV)
	Inside Cell	**Outside Cell**	
Na^+	15.0	150.0	+60
K^+	150.0	5.5	–90
Cl^-	9.0	125.0	–70

Resting membrane potential = –70 mV.

Note that in converting to the simplified expression the concentration ratio is reversed because the –1 valence of Cl^- has been removed from the expression.

The equilibrium potential for Cl^- (E_{Cl}) in the mammalian spinal neuron, calculated from the standard values listed in Table 1–1, is –70 mV, a value identical to the typical measured resting membrane potential of –70 mV. Therefore, no forces other than those represented by the chemical and electrical gradients need be invoked to explain the distribution of Cl^- across the membrane.

A similar equilibrium potential can be calculated for K^+ (E_K; Table 1–1). In this case, the concentration gradient is outward and the electrical gradient inward. In mammalian spinal motor neurons E_K is –90 mV. Because the resting membrane potential is –70 mV, there is somewhat more K^+ in the neurons that can be accounted for by the electrical and chemical gradients.

The situation for Na^+ in the mammalian spinal motor neuron is quite different from that for K^+ or Cl^-. The direction of the chemical gradient for Na^+ is inward, to the area where it is in lesser concentration, and the electrical gradient is in the same direction. E_{Na} is +60 mV (Table 1–1). Because neither E_K nor E_{Na} is equal to the membrane potential, one would expect the cell to gradually gain Na^+ and lose K^+ if only passive electrical and chemical forces were acting across the membrane. However, the intracellular concentration of Na^+ and K^+ remain constant because of selective permeability and because of the action of the Na, K ATPase that actively transports Na^+ out of the cell and K^+ into the cell (against their respective electrochemical gradients).

The distribution of ions across the cell membrane and the nature of this membrane provide the explanation for the membrane potential. The concentration gradient for K^+ facilitates its movement out of the cell via K^+ channels, but its electrical gradient is in the opposite (inward) direction. Consequently, an equilibrium is reached in which the tendency of K^+ to move out of the cell is balanced by its tendency to move into the cell, and at that equilibrium there is a slight excess of cations on the outside and anions on the inside. This condition is maintained by Na, K ATPase, which uses the energy of ATP to pump K^+ back into the cell and keeps the intracellular concentration of Na^+ low. Because the Na, K ATPase moves three Na^+ out of the cell for every two K^+ moved in, it also contributes to the membrane potential, and thus is termed an **electrogenic pump.** It should be emphasized that the number of ions responsible for the membrane potential is a minute fraction of the total number present and that the total concentrations of positive and negative ions are equal everywhere except along the membrane.

ENERGY PRODUCTION

ENERGY TRANSFER

Energy used in cellular processes is primarily stored in bonds between phosphoric acid residues and certain organic compounds. Because the energy of bond formation in some of these phosphates is particularly high, relatively large amounts of energy (10–12 kcal/mol) are released when the bond is hydrolyzed. Compounds containing such bonds are called **high-energy phosphate compounds.** Not all organic phosphates are of the high-energy type. Many, like glucose 6-phosphate, are low-energy phosphates that on hydrolysis liberate 2–3 kcal/mol. The most important high-energy phosphate compound is **adenosine triphosphate (ATP).** This ubiquitous molecule is the energy storehouse of the body. On hydrolysis to adenosine diphosphate (ADP), it liberates energy directly to such processes as muscle contraction, active transport, and the synthesis of many chemical compounds.

Another group of high-energy compounds are thioesters, the acyl derivatives of mercaptans. **Coenzyme A (CoA)** is a widely distributed mercaptan-containing adenine, ribose, pantothenic acid, and thioethanolamine. Reduced CoA (usually abbreviated HS-CoA) reacts with acyl groups (R–CO–) to form R–CO–S–CoA derivatives. A prime example is the reaction of HS-CoA with acetic acid to form acetylcoenzyme A (acetyl-CoA), a compound of pivotal importance in intermediary metabolism. Because acetyl-CoA has a much higher energy content than acetic acid, it combines readily with substances in reactions that would otherwise require outside energy. Acetyl-CoA is therefore often called "active acetate."

BIOLOGIC OXIDATIONS

Oxidation is the combination of a substance with O_2, or loss of hydrogen, or loss of electrons. The corresponding reverse processes are called **reduction.** Biologic oxidations are catalyzed by specific enzymes. Cofactors (simple ions) or coenzymes (organic, nonprotein substances) are accessory substances that usually act as carriers for products of the reaction. Unlike the enzymes, the coenzymes may catalyze a variety of reactions.

The principal process by which ATP is formed in the body is **oxidative phosphorylation.** This process harnesses the energy from a proton gradient across the mitochondrial membrane to produce the high-energy bond of ATP (see Figure 2–4 for details). Ninety percent of the O_2 consumption in the basal state is mitochondrial, and 80% of this is coupled to ATP synthesis. ATP is utilized throughout the cell, with the bulk used in a handful of processes: approximately 27% is used for protein synthesis, 24% by Na, K ATPase to help set membrane potential, 9% by gluconeogenesis, 6% by Ca^{2+} ATPase, 5% by myosin ATPase, and 3% by ureagenesis.

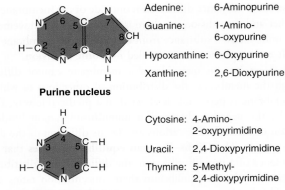

Purine nucleus

Adenine: 6-Aminopurine

Guanine: 1-Amino-
              6-oxypurine

Hypoxanthine: 6-Oxypurine

Xanthine: 2,6-Dioxypurine

Pyrimidine nucleus

Cytosine: 4-Amino-
           2-oxypyrimidine

Uracil: 2,4-Dioxypyrimidine

Thymine: 5-Methyl-
           2,4-dioxypyrimidine

FIGURE 1–3 Principal physiologically important purines and pyrimidines. Purine and pyrimidine structures are shown next to representative molecules from each group. Oxypurines and oxypyrimidines may form enol derivatives (hydroxypurines and hydroxypyrimidines) by migration of hydrogen to the oxygen substituents.

MOLECULAR BUILDING BLOCKS

NUCLEOSIDES, NUCLEOTIDES, & NUCLEIC ACIDS

Nucleosides contain a sugar linked to a nitrogen-containing base. The physiologically important bases, **purines** and **pyrimidines,** have ring structures (Figure 1–3). These structures are bound to ribose or 2-deoxyribose to complete the nucleoside. When inorganic phosphate is added to the nucleoside, a **nucleotide** is formed. Nucleosides and nucleotides form the backbone for RNA and DNA, as well as a variety of coenzymes and regulatory molecules of physiologic importance (eg, NAD^+, $NADP^+$, and ATP; Table 1–2). Nucleic acids in the diet are digested and their constituent purines and pyrimidines absorbed, but most of the purines and pyrimidines are synthesized from amino acids,

TABLE 1–2 Purine- and pyrimidine-containing compounds.

Type of Compound	Components
Nucleoside	Purine or pyrimidine plus ribose or 2-deoxyribose
Nucleotide (mononucleotide)	Nucleoside plus phosphoric acid residue
Nucleic acid	Many nucleotides forming double-helical structures of two polynucleotide chains
Nucleoprotein	Nucleic acid plus one or more simple basic proteins
Contain ribose	RNA
Contain 2-deoxyribose	DNA

principally in the liver. The nucleotides and RNA and DNA are then synthesized. RNA is in dynamic equilibrium with the amino acid pool, but DNA, once formed, is metabolically stable throughout life. The purines and pyrimidines released by the breakdown of nucleotides may be reused or catabolized. Minor amounts are excreted unchanged in the urine.

DNA

DNA is found in the cell nuclei and in mitochondria. It is made up of two extremely long nucleotide chains containing the bases adenine (typically abbreviated in sequence by the letter "A"), guanine (G), thymine (T), and cytosine (C). The chains are bound together by hydrogen bonding between the bases, with adenine bonding to thymine and guanine to cytosine. This stable association forms a double-helical structure. The double helical structure of DNA is compacted in the cell by association with **histones,** and further compacted into **chromosomes.** A diploid human cell contains 46 chromosomes.

A fundamental unit of DNA, or a **gene,** can be defined as the sequence of DNA nucleotides that contain the information for the production of an ordered amino acid sequence for a single polypeptide chain. The protein encoded by a single gene may be subsequently divided into several different physiologically active proteins. The basic structure of a typical eukaryotic gene is shown in diagrammatic form in **Figure 1–4.** It is made up of a strand of DNA that includes coding and noncoding regions. In eukaryotes the portions of the genes that dictate the formation of proteins are usually broken into several segments (**exons**) separated by segments that are not translated (**introns**). Near the transcription start site of the gene is a **promoter,** which is the site at which RNA polymerase and its cofactors bind. It often includes a thymidine–adenine–thymidine–adenine (TATA) sequence (**TATA box**), which ensures that transcription starts at the proper point. Farther out in the 5′ or 3′ regions are **regulatory elements,** which include enhancer and silencer sequences. Each gene can have multiple regulatory sites. In a diploid cell each gene will have two **alleles,** or versions of that gene. Each allele occupies the same position on the homologous chromosome. Individual alleles can confer slightly different properties of the gene when

fully transcribed. It is interesting to note that changes in single nucleotides within or outside coding regions of a gene (**single nucleotide polymorphisms; SNPs**) can have great consequences for gene function.

Gene mutations occur when the base sequence in the DNA is altered from its original sequence. Alterations can be through insertions, deletions, or duplications. Such alterations can affect protein structure and be passed on to daughter cells after cell division. The collection of genes within the full expression of DNA from an organism is termed its **genome.** An indication of the complexity of DNA in the human haploid genome (the total genetic message) is its size; it is made up of 3×10^9 base pairs that can code for approximately 30,000 genes. This genetic message is the blueprint for the heritable characteristics of the cell and its descendants. The proteins formed from the DNA blueprint include all the enzymes, and these in turn control the metabolism of the cell.

Each nucleated somatic cell in the body contains the full genetic message, yet there is great differentiation and specialization in the functions of the various types of adult cells. Only small parts of the message are normally transcribed. At the time of each somatic cell division (**mitosis**), the two DNA chains separate, each serving as a template for the synthesis of a new complementary chain. DNA polymerase catalyzes this reaction. One of the double helices thus formed goes to one daughter cell and one goes to the other, so the amount of DNA in each daughter cell is the same as that in the parent cell. The life cycle of the cell that begins after mitosis is highly regulated and is termed the **cell cycle** (**Figure 1–5**). The G_1 (or Gap 1) phase represents a period of cell growth and divides the end of mitosis from the DNA synthesis (or S) phase. Following DNA synthesis, the cell enters another period of cell growth, the G_2 (Gap 2) phase. The ending of G_2 is marked by chromosome condensation and the beginning of mitosis (M stage).

In germ cells, reductive division (**meiosis**) takes place during maturation. The net result is that one of each pair of chromosomes ends up in each mature germ cell; consequently, each mature germ cell contains half the amount of chromosomal material found in somatic cells. Therefore, when a sperm unites with an ovum, the resulting zygote has the full complement of DNA, half of which came from the father and half from the mother.

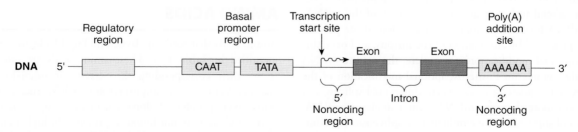

FIGURE 1–4 **Diagram of the components of a typical eukaryotic gene.** The region that produces introns and exons is flanked by noncoding regions. The 5′-flanking region contains stretches of DNA that interact with proteins to facilitate or inhibit transcription. The 3′-flanking region contains the poly(A) addition site. (Modified with permission from Murray RK et al: *Harper's Biochemistry,* 28th ed. New York, NY: McGraw-Hill; 2009.)

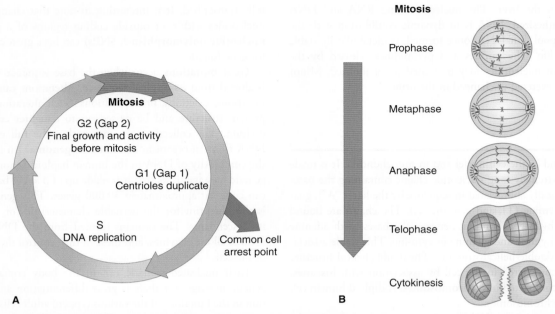

FIGURE 1–5   Sequence of events during the cell cycle. (A) Immediately following mitosis (M) the cell enters a gap phase (G1). At this point many cells will undergo cell arrest. G1 is followed by a DNA synthesis phase (S) a second gap phase (G2) and back to mitosis. **(B)** Stages of mitosis are highlighted.

RNA

The strands of the DNA double helix not only replicate themselves but also serve as templates by lining up complementary bases for the formation in the nucleus of **RNA.** RNA differs from DNA in that it is single-stranded, has **uracil** in place of thymine, and its sugar moiety is ribose rather than 2′-deoxyribose. The production of RNA from DNA is called **transcription.** Transcription can lead to several types of RNA including: **messenger RNA (mRNA), transfer RNA (tRNA), ribosomal RNA (rRNA),** and other RNAs. Transcription is catalyzed by various forms of **RNA polymerase.**

Typical transcription of an mRNA includes several unique steps. When suitably activated, transcription of the gene into a pre-mRNA starts at the **cap site** and ends about 20 bases beyond the AATAAA sequence. The RNA transcript is capped in the nucleus by addition of 7-methylguanosine triphosphate to the 5′ end; this cap is necessary for proper binding to the ribosome. A **poly(A) tail** of about 100 bases is added to the untranslated segment at the 3′-end to help maintain the stability of the mRNA. The pre-mRNA formed by capping and addition of the poly(A) tail is then processed by elimination of the introns, and once this posttranscriptional modification is complete, the mature mRNA moves to the cytoplasm. Posttranscriptional modification of the pre-mRNA is a regulated process where differential splicing can occur to form more than one mRNA from a single pre-mRNA. The introns of some genes are eliminated by **spliceosomes,** complex units that are made up of small RNAs and proteins. Other introns are eliminated by **self-splicing** by the RNA they contain. Because of introns and splicing, more than one mRNA can be formed from the same gene.

Most forms of RNA in the cell are involved in **translation,** or protein synthesis. A brief outline of the transition from transcription to translation is shown in **Figure 1–6.** In the cytoplasm, ribosomes provide a template for tRNA to deliver specific amino acids to a growing polypeptide chain based on specific sequences in mRNA. The mRNA molecules are smaller than the DNA molecules, and each represents a transcript of a small segment of the DNA chain. For comparison, the molecules of tRNA contain only 70–80 nitrogenous bases, compared with hundreds in mRNA and 3 billion in DNA. A newer class of RNA, **microRNAs,** have recently been reported. MicroRNAs measure approximately 21–25-nucleotides in length and have been shown to negatively regulate gene expression at the posttranscriptional level. It is expected that roles for these small RNAs will continue to expand as research into their function continues.

■ AMINO ACIDS & PROTEINS

AMINO ACIDS

Amino acids that form the basic building blocks for proteins are identified in **Table 1–3.** These amino acids are often referred to by their corresponding three-letter, or single-letter abbreviations. Various other important amino acids such as ornithine, 5-hydroxytryptophan, L-dopa, taurine, and thyroxine (T$_4$) occur in the body but are not found in proteins. In higher animals, the L isomers of the amino acids are the only naturally occurring forms in proteins. The amino acids are acidic, neutral, or basic, depending on the relative proportions of free acidic (–COOH) or basic (–NH$_2$) groups in the molecule. Some of the amino acids

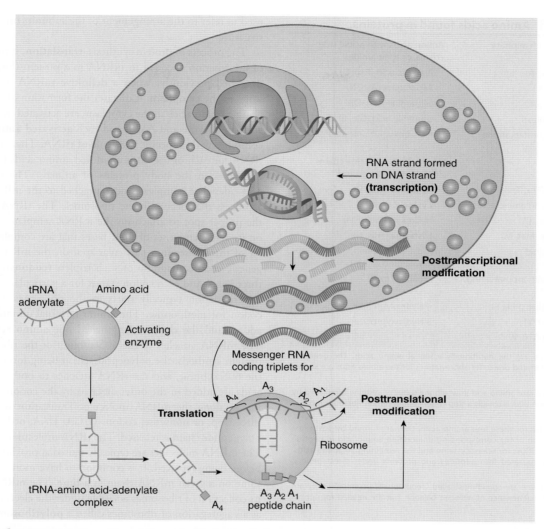

FIGURE 1–6 Diagrammatic outline of transcription to translation. In the nucleus, a messenger RNA is produced from the DNA molecule. This messenger RNA is processed and moved to the cytosol where it is presented to the ribosome. It is at the ribosome where charged tRNA match up with their complementary codons of mRNA to position the amino acid for growth of the polypeptide chain. The lines with multiple short projections in DNA and RNA represent individual bases. Small boxes labeled A represent individual amino acids.

are **nutritionally essential amino acids;** that is, they must be obtained in the diet, because they cannot be made in the body. Arginine and histidine must be provided through diet during times of rapid growth or recovery from illness and are termed **conditionally essential.** All others are **nonessential amino acids** in the sense that they can be synthesized in vivo in amounts sufficient to meet metabolic needs.

Most ingested proteins are digested into their constituent amino acids before absorption. The body's proteins are being continuously hydrolyzed to amino acids and resynthesized. The turnover rate of endogenous proteins averages 80–100 g/d, being highest in the intestinal mucosa and practically nil in the extracellular structural protein, collagen. The amino acids formed by endogenous protein breakdown are identical to those derived from ingested protein. Together, they form a common **amino acid pool** that supplies the needs of the body (**Figure 1–7**).

PROTEINS & PROTEIN SYNTHESIS

Proteins are made up of large numbers of amino acids linked into chains by **peptide bonds** joining the amino group of one amino acid to the carboxyl group of the next. In addition, some proteins contain carbohydrates (glycoproteins) and lipids (lipoproteins). Smaller chains of amino acids are called **peptides** or **polypeptides.** The order of the amino acids in the peptide chains is called the **primary structure** of a protein. The chains are twisted and folded in complex ways, and the term **secondary structure** of a protein refers to the spatial arrangement produced by the twisting and folding. Common secondary structures include the α-helix and β-sheet. The **tertiary structure** of a protein is the arrangement of the twisted chains into layers, crystals, or fibers. Many protein molecules are made of several proteins, or subunits (eg, hemoglobin), and the term **quaternary structure** is

TABLE 1–3 Amino acids found in proteins.

Amino acids with aliphatic side chains	Amino acids with acidic side chains, or their amides
Alanine (Ala, A)	Aspartic acid (Asp, D)
Valine (Val, V)	Asparagine (Asn, N)
Leucine (Leu, L)	Glutamine (Gln, Q)
Isoleucine (Ile, I)	Glutamic acid (Glu, E)
Hydroxyl-substituted amino acids	γ-Carboxyglutamic acid[b] (Gla)
Serine (Ser, S)	Amino acids with side chains containing basic groups
Threonine (Thr, T)	**Arginine**[c] (Arg, R)
Sulfur-containing amino acids	**Lysine** (Lys, K)
Cysteine (Cys, C)	Hydroxylysine[b] (Hyl)
Methionine (Met, M)	**Histidine**[c] (His, H)
Selenocysteine[a]	Imino acids (contain imino group but no amino group)
Amino acids with aromatic ring side chains	Proline (Pro, P)
Phenylalanine (Phe, F)	4-Hydroxyproline[b] (Hyp)
Tyrosine (Tyr, Y)	3-Hydroxyproline[b]
Tryptophan (Trp, W)	

Those in bold type are the nutritionally essential amino acids. The generally accepted three-letter and one-letter abbreviations for the amino acids are shown in parentheses.

[a]Selenocysteine is a rare amino acid in which the sulfur of cysteine is replaced by selenium. The codon UGA is usually a stop codon, but in certain situations it codes for selenocysteine.

[b]There are no tRNAs for these four amino acids; they are formed by posttranslational modification of the corresponding unmodified amino acid in peptide linkage. There are tRNAs for selenocysteine and the remaining 20 amino acids, and they are incorporated into peptides and proteins under direct genetic control.

[c]Arginine and histidine are sometimes called "conditionally essential"—they are not necessary for maintenance of nitrogen balance, but are needed for normal growth.

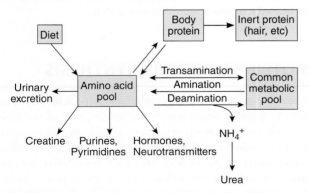

FIGURE 1–7 Amino acids in the body. There is an extensive network of amino acid turnover in the body. Boxes represent large pools of amino acids and some of the common interchanges are represented by arrows. Note that most amino acids come from the diet and end up in protein; however, a large portion of amino acids are interconverted and can feed into and out of a common metabolic pool through amination reactions.

used to refer to the arrangement of the subunits into a functional structure.

The process of protein synthesis, **translation,** is the conversion of information encoded in mRNA to a protein (Figure 1–6). As described previously, when a definitive mRNA reaches a ribosome in the cytoplasm, it dictates the formation of a polypeptide chain. Amino acids in the cytoplasm are activated by combination with an enzyme and AMP, and each **activated amino acid** then combines with a specific molecule of tRNA. There is at least one tRNA for each of the 20 unmodified amino acids found in large quantities in the body proteins of animals. The tRNA–amino acid–adenylate complex is next attached to the mRNA template, a process that occurs in the ribosomes. The tRNA "recognizes" the proper spot to attach on the mRNA template because it has on its active end a set of three bases that are complementary to a set of three bases in a particular spot on the mRNA chain. The genetic code is made up of such triplets (**codons**), sequences of three bases, and each codon stands for a particular amino acid.

Translation typically starts in the ribosomes with an AUG codon for methionine. The amino terminal amino acid is then added, and the chain is lengthened one amino acid at a time. The mRNA attaches to the 40S subunit of the ribosome during protein synthesis, the polypeptide chain being formed attaches to the 60S subunit, and the tRNA attaches to both. As the amino acids are added in the order dictated by the codon, the ribosome moves along the mRNA molecule. Translation stops at one of three stop, or nonsense, codons (UGA, UAA, or UAG), and the polypeptide chain is released. The tRNA molecules are used again. The mRNA molecules are typically reused approximately 10 times before being replaced. It is common to have more than one ribosome on a given mRNA chain at a time. The mRNA chain plus its collection of ribosomes is visible under the electron microscope as an aggregation of ribosomes called a **polyribosome.**

POSTTRANSLATIONAL MODIFICATION

After the polypeptide chain is formed, it "folds" into its biologic form and can be further modified to the final protein by one or more of a combination of reactions that include hydroxylation, carboxylation, glycosylation, or phosphorylation of amino acid residues; cleavage of peptide bonds that converts a larger polypeptide to a smaller form; and the further folding, packaging, or folding and packaging of the protein into its ultimate, often complex configuration. Protein folding is a complex process that is dictated primarily by the sequence of the amino acids in the polypeptide chain. In some instances, however, nascent proteins associate with other proteins called **chaperones.** Chaperones prevent inappropriate contacts with other proteins and ensure that the final "proper" conformation of the nascent protein is reached.

Proteins also contain information that helps direct them to individual cell compartments. Many proteins that are destined to be secreted or stored in organelles and most transmembrane proteins have at their amino terminal a **signal peptide** that guides them into the endoplasmic reticulum. The sequence is made up of 15–30 predominantly hydrophobic amino acid residues.

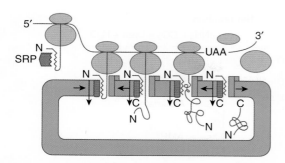

FIGURE 1–8 **Translation of protein into the endoplasmic reticulum according to the signal hypothesis.** The ribosomes synthesizing a protein move along the mRNA from the 5' to the 3' end. When the signal peptide of a protein destined for secretion, the cell membrane, or lysosomes emerges from the large unit of the ribosome, it binds to a signal recognition particle (SRP), and this arrests further translation until it binds to the translocon on the endoplasmic reticulum. N, amino end of protein; C, carboxyl end of protein. (Reproduced with permission from Perara E, Lingappa VR: Transport of proteins into and across the endoplasmic reticulum membrane. In: Das RC, Robbins PW: *Protein Transfer and Organelle Biogenesis.* Academic Press, 1988)

The signal peptide, once synthesized, binds to a **signal recognition particle (SRP),** a complex molecule made up of six polypeptides and 7S RNA, one of the small RNAs. The SRP stops translation until it binds to a **translocon,** a pore in the endoplasmic reticulum that is a heterotrimeric structure. The ribosome also binds, and the signal peptide leads the growing peptide chain into the cavity of the endoplasmic reticulum **(Figure 1–8)**. The signal peptide is next cleaved from the rest of the peptide by a signal peptidase while the rest of the peptide chain is still being synthesized. SRPs are not the only signals that help direct proteins to their proper place in or out of the cell; other signal sequences, posttranslational modifications, or both (eg, glycosylation) can serve this function.

UBIQUITINATION & PROTEIN DEGRADATION

Like protein synthesis, protein degradation is a carefully regulated, complex process. Abnormally produced proteins (up to 30% of newly produced proteins) and aged normal proteins need to be removed as they are replaced. Conjugation of proteins to the 74-amino-acid polypeptide **ubiquitin** marks them for degradation. This polypeptide is highly conserved across bacteria to humans. The process of binding ubiquitin is called **ubiquitination,** and in some instances, multiple ubiquitin molecules bind **(polyubiquitination)**. Ubiquitination of cytoplasmic proteins, including integral proteins of the endoplasmic reticulum, can mark the proteins for degradation in multisubunit proteolytic particles, or **proteasomes.** Ubiquitination of membrane proteins, such as the growth hormone receptors, also marks them for degradation; however, these can be degraded in lysosomes as well as via the proteasomes. Alteration of proteins by ubiquitin or the small

ubiquitin-related modifier **(SUMO)**, however, does not necessarily lead to degradation. More recently it has been shown that these posttranslational modifications can play important roles in protein–protein interactions and cellular signaling pathways. The rates at which individual proteins are metabolized vary, and the body has mechanisms by which abnormal proteins are recognized and degraded more rapidly than normal body constituents.

CATABOLISM OF AMINO ACIDS

The short-chain fragments produced by amino acid, carbohydrate, and fat catabolism are very similar and form a **common metabolic pool.** These fragments can also enter the citric acid cycle where they are broken down to hydrogen atoms and CO_2. Interconversion of amino acids involves transfer, removal, or formation of amino groups. **Transamination** reactions, conversion of one amino acid to the corresponding keto acid with simultaneous conversion of another keto acid to an amino acid, occur in many tissues. For example, alanine + α-ketoglutarate $\rightleftharpoons$ pyruvate + glutamate. Alternatively, **oxidative deamination** of amino acids occurs in the liver. In this two-step reaction, an imino acid is formed by dehydrogenation, and the imino acid is then hydrolyzed to the corresponding keto acid, with production of NH_4^+: amino acid + NAD^+ → imino acid + $NADH + H^+$; imino acid + H_2O → keto acid + NH_4^+. Most of the NH_4^+ formed by deamination of amino acids in the liver is converted to **urea**, and the urea is excreted in the urine (urea cycle; **Figure 1–9**). The NH_4^+ enters the mitochondria and forms carbamoyl phosphate where it is transferred to ornithine to form citrulline. The enzyme involved is ornithine carbamoyltransferase. Citrulline is converted to arginine, after which urea is split off and ornithine is regenerated. The overall reaction in the urea cycle consumes 3 ATP (not shown) and thus requires significant energy. Most of the urea is formed in the liver, and in severe liver disease the blood urea nitrogen (BUN) falls and blood NH_3 rises. Congenital deficiency of ornithine carbamoyltransferase can also lead to NH_3 intoxication.

■ CARBOHYDRATES

Carbohydrates are organic molecules made of equal amounts of carbon and H_2O. The simple sugars, or **monosaccharides,** including **pentoses** (five carbons; eg, ribose) and **hexoses** (six carbons; eg, glucose) perform both structural (eg, as part of nucleotides discussed previously) and functional roles (eg, inositol 1,4,5 trisphosphate acts as a cellular signaling molecules) in the body. Monosaccharides can be linked together to form disaccharides (eg, sucrose), or polysaccharides (eg, glycogen). The placement of sugar moieties onto proteins (glycoproteins) aids in cellular targeting, and in the case of some receptors, recognition of signaling molecules. In this section, the major role of carbohydrates in the production and storage of energy will be discussed.

Dietary carbohydrates are for the most part polymers of hexoses, of which the most important are glucose, galactose, and fructose. The principal product of carbohydrate digestion and

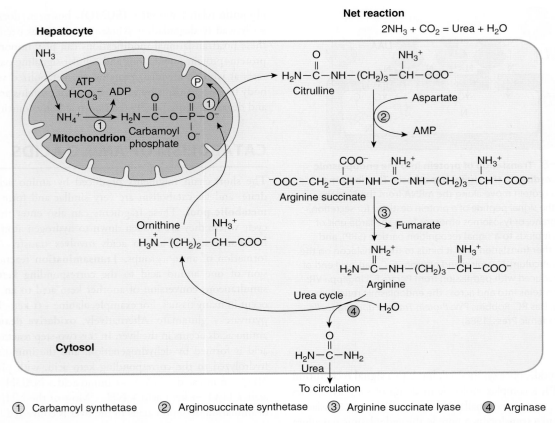

FIGURE 1–9 Urea cycle. The processing of NH_3 to urea for excretion contains coordinative steps in both the cytosol and the mitochondrion of a hepatocyte. Note that the production of carbamoyl phosphate and its conversion to citrulline occurs in the mitochondria, whereas other processes are in the cytoplasm.

the principal circulating sugar is glucose. The normal fasting level of plasma glucose in peripheral venous blood is 70–110 mg/dL (3.9–6.1 mmol/L). In arterial blood, the plasma glucose level is 15–30 mg/dL higher than in venous blood.

Once glucose enters cells, it is normally phosphorylated by **hexokinase**, forming glucose-6-phosphate. Glucokinase found in the liver has greater specificity for glucose, and unlike hexokinase, is increased by insulin and decreased in starvation and diabetes. The glucose-6-phosphate is either polymerized into glycogen or catabolized. The process of glycogen formation is called **glycogenesis**, and glycogen breakdown is called **glycogenolysis**. Glycogen, the storage form of glucose, is present in most body tissues, but the major supplies are in the liver and skeletal muscle. The breakdown of glucose to pyruvate or lactate (or both) is called **glycolysis**. Glucose catabolism proceeds via cleavage through fructose to trioses (**Embden–Meyerhof pathway**) or via oxidation and decarboxylation to pentoses (**direct oxidative pathway; hexose monophosphate shunt or pentose phosphate pathway**). Pyruvate is converted to acetyl-CoA. Interconversions between carbohydrate, fat, and protein include conversion of glycerol from fats to dihydroxyacetone phosphate and conversion of a number of amino acids with carbon skeletons resembling intermediates in the Embden–Meyerhof pathway and citric acid cycle by deamination.

In this way, and by conversion of lactate to glucose, nonglucose molecules can be converted to glucose (**gluconeogenesis**). Glucose can be converted to fats through acetyl-CoA, but because the conversion of pyruvate to acetyl-CoA, unlike most reactions in glycolysis, is irreversible, fats are not converted to glucose via this pathway.

CITRIC ACID CYCLE

The **citric acid cycle** (Krebs cycle, tricarboxylic acid cycle) is a sequence of reactions in which acetyl-CoA is metabolized to CO_2 and H atoms. Acetyl-CoA is first condensed with the anion of a four-carbon acid, oxaloacetate, to form citrate and HS-CoA. In a series of seven subsequent reactions, 2 CO_2 molecules are split off, regenerating oxaloacetate (**Figure 1–10**). Four pairs of H atoms are transferred to the flavoprotein–cytochrome chain, producing 12 ATP and 4 H_2O, of which 2 H_2O is used in the cycle. The citric acid cycle is the common pathway for oxidation to CO_2 and H_2O of carbohydrate, fat, and some amino acids. The major entry into it is through acetyl CoA, but a number of amino acids can be converted to citric acid cycle intermediates by deamination. The citric acid cycle requires O_2 and does not function under anaerobic conditions.

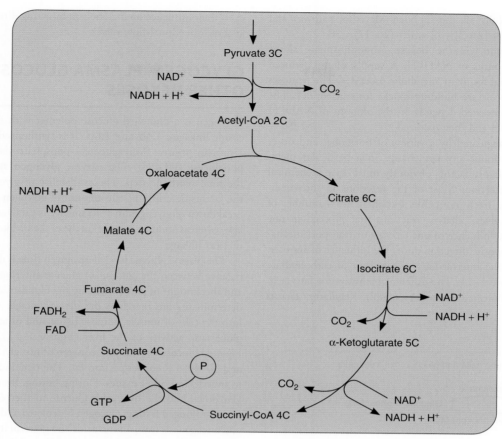

FIGURE 1–10 *Citric acid cycle.* The numbers (6C, 5C, etc.) indicate the number of carbon atoms in each of the intermediates. The conversion of pyruvate to acetyl-CoA and each turn of the cycle provide four NADH and one $FADH_2$ for oxidation via the flavoprotein-cytochrome chain plus formation of one GTP that is readily converted to ATP.

ENERGY PRODUCTION

The net production of energy-rich phosphate compounds during the metabolism of glucose and glycogen to pyruvate depends on whether metabolism occurs via the Embden–Meyerhof pathway or the hexose monophosphate shunt. By oxidation at the substrate level, the conversion of 1 mol of phosphoglyceraldehyde to phosphoglycerate generates 1 mol of ATP, and the conversion of 1 mol of phosphoenolpyruvate to pyruvate generates another. Because 1 mol of glucose-6-phosphate produces 2 mol of phosphoglyceraldehyde, 4 mol of ATP is generated per mole of glucose metabolized to pyruvate in the Embden–Meyerhof pathway. All these reactions occur in the absence of O_2 and consequently represent anaerobic production of energy. However, 1 mol of ATP is used in forming fructose 1,6-diphosphate from fructose 6-phosphate and 1 mol in phosphorylating glucose when it enters the cell. Consequently, when pyruvate is formed anaerobically from glycogen, there is a *net* production of 3 mol of ATP per mole of glucose-6-phosphate; however, when pyruvate is formed from 1 mol of blood glucose, the net gain is only 2 mol of ATP.

A supply of NAD⁺ is necessary for the conversion of phosphoglyceraldehyde to phosphoglycerate. Under anaerobic conditions,

a block of glycolysis at the phosphoglyceraldehyde conversion step might be expected to develop as soon as the available NAD⁺ is converted to NADH. However, pyruvate can accept hydrogen from NADH, forming NAD⁺ and lactate: pyruvate + NADH ⇌ lactate + NAD⁺. In this way, glucose metabolism and energy production can continue for a while without O_2. The lactate that accumulates is converted back to pyruvate when the O_2 supply is restored, with NADH transferring its hydrogen to the flavoprotein–cytochrome chain.

During aerobic glycolysis, the net production of ATP is 19 times greater than the 2 ATPs formed under anaerobic conditions. Six ATPs are formed by oxidation, via the flavoprotein–cytochrome chain, of the 2 NADHs produced when 2 molecules of phosphoglyceraldehyde is converted to phosphoglycerate (Figure 1–10), 6 ATPs are formed from the 2 NADHs produced when 2 molecules of pyruvate are converted to acetyl-CoA, and 24 ATPs are formed during the subsequent two turns of the citric acid cycle. Of these, 18 are formed by oxidation of 6 NADHs, 4 by oxidation of 2 $FADH_2$s, and 2 by oxidation at the substrate level, when succinyl-CoA is converted to succinate (this reaction actually produces guanosine triphosphate [GTP], but the GTP is converted to ATP). Thus, the net production of ATP per mol of blood glucose metabolized aerobically via the Embden–Meyerhof pathway and citric acid cycle is 2 + [2 × 3] + [2 × 3] + [2 × 12] = 38.

Glucose oxidation via the hexose monophosphate shunt generates large amounts of NADPH. A supply of this reduced coenzyme is essential for many metabolic processes. The pentoses formed in the process are building blocks for nucleotides. The amount of ATP generated depends on the amount of NADPH converted to NADH and then oxidized.

Metabolism is regulated by a variety of hormones and other factors. To bring about any net change in a particular metabolic process, regulatory factors obviously must drive a chemical reaction in one direction. Most of the reactions in intermediary metabolism are freely reversible, but there are a number of "directional-flow valves," that is, reactions that proceed in one direction under the influence of one enzyme or transport mechanism and in the opposite direction under the influence of another. Five examples in the intermediary metabolism of carbohydrate are shown in **Figure 1–11**. The different pathways for fatty acid synthesis and catabolism are another example. Regulatory factors exert their influence on metabolism by acting directly or indirectly at these directional-flow valves.

GLYCOGEN, PLASMA GLUCOSE & OTHER HEXOSES

Glycogen is a branched glucose polymer with two types of glycoside linkages: 1:4α and 1:6α. It is synthesized on **glycogenin**, a protein primer, from glucose-1-phosphate via uridine diphosphoglucose (UDPG). The enzyme **glycogen synthase** catalyzes the final synthetic step. The availability of glycogenin is one of the factors determining the amount of glycogen synthesized. The breakdown of glycogen in 1:4α linkage is catalyzed by phosphorylase, whereas another enzyme catalyzes the breakdown of glycogen in 1:6α linkage.

The plasma glucose level at any given time is determined by the balance between the amount of glucose entering the bloodstream and the amount of glucose leaving the bloodstream. The principal determinants are therefore the dietary intake; the rate of entry into the cells of muscle, adipose tissue, and other organs; and the glucostatic activity of the liver (**Figure 1–12**). Five percent of ingested glucose is promptly converted into glycogen in the liver, and 30–40% is converted into fat. The remainder is metabolized in muscle and other tissues. During fasting, liver glycogen is broken down and the liver adds glucose to the bloodstream. With more prolonged fasting, glycogen is depleted and there is increased gluconeogenesis from amino acids and glycerol in the liver. Plasma glucose declines modestly to about 60 mg/dL during prolonged starvation in normal individuals, but symptoms of hypoglycemia do not occur because gluconeogenesis prevents any further fall.

Other hexoses that are absorbed from the intestine include galactose, which is liberated by the digestion of lactose and converted to glucose in the body; and fructose, part of which is ingested and part produced by hydrolysis of sucrose. After phosphorylation, galactose reacts with UDPG to form uridine diphosphogalactose. The uridine diphosphogalactose is converted back to UDPG, and the UDPG functions in glycogen synthesis. This reaction is reversible, and conversion of UDPG to uridine

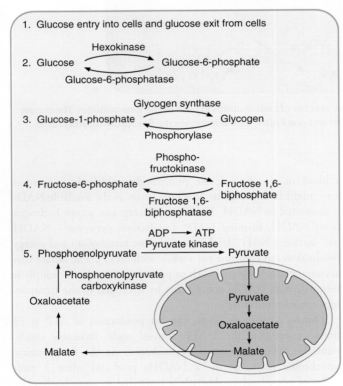

FIGURE 1–11 Directional-flow valves in energy production reactions. In carbohydrate metabolism there are several reactions that proceed in one direction by one mechanism and in the other direction by a different mechanism, termed "directional-flow valves." Five examples of these reactions are illustrated (numbered at left). The double line in example 5 represents the mitochondrial membrane. Pyruvate is converted to malate in mitochondria, and the malate diffuses out of the mitochondria to the cytosol, where it is converted to phosphoenolpyruvate.

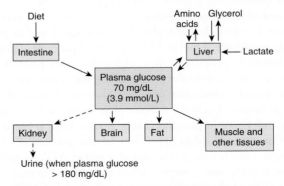

FIGURE 1–12 Plasma glucose homeostasis. Note the glucostatic function of the liver, as well as the loss of glucose in the urine when the renal threshold is exceeded (dashed arrows).

CLINICAL BOX 1–3

Galactosemia

In the inborn error of metabolism known as **galactosemia**, there is a congenital deficiency of galactose-1-phosphate uridyl transferase, the enzyme responsible for the reaction between galactose-1-phosphate and UDPG, so that ingested galactose accumulates in the circulation; serious disturbances of growth and development result.

THERAPEUTIC HIGHLIGHTS

Treatment with galactose-free diets improves galactosemia without leading to galactose deficiency. This occurs because the enzyme necessary for the formation of uridine diphosphogalactose from UDPG is present.

---

diphosphogalactose provides the galactose necessary for formation of glycolipids and mucoproteins when dietary galactose intake is inadequate. The utilization of galactose, like that of glucose, depends on insulin. The inability to make UDPG can have serious health consequences (**Clinical Box 1–3**).

Fructose is converted in part to fructose 6-phosphate and then metabolized via fructose 1,6-diphosphate. The enzyme catalyzing the formation of fructose 6-phosphate is hexokinase, the same enzyme that catalyzes the conversion of glucose to glucose-6-phosphate. However, much more fructose is converted to fructose 1-phosphate in a reaction catalyzed by fructokinase. Most of fructose 1-phosphate is then split into dihydroxyacetone phosphate and glyceraldehyde. The glyceraldehyde is phosphorylated, and it and the dihydroxyacetone phosphate enter the pathways for glucose metabolism. Fructose 6-phosphate can also be phosphorylated in the 2 position, forming fructose 2,6-diphosphate. This compound is an important regulator of hepatic gluconeogenesis. When the fructose 2,6-diphosphate level is high, conversion of fructose 6-phosphate to fructose 1,6-diphosphate is facilitated, and thus breakdown of glucose to pyruvate is increased. A decreased level of fructose 2,6-diphosphate facilitates the reverse reaction and consequently aids gluconeogenesis.

■ FATTY ACIDS & LIPIDS

The biologically important lipids are the fatty acids and their derivatives, the neutral fats (triglycerides), the phospholipids and related compounds, and the sterols. The triglycerides are made up of three fatty acids bound to glycerol (**Table 1–4**). Naturally occurring fatty acids contain an even number of carbon atoms. They may be saturated (no double bonds) or unsaturated (dehydrogenated, with various numbers of double bonds). The phospholipids are structural constituents of cell membranes and also provide an energy source and intracellular and intercellular signaling molecules.

TABLE 1–4 Lipids.

Typical fatty acids:

Palmitic acid: $CH_5(CH_2)_{14}-\overset{\overset{\displaystyle O}{\|}}{C}-OH$

Stearic acid: $CH_5(CH_2)_{16}-\overset{\overset{\displaystyle O}{\|}}{C}-OH$

Oleic acid: $CH_5(CH_2)_7CH=CH(CH_2)_7-\overset{\overset{\displaystyle O}{\|}}{C}-OH$
(Unsaturated)

Triglycerides (triacylglycerols): Esters of glycerol and three fatty acids

$$
\begin{array}{l}
CH_2-O-\overset{\overset{O}{\|}}{C}-R \\
CH_2-O-\overset{\overset{O}{\|}}{C}-R + 3H_2O \rightleftharpoons CHOH + 3HO-\overset{\overset{O}{\|}}{C}-R \\
CH_2-O-\overset{\overset{O}{\|}}{C}-R \\
\text{Triglyceride} \qquad\qquad \text{Glycerol}
\end{array}
$$

R = Aliphatic chain of various lengths and degrees of saturation

Phospholipids:

A. Esters of glycerol, two fatty acids, and

  1. Phosphate = phosphatidic acid

  2. Phosphate plus inositol = phosphatidylinositol

  3. Phosphate plus choline = phosphatidylcholine (lecithin)

  4. Phosphate plus ethanolamine = phosphatidyl-ethanolamine (cephalin)

  5. Phosphate plus serine = phosphatidylserine

B. Other phosphate-containing derivatives of glycerol

C. Sphingomyelins: Esters of fatty acid, phosphate, choline, and the amino alcohol sphingosine

Cerebrosides: Compounds containing galactose, fatty acid, and sphingosine

Sterols: Cholesterol and its derivatives, including steroid hormones, bile acids, and various vitamins

FATTY ACID OXIDATION & SYNTHESIS

In the body, fatty acids are broken down to acetyl-CoA, which enters the citric acid cycle. The main breakdown occurs in the mitochondria by β-oxidation. Fatty acid oxidation begins with activation (formation of the CoA derivative) of the fatty acid, a reaction that occurs both inside and outside the mitochondria. Medium- and short-chain fatty acids can enter the mitochondria without difficulty, but long-chain fatty acids must be bound to **carnitine** in ester linkage before they can cross the inner mitochondrial membrane. Carnitine is β-hydroxy-γ-trimethylammonium butyrate synthesized from lysine and methionine. A translocase moves the fatty acid–carnitine ester into the matrix space. The ester is hydrolyzed, and the carnitine recycles. β-Oxidation proceeds by serial removal of two carbon

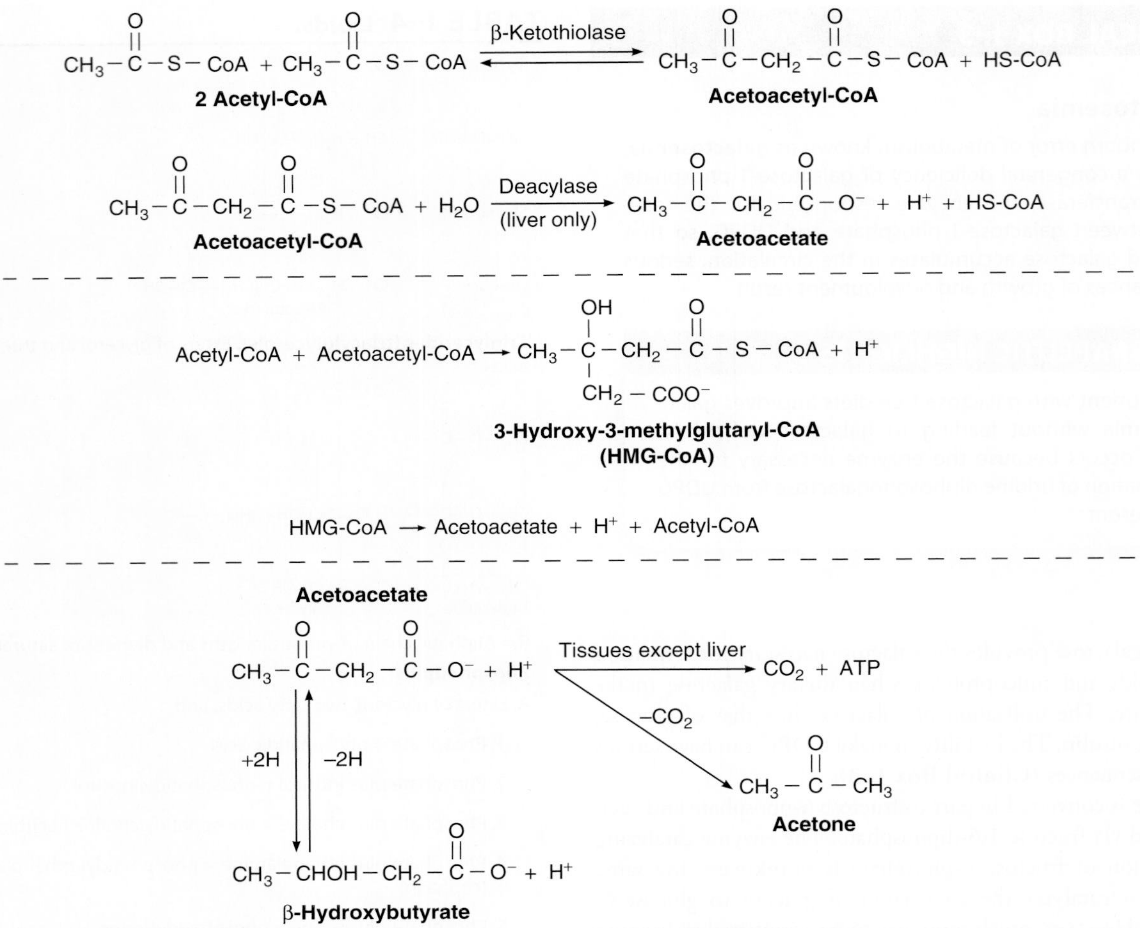

FIGURE 1–13 Formation and metabolism of ketone bodies. Note the two pathways for the formation of acetoacetate.

fragments from the fatty acid. The energy yield of this process is large. For example, catabolism of 1 mol of a six-carbon fatty acid through the citric acid cycle to CO_2 and H_2O generates 44 mol of ATP, compared with the 38 mol generated by catabolism of 1 mol of the six-carbon carbohydrate glucose.

KETONE BODIES

In many tissues, acetyl-CoA units condense to form acetoacetyl-CoA (**Figure 1–13**). Free acetoacetate is formed in the liver through the action of deacylase. This β-keto acid is converted to β-hydroxybutyrate and acetone, and because these compounds are metabolized with difficulty in the liver, they diffuse into the circulation. Acetoacetate is more prominently formed in the liver via the formation of 3-hydroxy-3-methylglutaryl-CoA. Acetoacetate, β-hydroxybutyrate, and acetone are called **ketone bodies.** Tissues other than liver transfer CoA from succinyl-CoA to acetoacetate and metabolize the "active" acetoacetate to CO_2 and H_2O via the citric acid cycle. Ketone bodies are also metabolized via other pathways. Acetone is discharged in the urine and expired air. An imbalance of ketone bodies can lead to serious health problems (**Clinical Box 1–4**).

CELLULAR LIPIDS

The lipids in cells are of two main types: **structural lipids,** which are an inherent part of the membranes and can serve as progenitors for cellular signaling molecules; and **neutral fat,** stored in the adipose cells of the fat depots. Neutral fat is mobilized during starvation, but structural lipid is preserved. The fat depots vary in size, but in non-obese individuals they make up about 15% of body weight in men and 21% in women. They are dynamic products undergoing continuous breakdown and resynthesis. In the depots, glucose is metabolized to fatty acids, and neutral fats are synthesized. Neutral fat is also broken down, and free fatty acids (FFAs) are released into the circulation.

A third, special type of lipid is **brown fat,** which makes up a small percentage of total body fat. Brown fat, which is somewhat more abundant in infants, is located between the scapulas, at the nape of the neck, along the great vessels in the thorax and abdomen, and in other scattered locations in the body. In brown fat depots, the fat cells as well as the blood vessels have an extensive sympathetic innervation. This is in contrast to white fat depots, in which some fat cells may be innervated but the principal sympathetic innervation is solely on blood vessels. Ordinary lipocytes have only a single large droplet of white fat, whereas brown fat

CLINICAL BOX 1–4

Diseases Associated with Imbalance of β-oxidation of Fatty Acids

Ketoacidosis

The normal blood ketone level in humans is low (about 1 mg/dL) and less than 1 mg is excreted per 24 h, because the ketones are normally metabolized as rapidly as they are formed. However, if the entry of acetyl-CoA into the citric acid cycle is depressed because of a decreased supply of the products of glucose metabolism, or if the entry does not increase when the supply of acetyl-CoA increases, acetyl-CoA accumulates, the rate of condensation to acetoacetyl-CoA increases, and more acetoacetate is formed in the liver. The ability of the tissues to oxidize the ketones is soon exceeded, and they accumulate in the bloodstream (ketosis). Two of the three ketone bodies, acetoacetate and β-hydroxybutyrate, are anions of the moderately strong acids acetoacetic acid and β-hydroxybutyric acid. Many of their protons are buffered, reducing the decline in pH that would otherwise occur. However, the buffering capacity can be exceeded, and the

metabolic acidosis that develops in conditions such as diabetic ketosis can be severe and even fatal. Three conditions lead to deficient intracellular glucose supplies, and hence to ketoacidosis: starvation; diabetes mellitus; and a high-fat, low-carbohydrate diet. The acetone odor on the breath of children who have been vomiting is due to the ketosis of starvation. Parenteral administration of relatively small amounts of glucose abolishes the ketosis, and it is for this reason that carbohydrate is said to be antiketogenic.

Carnitine Deficiency

Deficient β-oxidation of fatty acids can be produced by carnitine deficiency or genetic defects in the translocase or other enzymes involved in the transfer of long-chain fatty acids into the mitochondria. This causes cardiomyopathy. In addition, it causes **hypoketonemic hypoglycemia** with coma, a serious and often fatal condition triggered by fasting, in which glucose stores are used up because of the lack of fatty acid oxidation to provide energy. Ketone bodies are not formed in normal amounts because of the lack of adequate CoA in the liver.

cells contain several small droplets of fat. Brown fat cells also contain many mitochondria. In these mitochondria, an inward proton conductance that generates ATP takes places as usual, but in addition there is a second proton conductance that does not generate ATP. This "short-circuit" causes uncoupling of metabolism and the generation of ATP, resulting in increased heat production.

PLASMA LIPIDS & LIPID TRANSPORT

The major lipids are relatively insoluble in aqueous solutions and do not circulate in the free form. **FFAs** are bound to albumin, whereas cholesterol, triglycerides, and phospholipids are transported in the form of **lipoprotein** complexes. The complexes greatly increase the solubility of the lipids. The six families of

lipoproteins (**Table 1–5**) are graded in size and lipid content. The density of these lipoproteins is inversely proportionate to their lipid content. In general, the lipoproteins consist of a hydrophobic core of triglycerides and cholesteryl esters surrounded by phospholipids and protein. These lipoproteins can be transported from the intestine to the liver via an **exogenous pathway,** and between other tissues via an **endogenous pathway.**

Dietary lipids are processed by several pancreatic lipases in the intestine to form mixed micelles of predominantly FFA, **2-monoacylglycerols,** and cholesterol derivatives. These micelles additionally can contain important water-insoluble molecules such as **vitamins A, D, E, and K**. These mixed micelles are taken up into cells of the intestinal mucosa where large lipoprotein complexes, **chylomicrons,** are formed. The chylomicrons and their

TABLE 1–5 The principal lipoproteins.[a]

Lipoprotein	Size (nm)	Protein	Free Cholesteryl	Cholesterol Esters	Triglyceride	Phospholipid	Origin
Chylomicrons	75–1000	2	2	3	90	3	Intestine
Chylomicron remnants	30–80	…	…	…	…	…	Capillaries
Very low-density lipoproteins (VLDL)	30–80	8	4	16	55	17	Liver and intestine
Intermediate-density lipoproteins (IDL)	25–40	10	5	25	40	20	VLDL
Low-density lipoproteins (LDL)	20	20	7	46	6	21	IDL
High-density lipoproteins (HDL)	7.5–10	50	4	16	5	25	Liver and intestine

[a]The plasma lipids include these components plus free fatty acids from adipose tissue, which circulate bound to albumin.

remnants constitute a transport system for ingested exogenous lipids (exogenous pathway). Chylomicrons can enter the circulation via the lymphatic ducts. The chylomicrons are cleared from the circulation by the action of **lipoprotein lipase,** which is located on the surface of the endothelium of the capillaries. The enzyme catalyzes the breakdown of the triglyceride in the chylomicrons to FFA and glycerol, which then enter adipose cells and are reesterified. Alternatively, the FFA can remain in the circulation bound to albumin. Lipoprotein lipase, which requires heparin as a cofactor, also removes triglycerides from circulating **very low-density lipoproteins (VLDL).** Chylomicrons depleted of their triglyceride remain in the circulation as cholesterol-rich lipoproteins called **chylomicron remnants.** The remnants are carried to the liver, where they are internalized and degraded.

The endogenous system, made up of VLDL, **intermediate-density lipoproteins (IDL), low-density lipoproteins (LDL),** and **high-density lipoproteins (HDL),** also transports triglycerides and cholesterol throughout the body. VLDL are formed in the liver and transport triglycerides formed from fatty acids and carbohydrates in the liver to extrahepatic tissues. After their triglyceride is largely removed by the action of lipoprotein lipase, they become IDL. The IDL give up phospholipids and, through the action of the plasma enzyme **lecithin-cholesterol acyltransferase,** pick up cholesteryl esters formed from cholesterol in the HDL. Some IDL are taken up by the liver; the remaining IDL lose more triglyceride and protein, probably in the sinusoids of the liver, and become LDL. LDLs provide cholesterol to the tissues. The cholesterol is an essential constituent in cell membranes and is used by gland cells to make steroid hormones.

FREE FATTY ACID METABOLISM

In addition to the exogenous and endogenous pathways described above, FFAs are also synthesized in the fat depots in which they are stored. They can circulate as lipoproteins bound to albumin and are a major source of energy for many organs. They are used extensively in the heart, but probably all tissues can oxidize FFA to CO_2 and H_2O.

The supply of FFA to the tissues is regulated by two lipases. As noted above, lipoprotein lipase on the surface of the endothelium of the capillaries hydrolyzes the triglycerides in chylomicrons and VLDL, providing FFA and glycerol, which are reassembled into new triglycerides in the fat cells. The intracellular **hormone-sensitive lipase** of adipose tissue catalyzes the breakdown of stored triglycerides into glycerol and fatty acids, with the latter entering the circulation. Hormone-sensitive lipase is increased by fasting and stress and decreased by feeding and insulin. Conversely, feeding increases and fasting and stress decrease the activity of lipoprotein lipase.

CHOLESTEROL METABOLISM

Cholesterol is the precursor of the steroid hormones and bile acids and is an essential constituent of cell membranes. It is found only in animals. Related sterols occur in plants, but plant sterols are poorly absorbed from the gastrointestinal tract.

Cholesterol is absorbed from the intestine and incorporated into the chylomicrons formed in the intestinal mucosa. After the chylomicrons discharge their triglyceride in adipose tissue, the chylomicron remnants bring cholesterol to the liver. The liver and other tissues also synthesize cholesterol. Some of the cholesterol in the liver is excreted in the bile, both in the free form and as bile acids. Some of the biliary cholesterol is reabsorbed from the intestine. Most of the cholesterol in the liver is incorporated into VLDL and circulates in lipoprotein complexes.

Cholesterol is synthesized by a multistep reaction originating with acetyl-CoA, progressing to 3-hydroxy-3-methylglutaryl-coenzyme A (HMG-CoA) and mevalonic acid early in the reaction scheme. The enzyme that converts HMG-CoA to mevalonic acid, **HMG-CoA reductase,** is inhibited by cholesterol. Thus, when dietary cholesterol intake is high, hepatic cholesterol synthesis is decreased, and vice versa. However, the feedback compensation is incomplete, because a diet that is low in cholesterol and saturated fat leads to only a modest decline in circulating plasma cholesterol. The most effective and most commonly used cholesterol-lowering drugs are lovastatin and other **statins,** which reduce cholesterol synthesis by inhibiting HMG-CoA. The relationship between cholesterol and vascular disease is discussed in Clinical Box 1–5.

EICOSANOIDS

One of the reasons that fatty acids are necessary for health is that they are the precursors of prostaglandins, prostacyclin, thromboxanes, lipoxins, leukotrienes, and related compounds. These substances are called **eicosanoids,** reflecting their origin from the 20-carbon (eicosa-) polyunsaturated fatty acid **arachidonic acid (arachidonate)** and the 20-carbon derivatives of linoleic and linolenic acids.

The **prostaglandins** are a series of 20-carbon unsaturated fatty acids containing a cyclopentane ring. They were first isolated from semen but are synthesized in most and possibly in all organs in the body. Prostaglandin H_2 (PGH_2) is the precursor for various other prostaglandins, thromboxanes, and prostacyclin. Arachidonic acid is formed from tissue phospholipids by **phospholipase A_2.** It is converted to prostaglandin H_2 (PGH_2) by **prostaglandin G/H synthases** 1 and 2. These are bifunctional enzymes that have both cyclooxygenase and peroxidase activity, but they are more commonly known by the names cyclooxygenase 1 (**COX1**) and cyclooxygenase 2 (**COX2**). Their structures are very similar, but COX1 is constitutive whereas COX2 is induced by growth factors, cytokines, and tumor promoters. PGH_2 is converted to prostacyclin, thromboxanes, and prostaglandins by various tissue isomerases. The effects of prostaglandins are multitudinous and varied. They are particularly important in the female reproductive cycle, in parturition, in the cardiovascular system, in inflammatory responses, and in the causation of pain. Drugs that target production of prostaglandins are among the most common over the counter drugs available (Clinical Box 1–6).

Arachidonic acid also serves as a substrate for the production of several physiologically important **leukotrienes** and **lipoxins.**

Cholesterol & Atherosclerosis

The interest in cholesterol-lowering drugs stems from the role of cholesterol in the etiology and course of **atherosclerosis**. This extremely widespread disease predisposes to myocardial infarction, cerebral thrombosis, ischemic gangrene of the extremities, and other serious illnesses. It is characterized by infiltration of cholesterol and oxidized cholesterol into macrophages, converting them into foam cells in lesions of the arterial walls. This is followed by a complex sequence of changes involving platelets, macrophages, smooth muscle cells, growth factors, and inflammatory mediators that produces proliferative lesions that eventually ulcerate and may calcify. The lesions distort the vessels and make them rigid. In individuals with elevated plasma cholesterol levels, the incidence of atherosclerosis and its complications is increased. The normal range for plasma cholesterol is said to be 120–200 mg/dL, but in men, there is a clear, tight, positive correlation between the death rate from ischemic heart disease and plasma cholesterol levels above 180 mg/dL. Furthermore, it is now clear that lowering plasma cholesterol by diet and drugs slows and may even reverse the progression of atherosclerotic lesions and the complications they cause.

In evaluating plasma cholesterol levels in relation to atherosclerosis, it is important to analyze the LDL and HDL levels as well. LDL delivers cholesterol to peripheral tissues, including atheromatous lesions, and the LDL plasma concentration correlates positively with myocardial infarctions and ischemic strokes. On the other hand, HDL picks up cholesterol from peripheral tissues and transports it to the liver, thus lowering plasma cholesterol. It is interesting that women, who have a lower incidence of myocardial infarction than men, have higher HDL levels. In addition, HDL levels are increased in individuals who exercise and those who drink one or two alcoholic drinks per day, whereas they are decreased in individuals who smoke, are obese, or live sedentary lives. Moderate drinking decreases the incidence of myocardial infarction, and obesity and smoking are risk factors that increase it. Plasma cholesterol and the incidence of cardiovascular diseases are increased in **familial hypercholesterolemia**, due to various loss-of-function mutations in the genes for LDL receptors.

THERAPEUTIC HIGHLIGHTS

Although atherosclerosis is a progressive disease, it is also preventable in many cases by limiting risk factors, including lowering "bad" cholesterol through a healthy diet and exercise. Drug treatments for high cholesterol, including the statins among others, provide additional relief that can complement a healthy diet and exercise. If atherosclerosis is advanced, invasive techniques, such as angioplasty and stenting, can be used to unblock arteries.

Pharmacology of Prostaglandins

Because prostaglandins play a prominent role in the genesis of pain, inflammation, and fever, pharmacologists have long sought drugs to inhibit their synthesis. Glucocorticoids inhibit phospholipase A_2 and thus inhibit the formation of all eicosanoids. A variety of nonsteroidal anti-inflammatory drugs (NSAIDs) inhibit both cyclooxygenases, inhibiting the production of PGH_2 and its derivatives. Aspirin is the best known of these, but ibuprofen, indomethacin, and others are also used. However, there is evidence that prostaglandins synthesized by COX2 are more involved in the production of pain and inflammation, and prostaglandins synthesized by COX1 are more involved in protecting the gastrointestinal mucosa from ulceration. Several novel NSAIDs have been introduced in an attempt to specifically target COX enzymes. However in many cases significant side effects, including increased incidence of stroke and heart attack, have led to drug withdrawals from the market. More research is underway to better understand all the effects of the COX enzymes, their products, and their inhibitors.

The leukotrienes, thromboxanes, lipoxins, and prostaglandins have been called local hormones. They have short half-lives and are inactivated in many different tissues. They undoubtedly act mainly in the tissues at sites in which they are produced. The leukotrienes are mediators of allergic responses and inflammation. Their release is provoked when specific allergens combine with IgE antibodies on the surfaces of mast cells. They produce bronchoconstriction, constrict arterioles, increase vascular permeability, and attract neutrophils and eosinophils to inflammatory sites. Diseases in which they may be involved include asthma, psoriasis, acute respiratory distress syndrome, allergic rhinitis, rheumatoid arthritis, Crohn disease, and ulcerative colitis.

CHAPTER SUMMARY

- Cells contain approximately two-thirds of the body fluids, while the remaining extracellular fluid is found between cells (interstitial fluid) or in the circulating lymph and blood plasma.
- The number of molecules, electrical charges, and particles of substances in solution are important in physiology.
- Biologic buffers including bicarbonate, proteins, and phosphates can bind or release protons in solution to help maintain pH. Biologic buffering capacity of a weak acid or base is greatest when $pK_a = pH$.
- Although the osmolality of solutions can be similar across a plasma membrane, the distribution of individual molecules and distribution of charge across the plasma membrane can be quite different. The separation of concentrations of charged species sets up an electrical gradient at the plasma membrane

(inside negative). The electrochemical gradient is in large part maintained by the Na, K ATPase. These are affected by the Gibbs–Donnan equilibrium and can be calculated using the Nernst potential equation.

- Cellular energy can be stored in high-energy phosphate compounds, including adenosine triphosphate (ATP). Coordinated oxidation–reduction reactions allow for the production of a proton gradient at the inner mitochondrial membrane that ultimately yields to the production of ATP in the cell.

- Nucleotides made from purine or pyrimidine bases linked to ribose or 2-deoxyribose sugars with inorganic phosphates are the basic building blocks for nucleic acids, DNA, and RNA. The fundamental unit of DNA is the gene, which encodes information to make proteins in the cell. Genes are transcribed into messenger RNA, and with the help of ribosomal RNA and transfer RNAs, translated into proteins.

- Amino acids are the basic building blocks for proteins in the cell and can also serve as sources for several biologically active molecules. Translation is the process of protein synthesis. After synthesis, proteins can undergo a variety of posttranslational modifications prior to obtaining their fully functional cell state.

- Carbohydrates are organic molecules that contain equal amounts of C and H_2O. Carbohydrates can be attached to proteins (glycoproteins) or fatty acids (glycolipids) and are critically important for the production and storage of cellular and body energy. The breakdown of glucose to generate energy, or glycolysis, can occur in the presence or absence of O_2 (aerobic or anaerobically). The net production of ATP during aerobic glycolysis is 19 times higher than anaerobic glycolysis.

- Fatty acids are carboxylic acids with extended hydrocarbon chains. They are an important energy source for cells and fatty acid derivatives—including triglycerides, phospholipids and sterols—have additional important cellular applications.

MULTIPLE-CHOICE QUESTIONS

For all questions, select the single best answer unless otherwise directed.

1. In a patch clamp experiment on a neuron, a student is able to accurately measure membrane potential. At the start of the measurements, the student finds that the resting membrane potential is normal for a neuron, measuring –70 mV. The student manipulates the preparation to allow for membrane potential to stabilize at the K^+ equilibrium (E_K). In this preparation, the intracellular concentration for K^+ is 150 mmol/L and the extracellular concentration for K^+ is 5.5 mmol/L. Assuming the temperature of the experiment is 37°C, what is the equilibrium potential of the neuron in the experiment?
   A. –70 mV
   B. –90 mV
   C. +70 mV
   D. +90 mV

2. Parents of a child being treated for diabetes notice changes in their child that include a flushed face, a smell of acetone on his breath and a change in his breathing pattern that includes consistent sighs and deep breaths. They visit the family physician for tests and find excess sugars and ketones in the boy's urine, serum bicarbonate levels less than 15 mEq/L and blood pH less than 7.3. The doctor determines that the child is suffering from diabetic ketoacidosis and takes necessary steps to alter insulin, blood glucose and hydration. Note that a diagnosis of metabolic acidosis is determined even though the pH is 0.2 units less than normal. The difference in concentration of H^+ in a solution of pH 2.0 compared with one of pH 7.0 is
   A. 5-fold
   B. 1/5 as much
   C. 10^5-fold
   D. 10^{-5} as much

3. A woman with a family history of hemophilia brings her son to a hemophilia treatment center because she noticed excessive bruising in response to everyday activities and excessive bleeding after small cuts. At the center, it is discovered that the boy additionally displays hemarthroses and blood tests show that coagulation factor IX is very low. The family history includes an uncle that had similar bruising as a child but is now a healthy adult. He had been diagnosed with hemophilia B Leyden, a sex-linked inherited transcriptional defect of blood coagulation factor IX. The child is put on prophylactic treatment with recombinant factor IX to prevent bleeding and monitored for changes in coagulation factor IX as he enters adulthood. Transcription, abnormal in this patient, refers to
   A. the process where an mRNA is used as a template for protein production.
   B. the process where a DNA sequence is copied into RNA for the purpose of gene expression.
   C. the process where DNA wraps around histones to form a nucleosome.
   D. the process of replication of DNA prior to cell division.

4. In a mouse model of muscle development researchers found that insulin-like growth factor I (IGF-I) was not able to fully establish muscle development and growth. However, the mouse model contained a full and competent *Igf1* gene. Further study of the mouse showed that muscle fibers in the mouse contained an IGF-I-like peptide with an extended primary amino acid sequence. Further testing demonstrated that the mouse was deficient in a subtilisin-like peptidase that converted pro-IGF-I peptide to the fully active IGF-I peptide. The primary structure of this IGF-I peptide refers to which of the following:
   A. the twist, folds, or twist and folds of the amino acid sequence into stabilized structures within the protein (ie, α-helices and β-sheets).
   B. the arrangement of subunits to form a functional structure.
   C. the amino acid sequence.
   D. the arrangement of twisted chains and folds within a protein into a stable structure.

5. The parents of a developing infant bring their child to the family physician for a checkup. The doctor notices a low growth rate and a swollen abdomen and asks the parents if they have any concerns. The parents note that the child often seems to be hungry yet also seems tired and irritable. Blood tests indicate a low blood glucose concentration and higher than normal levels of lipids and uric acid. A genetic test reveals von Gierke disease, or type I glycogen storage disease (GSD I). In relation to glycogen storage, fill in the blanks to complete the following two sentences. _____ refers to the

process of making glycogen and _____ refers to the process of breakdown of glycogen.
  A. Glycogenolysis, glycogenesis
  B. Glycolysis, glycogenolysis
  C. Glycogenesis, glycogenolysis
  D. Glycogenolysis, glycolysis

6. A 44-year-old healthy, nonsmoking, physically active adult male visits his physician for a routine physical and has blood and urine analyzed. Because of a family history of heart disease, the patient pays special attention to his cholesterol levels. To his satisfaction, he finds that his cholesterol numbers are excellent: low-density lipoprotein (LDL) cholesterol is 90 mg/dL, high-density lipoprotein (HDL) is 60 mg/dL, triglycerides are 150 mg/dL and total cholesterol is 180 mg/dL. The major lipoprotein source of the cholesterol used in cells is
  A. chylomicrons.
  B. intermediate-density lipoproteins (IDL).
  C. albumin-bound free fatty acids.
  D. low-density lipoproteins (LDL).
  E. high-density lipoproteins (HDL).

7. In a biochemistry laboratory, an eager group of students discovered a way to quickly switch cells from aerobic to anaerobic metabolism and measure energy metabolism in response to the changes in substrate source. Their breakthrough came with a nanoparticle delivery system that allowed for instant delivery of sugars, amino acids and/or fatty acids to cells with near 100% transport to the energy metabolism machinery within the cells. They tested a variety of compounds under aerobic and anaerobic conditions. Which of the following substrate would produce the most high-energy phosphate compounds?
  A. Aerobic metabolism of 1 mol of glucose
  B. Anaerobic metabolism of 1 mol of glucose
  C. Aerobic metabolism of 1 mol of galactose
  D. Aerobic metabolism of 1 mol of amino acid
  E. Aerobic metabolism of 1 mol of long-chain fatty acid

8. A 25-year-old prospective father has a family history of myocardial infarction at less than 50 years of age and high serum levels of low-density lipoprotein (LDL) cholesterol. He attends genetic counseling with his wife and they are referred to a specialist in familial hypercholesterolemia. Following a genetic screen, the prospective father finds that he has a mutation in the LDL receptor that is likely the cause of his high LDL. He is prescribed a statin drug with the goal of reducing his LDL levels below 80 mg/dL. In this patient, when LDL binds to its receptor and enters cells by receptor-mediated endocytosis, which of the following does **NOT** occur?
  A. Decrease in the formation of cholesterol from mevalonic acid
  B. Increase in the intracellular concentration of cholesteryl esters
  C. Increase in the transfer of cholesterol from the cell to HDL
  D. Decrease in the rate of synthesis of LDL receptors
  E. Decrease in the amount of cholesterol in endosomes

9. You are interested in the differences in function of ordinary fat cells (lipocytes) from those found in brown fat. You know that catabolism of fat in brown fat cells can lead to increased heat generation when compared to similar reactions in white fat cells, and also are aware that brown fat cells contain larger fat droplets and increased mitochondria. However, you are unclear of the mechanism underlying these phenomena. In the laboratory, you are able to isolate mitochondria and fat droplets from each cell type, and place them into an artificial cell system that allows for full mitochondrial function. To evaluate if the mechanism of heat generation is from the type of fats stored, or mitochondrial differences, you conduct experiments that measure heat and ATP generation after mixing fat droplets and mitochondria from normal and brown fat cells in various combinations. Assuming you use equimolar fat in each experiment and hold mitochondrial function steady, which of the following outcomes is likely to occur.
  A. Combination of brown fat and brown mitochondria yields similar heat and ATP to white fat and brown mitochondria.
  B. Combination of brown fat and white mitochondria yields more heat and ATP to white fat and white mitochondria.
  C. Combination of white fat and white mitochondria yields similar heat and ATP to white fat and brown mitochondria.
  D. Combination of white fat and brown mitochondria yields similar heat and ATP to white fat and white mitochondria.
  E. Combination of white fat and brown mitochondria yields less heat and ATP than white fat and white mitochondria.

10. In a laboratory experiment designed to illustrate the necessity of Na, K ATPase in cells, students set up two liquid-containing chambers separated by a semipermeable membrane. The students half-filled both sides with H_2O. They labeled side A of the chamber as representing the intracellular side and side B of the chamber as the extracellular fluid. To side A they added a 120-mM solution of negatively charged, impermeable protein balanced with K^+ in an effort to mimic the increased protein concentration in the intracellular compartment. Based on the Donnan effect, what would be predicted to happen to K^+, Cl^- and H_2O in the two chambers?
  A. $[K^+]$ and $[Cl^-]$ would increase in side A and H_2O would also increase in side A.
  B. $[K^+]$ and $[Cl^-]$ would increase in side A and H_2O would move to side B.
  C. $[K^+]$ and $[Cl^-]$ would decrease in side A and H_2O would move to side B.
  D. $[K^+]$ and $[Cl^-]$ would decrease in side A and H_2O would increase in side A.
  E. $[K^+]$ and $[Cl^-]$ would not move, H_2O would increase in side A.

ANSWERS

1. The correct answer is **B.** The E_K can be calculated using the Nernst equation: $E_K = (RT/FZ_K) \ln [K^+_o]/[K^+_i]$. Converting to log and substituting for RT/FZ_K yields: $61.5 \log [K^+_o]/[K^+_i]$. Using the numbers above yields: $61.5 \log (150/5.5) = -90$ mV. **A** represents a typical resting potential for a neuron, close to, but slightly different than the E_K; **C** and **D** represent values for E_K if valence of K^+ were (−), or, if the intracellular and extracellular concentrations were reversed.

2. The correct answer is **C**. The biological H^+ concentration ($[H^+]$), critical for the proper function of proteins and enzymes in the body, is measured on a logarithmic scale. Thus, a difference of 5 units of pH is equivalent to a 5-log difference, or 10^5-fold change. **A** and **B** represent changes measured on a straight multiplicative scale and are ruled out. Since pH is the $-$log of the $[H^+]$, the concentration is much higher at the lower pH, and so **D** can be ruled out.

3. The correct answer is **B**. Improper transcription such as that observed in hemophilia B Leyden can occur from mutations in promoter regions that prevent mRNA production and downstream protein production. Protein production from mRNA **A** is translation and can be ruled out as an answer. The condensation of DNA around histones **C** is necessary for the compacting of DNA when it is not undergoing transcription or replication and so can be ruled out. Replication of DNA **D** is also separate from the production of mRNA, and thus, can be ruled out.

4. The correct answer is **C**. Active IGF-I is a product of several posttranslational modifications of the originally transcribed protein. IGF-I is initially translated as a pre-pro-peptide. The N-terminal "pre" sequence is used as a signaling peptide to direct IGF-I for secretion and is cleaved by signal peptidases. The "pro" sequence is a C-terminal peptide that is cleaved by subtilisin-like peptidases to complete posttranslational cleavage processing of the signaling molecule. The primary amino acid sequence, whether it is that of the functional peptide or the pre-processed peptide, refers to amino acid content and their specific order from the amino- to the carboxy-terminus. The twists and folds **A** of these peptides/proteins are the secondary structure, and can be ruled out. The arrangements of multiple subunits of a protein refers to the quaternary structure, and so **B** can be eliminated. The arrangement of twisted changes and folds within a protein refers to the tertiary structure, eliminating **D**.

5. The correct answer is **C**. When glucose is in excess (eg, after meals) it is stored as glycogen in the liver until needed. In GSD I, the stored glycogen cannot be broken down into glucose when needed due to an enzyme deficiency. This prevents proper blood glucose level maintenance and results in hypoglycemia within a few hours after eating. Glycogenesis refers to the forming of the glycogen from glucose and glycogenolysis is the breakdown of glycogen to form glucose that can be used for energy production. **A** has the terms reversed and can be ruled out. Glycolysis specifically refers to the breakdown of glucose and eventual formation of energy, ruling out **B** and **D**.

6. The correct answer is **D**. Cholesterol can be made within cells and also carried in the blood through a variety of lipoproteins. LDLs have a high percentage of cholesterol and represent the major carrier in the serum that can disperse cholesterol made in the liver to various cells in the body. Chylomicrons **A** are rich in triglycerides. They represent the least dense of the cholesterol transport molecules and can be ruled out as the major source for cellular delivery. IDLs have a moderate amount of cholesterol. Their fate is to be taken up by liver cells, or to lose triglycerides in the bloodstream until they become LDL molecules. Thus, IDLs **B** can be ruled out as the major lipoprotein source of cholesterol used in cells. Albumin is a common blood protein that is frequently used by hydrophic proteins or fatty acids as a carrier in the blood; however, albumin-bound fatty acids **C** do not account for serum cholesterol transport. HDLs **E** contain a higher percentage of proteins than cholesterol and tend to carry cholesterol back to the liver, and thus can be ruled out.

7. The correct answer is **E**. Catabolism of a 6 carbon fatty acid to CO_2 and H_2O through the citric acid cycle yields 44 mol of ATP. In contrast, catabolism of 1 mol of the more common substrate, glucose **A** to CO_2 and H_2O through the citric acid cycle will yield 38 mol of ATP. Anaerobic metabolism of 1 mol of glucose via the Embden–Meyerhof pathway yields only 3 mol of ATP, ruling out **B**. For galactose to be metabolized to ATP, it first has to be converted to glucose. This necessary step requires energy and thus will yield less energy than glucose such that **C** can be ruled out. When required, proteins can be broken down into amino acids that can be further catabolized, with energy produced. However, the many biochemical steps necessary to produce a sugar that can then enter the energy-producing pathway are costly and rule out **D**.

8. The correct answer is **E**. Metabolic pathways and receptor-mediated uptake of cholesterol in the cell are subject to negative feedback; that is, as the concentrations of their products increase, the reactions that produce the product are negatively regulated. Because LDL receptor-mediated endocytosis results in an immediate increase in intracellular cholesterol concentration, there is a decrease in cell-based cholesterol metabolism and a decrease in LDL receptor synthesis, eliminating **A** and **D**. The internalization of LDLs into the cell necessarily increases cholesteryl delivery to the cell and upregulates movement of excess cholesterol to HDL to leave the cell, eliminating both **B** and **C**.

9. The correct answer is **A**. While brown fat cells have larger lipid droplets than normal lipocytes, it is a defect in the mitochondrial transport chain such that the proton conductance is compromised, leading to greater heat and less ATP production than would be seen if the mitochondrial reactions were fully conserved. The large numbers of mitochondria in these cells further amplifies this difference. Thus, there should be no differences between comparisons of fats from the brown fat cells and normal lipocytes, ruling out **B**. Likewise, there should be increased heat and reduced ATP in brown mitochondria from normal mitochondria when comparing similar fats, ruling out **C**, **D**, and **E**.

10. The correct answer is **A**. The Gibbs–Donnan equation states that at equilibrium $[K^+_A][Cl^-_A] = [K^+_B][Cl^-_B]$, while the protein will remain in side A. This results in a net movement of both K^+ and Cl^- to side A and rules out **C**, **D**, and **E**. H_2O follows the salts, moving down its concentration gradient to side A, eliminating **B**. In a cell system, this added osmotic pressure would cause a cell to swell; however, the action of Na, K ATPase uses the energy of ATP to maintain salt concentrations and reduce osmotic pressure.

Overview of Cellular Physiology in Medical Physiology

CHAPTER

2

OBJECTIVES

After studying this chapter, you should be able to:

- Name the prominent cellular organelles and state their functions in cells.
- Name the building blocks of the cellular cytoskeleton and state their contributions to cell structure and function.
- Name the intercellular and cellular to extracellular connections.
- Define the processes of exocytosis and endocytosis, and describe the contribution of each to normal cell function.
- Define proteins that contribute to membrane permeability and transport.
- Recognize various forms of intercellular communication and describe ways in which chemical messengers (including second messengers) affect cellular physiology.

INTRODUCTION

The cell is the fundamental working unit of all organisms. In humans, cells can be highly specialized in both structure and function; alternatively, cells from different organs can share features and function. A basic knowledge of cell biology is essential to an understanding of the organ systems and the way they function in the body. The fundamental aspects of cellular and molecular physiology will be reviewed in this chapter.

■ FUNCTIONAL MORPHOLOGY OF THE CELL

A key tool for examining cellular constituents is the microscope. A light microscope can resolve structures as close as 0.2 μm, while an electron microscope can resolve structures as close as 0.002 μm. The advent of common access to phase contrast, fluorescent, confocal, and many other microscopy techniques along with specialized probes for both static and dynamic cellular structures further expanded the examination of cell structure and function. Equally revolutionary advances in modern biophysical, biochemical, and molecular biological techniques have also greatly contributed to our knowledge of the cell. The specialization of the cells in the various organs is considerable, and no cell can be called "typical" of all cells in the body. However, a number of structures (**organelles**) are common to most cells. These structures are shown in **Figure 2–1**.

CELL MEMBRANES

The membrane that surrounds the cell, the **plasma membrane**, is made up of lipids and proteins and is semipermeable, allowing some substances to pass through it while excluding others. Its permeability can also be varied because it contains numerous regulated ion channels and transport proteins that can change the amounts of substances moving across it. The nucleus and other organelles in the cell are bound by similar membranous structures.

General features among the cellular membranes include their size and lipid makeup. They are generally about 7.5 nm (75 angstroms [Å]) thick. The major lipids are phospholipids such as phosphatidylcholine, phosphatidylserine, and phosphatidylethanolamine. The shape of the phospholipid molecule reflects its solubility properties: the "head" end of the molecule contains the phosphate portion and is relatively soluble in water (polar,

25

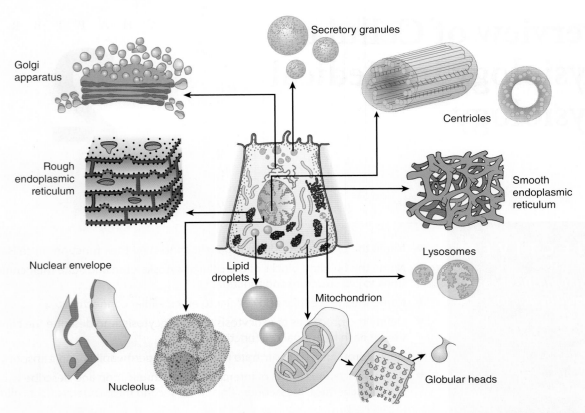

FIGURE 2–1 **Cross-sectional diagram of a hypothetical cell as seen with the light microscope.** Individual organelles are expanded for closer examination. (Modified with permission from Bloom W, Fawcett DW: A Textbook of Histology, 9th ed. Philadelphia: Saunders; 1968)

hydrophilic) and the "tail" ends are relatively insoluble (nonpolar, **hydrophobic**). The possession of both hydrophilic and hydrophobic properties makes the lipid an **amphipathic** molecule. In the membrane, the hydrophilic ends of the molecules are exposed to the aqueous environment that bathes the exterior of the cells and the aqueous cytoplasm; the hydrophobic ends meet in the water-poor interior of the membrane (**Figure 2–2**). Cell membranes additionally can contain various glycosphingolipids, sphingomyelin, and cholesterol, depending on their structure and function.

Many different proteins are embedded in the membrane **(integral proteins),** whereas others **(peripheral proteins)** are associated with the inside or outside of the membrane (Figure 2–2). The amount of protein varies significantly with the function of the cell but makes up on average 50% of the mass of the membrane which amounts to approximately one protein molecule per 50 of the much smaller phospholipid molecules. The proteins in the membrane carry out many functions. Some are **cell adhesion molecules (CAMs)** that anchor cells to their neighbors or to basal laminas. Some proteins function as **pumps,** actively transporting ions across the membrane. Other proteins function as **carriers,** transporting substances down electrochemical gradients by facilitated diffusion. Still others are **ion channels,** which, when activated, permit the passage of ions into or out of the cell. Specialized proteins termed **receptors** can bind **ligands** or messenger molecules, initiating physiologic changes inside

the cell. Proteins also function as **enzymes,** catalyzing reactions at the surfaces of the membrane.

The hydrophobic portions of the proteins are usually located in the interior of the membrane, whereas the charged, hydrophilic portions are located on the surfaces. Peripheral proteins are attached to the surfaces of the membrane in various ways. One common way is attachment to glycosylated forms of phosphatidylinositol. Proteins held by these **glycosylphosphatidylinositol (GPI) anchors** (**Figure 2–3**) include enzymes, various antigens, a number of CAMs, and proteins that combat cell lysis by complement. Other membrane associated proteins are **lipidated** (Figure 2–3) with **myristoyl, palmitoyl,** or **prenyl** groups (ie, attached to geranylgeranyl or farnesyl groups).

The protein structure of biologic membranes varies not only from cell to cell, but also within the same cell. For example, some of the enzymes embedded in cell membranes are different from those in mitochondrial membranes. In epithelial cells, the enzymes in the cell membrane on the mucosal surface differ from those in the cell membrane on the basal and lateral margins of the cells; that is, the cells are **polarized.** Such polarization makes directional transport across epithelia possible. The membranes are dynamic structures, and their constituents are being constantly renewed at different rates. Some proteins are anchored to the cytoskeleton, but others move laterally in the membrane.

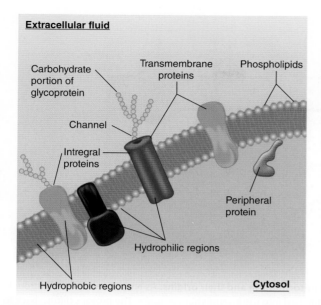

FIGURE 2–2 Organization of the phospholipid bilayer and associated proteins in a biologic membrane. The phospholipid molecules that make up the membrane each have two hydrophobic fatty acid chains attached to a hydrophilic phosphate head. Individual proteins take on different shapes and positions in the cell. Many are integral proteins, extending into the membrane or peripheral proteins that are attached to the inside or outside (not shown) of the membrane. Proteins can be modified (eg, with carbohydrate chains). Many specific protein attachments and cholesterol that are commonly found in the bilayer are omitted for clarity.

Underlying most cells is a thin **basement membrane** or, more properly, the **basal lamina.** The basal lamina is an extracellular matrix made up of many proteins that hold cells together, regulate their development, and determine their growth. These include collagens, laminins, fibronectin, tenascin, and various proteoglycans.

MITOCHONDRIA

Mitochondria provide eukaryotic cells with the ability to form the energy-rich compound ATP by **oxidative phosphorylation** and **apoptosis** (programmed cell death), among other functions. Each eukaryotic cell can have hundreds to thousands of mitochondria. Each mitochondrion has an outer membrane, an intermembrane space, an inner membrane, which is folded to form shelves **(cristae),** and a central matrix space. The enzyme complexes responsible for oxidative phosphorylation are lined up on the cristae (**Figure 2–4**).

Mitochondria have their own genome. Human mitochondrial DNA is a double-stranded circular molecule containing approximately 16,500 base pairs (compared with over a billion in nuclear DNA). It codes for 13 protein subunits that are associated with proteins encoded by nuclear genes to form four enzyme complexes plus two ribosomal and 22 transfer RNAs that are needed for protein production by the intramitochondrial ribosomes. Mitochondria have an ineffective DNA repair system; the mutation rate for mitochondrial DNA is over 10 times the rate for nuclear DNA. A large number of relatively rare diseases have been traced to mutations in mitochondrial DNA. These include disorders of

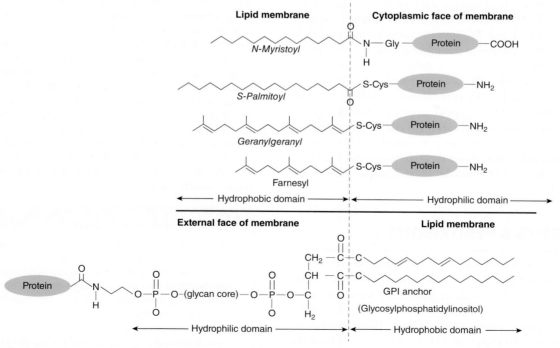

FIGURE 2–3 Protein linkages to membrane lipids. A variety of lipid modifications can occur at amino or carboxy terminals of proteins attached to cytosolic side of the plasma membrane. Many proteins associated with the external side of the plasma membrane can be attached via glycosylated forms of phosphatidylinositol (eg, GPI anchors).

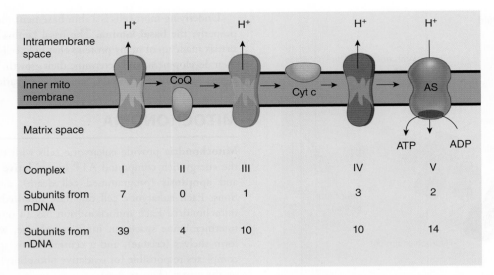

Complex	I	II	III	IV	V
Subunits from mDNA	7	0	1	3	2
Subunits from nDNA	39	4	10	10	14

FIGURE 2–4 **Components involved in oxidative phosphorylation in mitochondria and their origins.** As enzyme complexes I through IV convert 2-carbon metabolic fragments to CO_2 and H_2O, protons (H^+) are pumped into the intermembrane space. The protons diffuse back to the matrix space via complex V, ATP synthase (AS), in which ADP is converted to ATP. The enzyme complexes are made up of subunits coded by mitochondrial DNA (mDNA) and nuclear DNA (nDNA), and the figures document the contribution of each DNA to the complexes.

tissues with high metabolic rates in which energy production is defective as a result of abnormalities in the production of ATP, as well as other disorders (**Clinical Box 2–1**).

The enzyme complexes responsible for oxidative phosphorylation illustrate the interactions between the products of the mitochondrial genome and the nuclear genome. For example, complex I, reduced nicotinamide adenine dinucleotide dehydrogenase (NADH), is made up of 7 protein subunits coded by mitochondrial DNA and 39 subunits coded by nuclear DNA. The origin of the subunits in the other complexes is shown in Figure 2–4. Complex II, succinate dehydrogenase-ubiquinone oxidoreductase; complex III, ubiquinonecytochrome c oxidoreductase; and complex IV, cytochrome c oxidase, act with complex I, coenzyme Q, and cytochrome c to convert metabolites to CO_2 and water. Complexes I, III, and IV pump protons (H^+) into the intermembrane space during this electron transfer. The protons then flow down their electrochemical gradient through complex V, ATP synthase, which harnesses this energy to generate ATP.

LYSOSOMES & PEROXISOMES

Lysosomes are somewhat irregular cytoplasmic structures surrounded by membranes. The interior of these structures is more acidic than the rest of the cytoplasm, providing a degradation environment for endocytosed material. The interior is kept acidic by the action of a **proton pump,** or **H^+ ATPase.** This integral membrane protein uses the energy of ATP to move protons from the cytosol up their electrochemical gradient and keep the lysosome near pH 5.0. Lysosomes can contain over 40 types of hydrolytic enzymes, some of which are listed in **Table 2–1**. These enzymes

TABLE 2–1 Some of the enzymes found in lysosomes and the cell components that are their substrates.

Enzyme	Substrate
Ribonuclease	RNA
Deoxyribonuclease	DNA
Phosphatase	Phosphate esters
Glycosidases	Complex carbohydrates: glycosides and polysaccharides
Arylsulfatases	Sulfate esters
Collagenase	Collagens
Cathepsins	Proteins

function best at the acidic pH of the lysosomal compartment. This can be a safety feature for the cell; if the lysosomes were to break open and release their contents, the enzymes would not be efficient at the near neutral cytosolic pH 7.2, and thus would be unable to digest cytosolic targets they may encounter. Diseases associated with lysosomal dysfunction are discussed in Clinical Box 2–2.

Peroxisomes are 0.5 μm in diameter, are surrounded by a membrane, and contain enzymes that can either produce H_2O_2 (**oxidases**) or break it down (**catalases**). Proteins are directed to the peroxisome by a unique signal sequence with the help of protein chaperones, **peroxins.** The peroxisome membrane contains a number of peroxisome-specific proteins for specialized transport. The peroxisome matrix contains more than 40 enzymes which operate in concert with enzymes outside the peroxisome to catalyze a variety of anabolic and catabolic reactions (eg, breakdown of lipids). Peroxisomes can form by budding of the endoplasmic reticulum, or by division.

CYTOSKELETON

All cells have a **cytoskeleton,** a system of fibers that not only maintains the structure of the cell but also permits it to change shape and move. The cytoskeleton is made up primarily of **microtubules, intermediate filaments,** and **microfilaments** (Figure 2–5), along with proteins that anchor them and tie them together. Specialized molecular motors can move proteins and organelles along microtubules and microfilaments.

Microtubules (Figure 2–5) are long, hollow structures with 5 nm walls surrounding a cavity 15 nm in diameter. They are made up of two globular protein subunits: α- and β-tubulin. A third subunit, γ-tubulin, is associated with the production of microtubules by the centrosomes. The α and β subunits form heterodimers, which aggregate to form long tubes made up of stacked rings, with each ring usually containing 13 subunits. The tubules interact with guanosine triphosphate (GTP) to facilitate their formation. Although microtubule subunits can be added to either end, microtubules are polar with assembly predominating at the "+" end and disassembly predominating at the "−" end. Both processes occur simultaneously in vitro. The growth of microtubules is under the control of a variety of physical (eg, temperature) and cellular factors that can directly interact with microtubules.

Because of their constant assembly and disassembly, microtubules are a dynamic portion of the cytoskeleton. They provide

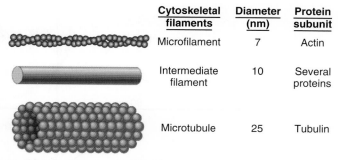

Cytoskeletal filaments	Diameter (nm)	Protein subunit
Microfilament	7	Actin
Intermediate filament	10	Several proteins
Microtubule	25	Tubulin

FIGURE 2–5 Cytoskeletal elements of the cell. Artistic impressions that depict the major cytoskeletal elements are shown on the left, with approximate diameters and protein subunits of these elements are listed for comparison. (Reproduced with permission from Widmaier EP, Raff H, Strang KT: *Vander's Human Physiology: The Mechanisms of Body Function*, 11th ed. New York, NY: McGraw-Hill; 2008.)

the tracks along which several different molecular motors move transport vesicles, organelles such as secretory granules, and mitochondria from one part of the cell to another. They also form the spindle, which moves the chromosomes in mitosis. Cargo can be transported in either direction on microtubules. Microtubule assembly is prevented by several drugs including colchicine and vinblastine. The anticancer drug **paclitaxel (Taxol)** binds to microtubules and makes them so stable that organelles cannot move, mitotic spindles cannot form, and the cells die.

Intermediate filaments (Figure 2–5) are 8–14 nm in diameter and are made up of various subunits. Some of these filaments connect the nuclear membrane to the cell membrane. They form a flexible scaffolding for the cell and help it resist external pressure. In their absence, cells rupture more easily, and when they are abnormal in humans, blistering of the skin is common. The proteins that make up intermediate filaments are cell-type specific, and are thus frequently used as cellular markers. For example, vimentin is a major intermediate filament in fibroblasts, whereas cytokeratin is expressed in epithelial cells.

Microfilaments (Figure 2–5) are long solid fibers with a 5- to 9-nm diameter that are made up of **actin.** Although actin is most often associated with muscle contraction, it is present in all types of cells. It is the most abundant protein in mammalian cells, and can account for as much as 15% of the total cellular protein. Its structure is highly conserved; for example, 88% of the amino acid sequences in yeast and rabbit actin are identical. Actin filaments polymerize and depolymerize in vivo, and it is not uncommon to find polymerization occurring at one end of the filament while depolymerization is occurring at the other end. **Filamentous (F) actin** refers to intact microfilaments and **globular (G) actin** refers to the unpolymerized protein actin subunits. F-actin fibers attach to various parts of the cytoskeleton and can interact directly or indirectly with membrane-bound proteins. They reach to the tips

of the microvilli on the epithelial cells of the intestinal mucosa. They are also abundant in the lamellipodia that cells put out when they crawl along surfaces. The actin filaments interact with integrin receptors and form **focal adhesion complexes,** which serve as points of traction with the surface over which the cell pulls itself. Some molecular motors use microfilaments as tracks.

MOLECULAR MOTORS

The molecular motors that move proteins, organelles, and other cell parts (collectively referred to as "cargo") to all parts of the cell are 100–500 kDa ATPases. They attach to their cargo at one end of the molecule and to microtubules or actin polymers with the other end, sometimes referred to as the "head." They convert the energy of ATP into movement along the cytoskeleton, taking their cargo with them. There are three super families of molecular motors: **kinesin, dynein,** and **myosin.** Examples of individual proteins from each superfamily are shown in **Figure 2–6.** It is important to note that there is extensive variation among superfamily members, allowing for the specialization of function (eg, choice of cargo, cytoskeletal filament type, and/or direction of movement).

The conventional form of **kinesin** is a double-headed molecule that tends to move its cargo toward the "+" ends of microtubules. One head binds to the microtubule and then bends its neck while the other head swings forward and binds, producing almost continuous movement. Some kinesins are associated with mitosis and meiosis. Other kinesins perform different functions, including moving cargo to the "–" end of microtubules. **Dyneins** have two heads, with their "neck" pieces embedded in a complex of proteins. **Cytoplasmic dyneins** have a function like that of conventional kinesin, except they tend to move particles and

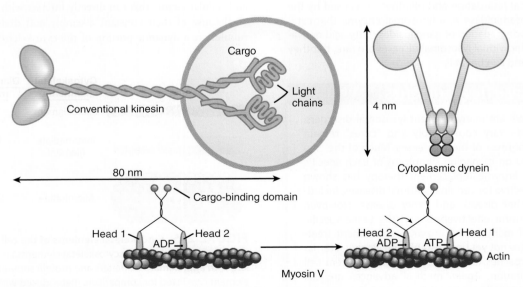

FIGURE 2–6 Examples of molecular motors. Conventional kinesin is shown attached to cargo, in this case a membrane-bound organelle (light blue). Cytoplasmic dynein is shown in isolation. Myosin V and its ability to "walk" along a microfilament are displayed in a two-part sequence. Note that the "heads" of each of the motors hydrolyze ATP and use the energy to produce motion.

membranes to the "–" end of the microtubules. The multiple forms of **myosin** in the body are divided into 18 classes. The heads of myosin molecules bind to actin and produce motion by bending their neck regions (myosin II) or walking along microfilaments, one head after the other (myosin V). In these ways, they perform functions as diverse as contraction of muscle and cell migration.

MICROTUBULE STRUCTURES: CENTROSOMES & CILIA

Near the nucleus in the cytoplasm of eukaryotic animal cells is a **centrosome.** The centrosome is made up of two **centrioles** and surrounding amorphous **pericentriolar material.** The centrioles are short cylinders arranged so that they are at right angles to each other. Microtubules in groups of three run longitudinally in the walls of each centriole (Figure 2–1). Nine of these triplets are spaced at regular intervals around the circumference. The centrosomes are **microtubule-organizing centers (MTOCs)** that contain γ-tubulin. The microtubules grow out of this γ-tubulin in the pericentriolar material. When a cell divides, the centrosomes duplicate themselves, and the pairs move apart to the poles of the mitotic spindle, where they monitor the steps in cell division. In multinucleate cells, a centrosome is near each nucleus.

Cilia are specialized cellular projections that are used by multicellular organisms to propel mucus and other substances over the surface of various epithelia. Additionally, virtually all cells in the human body contain a primary cilium that emanates from the surface. The primary cilium serves as a sensory organelle that receives both mechanical and chemical signals from other cells and the environment. Cilia are functionally indistinct from the eukaryotic flagella of sperm cells. Within the cilium there is an **axoneme** that comprises a unique arrangement of nine outer microtubule doublets and two inner microtubules ("9+2" arrangement). Along this cytoskeleton is **axonemal dynein.** Coordinated dynein–microtubule interactions within the axoneme are the basis of ciliary and sperm movement. At the base of the axoneme and just inside lies the **basal body.** It has nine circumferential triplet microtubules, like a centriole, and there is evidence that basal bodies and centrioles are interconvertible. A wide variety of diseases and disorders arise from dysfunctional cilia (**Clinical Box 2–3**).

CELL ADHESION MOLECULES

Cells are attached to the basal lamina and to each other by cell adhesion molecules (**CAMs**). The unique structural and signaling functions of these adhesion proteins have been found to be important in embryonic development for formation of the nervous system and other tissues, in holding tissues together in adults, in inflammation and wound healing, and in the metastasis of tumors. Many CAMs pass through the cell membrane and are anchored to the cytoskeleton inside the cell. Some bind to like molecules on other cells (homophilic binding), whereas others bind to nonself molecules (heterophilic binding). Many bind to

laminins, a family of large cross-shaped molecules with multiple receptor domains in the extracellular matrix.

CAMs can be divided into four broad families: (1) **integrins,** heterodimers that bind to various receptors; (2) adhesion molecules of the **IgG superfamily** of immunoglobulins; (3) **cadherins,** Ca^{2+}-dependent molecules that mediate cell-to-cell adhesion by homophilic reactions; and (4) **selectins,** which have lectin-like domains that bind carbohydrates. CAMs can provide structure as well as transmit signals into and out of the cell. For example, cells that lose their contact with the extracellular matrix via integrins have a higher rate of apoptosis than anchored cells, and interactions between integrins and the cytoskeleton are involved in cell movement.

INTERCELLULAR CONNECTIONS

Intercellular junctions that form between the cells in tissues can be broadly split into two groups: junctions that fasten the cells to one another and to surrounding tissues, and junctions that permit transfer of ions and other molecules from one cell to another. The types of junctions that tie cells together and endow tissues

---

CLINICAL BOX 2–3

Ciliary Diseases

Primary ciliary dyskinesia refers to a set of inherited disorders that limit ciliary structure and/or function. Disorders associated with ciliary dysfunction have long been recognized in the conducting airway. Altered ciliary function in the conducting airway can slow the mucociliary escalator and result in airway obstruction and increased infection. Dysregulation of ciliary function in sperm cells has also been well characterized to result in loss of motility and infertility. Ciliary defects in the function or structure of primary cilia have been shown to have effects on a variety of tissues/organs. As would be expected, such diseases are quite varied in their presentation, largely due to the affected tissue, and include mental retardation, retinal blindness, obesity, polycystic kidney disease, liver fibrosis, ataxia, and some forms of cancer.

THERAPEUTIC HIGHLIGHTS

The severity in ciliary disorders can vary widely, and treatments targeted to individual organs also vary. Treatment of ciliary dyskinesia in the conducting airway is focused on keeping the airways clear and free of infection. Strategies include routine washing and suctioning of the sinus cavities and ear canals and liberal use of antibiotics. Other treatments that keep the airway from being obstructed (eg, bronchodilators, mucolytics, and corticosteroids) are also commonly used.

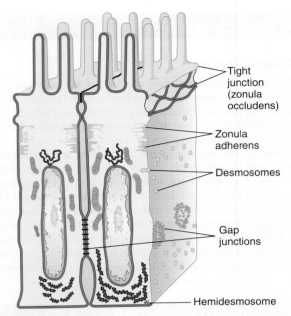

FIGURE 2–7 Intercellular junctions in the mucosa of the small intestine. Tight junctions (zonula occludens), adherens junctions (zonula adherens), desmosomes, gap junctions, and hemidesmosomes are all shown in relative positions in a polarized epithelial cell.

with strength and stability include **tight junctions,** which are also known as the **zonula occludens** (Figure 2–7). The **desmosome** and **zonula adherens** also help hold cells together, and the **hemidesmosome** and **focal adhesions** attach cells to their basal laminas. The **gap junction** forms a cytoplasmic "tunnel" for regulated diffusion of small molecules (< 1000 Da) between two neighboring cells.

Tight junctions characteristically surround the apical margins of the cells in epithelia such as the intestinal mucosa, the walls of the renal tubules, and the choroid plexus. They are also important to endothelial barrier function. They are made up of ridges—half from one cell and half from the other—which adhere so strongly at cell junctions that they almost obliterate the space between the cells. There are three main families of transmembrane proteins that contribute to tight junctions: **occludin, junctional adhesion molecules,** and **claudins;** there are several more proteins that interact from the cytosolic side. Tight junctions permit the passage of some ions and solute in between adjacent cells (**paracellular pathway**) and the degree of this "leakiness" varies, depending in part on the protein makeup of the tight junction. Extracellular fluxes of ions and solute across epithelia at these junctions are a significant part of overall ion and solute flux. Tight junctions also prevent the movement of proteins in the plane of the membrane, helping maintain the different distribution of transporters and channels in the apical and basolateral cell membranes that make transport across epithelia possible.

In epithelial cells, each zonula adherens is usually a continuous structure on the basal side of the zonula occludens, and it is a major site of attachment for intracellular microfilaments. It contains cadherins. Desmosomes are patches characterized by apposed thickenings of the membranes of two adjacent cells.

Attached to the thickened area in each cell are intermediate filaments, some running parallel to the membrane and others radiating away from it. Between the two membrane thickenings, the intercellular space contains filamentous material that includes cadherins and the extracellular portions of several other transmembrane proteins. Hemidesmosomes look like half-desmosomes that attach cells to the underlying basal lamina and are connected intracellularly to intermediate filaments. However, they contain integrins rather than cadherins. Focal adhesions also attach cells to their basal laminas. As noted previously, they are labile structures associated with actin filaments inside the cell, and they play an important role in cell movement.

GAP JUNCTIONS

The intercellular space is up to 4 nm at gap junctions. Here, units called **connexons** in the membrane of each cell are lined up with one another to form the dodecameric gap junction. Each connexon is made up of six protein subunits called **connexins.** They surround a channel that, when lined up with the channel in the corresponding connexon in the adjacent cell, permits substances to pass between the cells without entering the extracellular fluid (ECF). The pore diameter in the channel is estimated between 0.8 and 1.4 nm, which permits the passage of ions, sugars, amino acids, and other solutes with molecular weights up to about 1000 Da. Gap junctions thus permit the rapid propagation of electrical activity from cell to cell, as well as the exchange of various chemical messengers. However, the gap junction channels are not simply passive, nonspecific conduits. At least 20 different gene codes for connexins in humans, and mutations in these genes can lead to diseases that are highly selective in terms of the tissues involved and the type of communication between cells produced (**Clinical Box 2–4**). It should be noted that connexons can also provide a conduit for regulated passage of small molecules between the cytoplasm and the ECF. Such movement can allow autocrine and/or paracrine signaling between and among cells in a tissue.

NUCLEUS & RELATED STRUCTURES

A nucleus is present in all eukaryotic cells that divide. The nucleus is made up in large part of the **chromosomes,** the structures in the nucleus that carry a complete blueprint for all the heritable species and individual characteristics of the animal. Except in germ cells, the chromosomes occur in pairs, one originally from each parent. Each chromosome is made up of a giant molecule of **DNA.** The DNA strand is about 2 m long, but it can fit in the nucleus because at intervals it is wrapped around a core of histone proteins to form a **nucleosome.** There are about 25 million nucleosomes in each nucleus. The whole complex of DNA and proteins is called **chromatin.** During cell division, the coiling around histones is loosened and pairs of chromosomes become visible, but between cell divisions only clumps of chromatin can be discerned in the nucleus.

The nucleus of most cells contains a **nucleolus** (Figure 2–1), a patchwork of granules rich in **RNA.** In some cells, the nucleus

Connexins in Disease

There is extensive information related to the in vivo functions of connexins, growing out of work on connexin knockouts in mice and the analysis of mutations in human connexins. The mouse knockouts demonstrated that connexin deletions lead to electrophysiologic defects in the heart and predisposition to sudden cardiac death, female sterility, abnormal bone development, abnormal growth in the liver, cataracts, hearing loss, and a host of other abnormalities. Information from these and other studies has allowed for the identification of several connexin mutations known to be responsible for almost 20 different human diseases. These diseases include several skin disorders such as Clouston syndrome (a connexin 30 (Cx30) defect) and erythrokeratoderma variabilis (Cx30.3 and Cx31); inherited deafness (Cx26, Cx30, and Cx31); predisposition to myoclonic epilepsy (Cx36); predisposition to arteriosclerosis (Cx37); cataract (Cx46 and Cx50); idiopathic atrial fibrillation (Cx40); and X-linked Charcot-Marie-Tooth disease (Cx32). It is interesting to note that each of these target tissues for disease contain other connexins that do not fully compensate for loss of the crucial connexins in disease development. Understanding how loss of individual connexins alters cell physiology to contribute to these and other human diseases is an area of intense research.

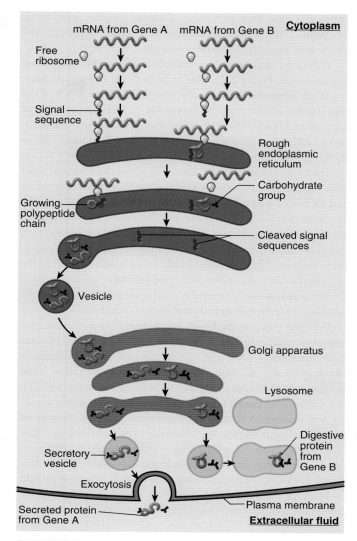

FIGURE 2–8 Rough endoplasmic reticulum and protein translation. Messenger RNA and ribosomes meet up in the cytosol for translation. Proteins that have appropriate signal peptides begin translation, and then associate with the endoplasmic reticulum (ER) to complete translation. The association of ribosomes is what gives the ER its "rough" appearance. (Reproduced with permission from Widmaier EP, Raff H, Strang KT: *Vander's Human Physiology: The Mechanisms of Body Function,* 11th ed. New York, NY: McGraw-Hill; 2008.)

contains several of these structures. Nucleoli are most prominent and numerous in growing cells. They are the site of synthesis of ribosomes, the structures in the cytoplasm in which proteins are synthesized. The interior of the nucleus has a skeleton of fine filaments that are attached to the **nuclear membrane,** or **envelope** (Figure 2–1), which surrounds the nucleus. This membrane is a double membrane, and spaces between the twofolds are called **perinuclear cisterns.** The membrane is permeable only to small molecules. However, it contains **nuclear pore complexes,** which allows for transport of proteins and mRNA.

ENDOPLASMIC RETICULUM & GOLGI APPARATUS

The **endoplasmic reticulum** is a complex series of tubules in the cytoplasm of the cell (**Figures** 2–1 and **2–8**). The inner limb of its membrane is continuous with a segment of the nuclear membrane, so in effect this part of the nuclear membrane is a cistern of the endoplasmic reticulum. The tubule walls are made up of membrane. In **rough (granular) endoplasmic reticulum,** ribosomes are attached to the cytoplasmic side of the membrane, whereas in **smooth (agranular) endoplasmic reticulum,** ribosomes are absent. Free ribosomes are also found in the cytoplasm. The granular endoplasmic reticulum is concerned with protein synthesis and the initial folding of polypeptide chains with the formation of disulfide bonds. The agranular endoplasmic reticulum is the site of steroid synthesis in steroid-secreting cells and the site of detoxification processes in other cells. A modified endoplasmic

reticulum, the sarcoplasmic reticulum, plays an important role in skeletal and cardiac muscle. In particular, the endoplasmic or sarcoplasmic reticulum can sequester Ca^{2+} ions and allow for their release as signaling molecules in the cytosol.

The ribosomes in eukaryotes measure approximately 22 × 32 nm. Each is made up of a large (60S) and a small (40S) subunit. The ribosomes are complex structures, containing many different proteins and at least three ribosomal RNAs. They are the sites of protein synthesis. The ribosomes that become attached to the endoplasmic reticulum synthesize all transmembrane proteins, most secreted proteins, and most proteins that are stored in the **Golgi apparatus,** lysosomes, and endosomes. These proteins typically have a hydrophobic **signal peptide** at one end (Figure 2–8). The polypeptide chains that form these proteins are extruded into the endoplasmic reticulum. The free ribosomes synthesize cytoplasmic proteins and the proteins found in peroxisomes and mitochondria.

The Golgi apparatus is a collection of membrane-enclosed sacs (cisternae; Figure 2–1). One or more Golgi apparati are present in all eukaryotic cells, usually near the nucleus. Much of the organization of the Golgi is directed at proper glycosylation of proteins and lipids. There are more than 200 enzymes that function to add, remove, or modify sugars from proteins and lipids in the Golgi apparatus.

The Golgi apparatus is a polarized structure, with cis and trans sides. Membranous vesicles containing newly synthesized proteins bud off from the granular endoplasmic reticulum and fuse with the cistern on the cis side of the apparatus. The proteins are then passed via other vesicles to the middle cisterns and finally to the cistern on the trans side, from which vesicles branch off into the cytoplasm. From the trans Golgi, vesicles shuttle to the lysosomes and to the cell exterior via constitutive and nonconstitutive pathways, both involving **exocytosis.** Conversely, vesicles are pinched off from the cell membrane by **endocytosis** and pass to endosomes.

Vesicular traffic in the Golgi, and between other membranous compartments in the cell, is regulated by a combination of common mechanisms along with special mechanisms that determine where inside the cell they will go. One prominent feature is the involvement of a series of regulatory proteins controlled by GTP or GDP binding (**small G proteins**) associated with vesicle assembly and delivery. A second prominent feature is the presence of proteins called **SNAREs** (for soluble N-ethylmaleimide-sensitive factor attachment receptor). The v- (for vesicle) SNAREs on vesicle membranes interact in a lock-and-key fashion with t- (for target) SNAREs. Individual vesicles also contain structural protein or lipids in their membrane that help target them for specific membrane compartments (eg, Golgi sacs, cell membranes).

APOPTOSIS

In addition to dividing and growing, cells can die and be absorbed under genetic control. This process is called **programmed cell death,** or **apoptosis.** It should be distinguished from necrosis, in which healthy cells are destroyed by external processes such as inflammation. Apoptosis is a very common process during development and in adulthood. In the central nervous system (CNS), large numbers of neurons are produced and then die during the remodeling that occurs during development and synapse formation. In the immune system, apoptosis gets rid of inappropriate clones of immunocytes and is responsible for the lytic effects of glucocorticoids on lymphocytes. Apoptosis is also an important factor in processes such as removal of the webs between the fingers in fetal life and regression of duct systems in the course of sexual development in the fetus. In adults, it participates in the cyclic breakdown of the endometrium that leads to menstruation. In epithelia, such as enterocytes sloughed off the tips of intestinal villi, cells that lose their connections to the basal lamina and neighboring cells undergo apoptosis. Abnormal apoptosis can occur in autoimmune diseases, neurodegenerative diseases, and cancer.

One final common pathway bringing about apoptosis is activation of **caspases,** a group of cysteine proteases. Many of these have been characterized to date in mammals; 11 have been found in humans. They exist in cells as inactive proenzymes until activated by the cellular machinery. The net result is DNA fragmentation, cytoplasmic and chromatin condensation, and eventually membrane bleb formation, with cell breakup and removal of the debris by phagocytes (**Clinical Box 2–5**).

CLINICAL BOX 2–5

Molecular Medicine

Fundamental research on molecular aspects of genetics, regulation of gene expression, and protein synthesis has been paying off in clinical medicine at a rapidly accelerating rate.

One early dividend was an understanding of the mechanisms by which antibiotics exert their effects. Almost all act by inhibiting protein synthesis at one or another of the steps described previously. Antiviral drugs act in a similar way; for example, acyclovir and ganciclovir act by inhibiting DNA polymerase. Some of these drugs have this effect primarily in bacteria, but others inhibit protein synthesis in the cells of other animals, including mammals. This fact makes antibiotics of great value for research as well as for treatment of infections. Single genetic abnormalities that cause over 600 human diseases have been identified. Many of the diseases are rare, but others are more common and some cause conditions that are severe and eventually fatal. Examples include the defectively regulated Cl⁻ channel in cystic fibrosis and the unstable **trinucleotide repeats** in various parts of the genome that cause Huntington disease, the fragile X syndrome, and several other neurologic diseases. Abnormalities in mitochondrial DNA can also cause human diseases such as Leber hereditary optic neuropathy and some forms of cardiomyopathy. Not surprisingly, genetic aspects of cancer are probably receiving the greatest current attention. Some cancers are caused by **oncogenes,** genes that are carried in the genomes of cancer cells and are responsible for producing their malignant properties. These genes are derived by somatic mutation from closely related **proto-oncogenes,** which are normal genes that control growth. Over 100 oncogenes have been described. Another group of genes produce proteins that suppress tumors, and more than 10 of these **tumor suppressor genes** have been described. The most studied of these is the p53 gene on human chromosome 17. The p53 protein produced by this gene triggers apoptosis. It is also a nuclear transcription factor that appears to increase production of a 21-kDa protein that blocks two-cell cycle enzymes, slowing the cycle and permitting repair of mutations and other defects in DNA. The p53 gene is mutated in up to 50% of human cancers, with the production of p53 proteins that fail to slow the cell cycle and permit other mutations in DNA to persist. The accumulated mutations eventually cause cancer.

■ TRANSPORT ACROSS CELL MEMBRANES

EXOCYTOSIS & ENDOCYTOSIS

Vesicles containing material for export are targeted to the cell membrane (Figure 2–9), where they bond in a similar manner to that discussed in vesicular traffic between Golgi stacks, via the v-SNARE/t-SNARE arrangement. The area of fusion then breaks down, leaving the contents of the vesicle outside and the cell membrane intact. This is the Ca^{2+}-dependent process of **exocytosis**. Note that exocytotic secretion from the cell occurs via two pathways (Figure 2–9). In the **nonconstitutive pathway,** proteins from the Golgi apparatus initially enter secretory granules, where processing of prohormones to the mature hormones occurs before exocytosis. The other pathway, the **constitutive pathway,** involves the prompt transport of proteins to the cell membrane in vesicles, with little or no processing or storage. The nonconstitutive pathway is sometimes called the **regulated pathway,** but this term is misleading because the output of proteins by the constitutive pathway is also regulated. It is apparent that exocytosis adds to the total amount of membrane surrounding the cell, and if membrane were not removed elsewhere at an equivalent rate, the cell would enlarge. However, removal of cell membrane occurs by **endocytosis**, and such exocytosis–endocytosis coupling maintains the surface area of the cell at its normal size.

There are various types of endocytosis named for the size of particles being ingested as well as the regulatory requirements for the particular process. These include **phagocytosis, pinocytosis, clathrin-mediated endocytosis, caveolae-dependent uptake,** and **nonclathrin/noncaveolae endocytosis.**

Phagocytosis ("cell eating") is the process by which bacteria, dead tissue, or other bits of microscopic material are engulfed by cells such as the polymorphonuclear leukocytes of the blood. The material makes contact with the cell membrane, which then invaginates. The invagination is pinched off, leaving the engulfed material in the membrane-enclosed vacuole and the cell membrane intact. **Pinocytosis** ("cell drinking") is a similar process with the vesicles much smaller in size and the substances ingested are in solution. The small size membrane that is ingested with each event should not be misconstrued; cells undergoing active pinocytosis (eg, macrophages) can ingest the equivalent of their entire cell membrane in just 1 h.

Clathrin-mediated endocytosis occurs at membrane indentations where the protein **clathrin** accumulates. As endocytosis progresses, the clathrin molecules form a protein array that surrounds the endocytotic vesicle. At the neck of the vesicle, the GTP binding protein **dynamin** is involved in pinching off the vesicle. Once the complete vesicle is formed, the clathrin falls off and is recycled to form another vesicle. The vesicle fuses with and dumps its contents into an **early endosome** (Figure 2–9). From the early endosome, a new vesicle can bud off and return to the cell membrane. Alternatively, the early endosome can become a **late endosome** and fuse with a lysosome (Figure 2–9) in which the contents are digested by the lysosomal proteases. Clathrin-mediated endocytosis is responsible for the internalization of many receptors and the ligands bound to them and plays a major role in synaptic function.

Some areas of the cell membrane are especially rich in cholesterol and sphingolipids and have been called **rafts.** These rafts are probably the precursors of flask-shaped membrane depressions called **caveolae** when their walls become infiltrated with a protein called **caveolin.** Cholesterol can interact directly with caveolin, effectively limiting the protein's ability to move around in the membrane. Internalization via caveolae involves binding of cargo to caveolin and regulation by dynamin. Caveolae are prominent in endothelial cells, where they help in the uptake of nutrients from the blood.

It now appears that all vesicles involved in transport have protein coats. In humans, over 50 coat complex subunits have been identified. Vesicles that transport proteins from the trans Golgi to lysosomes have assembly protein 1 (AP-1) clathrin coats, and endocytotic vesicles that transport to endosomes have AP-2 clathrin coats. Vesicles that transport between the endoplasmic reticulum and the

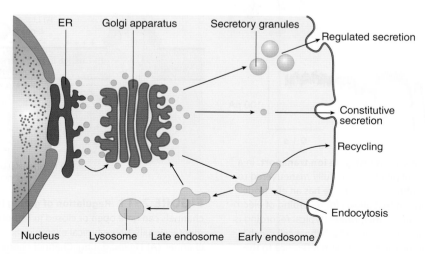

FIGURE 2–9 Cellular structures involved in protein processing. Structures involved in protein processing, from transcription to secretion, are shown. See text for details.

Golgi have coat proteins I and II (COPI and COPII). Certain amino acid sequences or attached groups on the transported proteins can target the proteins for particular locations. For example, mannose-6-phosphate groups target transfer from the Golgi to mannose-6-phosphate receptors (MPR) on the lysosomes.

Various small G proteins of the Rab family are especially important in vesicular traffic. They guide and facilitate orderly attachments of these vesicles. To illustrate the complexity of directing vesicular traffic, humans have 60 Rab proteins and 35 SNARE proteins.

MEMBRANE PERMEABILITY & MEMBRANE TRANSPORT PROTEINS

An important technique that has permitted major advances in our knowledge about transport proteins is **patch clamping.** A micropipette is placed on the membrane of a cell and forms a tight seal to the membrane. The patch of membrane under the pipette tip usually contains only a few transport proteins, allowing for their detailed biophysical study (**Figure 2–10**). The cell can be

left intact (**cell-attached patch clamp**). Alternatively, the patch can be pulled loose from the cell, forming an **inside-out patch.** A third alternative is to suck out the patch with the micropipette still attached to the rest of the cell membrane, providing direct access to the interior of the cell (**whole cell recording**).

Small, nonpolar molecules (including O_2 and N_2) and small uncharged polar molecules such as CO_2 diffuse across the lipid membranes of cells. However, the membranes have very limited permeability to other substances. Instead, they cross the membranes by endocytosis and exocytosis and by passage through highly specific **transport proteins,** transmembrane proteins that form channels for ions or transport substances such as glucose, urea, and amino acids. The limited permeability applies even to water, with simple diffusion being supplemented throughout the body with various water channels (**aquaporins**).

Some transport proteins are simple aqueous **ion channels,** though many of these have special features that make them selective for a given substance such as Ca^{2+} or, in the case of aquaporins, for water. These membrane-spanning proteins (or collections of proteins) have tightly regulated pores that can be **gated** opened or closed in response to local changes (**Figure 2–11**). Some are gated by alterations in membrane potential (**voltage-gated**), whereas others are opened or closed in response to a ligand (**ligand-gated**). The ligand is often external (eg, a neurotransmitter or a hormone). However, it can also be internal; intracellular Ca^{2+}, cyclic adenosine 3′,5′-monophosphate (cAMP), lipids, or one of the G proteins produced in cells can bind directly to channels and activate them. Some channels are also opened by mechanical stretch, and these **mechanosensitive channels** play an important role in cell movement.

Other transport proteins are **carriers** that bind ions and other molecules and then change their configuration, moving the bound molecule from one side of the cell membrane to the other. Molecules move from areas of high concentration to areas of low

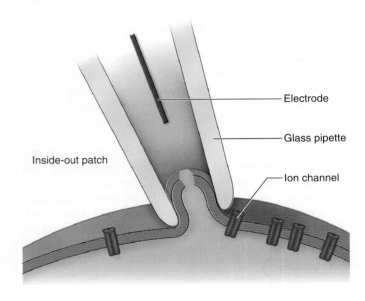

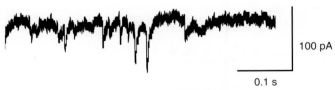

100 pA

0.1 s

FIGURE 2–10   Patch clamp to investigate ion transport. In a patch clamp experiment, a small pipette is carefully maneuvered to seal off a portion of a cell membrane. The pipette has an electrode bathed in an appropriate solution that allows for recording of electrical changes through any pore in the membrane (typical recording is shown below). The illustrated setup is termed a "whole cell patch" because of the orientation of the membrane with reference to the electrode. Other configurations include cell attached, inside-out, and outside-out patches. (Whole cell recording used with permission from Lila Wollman.)

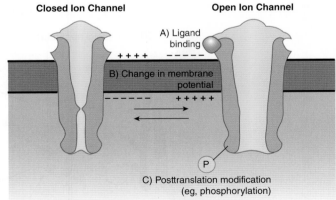

FIGURE 2–11   Regulation of gating in ion channels. Ion channels can gate open or closed in response to several environmental signals. Some typical examples are shown in an idealized channel. **(A)** Ligand gating: Channel opens in response to ligand binding. **(B)** Voltage gating: Channel opens in response to a change in membrane potential. **(C)** Posttranslational modification: Channel gates in response to modification such as phosphorylation.

concentration (down their **chemical gradient**), and cations move to negatively charged areas whereas anions move to positively charged areas (down their **electrical gradient**). When carrier proteins move substances in the direction of their chemical or electrical gradients, no energy input is required and the process is called **facilitated diffusion.** A typical example is glucose transport by the glucose transporter, which moves glucose down its concentration gradient from the ECF to the cytoplasm of the cell. Other carriers transport substances against their electrical and chemical gradients. This form of transport requires energy and is called **active transport.** In animal cells, the energy is provided almost exclusively by hydrolysis of ATP. Not surprisingly, therefore, many carrier molecules are ATPases, enzymes that catalyze the hydrolysis of ATP. One of these ATPases is **sodium–potassium adenosine triphosphatase (Na, K ATPase),** which is also known as the **Na, K pump.** There are also H, K ATPases in the gastric mucosa and the renal tubules. Ca^{2+} ATPase pumps Ca^{2+} out of cells. Proton ATPases acidify many intracellular organelles, including parts of the Golgi complex and lysosomes.

Some of the transport proteins are called **uniports** because they transport only one substance. Others are called **symports** because transport requires the binding of more than one substance to the transport protein and the substances are transported across the membrane together. An example is the symport in the intestinal mucosa that is responsible for the cotransport of Na^+ and glucose from the intestinal lumen into mucosal cells. Other transporters are called **antiports** because they exchange one substance for another.

ION CHANNELS

There are ion channels specific for K^+, Na^+, Ca^{2+}, and Cl^-, as well as channels that are nonselective for cations or anions. Each type of channel exists in multiple forms with diverse properties. Channels can be made up of identical subunits, combinations of very similar subunits, or combinations of asimilar subunits. Most K^+ channels are tetramers, with each of the four subunits forming part of the pore through which K^+ ions pass. Structural analysis of a bacterial voltage-gated K^+ channel indicates that each of the four subunits have a paddle-like extension containing four charges. When the channel is closed, these extensions are near the negatively charged interior of the cell. When the membrane potential is reduced, the paddles containing the charges bend through the membrane to its exterior surface, causing the channel to open. In the acetylcholine ion channel and other ligand-gated cation or anion channels, five subunits make up the pore. Members of the ClC family of Cl^- channels are dimers, but they have two pores, one in each subunit. Finally, aquaporins are tetramers with a water pore in each of the subunits.

Another family of Na^+ channels with a different structure has been found in the apical membranes of epithelial cells in the kidneys, colon, lungs, and brain. The **epithelial sodium channels (ENaCs)** are made up of three subunits encoded by three different genes. Each of the subunits probably spans the membrane twice, and the amino terminal and carboxyl terminal are located inside the cell. The α subunit transports Na^+, whereas the β and

γ subunits do not. However, the addition of the β and γ subunits increases Na^+ transport through the α subunit.

Humans have several types of Cl^- channels. The ClC dimeric channels are found in plants, bacteria, and animals, and there are nine different ClC genes in humans. Other Cl^- channels have the same pentameric form as the acetylcholine receptor; examples include the γ-aminobutyric acid A (GABA$_A$) and glycine receptors in the CNS. The cystic fibrosis transmembrane conductance regulator (CFTR) that is mutated in cystic fibrosis is also a Cl^- channel. Ion channel mutations cause a variety of **channelopathies**—diseases that mostly affect muscle and brain tissue and produce episodic paralyses or convulsions, but are also observed in nonexcitable tissues (Clinical Box 2–6).

Na, K ATPase

Na, K ATPase catalyzes the hydrolysis of ATP to adenosine diphosphate (ADP) and uses the energy to extrude three Na^+ from the cell and take two K^+ into the cell for each molecule of ATP hydrolyzed. It is an **electrogenic pump** in that it moves three positive charges out of the cell for each two that it moves in. It is found in all parts of the body. Its activity is inhibited by ouabain and related digitalis glycosides used in the treatment of heart failure. It is a heterodimer made up of α and β subunits both of which extend through the cell membrane (Figure 2–12). Separation of the subunits eliminates activity. The β subunit is a glycoprotein, whereas Na^+ and K^+ transport occur through the α subunit. The β subunit has a single membrane-spanning domain and is glycosylated. The α subunit probably spans the cell membrane 10 times, with the amino and carboxyl terminals both located intracellularly. This subunit has intracellular Na^+ and ATP binding sites and a phosphorylation site; it also has an

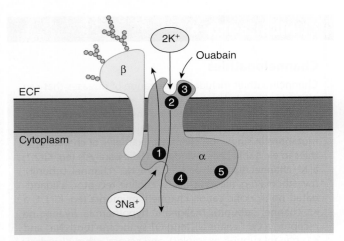

FIGURE 2–12   Na, K ATPase. The intracellular portion of the α subunit has a Na^+-binding site **(1)**, a phosphorylation site **(4)**, and an ATP-binding site **(5)**. The extracellular portion has a K^+-binding site **(2)** and an ouabain-binding site **(3)**. (Reproduced with permission from Horisberger JD, Lemas V, Kraehenbühl JP et al: Structure–function relationship of Na, K-ATPase, *Annu Rev Physiol.* 1991;53:565-584.)

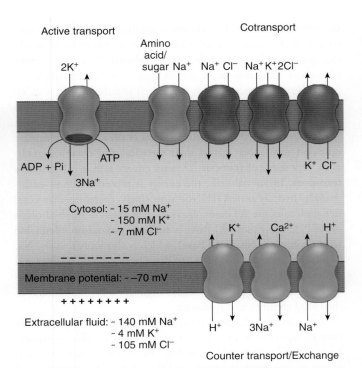

FIGURE 2–13   Composite diagram of main secondary effects of active transport of Na^+ and K^+. Na, K ATPase converts the chemical energy of ATP hydrolysis into maintenance of an inward gradient for Na^+ and an outward gradient for K^+. The energy of the gradients is used for countertransport, cotransport, and maintenance of the membrane potential. Some examples of cotransport and countertransport that use these gradients are shown.

extracellular binding site for K^+ When Na^+ binds to the α subunit, ATP also binds and is converted to ADP, with a phosphate being transferred to Asp 376. This causes a change in the configuration of the protein, extruding Na^+ into the ECF. K^+ then binds extracellularly, dephosphorylating the α subunit, which returns to its previous conformation, releasing K^+ into the cytoplasm.

The α and β subunits are heterogeneous, with $α_1$, $α_2$, and $α_3$ subunits and $β_1$, $β_2$, and $β_3$ subunits described so far. The $α_1$ isoform is found in the membranes of most cells, whereas $α_2$ is present in muscle, heart, adipose tissue, and brain, and $α_3$ is present in heart and brain. The $β_1$ subunit is widely distributed but is absent in certain astrocytes, vestibular cells of the inner ear, and glycolytic fast-twitch muscles. The fast-twitch muscles contain only $β_2$ subunits. The different α and β subunit structures of Na, K ATPase in various tissues allow for fine-tuning tissue functions.

The amount of Na^+ normally found in cells is not enough to saturate the pump, so if the Na^+ increases, more is pumped out. Pump activity is affected by second messenger molecules (eg, cAMP and diacylglycerol [DAG]). Thyroid hormones increase pump activity by a genomic action to increase the formation of Na, K ATPase molecules. Aldosterone also increases the number of pumps, although this effect is probably secondary. Dopamine in the kidney inhibits the pump via a phosphorylation and resulting in a natriuresis. Insulin increases pump activity by a variety of different mechanisms.

SECONDARY ACTIVE TRANSPORT

In many situations, the active transport of Na^+ is coupled to the transport of other substances (**secondary active transport**). For example, the luminal membranes of mucosal cells in the small intestine contain a symport that transports glucose into the cell

only if Na^+ binds to the protein and is transported into the cell at the same time. From the cells, the glucose enters the blood. The electrochemical gradient for Na^+ is maintained by the active transport of Na^+ out of the mucosal cell into ECF. Other examples are shown in **Figure 2–13**. In the heart, Na, K ATPase indirectly affects Ca^{2+} transport. An antiport in the membranes of cardiac muscle cells normally exchanges intracellular Ca^{2+} for extracellular Na^+.

Active transport of Na^+ and K^+ is one of the major energy-using processes in the body. On the average, it accounts for about 24% of the energy utilized by cells, and in neurons it accounts for 70%. Thus, it accounts for a large part of the basal metabolism. A major payoff for this energy use is the establishment of the electrochemical gradient in cells.

TRANSPORT ACROSS EPITHELIUM & ENDOTHELIUM

In the gastrointestinal tract, the pulmonary airways, the renal tubules, and other structures lined with polarized epithelial cells, as well as in lumen of blood and lymph vessels lined with endothelial cells, substances enter one side of a cell and exit another. This produces net movement of the substance from one side of the epithelium/endothelium to the other. For transepithelial/transendothelial transport to occur, the cells need to be bound by tight junctions and, obviously, have different ion channels and transport proteins in different parts of their membranes. Most of the instances of secondary active transport cited in the preceding paragraph involve transepithelial movement of ions and other molecules.

The capillary wall separating plasma from interstitial fluid is different from the cell membranes separating interstitial fluid from intracellular fluid because the pressure difference across it makes **filtration** a significant factor in producing movement of water and solute. By definition, filtration is the process by which fluid is forced through a membrane or other barrier because of a difference in pressure on the two sides. The structure of the capillary wall varies from one vascular bed to another. However, near skeletal muscle and many other organs, water and relatively small solutes are the only substances that cross the wall with ease. The apertures in the junctions between the endothelial cells are too small to permit plasma proteins and other colloids to pass through in significant quantities. The colloids have a high molecular weight but are present in large amounts. Small amounts cross the capillary wall by vesicular transport, but their effect is slight. Therefore, the capillary wall behaves like a membrane impermeable to colloids, and these exert an osmotic pressure of about 25 mmHg. The colloid osmotic pressure due to the plasma colloids is called the **oncotic pressure.** Filtration across the capillary membrane as a result of the hydrostatic pressure head in the vascular system is opposed by the oncotic pressure.

■ INTERCELLULAR COMMUNICATION

Cells communicate with one another primarily via chemical messengers. Within a given tissue, some messengers move from cell to cell via gap junctions without entering the ECF. In addition, cells are affected by chemical messengers secreted into the ECF, or by direct cell–cell contacts. Chemical messengers typically bind to protein receptors on the surface of the cell or, in some instances, in the cytoplasm or the nucleus, triggering sequences of intracellular changes that produce their physiologic effects. Three general types of intercellular communication are mediated by messengers in the ECF: (1) **neural communication,** in which neurotransmitters are released at synaptic junctions from nerve cells and act across a narrow synaptic cleft on a postsynaptic cell; (2) **endocrine communication,** in which hormones and growth factors reach cells via the circulating blood or the lymph; and (3) **paracrine communication,** in which the products of cells diffuse in the ECF to affect neighboring cells that may be some distance away (**Figure 2–14**). In addition, cells secrete chemical messengers that in some situations bind to receptors on the same cell, that is, the cell that secreted the messenger (**autocrine communication).** The chemical messengers include amines, amino acids, steroids, polypeptides, and in some instances, lipids, purine nucleotides, and pyrimidine nucleotides.

RECEPTORS FOR CHEMICAL MESSENGERS

The recognition of chemical messengers by cells typically begins by interaction with a receptor at that cell. There are over 20 families of receptors for chemical messengers characterized. These proteins are not static components of the cell; their numbers increase and decrease in response to various stimuli, and their properties change with changes in physiologic conditions. When a hormone or neurotransmitter is present in excess, the number of active receptors generally decreases (**downregulation**), whereas in the presence of a deficiency of the chemical messenger, there is an increase in the number of active receptors (**upregulation**). In the case of receptors in the membrane, receptor-mediated endocytosis is responsible for down-regulation in some instances; ligands bind to their receptors, and the ligand-receptor complexes move laterally in the membrane to coated pits, where they are taken into the cell by endocytosis (**internalization**). This decreases the number of receptors in the membrane. Some receptors are recycled after

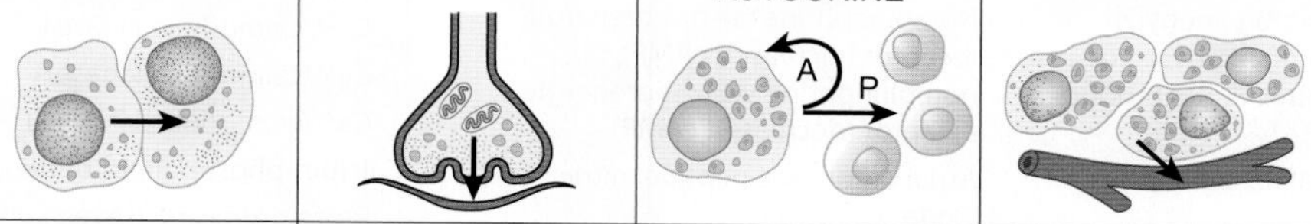

	GAP JUNCTIONS	SYNAPTIC	PARACRINE AND AUTOCRINE	ENDOCRINE
Message transmission	Directly from cell to cell	Across synaptic cleft	By diffusion in interstitial fluid	By circulating body fluids
Local or general	Local	Local	Locally diffuse	General
Specificity depends on	Anatomic location	Anatomic location and receptors	Receptors	Receptors

FIGURE 2–14 Intercellular communication by chemical mediators. Several common forms of cellular communication are illustrated. A, autocrine; P, paracrine.

internalization, whereas others are replaced by de novo synthesis in the cell. Another type of downregulation is **desensitization,** in which receptors are chemically modified in ways that make them less responsive.

MECHANISMS BY WHICH CHEMICAL MESSENGERS ACT

Receptor–ligand interaction is usually just the beginning of the cell response. This event is transduced into secondary responses within the cell that can be divided into four broad categories: (1) ion channel activation, (2) **G proteins** activation, (3) activation of enzyme activity within the cell, or (4) direct activation of transcription. Within each of these groups, responses can be quite varied. Some of the common mechanisms by which chemical messengers exert their intracellular effects are summarized in Table 2–2. Ligands such as acetylcholine bind directly to ion channels in the cell membrane, changing their conductance. Thyroid and steroid hormones, 1,25-dihydroxycholecalciferol, and retinoids enter cells and act on one or another member of a family of structurally related cytoplasmic or nuclear receptors. The activated receptor binds to DNA and increases transcription of selected mRNAs. Many other ligands in the ECF bind to receptors on the surface of cells and trigger the release of intracellular mediators such as cAMP, inositol trisphosphate (IP_3),

and DAG that initiate changes in cell function. Consequently, the extracellular ligands are called **"first messengers"** and the intracellular mediators are called **"second messengers."** Second messengers bring about many short-term changes in cell function by altering enzyme function, triggering exocytosis, and so on, but they also can lead to the alteration of transcription of various genes. A variety of enzymatic changes, protein–protein interactions, or second messenger changes can be activated within a cell in an orderly fashion following receptor recognition of the primary messenger. The resulting **cell signaling pathway** provides amplification of the primary signal and distribution of the signal to appropriate targets within the cell. Extensive cell signaling pathways also provide opportunities for feedback and regulation that can fine-tune the signal for the correct physiologic response by the cell.

The most predominant posttranslation modification of proteins, phosphorylation, is a common theme in cell signaling pathways. Cellular phosphorylation is under the control of two groups of proteins: **kinases,** enzymes that catalyze the phosphorylation of tyrosine or serine and threonine residues in proteins (or in some cases, in lipids); and **phosphatases,** proteins that remove phosphates from proteins (or lipids). Some of the larger receptor families are themselves kinases. Tyrosine kinase receptors initiate phosphorylation on tyrosine residues on complementary receptors following ligand binding. Serine/threonine kinase receptors initiate phosphorylation on serines or threonines in complementary receptors following ligand binding. Cytokine receptors are directly associated with a group of protein kinases that are activated following cytokine binding. Alternatively, second messenger changes can lead to phosphorylation further downstream in the signaling pathway. More than 500 protein kinases have been described. Some of the principal ones that are important in mammalian cell signaling are summarized in Table 2–3. In general, addition of phosphate groups changes the conformation of a targeted protein,

TABLE 2–2 Common mechanisms by which chemical messengers in the ECF bring about changes in cell function.

Mechanism	Examples
Open or close ion channels in cell membrane	Acetylcholine on nicotinic cholinergic receptor; norepinephrine on K^+ channel in the heart
Act via cytoplasmic or nuclear receptors to increase transcription of selected mRNAs	Thyroid hormones, retinoic acid, steroid hormones
Activate phospholipase C with intracellular production of DAG, IP_3, and other inositol phosphates	Angiotensin II, norepinephrine via α_1-adrenergic receptor, vasopressin via V_1 receptor
Activate or inhibit adenylyl cyclase, causing increased or decreased intracellular production of cAMP	Norepinephrine via β_1-adrenergic receptor (increased cAMP), norepinephrine via α_2-adrenergic receptor (decreased cAMP)
Increase cGMP in cell	Atrial natriuretic peptide, nitric oxide
Increase tyrosine kinase activity of cytoplasmic portions of transmembrane receptors	Insulin, EGF, PDGF, M-CSF
Increase serine or threonine kinase activity	TGF-β, activin, inhibin

cAMP, cyclic adenosine 3′,5′-monophosphate; cGMP, cyclic guanosine monophosphate; DAG, diacylglycerol; ECF, extracellular fluid; EGF, epidermal growth factor; IP_3, inositol triphosphate; M-CSF, monocyte colony-stimulating factor; PDGF, platelet-derived growth factor; TGF-β, transforming growth factor β.

TABLE 2–3 Sample protein kinases.

Phosphorylate serine or threonine residues, or both
Calmodulin-dependent
Myosin light-chain kinase
Phosphorylase kinase
Ca^{2+}/calmodulin kinase I
Ca^{2+}/calmodulin kinase II
Ca^{2+}/calmodulin kinase III
Calcium-phospholipid-dependent
Protein kinase C (seven subspecies)
Cyclic nucleotide-dependent
cAMP-dependent kinase (protein kinase A; two subspecies)
cGMP-dependent kinase
Phosphorylate tyrosine residues
Insulin receptor, EGF receptor, PDGF receptor, and M-CSF receptor

cAMP, cyclic adenosine 3′,5′-monophosphate; cGMP, cyclic guanosine monophosphate; EGF, epidermal growth factor; M-CSF, monocyte colony-stimulating factor; PDGF, platelet-derived growth factor.

Kinases in Cancer: Chronic Myeloid Leukemia

Kinases frequently play important roles in regulating cellular physiology outcomes, including cell growth and cell death. Dysregulation of cell proliferation or cell death is a hallmark of cancer. Although cancer can have many causes, a role for kinase dysregulation is exemplified in chronic myeloid leukemia (CML). CML is a pluripotent hematopoietic stem cell disorder characterized by the Philadelphia (Ph) chromosome translocation. The Ph chromosome is formed following a translocation of chromosomes 9 and 22, resulting in a shortened chromosome 22 (Ph chromosome). At the point of fusion, a novel gene (*bcr-abl*) encoding the active tyrosine kinase domain from a gene on chromosome 9 (Abelson tyrosine kinase; c-Abl) is fused to novel regulatory region of a separate gene on chromosome 22 (breakpoint cluster region; bcr). The *bcr-abl* fusion gene encodes a cytoplasmic protein with constitutively active tyrosine kinase. The dysregulated kinase activity in bcr-abl protein effectively limits white blood cell death signaling pathways while promoting cell proliferation and genetic instability. Experimental models have shown that translocation to produce the fusion bcr-abl protein is sufficient to produce CML in animal models.

THERAPEUTIC HIGHLIGHTS

The identification of *bcr-abl* as the initial transforming event in CML provided an ideal target for drug discovery. The drug imatinib was developed to specifically block the tyrosine kinase activity of the bcr-abl protein. Imatinib has proven to be an effective agent for treating chronic phase CML.

altering its functions and consequently the functions of the cell. The close relationship between phosphorylation and dephosphorylation of cellular proteins allows for a temporal control of activation of cell signaling pathways. The dysregulation of the phosphorylation and subsequent cellular signaling in a cell can lead to disease (Clinical Box 2–7).

STIMULATION OF TRANSCRIPTION

The activation of transcription, and subsequent translation, is a common outcome of cellular signaling. There are three distinct pathways for primary messengers to alter transcription of cells. First, as is the case with steroid or thyroid hormones, the primary messenger is able to cross the cell membrane and bind to a nuclear receptor, which then can directly interact with DNA to alter gene expression. A second pathway to gene transcription is the activation of cytoplasmic protein kinases that can move to the nucleus to phosphorylate a latent transcription factor for activation.

This pathway is a common end point of signals that go through the **mitogen activated protein (MAP) kinase** cascade. MAP kinases can be activated following a variety of receptor–ligand interactions through second messenger signaling. They comprise a series of three kinases that coordinate a stepwise phosphorylation to activate each protein in series in the cytosol. Phosphorylation of the last MAP kinase in series allows it to migrate to the nucleus where it phosphorylates a latent transcription factor. A third common pathway is the activation of a latent transcription factor in the cytosol, which then migrates to the nucleus and alters transcription. This pathway is shared by a diverse set of transcription factors that include **nuclear factor kappa B (NFκB**; activated following tumor necrosis family receptor binding and others) and **signal transducers of activated transcription (STATs**; activated following cytokine receptor binding). In all cases, the binding of the activated transcription factor to DNA increases (or in some cases, decreases) the transcription of mRNAs encoded by the gene to which it binds. The mRNAs are translated in the ribosomes, with the production of increased quantities of proteins that alter cell function.

INTRACELLULAR Ca²⁺ AS A SECOND MESSENGER

Ca^{2+} regulates a very large number of physiologic processes that are as diverse as proliferation, neural signaling, learning, contraction, secretion, and fertilization, so regulation of intracellular Ca^{2+} is of great importance. The free Ca^{2+} concentration in the cytoplasm at rest is maintained at about 100 nmol/L. The Ca^{2+} concentration in the interstitial fluid is about 12,000 times the cytoplasmic concentration (ie, 1,200,000 nmol/L), so there is a marked inwardly directed concentration gradient as well as an inwardly directed electrical gradient. Much of the intracellular Ca^{2+} is stored at relatively high concentrations in modified endoplasmic reticulum and other organelles (Figure 2–15), and these organelles provide a store from which Ca^{2+} can be mobilized via ligand-gated channels to increase the concentration of free Ca^{2+} in the cytoplasm. Increased cytoplasmic Ca^{2+} binds to and activates calcium-binding proteins. These proteins can have direct effects in cellular physiology, or can activate other proteins, commonly protein kinases, to further cell signaling pathways.

Ca^{2+} can enter the cell from the ECF, down its electrochemical gradient, through many different Ca^{2+} channels. Some of these are ligand-gated and others are voltage-gated. Stretch-activated-channels exist in some cells as well.

Many second messengers act by increasing the cytoplasmic Ca^{2+} concentration. The increase is produced by releasing Ca^{2+} from intracellular stores or by increasing the entry of Ca^{2+} into cells, or by both. IP_3 is the major second messenger that causes Ca^{2+} release from the endoplasmic reticulum through the direct activation of a ligand-gated channel, the IP_3 receptor. In effect, the generation of one second messenger (IP_3) can lead to the release of another second messenger (Ca^{2+}). In many tissues, transient release of Ca^{2+} from internal stores into the cytoplasm triggers opening of a population of Ca^{2+} channels in the cell membrane

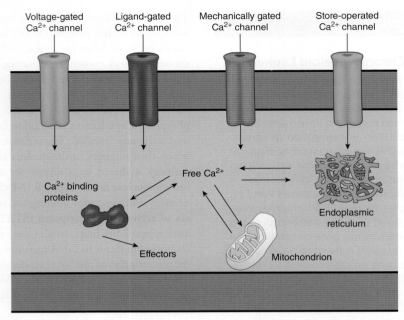

FIGURE 2–15 **Ca²⁺ handling in mammalian cells.** Ca²⁺ can enter the cell via a variety of channel types. In addition, Ca²⁺ is stored in the endoplasmic reticulum (and, to a lesser extent in the mitochondrion) where it can be released to alter free Ca²⁺ concentration in the cytoplasm. Free Ca²⁺ can be bound by proteins that then have a variety of downstream physiologic effects. Ca²⁺ can be removed from the cytoplasm by ATPases in the endoplasmic reticulum or at the plasma membrane, or via Na, Ca exchangers (not shown).

(store-operated Ca²⁺ channels; SOCCs). The resulting Ca²⁺ influx replenishes the total intracellular Ca²⁺ supply and refills the endoplasmic reticulum. Recent research has identified the physical relationships between SOCCs and regulatory interactions of proteins from the endoplasmic reticulum that gate these channels.

As with other second messenger molecules, the increase in Ca²⁺ within the cytosol is rapid, and is followed by a rapid decrease. Because the movement of Ca²⁺ outside of the cytosol (ie, across the plasma membrane or the membrane of the internal store) requires that it move up its electrochemical gradient, it requires energy. Ca²⁺ movement out of the cell is facilitated by the plasma membrane Ca²⁺ ATPase. Alternatively, it can be transported by an antiport that exchanges three Na⁺ for each Ca²⁺ driven by the energy stored in the Na⁺ electrochemical gradient. Ca²⁺ movement into the internal stores is through the action of the **sarcoplasmic** or **endoplasmic reticulum Ca²⁺ ATPase,** also known as the **SERCA pump.**

Many different Ca²⁺-binding proteins have been described, including **troponin, calmodulin,** and **calbindin.** Troponin is the Ca²⁺-binding protein involved in contraction of skeletal muscle. Calmodulin contains 148 amino acid residues and has four Ca²⁺-binding domains. When calmodulin binds Ca²⁺, it is capable of activating five different calmodulin-dependent kinases (CaMKs; Table 2–3), among other proteins. One of the kinases is **myosin light-chain kinase,** which phosphorylates myosin. This brings about contraction in smooth muscle. CaMKI and CaMKII are concerned with synaptic function, and CaMKIII is concerned with protein synthesis. Another calmodulin-activated protein is **calcineurin,** a phosphatase that inactivates Ca²⁺ channels by dephosphorylating them. It also plays a prominent role in activating T cells and is inhibited by some immunosuppressants.

G PROTEINS

A common way to translate a signal to a biologic effect inside cells is by way of nucleotide regulatory proteins that are activated after binding GTP **(G proteins).** When an activating signal reaches a G protein, the protein exchanges GDP for GTP. The GTP–protein complex brings about the activating effect of the G protein. The inherent GTPase activity of the protein then converts GTP to GDP, restoring the G protein to an inactive resting state. G-proteins can be divided into two principal groups involved in cell signaling: **small G proteins** and **heterotrimeric G proteins.** Other groups that have similar regulation and are also important to cell physiology include elongation factors, dynamin, and translocation GTPases.

There are several different families of small G proteins (or **small GTPases**) that are all highly regulated. **GTPase activating proteins (GAPs)** tend to inactivate small G proteins by encouraging hydrolysis of GTP to GDP in the central binding site. **Guanine exchange factors (GEFs)** tend to activate small G proteins by encouraging exchange of GDP for GTP in the active site. Some of the small G proteins contain lipid modifications that help anchor them to membranes, while others are free to diffuse throughout the cytosol. Small G proteins are involved in many cellular functions. Members of the Rab family regulate the rate of vesicle traffic between the endoplasmic reticulum, the Golgi apparatus, lysosomes, endosomes, and the cell membrane. Another family of small GTP-binding proteins, the Rho/Rac family, mediates interactions between the cytoskeleton and cell membrane. The Ras family regulates growth by transmitting signals from the cell membrane to the nucleus.

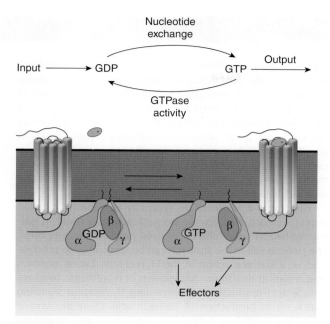

Nucleotide exchange

Input → GDP → GTP → Output

GTPase activity

Effectors

FIGURE 2–16 **Heterotrimeric G proteins. Top:** Summary of overall reaction that occurs in the Gα subunit. **Bottom:** When the ligand (red oval) binds to the G protein–coupled receptor in the cell membrane, GTP replaces GDP on the α subunit. GTP-α separates from the βγ subunit and GTP-α and βγ both activate various effectors, producing physiologic effects. The intrinsic GTPase activity of GTP-α then converts GTP to GDP, and the α, β, and γ subunits reassociate.

Another family of G proteins, the larger **heterotrimeric G proteins,** couple cell surface receptors to catalytic units that catalyze the intracellular formation of second messengers or couple the receptors directly to ion channels. Despite the knowledge of the small G proteins described above, the heteromeric G proteins are frequently referred to in the shortened "G protein" form because they were the first to be identified. Heterotrimeric G proteins are made up of three subunits designated α, β, and γ (Figure 2–16). Both the α and the γ subunits have lipid modifications that anchor these proteins to the plasma membrane. The α subunit is bound to GDP. When a ligand binds to a G protein–coupled receptor (GPCR), the α subunit GDP is exchanged for GTP and the α subunit separates from the combined β and γ subunits. The separated α subunit brings about many biologic effects. The β and γ subunits are tightly bound in the cell and together form a signaling molecule that can also activate a variety of effectors. The intrinsic GTPase activity of the α subunit then converts GTP to GDP, and this leads to reassociation of the α with the βγ subunit and termination of effector activation. The GTPase activity of the α subunit can be accelerated by a family of **regulators of G protein signaling (RGS).**

Heterotrimeric G proteins relay signals from over 1000 GPCRs, and their effectors in the cells include ion channels and enzymes. There are 20 α, 6 β, and 12 γ genes, which allow for over 1400 α, β, and γ combinations. Not all combinations occur in the cell, but over 20 different heterotrimeric G proteins have

been well documented in cell signaling. They can be divided into five families, each with a relatively characteristic set of effectors.

G PROTEIN–COUPLED RECEPTORS

All the **GPCRs** that have been characterized to date are proteins that span the cell membrane seven times. Because of this structure they are alternatively referred to as **seven-helix receptors** or **serpentine receptors.** GPCR functions are multiple and diverse; this is emphasized by the extensive variety of ligands that target GPCRs (Table 2–4). Upon ligand binding, a conformational change activates a resting heterotrimeric G protein associated with the cytoplasmic leaf of the plasma membrane. Activation of a single receptor can result in 1, 10, or more active heterotrimeric G proteins, providing amplification as well as transduction of the first messenger. Bound receptors can be inactivated to limit the amount of cellular signaling. This frequently occurs through phosphorylation of the cytoplasmic side of the receptor. Because of their diversity and importance in cellular signaling pathways, GPCRs are prime targets for drug discovery (Clinical Box 2–8).

TABLE 2–4 Examples of ligands for G protein–coupled receptors.

Class	Ligand
Neurotransmitters	Epinephrine
	Norepinephrine
	Dopamine
	5-Hydroxytryptamine
	Histamine
	Acetylcholine
	Adenosine
	Opioids
Tachykinins	Substance P
	Neurokinin A
	Neuropeptide K
Other peptides	Angiotensin II
	Arginine vasopressin
	Oxytocin
	VIP, GRP, TRH, PTH
Glycoprotein hormones	TSH, FSH, LH, hCG
Arachidonic acid derivatives	Thromboxane A_2
Other	Odorants
	Tastants
	Endothelins
	Platelet-activating factor
	Cannabinoids
	Light

FSH, follicle-stimulating hormone; GRP, gastrin-releasing hormone; hCG, human chorionic gonadotropin; LH, luteinizing hormone; PTH, parathyroid hormone; TRH, thyrotropin-releasing hormone; TSH, thyroid-stimulating hormone; VIP, vasoactive intestinal peptide.

CLINICAL BOX 2–8

Drug Development: Targeting the G protein–Coupled Receptors (GPCRs)

GPCRs are among the most heavily investigated drug targets in the pharmaceutical industry, representing approximately 40% of all the drugs in the marketplace today. These proteins are active in just about every organ system and present a wide range of opportunities as therapeutic targets in areas including cancer, cardiac dysfunction, diabetes, central nervous system disorders, obesity, inflammation, and pain. Features of GPCRs that allow them to be drug targets are their specificity in recognizing extracellular ligands to initiate cellular response, the cell surface location of GPCRs that make them accessible to novel ligands or drugs, and their prevalence in leading to human pathology and disease.

Specific examples of successful GPCR drug targets are noted with two types of **histamine receptors.**

Histamine-1 receptor (H_1-receptor) antagonists: allergy therapy. Allergens can trigger local mast cells or basophils to release histamine in the airway. A primary target for histamine is the H_1-receptor in several airway cell types and this can lead to transient itching, sneezing, rhinorrhea, and nasal congestion.

There are a variety of medications with improved peripheral H_1-receptor selectivity that are currently used to block histamine activation of the H_1-receptor and thus limit allergen effects in the upper airway. H_1-receptor antagonists on the market include loratadine, fexofenadine, cetirizine, and desloratadine. These "second" and "third" generation medications have improved specificity and reduced adverse side effects (eg, drowsiness and central nervous system dysfunction) associated with some of the "first" generation drugs first introduced in the late 1930s and widely developed over the next 40 years.

Histamine-2 receptor (H_2-receptor) antagonists: treating excess stomach acid. Excess stomach acid can result in gastroesophageal reflux disease or even peptic ulcer symptoms. The parietal cell in the stomach can be stimulated to produce acid via histamine action at the H_2-receptor. Excess stomach acid results in heartburn. Antagonists or H_2-receptor blockers, reduce acid production by preventing H_2-receptor signaling that leads to production of stomach acid. There are several drugs (eg, ranitidine, famotidine, cimetidine, and nizatidine) that specifically block the H_2-receptor and thus reduce excess acid production.

INOSITOL TRISPHOSPHATE & DIACYLGLYCEROL AS SECOND MESSENGERS

The link between membrane binding of a ligand that acts via Ca^{2+} and the prompt increase in the cytoplasmic Ca^{2+} concentration is often **IP₃.** When one of these ligands binds to its receptor, activation of the receptor produces activation of phospholipase C (PLC) on the inner surface of the membrane. Ligands bound to GPCR can do this through the G_q heterotrimeric G proteins, while ligands bound to tyrosine kinase receptors can do this through other cell signaling pathways. PLC has at least eight isoforms; PLC_β is activated by heterotrimeric G proteins, while $PLC\gamma$ forms are activated through tyrosine kinase receptors. PLC isoforms can catalyze the hydrolysis of the membrane lipid phosphatidylinositol 4,5-diphosphate (PIP_2) to form IP_3 and **DAG (Figure 2–17).** The IP_3 diffuses to the endoplasmic reticulum where it triggers the release of Ca^{2+} into the cytoplasm by binding the IP_3 receptor,

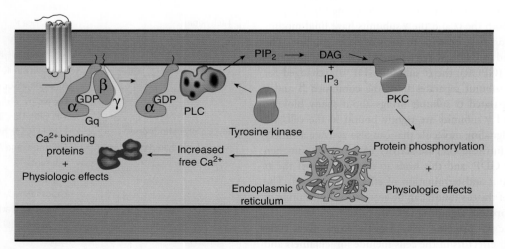

FIGURE 2–17 **Diagrammatic representation of release of inositol trisphosphate (IP_3) and diacylglycerol (DAG) as second messengers.** Binding of ligand to G-protein–coupled receptor activates phospholipase C (PLC)$_\beta$. Alternatively, activation of receptors with intracellular tyrosine kinase domains can activate $PLC\gamma$. The resulting hydrolysis of phosphatidylinositol 4,5-diphosphate (PIP_2) produces IP_3, which releases Ca^{2+} from the endoplasmic reticulum (ER), and DAG, which activates protein kinase C (PKC). CaBP, Ca^{2+}-binding proteins; ISF, interstitial fluid.

a ligand-gated Ca^{2+} channel. DAG is also a second messenger; it stays in the cell membrane where it activates one of several isoforms of **protein kinase C.**

CYCLIC NUCLEOTIDES AS SECOND MESSENGERS

Another important second messenger is cyclic adenosine mono phosphate, (**cyclic AMP or cAMP**). cAMP is formed from ATP by the action of the enzyme **adenylyl cyclase** and converted to physiologically inactive 5′ AMP by the action of the enzyme **phosphodiesterase.** cAMP activates one of the cyclic nucleotide-dependent protein kinases (**protein kinase A, PKA**) that, like protein kinase C, catalyzes the phosphorylation of proteins, changing their conformation and altering their activity. In addition, the active catalytic subunit of PKA moves to the nucleus and phosphorylates the **cAMP-responsive element-binding protein (CREB).** This transcription factor then binds to DNA and alters transcription of a number of genes.

Adenylyl cyclase is a membrane bound protein with 12 transmembrane regions. Ten isoforms of this enzyme have been described and each can have distinct regulatory properties, permitting the cAMP pathway to be customized to specific tissue needs. Notably, stimulatory heterotrimeric G proteins (G_s) activate, while inhibitory heterotrimeric G proteins (G_i) inactivate adenylyl cyclase (**Figure 2–18**). In addition, cross-talk occurs between the phospholipase C system and the adenylyl cyclase system, as several of the isoforms of adenylyl cyclase are stimulated by calmodulin. Finally, the effects of protein kinase A and protein kinase C are very widespread and can also affect directly, or indirectly, the activity at adenylyl cyclase. The close relationship between activation of G proteins and adenylyl cyclases also allows for spatial regulation of cAMP production. All of these events, and others, allow for fine-tuning the cAMP response for a particular physiologic outcome in the cell.

Two bacterial toxins have important effects on adenylyl cyclase that are mediated by G proteins. The A subunit of **cholera toxin** catalyzes the transfer of ADP ribose to an arginine residue in the middle of the α subunit of G_s. This inhibits its GTPase activity, producing prolonged stimulation of adenylyl cyclase. **Pertussis toxin** catalyzes ADP-ribosylation of a cysteine residue near the carboxyl terminal of the α subunit of G_i. This inhibits the function of G_i. In addition to the implications of these alterations in disease, both toxins are used for fundamental research on G protein function. The compound forskolin also stimulates adenylyl cyclase activity by a direct action on the enzyme, and is commonly used in research studies to evaluate adenylyl cyclase/cAMP contributions to cellular physiology.

Another cyclic nucleotide of physiologic importance is **cyclic guanosine monophosphate (cyclic GMP or cGMP).** cGMP is important in vision in both rod and cone cells. In addition, there are cGMP-regulated ion channels, and cGMP activates cGMP-dependent kinase, producing a number of physiologic effects. Guanylyl cyclases are a family of enzymes that catalyze the formation of cGMP. They exist in two forms (**Figure 2–19**). One form has an extracellular amino terminal domain that is a receptor, a single transmembrane domain, and a cytoplasmic portion with guanylyl cyclase catalytic activity. Several such guanylyl cyclases have been characterized. Two are receptors for atrial natriuretic peptide (ANP), and a third binds an *Escherichia coli* enterotoxin and the gastrointestinal polypeptide guanylin. The other form of guanylyl cyclase is soluble, contains heme, and is not bound to the membrane. There appear to be several isoforms of the intracellular enzyme. They are activated by nitric oxide (NO) and NO-containing compounds.

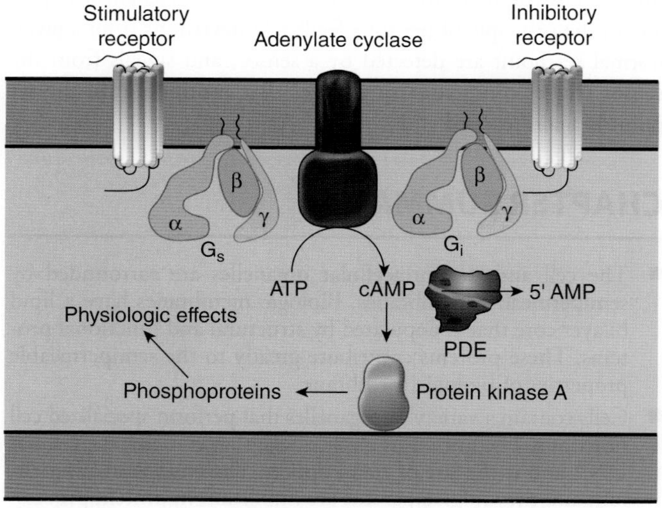

FIGURE 2–18 **The cAMP system.** Activation of adenylyl cyclase catalyzes the conversion of ATP to cAMP. Cyclic AMP activates protein kinase A, which phosphorylates proteins, producing physiologic effects. Stimulatory ligands bind to stimulatory receptors and activate adenylyl cyclase via G_s. Inhibitory ligands inhibit adenylyl cyclase via inhibitory receptors and G_i.

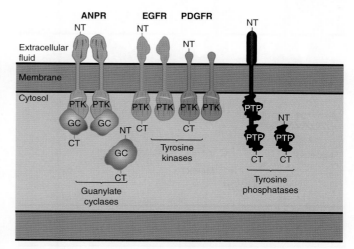

FIGURE 2–19 **Diagrammatic representation of guanylyl cyclases, tyrosine kinases, and tyrosine phosphatases.** NT refers to the amino (NH$_2$) terminus and CT to the carboxyl terminus of each protein. Individual molecules are as follows: ANP, atrial natriuretic peptide; GC, guanylyl cyclase domain; EGFR, epidermal growth factor receptor; PDGFR, platelet-derived growth factor receptor; PTK, protein tyrosine kinase domain (PTK is inactive in guanylyl cyclase); PTP, tyrosine phosphatase domain.

GROWTH FACTORS

Growth factors are polypeptides and proteins that are conveniently divided into three groups. One group is made up of agents that foster the multiplication or development of various types of cells; NGF, insulin-like growth factor I (IGF-I), activins and inhibins, and epidermal growth factor (EGF) are examples. More than 20 have been described. The cytokines are a second group. These factors are produced by macrophages and lymphocytes, as well as other cells, and are important in regulation of the immune system. Again, more than 20 have been described. The third group is made up of the colony-stimulating factors that regulate proliferation and maturation of red and white blood cells.

Receptors for EGF, platelet-derived growth factor (PDGF), and many of the other factors that foster cell multiplication and growth have a single membrane-spanning domain with an intracellular tyrosine kinase domain (Figure 2–19). When ligand binds to a tyrosine kinase receptor, it first causes a dimerization of two similar receptors. The dimerization results in partial activation of the intracellular tyrosine kinase domains and a cross-phosphorylation to fully activate each other. One of the pathways activated by phosphorylation leads, through the small G protein Ras, to MAP kinases, and eventually to the production of transcription factors in the nucleus that alter gene expression (Figure 2–20).

Receptors for cytokines and colony-stimulating factors differ from the other growth factors in that most of them do not have tyrosine kinase domains in their cytoplasmic portions and some have little or no cytoplasmic tail. However, they do initiate tyrosine kinase activity in the cytoplasm. In particular, they activate the so-called Janus tyrosine kinases (**JAKs**) in the cytoplasm (Figure 2–21). These in turn phosphorylate **STAT** proteins. The phosphorylated STATs form homo- and heterodimers and move to the nucleus, where they act as transcription factors. There are four known mammalian JAKs and seven known STATs. Interestingly, the JAK–STAT pathway can also be activated by growth hormone and is another important direct path from the cell surface to the nucleus. However, it should be emphasized that both the Ras and the JAK–STAT pathways are complex and there is cross-talk between them and other signaling pathways discussed previously.

Finally, note that the whole subject of second messengers and intracellular signaling has become immensely complex, with multiple pathways and interactions. It is only possible in a book such as this to list highlights and present general themes that will aid the reader in understanding the rest of physiology (Clinical Box 2–9).

HOMEOSTASIS

The actual environment of the cells of the body is the interstitial component of the ECF. Because normal cell function depends on the constancy of this fluid, it is not surprising that in multicellular animals, an immense number of regulatory mechanisms have evolved to maintain it. To describe "the various physiologic arrangements which serve to restore the normal state, once it has been disturbed," W.B. Cannon coined the term **homeostasis.** The buffering properties of the body fluids and the renal and respiratory adjustments to the presence of excess acid or alkali are examples of homeostatic mechanisms. There are countless other examples, and a large part of physiology is concerned with regulatory mechanisms that act to maintain the constancy of the internal environment. Many of these regulatory mechanisms operate on the principle of negative feedback; deviations from a given normal set point are detected by a sensor, and signals from the sensor trigger compensatory changes that continue until the set point is again reached.

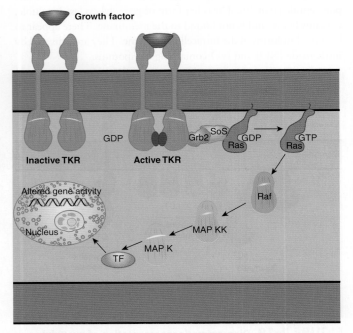

CHAPTER SUMMARY

- The cell and the intracellular organelles are surrounded by semipermeable membranes. Biologic membranes have a lipid bilayer core that is populated by structural and functional proteins. These proteins contribute greatly to the semipermeable properties of biologic membrane.

- Cells contain a variety of organelles that perform specialized cell functions. The nucleus is an organelle that contains the cellular DNA and is the site of transcription. The endoplasmic reticulum and the Golgi apparatus are important in protein processing and the targeting of proteins to correct compartments within the cell. Lysosomes and peroxisomes are membrane-bound organelles that contribute to protein and lipid processing. Mitochondria are organelles that allow for oxidative phosphorylation in eukaryotic cells and also are important in specialized cellular signaling.

FIGURE 2–20 One of the direct pathways by which growth factors alter gene activity. TKR, tyrosine kinase domain; Grb2, Ras activator/controller; Sos, Ras activator; Ras, product of the *ras* gene; MAP K, mitogen-activated protein kinase; MAP KK, MAP kinase kinase; TF, transcription factors. There is a cross-talk between this pathway and the cAMP pathway, as well as a cross-talk with the IP$_3$–DAG pathway.

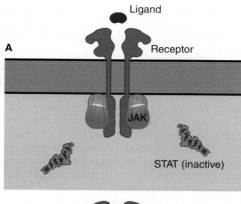

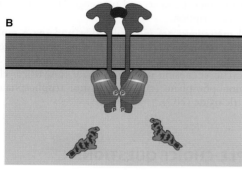

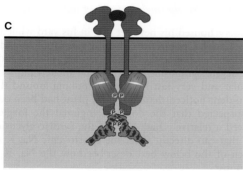

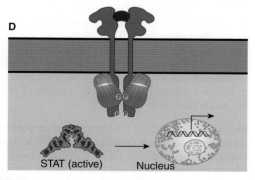

FIGURE 2–21 Signal transduction via the JAK–STAT pathway. (**A**) Inactive JAKs are associated with individual receptors. (**B**) Ligand binding leads to dimerization of receptor and activation JAKs that phosphorylate tyrosine residues on opposing receptors and their associated JAK. (**C**) STATs then associate with the phosphorylated receptors and JAKs in turn phosphorylate these STATs. (**D**) Phosphorylated STATs dimerize and move to nucleus, where they bind to response elements on DNA.

■ The cytoskeleton is a network of three types of filaments that provide structural integrity to the cell as well as a means for trafficking of organelles and other structures around the cell. Actin filaments are important in cellular contraction, migration, and signaling. Actin filaments also provide the backbone for muscle contraction. Intermediate filaments are primarily structural. Microtubules provide a dynamic structure in cells that allows for the movement of cellular components around the cell.

■ There are three superfamilies of molecular motor proteins in the cell that use the energy of ATP to generate force, movement, or both. Myosin is the force generator for muscle

---

CLINICAL BOX 2–9

Receptor & G protein Diseases

Many diseases are being traced to mutations in the genes for receptors. For example, loss-of-function receptor mutations that cause disease have been reported for the 1,25-dihydroxycholecalciferol receptor and the insulin receptor. Certain other diseases are caused by production of antibodies against receptors. Thus, antibodies against thyroid-stimulating hormone (TSH) receptors cause Graves disease, and antibodies against nicotinic acetylcholine receptors cause myasthenia gravis.

An example of loss of function of a receptor is the type of nephrogenic diabetes insipidus that is due to loss of the ability of mutated V_2 vasopressin receptors to mediate concentration of the urine. Mutant receptors can gain as well as lose function. A gain-of-function mutation of the Ca^{2+} receptor causes excess inhibition of parathyroid hormone secretion and familial hypercalciuric hypocalcemia. G proteins can also undergo loss-of-function or gain-of-function mutations that cause disease (Table 2–5). In one form of pseudohypoparathyroidism, a mutated $G_s\alpha$ fails to respond to parathyroid hormone, producing the symptoms of hypoparathyroidism without any decline in circulating parathyroid hormone. Testotoxicosis is an interesting disease that combines gain and loss of function. In this condition, an activating mutation of $G_s\alpha$ causes excess testosterone secretion and prepubertal sexual maturation. However, this mutation is temperature-sensitive and is active only at the relatively low temperature of the testes (33°C). At 37°C, the normal temperature of the rest of the body, it is replaced by loss of function, with the production of hypoparathyroidism and decreased responsiveness to TSH. A different activating mutation in Gsα is associated with the rough-bordered areas of skin pigmentation and hypercortisolism of the McCune–Albright syndrome. This mutation occurs during fetal development, creating a mosaic of normal and abnormal cells. A third mutation in $G_s\alpha$ reduces its intrinsic GTPase activity. As a result, it is much more active than normal, and excess cAMP is produced. This causes hyperplasia and eventually neoplasia in somatotrope cells of the anterior pituitary. Forty percent of somatotrope tumors causing acromegaly have cells containing a somatic mutation of this type.

TABLE 2–5 Examples of abnormalities caused by loss- or gain-of-function mutations of heterotrimeric G protein–coupled receptors and G proteins.

Site	Type of Mutation	Disease
Receptor		
Cone opsins	Loss	Color blindness
Rhodopsin	Loss	Congenital night blindness; two forms of retinitis pigmentosa
V_2 vasopressin	Loss	X-linked nephrogenic diabetes insipidus
ACTH	Loss	Familial glucocorticoid deficiency
LH	Gain	Familial male precocious puberty
TSH	Gain	Familial nonautoimmune hyperthyroidism
TSH	Loss	Familial hypothyroidism
Ca^{2+}	Gain	Familial hypercalciuric hypocalcemia
Thromboxane A_2	Loss	Congenital bleeding
Endothelin B	Loss	Hirschsprung disease
G protein		
$G_s \alpha$	Loss	Pseudohypothyroidism type 1a
$G_s \alpha$	Gain/loss	Testotoxicosis
$G_s \alpha$	Gain (mosaic)	McCune-Albright syndrome
$G_s \alpha$	Gain	Somatotroph adenomas with acromegaly
$G_i \alpha$	Gain	Ovarian and adrenocortical tumors

ACTH, adrenocorticotropic hormone; LH, luteinizing hormone; TSH, thyroid-stimulating hormone.

cell contraction. Cellular myosins can also interact with the cytoskeleton (primarily thin filaments) to participate in contraction as well as movement of cell contents. Kinesins and cellular dyneins are motor proteins that primarily interact with microtubules to move cargo around the cells.

■ Cellular adhesion molecules aid in tethering cells to each other or to the extracellular matrix as well as providing for initiation of cellular signaling. There are four main families of these proteins: integrins, immunoglobulins, cadherins, and selectins.

■ Cells contain distinct protein complexes that serve as cellular connections to other cells or the extracellular matrix. Tight junctions provide intercellular connections that link cells into a regulated tissue barrier and also provide a barrier to movement of proteins in the cell membrane. Gap junctions provide contacts between cells that allow for direct passage of small molecules between two cells. Desmosomes and adherens junctions are specialized structures that hold cells together. Hemidesmosomes and focal adhesions attach cells to their basal lamina.

■ Exocytosis and endocytosis are vesicular fusion events that allow for movement of proteins and lipids between the cell interior, the plasma membrane, and the cell exterior. Exocytosis can be constitutive or nonconstitutive; both are regulated processes that require specialized proteins for vesicular fusion. Endocytosis is the formation of vesicles at the plasma membrane to take material from the extracellular space into the cell interior.

■ Cells can communicate with one another via chemical messengers. Individual messengers (or ligands) typically bind to a plasma membrane receptor to initiate intracellular changes that lead to physiologic changes. Plasma membrane receptor families include ion channels, G protein–coupled receptors, or a variety of enzyme-linked receptors (eg, tyrosine kinase receptors). There are additional cytosolic receptors (eg, steroid receptors) that can bind membrane-permeant compounds. Activation of receptors leads to cellular changes that include changes in membrane potential, activation of heterotrimeric G proteins, increase in second messenger molecules, or initiation of transcription.

■ Second messengers are molecules that undergo a rapid concentration changes in the cell following primary messenger recognition. Common second messenger molecules include Ca^{2+}, cyclic adenosine monophosphate (cAMP), cyclic guanine monophosphate (cGMP), inositol trisphosphate (IP_3), and nitric oxide (NO).

MULTIPLE-CHOICE QUESTIONS

For all questions, select the single best answer unless otherwise directed.

1. A student housed his new pet dog in his yard while he went off to school. Upon return, the dog was drooling and vomiting. Upon tending to the dog, the student noticed additional, more severe symptoms that included dilated pupils and an irregular and very fast heartbeat. Looking around the yard, the student noticed that a foxglove plant had been damaged. He suspected that the dog had ingested the foxglove and received a relatively high dose of the cardiac glycoside digitalin that can directly affect the electrogenic Na, K ATPase. Which of the below best describes how the Na, K ATPase functions?
   A. It uses the energy in ATP to extrude 3 Na^+ out of the cell in exchange for taking two K^+ into the cell.
   B. It uses the energy in ATP to extrude 3 K^+ out of the cell in exchange for taking two Na^+ into the cell.
   C. It uses the energy in moving Na^+ into the cell or K^+ outside the cell to make ATP.
   D. It uses the energy in moving Na^+ outside of the cell or K^+ inside the cell to make ATP.

2. Students in an introductory laboratory class are able to isolate apical and basolateral membranes from undifferentiated and differentiated gut epithelial cells. Following isolation, the students can categorize the protein, lipid and carbohydrate makeup of each batch of isolated membranes. Results from these experiments help them to draw which of the following conclusions about cell membranes?
   A. Cell membranes contain relatively few protein molecules.
   B. Cell membranes contain mostly carbohydrate molecules.
   C. Cell membranes are freely permeable to electrolytes but not to proteins.
   D. Cell membranes have variable protein and lipid contents depending on their location in the cell.
   E. Cell membranes have a stable composition throughout the life of the cell.

3. In an airway epithelial preparation, Cl⁻ current could be manipulated and resulting airway surface liquid changes could be monitored. It was noted that both the β-adrenergic receptor agonist salbutamol and the purinergic receptor agonist ATP acted to increase Cl⁻ current and airway surface liquid. If intracellular [cAMP] was held constant in the airway epithelial cells, salbutamol was ineffective, however, ATP remained effective in increasing the airway surface liquid. If intracellular $[Ca^{2+}]$ was held constant, salbutamol was effective, but ATP was ineffective in increasing airway surface liquid. In these experiments both cAMP and Ca^{2+} could be said to be as second messengers. Which of the following statements are consistent with the definition of second messengers?

   A. Second messengers are substances that interact with first messengers outside cells.
   B. Second messengers are substances that bind to first messengers in the cell membrane.
   C. Second messengers are hormones secreted by cells in response to stimulation by another hormone.
   D. Second messengers mediate the intracellular responses to many different hormones and neurotransmitters.
   E. Second messengers are not formed in the brain.

4. A researcher uses an experimental cell model to apply a drug that alters hydration characteristics of the extracellular surface of the treated cells. However, examination of the membrane area showed no indication that his drug was interacting with the plasma membrane. After several experiments using markers for specific cellular organelles, he noticed slight changes in the morphology of the Golgi apparatus. Using pH sensitive dyes, he was able to determine altered pH in the Golgi. He postulated that a dysfunctional Golgi apparatus was the cause of the observed changes in the cell plasma membranes. He postulated this in part on the knowledge that the Golgi complex

   A. is an organelle that participates in the breakdown of proteins and lipids.
   B. is an organelle that participates in posttranslational processing of proteins and modification of lipids.
   C. is an organelle that participates in energy production.
   D. is an organelle that participates in transcription and translation.
   E. is a subcellular compartment that stores proteins for trafficking to the nucleus.

5. Several students were conducting experiments on constitutive exocytosis in their biology laboratory. Despite their ability to use fluorescent tracking to monitor vesicle and protein movement from the Golgi complex to the plasma membrane and protein secretion into the extracellular space, they noticed that the overall size of the cell did not change. They were able to show through fluorescent microscopy that plasma membrane was taken up into the cell at a balanced rate through the process of endocytosis. Which of the following statements are consistent with endocytosis?

   A. Endocytosis includes phagocytosis and pinocytosis, but not clathrin-mediated or caveolae-dependent uptake of extracellular contents.
   B. Endocytosis refers to the merging of an intracellular vesicle with the plasma membrane to deliver intracellular contents to the extracellular milieu.
   C. Endocytosis refers to the invagination of the plasma membrane to uptake extracellular contents into the cell.
   D. Endocytosis refers to vesicular trafficking between Golgi stacks.

6. A new assistant professor with an established background in cell biology and pharmacology decides to switch her laboratory research focus toward drug discovery. She knows that G protein–coupled receptors (GPCRs) represent the largest collection of genes expressed in the human genome. Further, GPCRs represent the most frequently targeted protein for established and novel drugs. She chooses to organize her laboratory around GPCR drug discovery and sets out to determine an acceptable target for her research. GPCRs can best be described as

   A. intracellular membrane proteins that help regulate movement within the cell.
   B. plasma membrane proteins that couple the extracellular binding of primary signaling molecules to exocytosis.
   C. plasma membrane proteins that couple the extracellular binding of primary signaling molecules to the activation of heterotrimeric G proteins.
   D. intracellular proteins that couple the binding of primary messenger molecules with transcription.

7. Parents of an active family with three daughters and a son had always noticed that the son had a history of clumsiness that showed up in adolescence and into early adulthood. As he got older, the clumsiness progressed toward weakness and muscle atrophy, especially evident in the hands, where fine motor skills were compromised. The family doctor suggested the possibility of a hereditary peripheral neuropathy and the son was screened for Charcot Marie Tooth disease. The results showed a mutation in the *GJB1* gene that codes for the gap junction connexin 32 protein. Gap junctions are intercellular connections that

   A. primarily serve to keep cells separated and allow for transport across a tissue barrier.
   B. serve as a regulated cytoplasmic bridge for sharing of small molecules between cells.
   C. serve as a barrier to prevent protein movement within the cellular membrane.
   D. are cellular components for constitutive exocytosis that occurs between adjacent cells.

8. Two undergraduate students are part of a mycology class visiting the California coast for an overnight adventure of mushroom hunting. One of their finds includes a white mushroom with a discolored green cap growing next to an oak tree. They place the mushroom in their bag and head back to meet up with the class instructor for identification. Upon arrival they are told they have found an *Amanita phalloides*, or a "death cap" mushroom. The death cap is associated with liver hemorrhage and acts in part by stabilizing F-actin and preventing normal cycling between F-actin and G-actin within the cell. F-actin is a component of the cellular cytoskeleton that

   A. provides a structural component for cell movement.
   B. is defined as the "functional" form of actin in the cell.
   C. refers to the actin subunits that provide the molecular building blocks of the extended actin molecules found in the cell.
   D. provides the molecular architecture for cell to cell communication.

9. A patient was diagnosed with pancreatic cancer with tumors that could not be surgically removed. The patient was given the option of standard chemotherapy using gemcitabine, or he could be placed in a new clinical trial that combined gemcitabine with a nanoparticle albumin-bound (nab)-paclitaxel. The nab-paclitaxel drug is a taxol derivative that works by

altering microtubule dynamics. How does altering microtubule dynamics affect cancer progression?

A. Disruption of microtubules alters rough endoplasmic reticulum structure and limits production of cytosolic proteins.

B. Disruption of microtubules prevents translation and halts cell cycle progression.

C. Disruption of microtubules prevents proper assembly of a spindle fiber necessary for cell division, effectively halting cancer cell progression.

D. Disruption of microtubules allows for better secretion of insulin from pancreatic islet β cells and restores pancreatic function.

E. Disruption of microtubules breaks down the ability for cells to migrate and shuts down metastatic potential of cancer cells.

10. A 42-year-old, nonsmoking and nonasthmatic female patient visits her family care physician with complaints of repeated heartburn. After examination it is deduced that she is suffering from gastroesophageal reflux disease (GERD) and would benefit from a reduction in stomach acid. She is asked about her diet and declares that she does not enjoy acidic foods, including citrus and tomatoes, and drinks very little. Absent many triggers for increased stomach acid, it is suggested she try an over the counter proton pump inhibitor (eg, esomeprazole, lansoprazole, omeprazole) to block H^+/K^+ ATPase in the parietal cells of the stomach that contribute to increased stomach acid. The H^+/K^+ ATPase is an example of

A. tyrosine kinase receptor.

B. H_2 receptor.

C. ion channel.

D. cotransporter.

E. counter transporter.

ANSWERS

1. The correct answer is **A.** The foxglove plant, and more specifically the inhibitory cardiac glycoside contained in the foxglove that interrupts Na, K ATPase activity, has been used for over two centuries to manage certain heart malfunctions. However, excessive doses of these cardiac glycosides such as can occur after uncontrolled eating of the plant can cause significant pathology. Under normal circumstances, Na, K ATPase moves 3 Na^+ out of the cell for every two K^+ that move in, ruling out **B.** While the Na, K ATPase is electrogenic, Na^+ and K^+ both move "up" their electrochemical gradients and require energy for this movement, ruling out **C** and **D.**

2. The correct answer is **D.** Cell membranes are varied structures that commonly have significantly different lipid and protein makeups depending on their placement in the cell and the developmental state of the cell (ruling out option **E**). The experiments would yield a significant amount of protein as they make up a large portion of the membrane preparations, eliminating **A.** While carbohydrates can be important components of plasma membrane proteins and lipids, there are many more protein and lipid components in each of the membrane preparations, eliminating **B.** Although plasma membranes are not permeable to electrolytes or proteins, this knowledge could not be obtained from the experiments described and **C** can be eliminated.

3. The correct answer is **D.** In a typical signaling cascade the primary messenger is the ligand (eg, salbutamol or ATP) that binds to a receptor to initiate signal transduction. The second messenger is an intracellular messenger (eg, cAMP or Ca^{2+}) that triggers a cellular response (eg, binding to cAMP-gated or Ca^{2+}-gated Cl^- channels). The outside messenger (or ligand) binds to a receptor and is independent of the second messenger produced inside the cell, eliminating **A** and **B.** Hormones are primary messengers that require signal transduction for their physiologic response, eliminating **C.** Second messengers are used in most cells in the body, including those in the brain, eliminating **E.**

4. The correct answer is **B.** A primary function of the Golgi complex is the processing of proteins and lipids. This includes glycosylation of proteins and lipids that are transported to the outer leaflet of the plasma membrane. Reduced glycosylation of these proteins and lipids would significantly affect hydration properties of the membrane. Breakdown of proteins and lipids takes place in the lysosome and/or proteasome and not in the Golgi, eliminating **A.** Energy production is a feature of mitochondria and not the Golgi, ruling out **C.** Transcription and translation are not part of the Golgi complex function and so **D** can be eliminated. Proteins that traffic into the nucleus go through nuclear pores that are independent of the Golgi complex, ruling out **E.**

5. The correct answer is **C.** Endocytosis refers to the uptake or transport of extracellular material into the cell through a process of plasma membrane invagination. It includes phagocytosis, pinocytosis as well as clathrin-mediated and caveolae-dependent uptake, eliminating **A.** The process described in **B** refers to the exocytosis being studied by the students and can be eliminated. While vesicles do move between Golgi stacks **D**, this movement does not cover transport of material from outside the cell to inside, and thus is not considered endocytosis.

6. The correct answer is **C.** GPCRs are a group of proteins that link extracellular signals to intracellular changes by the activation of intracellular trimeric G proteins. Option **A** can be ruled out because GPCRs cross the cytoplasmic membrane and are not classified as intracellular proteins. GPCRs are quite diverse and dependent on the extracellular ligand, the specific GPCR and intracellular signaling mechanisms. These functions are not limited to intracellular movement **A**, exocytosis **B** or downstream transcription changes **D**, and thus all three of these answers are ruled out.

7. The correct answer is **B.** Gap junctions are communication channels that allow for regulated traffic of small molecules between cells. The connexin 32 protein can contribute to gap junctional communication in myelin sheaths. When mutated, myelin is compromised and peripheral neuropathies can occur. Tight junctions are the intercellular components that serve as a physical barrier between cells **A** and help keep proteins from moving from the basolateral to apical membrane **C**, eliminating these two answers. While hemichannels or connexons can serve as pores for release of signaling compounds to the extracellular space, neither these structures, nor the full gap junction, participate in exocytosis, ruling out **D.**

8. The correct answer is **A.** The phalloidin toxin found in death cap mushrooms is a heat labile protein that directly interacts with filamentous or F-actin, and not the globular or G-actin

forms. This interaction leads to highly stabilized actin filaments, which resist depolymerization and disassembly. Both F-actin and G-actin have cellular function, eliminating **B.** Under normal conditions, F-actin is built up from cycling of G-actin at the ends of the filaments, eliminating **C.** Cell-to-cell communication, such as paracrine, autocrine, endocrine, gap junctional or synaptic signaling require diverse components that can include but are largely independent of F-actin, eliminating **D.**

9. The correct answer is **C.** Microtubules are the key cytoskeletal component in the spindle fiber, allowing for chromosome alignment and cell division. Disrupting microtubules limits the ability of a cell to divide. Although protein synthesis is essential for cell health, microtubules are not directly involved in translation at the rough endoplasmic reticulum, ruling out **A** or translation in general, ruling out **B.** Regulated secretion of insulin from pancreatic islet β cells requires microtubules for vesicular movement. Thus, disruption of microtubules would not improve insulin secretion, ruling out **D,** nor would this likely have an effect on the cell division that underlies cancer progression. While cell migration is important for metastasis, actin is the primary cytoskeletal component for such cell movement, and microtubules disruption would not affect cancer progression through this mechanism, ruling out **E.**

10. The correct answer is **E.** The H^+/K^+ ATPase uses the energy of ATP to actively transport H^+ into the gastric lumen while moving K^+ into the cell. Tyrosine Kinase Receptors are a class of plasma membrane molecules that bind external ligands and transduce their signals into the cell by the activation of intracellular kinase domains and so **A** can be eliminated. H_2 Receptors are G protein–coupled receptors that bind histamine and activate cAMP-dependent regulation of H^+/K^+ ATPases in the parietal cell. While H_2 inhibitors are also used to combat increased stomach acid, the H_2 Receptor is upstream in signaling and so **B** can be eliminated. Ion channels allow for the movement of ions down their electrochemical gradient without the direct use of ATP. In contrast, the H^+/K^+ ATPase requires energy and has specific binding pockets for the exchange of two ions, eliminating **C.** Cotransporters work similarly to counter transporters, however, they move ions in the same direction across a membrane. Since H^+ and K^+ are moving in opposite directions, **D** can be eliminated.

Immunity, Infection, & Inflammation

OBJECTIVES	
After studying this chapter, you should be able to:	■ Understand the significance of immunity for defending the body against microbial invaders. ■ Define the cell types that contribute to immune and inflammatory responses. ■ Describe how phagocytes kill internalized bacteria. ■ Identify the functions of hematopoietic growth factors, cytokines, and chemokines. ■ Delineate the roles and mechanisms of innate, acquired, humoral, and cellular immunity. ■ Understand the basis of inflammatory responses and wound healing.

INTRODUCTION

As an open system, the body is continuously called upon to defend itself from potentially harmful invaders. This is accomplished by the immune system, subdivided into innate and adaptive branches. The immune system is composed of specialized cells that sense and respond to nonhost molecular patterns. Likewise, the immune system clears the body's own cells that have become senescent or abnormal. Finally, normal host tissues occasionally become the subject of inappropriate immune attack. The student of physiology should have a working knowledge of immune functions because the immune system contributes to normal physiologic regulation as well as pathophysiology.

■ IMMUNE EFFECTOR CELLS

Many immune cells circulate in the blood as the white blood cells. In addition, the blood delivers precursors that develop into tissue immune cells. Circulating immunologic cells include **granulocytes (polymorphonuclear leukocytes, PMNs)**, comprising **neutrophils, eosinophils**, and **basophils; lymphocytes**; and **monocytes.** Immune responses in the tissues are further amplified by these cells following their extravascular migration, as well as tissue **macrophages** (derived from monocytes) and **mast cells** (related to basophils). Acting together, these cells provide the body with powerful defenses.

GRANULOCYTES

All granulocytes have cytoplasmic granules that contain biologically active substances involved in inflammatory and allergic reactions.

The average half-life of a neutrophil in the circulation is only 6 h. Many neutrophils enter the tissues. They are attracted to the endothelial surface by cell adhesion molecules known as selectins, and they roll along it. They then bind firmly to integrins and insinuate themselves through the walls of the capillaries by **diapedesis.** Many of those that leave the circulation enter the gastrointestinal tract and are eventually lost from the body.

Invasion of the body by bacteria triggers the **inflammatory response.** Bacterial products trigger production of agents that attract neutrophils to the area **(chemotaxis).** Chemotactic agents include a component of the complement system (C5a); leukotrienes; and **chemokine** polypeptides from lymphocytes, mast cells, and basophils. Other plasma factors coat the bacteria to make them "tasty" to the phagocytes **(opsonization).** The principal opsonins are immunoglobulin G and complement proteins. The coated bacteria then bind to G-protein–coupled receptors on the neutrophil membrane. This triggers increased motor activity of the cell, exocytosis, and the respiratory burst. Increased motor activity leads to ingestion of the bacteria by endocytosis **(phagocytosis).** By **exocytosis,** neutrophil granules discharge their contents into phagocytic vacuoles containing bacteria and also into the interstitial space **(degranulation).** The granules contain various proteases plus antimicrobial proteins called **defensins.** In addition, the cell membrane-bound enzyme **nicotinamide adenine dinucleotide phosphate (NADPH) oxidase** is activated, with the production of toxic oxygen metabolites. The combination of the toxic oxygen metabolites and the proteolytic enzymes from the granules makes the neutrophil a very effective killing machine for bacteria, but may also cause local destruction of host tissue.

NADPH oxidase generates O_2^- by the following reaction:

$$NADPH + H^+ + 2O_2 \rightarrow NADP^+ + 2H^+ + 2O_2^-$$

O_2^- is a **free radical** formed by the addition of one electron to O_2. Two O_2^- react with two H^+ to form H_2O_2 in a reaction catalyzed by superoxide dismutase (SOD-1):

$$2O_2^- + 2H^+ \xrightarrow{SOD-1} H_2O_2 + O_2$$

O_2^- and H_2O_2 are bactericidal oxidants, but H_2O_2 is converted to H_2O and O_2 by the enzyme **catalase.**

Neutrophils also discharge the enzyme **myeloperoxidase,** which catalyzes conversion of Cl^-, Br^-, I^-, and SCN^- to the corresponding acids ($HOCl$, $HOBr$, etc) that are also potent oxidants.

Like neutrophils, **eosinophils** have a short half-life in the circulation, are attracted to the surface of endothelial cells by selectins, bind to integrins, and enter the tissues by diapedesis. Like neutrophils, they release proteins, cytokines, and chemokines that produce inflammation but are capable of killing invading organisms. However, eosinophils have some selectivity in the way in which they respond and in the killing molecules they secrete. Their maturation and activation in tissues is particularly stimulated by IL-3, IL-5, and granulocyte-macrophage colony-stimulating factor (GM-CSF). They are especially abundant in the mucosa of the gastrointestinal, respiratory and urinary tracts, and are increased in allergic diseases such as asthma.

Basophils also enter tissues and release proteins and cytokines. They resemble mast cells, and like mast cells they release histamine and other inflammatory mediators when activated by binding of antigens to cell-fixed IgE molecules, and participate in immediate-type hypersensitivity (allergic) reactions. The antigens that trigger IgE formation are innocuous to most individuals and referred to as allergens.

MAST CELLS

Mast cells are heavily granulated connective tissue cells that are abundant beneath epithelial surfaces. Their granules contain proteoglycans, histamine, and many proteases. They are involved in inflammatory responses initiated by immunoglobulins IgE and IgG and release TNF-α in response to bacterial products by an antibody-independent mechanism, thus participating in **innate immunity**.

MONOCYTES

Monocytes enter the blood from the bone marrow and circulate for about 72 h. They then enter the tissues and become **tissue macrophages**. These persist in tissues for about 3 months. Some may end up as the multinucleated giant cells seen in chronic inflammatory diseases such as tuberculosis. Tissue macrophages include Kupffer cells of the liver, pulmonary alveolar macrophages (see Chapter 34), and microglia in the brain.

Macrophages are activated by cytokines released from T lymphocytes, among others. Activated macrophages migrate in response to chemotactic stimuli and engulf and kill bacteria by processes generally similar to those occurring in neutrophils. They play a key role in innate immunity. They also secrete factors that affect lymphocytes and other cells, prostaglandins of the E series, and clot-promoting factors.

LYMPHOCYTES

Lymphocytes are key elements in acquired immunity. After birth, most are formed in the lymph nodes, thymus, and spleen from bone marrow precursor cells that were processed in the thymus (T cells) or bone marrow (B cells). Lymphocytes enter the bloodstream for the most part via the lymphatics. At any given time, only about 2% of lymphocytes are in the peripheral blood. Most of the rest are in the lymphoid organs.

During fetal development, and to a lesser extent during adult life, lymphocyte precursors come from the bone marrow. Those that populate the thymus (Figure 3–1) become transformed into T lymphocytes. Another lymphoid subset that forms in the thymus is the NKT cell, so-called because it shares features of both T lymphocytes and **natural killer** (NK) cells. Transformation to B lymphocytes occurs in the fetal liver and, after birth, the bone marrow. NK cells also form in these sites. After residence in the thymus, liver, or bone marrow, many T and B lymphocytes migrate to the lymph nodes.

T and B lymphocytes are morphologically indistinguishable but can be identified by markers on their cell membranes. B cells differentiate sequentially into cells capable of production of the various classes of immunoglobulins and thereafter into **plasma cells.** There are two major types of T cells: **cytotoxic T cells** and **helper/effector T cells.** Cytotoxic T cells destroy transplanted

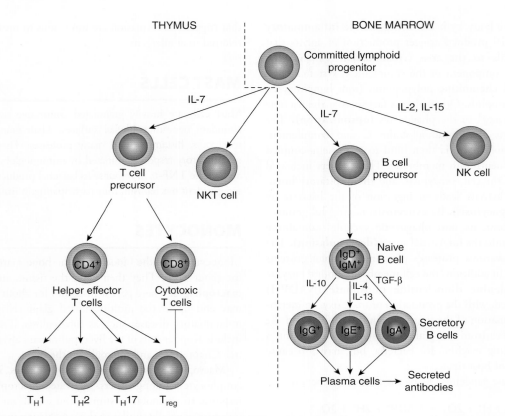

FIGURE 3–1 Development of the system mediating acquired immunity. Committed lymphoid progenitors arise in the bone marrow. Maturation into the B and NK cell lineages occurs in this site, whereas development into T and NKT cells takes place after lymphoid progenitors migrate to the thymus. NK, natural killer.

cells and those expressing foreign antigens (eg, virally infected targets), with their development aided and directed by helper T cells. There are at least four subtypes of helper T cells: T helper 1 (T_H1) cells secrete IL-2 and γ-interferon and are concerned primarily with stimulating cellular immunity; T_H2 cells secrete IL-4 and IL-5 and interact primarily with B cells in relation to humoral immunity. T_H17 cells are induced in response to bacterial infections, produce IL-6 and IL-17, and help recruit neutrophils. They are also implicated in inflammatory responses. Finally, T_{reg} cells produce IL-10 to dampen T-cell-driven responses.

Most cytotoxic T cells display the glycoprotein cluster of differentiation (CD) 8, and helper T cells display the glycoprotein CD4. These proteins are closely associated with T cell receptors and may function as coreceptors. On the basis of differences in their receptors and functions, cytotoxic T cells are divided into αβ and γδ types. NK and NKT cells (see above) are also cytotoxic. Thus, there are four main types of cytotoxic lymphocytes in the body: αβ T cells, γδ T cells, NK cells, and NKT cells.

MEMORY B CELLS & T CELLS

After exposure to a given antigen, a small number of activated B and T cells persist as memory cells. These cells are readily converted to effector cells by a later encounter with the same antigen.

This accelerated response to a second antigen is a key characteristic of acquired immunity. The ability persists for long periods of time, and can even be life-long.

After activation in lymph nodes, lymphocytes disperse widely and are especially plentiful in areas where invading organisms enter the body. This puts memory cells close to sites of reinfection and may account in part for the rapidity and strength of their response.

COLONY-STIMULATING FACTORS

The production of white blood cells is regulated with great precision, and rapidly increased in infections. The proliferation and self-renewal of hematopoietic stem cells (HSCs) depends on **stem cell factor (SCF).** Other factors specify particular lineages (Table 3–1). The regulation of erythrocyte production by **erythropoietin** is discussed in Chapter 38. Other growth factors include **granulocyte/ macrophage colony-stimulating factor (GM-CSF), granulocyte CSF (G-CSF),** and **macrophage CSF (M-CSF).** Interleukins **IL-1** and **IL-6** followed by **IL-3** (Table 3–1) act in sequence to convert pluripotential stem cells to committed progenitor cells. IL-3 is also known as **multi-CSF.** Each of the CSFs has a predominant action, but also has other overlapping actions. In addition, they activate and sustain mature blood cells.

TABLE 3–1 Hematopoietic growth factors.

Cytokine	Cell Lines Stimulated	Cytokine Source
IL-1	Erythrocyte Granulocyte Megakaryocyte Monocyte	Multiple cell types
IL-3	Erythrocyte Granulocyte Megakaryocyte Monocyte	T lymphocytes
IL-4	Basophil	T lymphocytes
IL-5	Eosinophil	T lymphocytes
IL-6	Erythrocyte Granulocyte Megakaryocyte Monocyte	Endothelial cells, fibroblasts, Macrophages
IL-11	Erythrocyte Granulocyte Megakaryocyte	Fibroblasts, Osteoblasts
Erythropoietin	Erythrocyte	Kidney Kupffer cells of liver
SCF	Erythrocyte Granulocyte Megakaryocyte Monocyte	Multiple cell types
G-CSF	Granulocyte	Endothelial cells, fibroblasts, Monocytes
GM-CSF	Erythrocyte Granulocyte Megakaryocyte	Endothelial cells, fibroblasts, monocytes, T lymphocytes
M-CSF	Monocyte	Endothelial cells, fibroblasts, monocytes,
Thrombopoietin	Megakaryocyte	Liver, kidney

CSF, colony-stimulating factor; G, granulocyte; IL, interleukin; M, macrophage; SCF, stem cell factor.

Reproduced with permission from McPhee SJ, Lingappa VR, Ganong WF (editors): *Pathophysiology of Disease*, 6th ed. New York, NY: McGraw-Hill; 2010.

As noted in Chapter 38, erythropoietin is produced mainly by kidney cells and is a circulating hormone. The other factors are produced by macrophages, activated T cells, fibroblasts, and endothelial cells. For the most part, the factors act locally in the bone marrow (Clinical Box 3–1).

■ IMMUNITY

OVERVIEW

The **innate immune system** is triggered by receptors for structures that are common on bacteria and other microorganisms, but are not found in eukaryotic cells. These receptors, in turn, activate various defense mechanisms including release of interferons, phagocytosis, production of antibacterial peptides, activation of the complement system, and several proteolytic

CLINICAL BOX 3–1

Disorders of Phagocytic Function

Many primary and secondary defects in neutrophil function have been described. Patients with these diseases are prone to infections that are relatively mild when only the neutrophil system is involved, but which can be severe when the monocyte-tissue macrophage system is also defective. In one syndrome (neutrophil hypomotility), actin in neutrophils does not polymerize normally, and the neutrophils move slowly. In another, there is a congenital deficiency of leukocyte integrins. In a more serious disease (chronic granulomatous disease), there is a failure to generate O_2^- in both neutrophils and monocytes and consequent inability to kill many bacteria. In severe congenital glucose-6-phosphate dehydrogenase deficiency, multiple infections occur due to an inability to generate NADPH. In myeloperoxidase deficiency, microbial killing power is reduced because hypochlorous acid is not formed.

THERAPEUTIC HIGHLIGHTS

Disorders of phagocytic function require scrupulous efforts to avoid infections, and antibiotic and antifungal prophylaxis, along with aggressive therapy if infections occur. Sometimes, surgery is needed to excise and/or drain abscesses and relieve obstructions. Hematopoietic stem cell transplantation may offer the hope of a definitive cure for severe conditions, such as chronic granulomatous disease. Sufferers of this condition have a significantly reduced life, and so the risks of bone marrow transplantation may be deemed acceptable.

cascades. In vertebrates, innate immunity is complemented by **adaptive** or **acquired immunity**, in which T and B lymphocytes are activated by specific antigens. T cells bear receptors related to antibody molecules. When these receptors encounter their cognate antigen, the cells proliferate and produce cytokines that orchestrate the immune response, including that of B cells. Activated B lymphocytes produce secreted antibodies, which attack foreign proteins.

Innate immunity provides the first line of defense against infections, but it also triggers the slower but more specific acquired immune response. Natural and acquired immune mechanisms also attack tumors and tissue transplanted from other animals.

CYTOKINES

Cytokines are hormone-like molecules that act—generally in a paracrine fashion—to regulate immune responses.

One superfamily of cytokines is the **chemokine** family. Chemokines are substances that attract neutrophils and other white blood cells to areas of inflammation or immune response.

They also play a role in the regulation of cell growth and angiogenesis. The chemokine receptors are G-protein–coupled receptors that cause, among other things, extension of pseudopodia with migration of the cell toward the source of the chemokine.

THE COMPLEMENT SYSTEM

The cell-killing effects of innate and acquired immunity are mediated in part by plasma proteins named the **complement system.** Three different pathways or enzyme cascades activate the system: the **classic pathway**, triggered by immune complexes; the **mannose-binding lectin pathway**, triggered when this lectin binds mannose groups in bacteria; and the **alternative** or **properdin pathway**, triggered by contact with various viruses, bacteria, fungi, and tumor cells. Complement proteins have three functions: they help kill invading bacteria; they serve as a bridge from innate to acquired immunity by activating B cells and aiding immune memory; and they help dispose of waste products after apoptosis. Cell lysis, one of the principal ways the complement system kills cells, is brought about by inserting pore-forming proteins called **perforins** into their cell membranes.

INNATE IMMUNITY

Cells mediating innate immunity include neutrophils, macrophages, and **NK cells.** Cells that are not professional immunocytes may also contribute. The activated cells produce their effects via the release of cytokines, as well as, in some cases, complement and other systems.

Innate immunity in *Drosophila* centers around a receptor named **toll**, which binds fungal antigens and triggers genes coding for antifungal proteins. Toll-like receptors (TLRs) have been identified in humans and other vertebrates. One of these, TLR4, binds bacterial lipopolysaccharide and a protein called CD14, and activates transcription of genes for proteins involved in innate immune responses. TLR2 mediates the response to microbial lipoproteins, TLR6 cooperates with TLR2 in recognizing certain peptidoglycans, TLR5 recognizes flagellin in bacterial flagella, and TLR9 recognizes bacterial DNA. TLRs are referred to as **pattern recognition receptors (PRRs)** because they recognize and respond to the molecular patterns expressed by pathogens. Other PRRs may be intracellular, such as the so-called NOD proteins. NOD2 has received attention as a candidate gene in Crohn disease (**Clinical Box 3–2**).

ACQUIRED IMMUNITY

The key to acquired immunity is the ability of lymphocytes to produce antibodies (in the case of B cells) or cell-surface receptors (in the case of T cells) that are specific for one of the many millions of foreign agents that may invade the body. Acquired immunity has two components: humoral immunity and cellular immunity. **Humoral immunity** is mediated by immunoglobulins, which are produced by plasma cells and activate the complement system and attack and neutralize antigens.

Humoral immunity is a major defense against bacterial infections. **Cellular immunity** is mediated by T lymphocytes. It is responsible for delayed allergic reactions and rejection of transplants of foreign tissue. Cytotoxic T cells attack and destroy cells bearing the antigen that activated them. Cellular immunity constitutes a major defense against infections due to viruses, fungi, and a few bacteria such as the tubercle bacillus. It also helps defend against tumors.

ANTIGEN RECOGNITION

The number of different antigens recognized by lymphocytes is extremely large. Stem cells differentiate into many million different T and B lymphocytes, each with the ability to respond to a particular antigen. When the antigen first enters the body, it can bind directly to the appropriate receptors on B cells. However, a full antibody response requires that the B cells contact helper T cells. In the case of T cells, the antigen is taken up by an antigen-presenting cell (APC) and partially digested. A peptide fragment of it is presented to the appropriate receptors on T cells. In either case, the lymphocytes are stimulated to divide, forming **clones** of cells that respond to this antigen (**clonal selection**). Effector cells are also subject to **negative selection**, during which precursors reactive with self-antigens are deleted. This results in immune **tolerance.**

ANTIGEN PRESENTATION

APCs include specialized **dendritic cells** in the lymph nodes and spleen and the Langerhans dendritic cells in the skin. Macrophages and B cells themselves, and likely many other cell types, can also function as APCs. In APCs, polypeptide products of antigen digestion are coupled to the HLA protein products of the **major histocompatibility complex (MHC)** genes and presented on the surface of the cell.

The genes of the MHC encode glycoproteins that are divided into two classes. Class I proteins (MHC-I) are composed of a heavy chain associated noncovalently with β_2-microglobulin. They are found on all nucleated cells. Class II proteins (MHC-II) are heterodimers made up of an α chain associated noncovalently with a β chain. They are present in "professional" APCs and in activated T cells.

MHC-I proteins are coupled primarily to peptide fragments generated from proteins synthesized within cells. Peptides to which the host is not tolerant (eg, those from mutant or viral proteins) are recognized by T cells. The digestion of these proteins occurs in complexes of proteolytic enzymes known as **proteasomes**, and the peptide fragments bind to MHC proteins in the endoplasmic reticulum. MHC-II proteins are concerned primarily with peptide products of extracellular antigens, such as bacteria, that enter the cell by endocytosis and are digested in the late endosomes.

T-CELL RECEPTORS

MHC protein–peptide complexes on the surface of APCs bind to appropriate T cells. Therefore, T-cell receptors recognize a very wide variety of complexes. Most of the receptors on circulating T cells are made up of polypeptide units designated α and β ($\alpha\beta$ T cells). They form heterodimers that recognize MHC proteins and the antigen fragments with which they are combined. On the other hand, about 10% of circulating T cells have receptors made up of γ and δ chains ($\gamma\delta$ T cells). These T cells are prominent in the mucosa of the gastrointestinal tract, and may link innate and acquired immune systems by way of the cytokines they secrete (Figure 3–1).

CD8 and CD4 occur on the surface of T cells that bind MHC-I or MHC-II proteins, respectively. CD8 and CD4 facilitate binding of MHC proteins to the T-cell receptors. Activated CD8 cytotoxic T cells kill their targets directly, whereas activated CD4 helper T cells secrete cytokines that activate other lymphocytes.

The T-cell receptors are surrounded by adhesion molecules and proteins that bind to complementary proteins on the APC when the two cells transiently form the "immunologic synapse." It is now generally accepted that two signals are necessary to produce activation. One is produced by the binding of the digested antigen to the T-cell receptor. The other is produced by the joining of the surrounding proteins in the "synapse." If the first signal occurs but the second does not, the T cell is inactivated and becomes unresponsive.

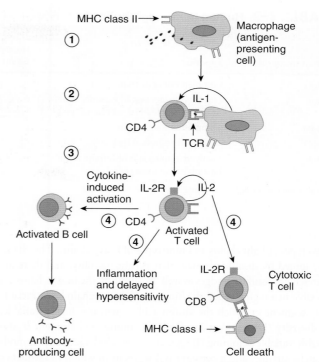

FIGURE 3–2   Summary of acquired immunity. (1) An antigen-presenting cell (depicted here as a macrophage, but other cell types, including dendritic cells, are important) ingests and partially digests an antigen, then presents part of the antigen along with MHC peptides (in this case, MHC II peptides on the cell surface). **(2)** An "immune synapse" forms with a naive CD4 T cell, which is activated to produce IL-2. **(3)** IL-2 acts in an autocrine fashion to cause the cell to multiply, forming a clone. **(4)** The activated CD4 cell may promote B cell activation and the proliferation of plasma cells that produce antibodies or it may activate a cytotoxic CD8 cell. The CD8 cell can also be activated by forming a synapse with an MCH I antigen-presenting cell. MHC, major histocompatibility complex. (Reproduced with permission from McPhee SJ, Lingappa VR, Ganong WF [editors]: *Pathophysiology of Disease,* 6th ed. New York, NY: McGraw-Hill; 2010.)

B CELLS

B cells can bind antigens directly, but they must contact helper T cells to produce full activation and antibody formation. It is the $T_{H}2$ subtype that is mainly involved. The role of various cytokines in B cell and T cell activation is summarized in **Figure 3–2.** Activated B cells proliferate and transform into **memory B cells** (see above) and **plasma cells.**

IMMUNOGLOBULINS

Five classes of circulating antibodies protect their host by binding to and neutralizing some toxins, by blocking attachment of viruses and bacteria to cells, by opsonizing bacteria, and by activating complement. The basic immunoglobulin component contains four polypeptide chains—two **heavy chains** and two **light chains.** There are

TABLE 3–2 Human immunoglobulins.[a]

Immunoglobulin	Function	Heavy Chain	Additional Chain	Structure	Plasma Concentration (mg/dL)
IgG	Complement activation	$\gamma_1, \gamma_2, \gamma_3, \gamma_4$		Monomer	1000
IgA	Localized protection in external secretions (tears, intestinal secretions, etc)	α_1, α_2	J, SC	Monomer; dimer with J or SC chain; trimer with J chain	200
IgM	Complement activation	μ	J	Pentamer with J chain	120
IgD	Antigen recognition by B cells	δ		Monomer	3
IgE	Involved in releasing histamine from basophils and mast cells	ε		Monomer	0.05

[a]In all instances, the light chains are k or γ.

two types of light chains and nine types of heavy chains. The chains are joined by disulfide bridges that permit mobility, and there are intrachain disulfide bridges as well. In addition, the heavy chains are flexible in a region called the hinge. Each heavy chain has a variable (V) segment in which the amino acid sequence is highly variable, a diversity (D) segment in which the amino acid segment is also highly variable, a joining (J) segment in which the sequence is moderately variable, and a constant (C) segment in which the sequence is constant. Each light chain has a V, J, and C segment. The V segments form part of the antigen-binding sites (Fab portion of the molecule). The Fc portion of the molecule is the effector portion.

Two classes of immunoglobulins contain additional polypeptide components (Table 3–2). In IgM, five immunoglobulin units join around a polypeptide called the J chain to form a pentamer. In IgA, the immunoglobulin units form dimers around a J chain and a polypeptide that comes from epithelial cells, the secretory component (SC). This secretory IgA is important in protecting mucosal surfaces.

GENETIC BASIS OF DIVERSITY IN THE IMMUNE SYSTEM

Production of the immensely large number of different immunoglobulins produced by human B cells is brought about in part by the various heavy and light chains in immunoglobulin molecules. There are also areas of great variability (**hypervariable regions**) in each chain. During B cell development, one each of many V, D, and J heavy chain coding regions are selected at random and recombined to form the gene that produces that particular variable portion. A similar variable recombination takes place for the light chain. In addition, the J segments vary further because the gene segments join in an imprecise and variable fashion (junctional site diversity) and nucleotides are sometimes added (junctional insertion diversity). It has been calculated that these mechanisms permit the production of about 10^{15} different immunoglobulin molecules. Similar gene rearrangement and joining mechanisms operate to produce an estimated 10^{15} different T-cell receptors (**Clinical Boxes 3–3** and **3–4**).

More than 300 primary immunodeficiency states are now known to arise from defects in these various stages of B and T lymphocyte maturation (**Clinical Box 3–5**).

CLINICAL BOX 3–3

Autoimmunity

Sometimes the processes that eliminate antibodies against self-antigens fail resulting in **autoimmune diseases.** They include type 1 diabetes mellitus (antibodies against pancreatic islet B cells), myasthenia gravis (antibodies against nicotinic cholinergic receptors), and multiple sclerosis (antibodies against myelin basic protein and several other components of myelin). Antibodies against invading organisms may also cross-react with normal body constituents (**molecular mimicry**). Some conditions may be due to **bystander effects**, in which inflammation sensitizes T cells in the neighborhood, causing them to become activated when otherwise they would not respond.

THERAPEUTIC HIGHLIGHTS

The therapy of autoimmune disorders rests on efforts to replace or restore the damaged function (eg, provision of exogenous insulin in type 1 diabetes) as well as nonspecific efforts to reduce inflammation (using corticosteroids) or to suppress immunity. Recently, agents that deplete or dampen the function of B cells have been shown to have some efficacy, most likely by interrupting the production of autoantibodies.

■ PLATELETS

Platelets are circulating mediators of hemostasis and participate in the response to tissue injury. Their membranes contain receptors for collagen, ADP, von Willebrand factor (see below), and fibrinogen. Their cytoplasm contains actin, myosin, glycogen, lysosomes, and two types of granules: (1) dense granules, which contain nonprotein substances that are secreted in response to platelet activation, including serotonin, ADP, and other adenine nucleotides; and (2) α-granules, which contain secreted proteins. These proteins include

Tissue Transplantation

The T lymphocyte system is responsible for the rejection of transplanted tissue. When tissues such as skin and kidneys are transplanted from a donor to a recipient of the same species, the transplants function for a while but are "rejected" because an immune response to the transplanted tissue develops. This is generally true even if the donor and recipient are close relatives, and the only transplants that are never rejected are those from an identical twin. Nevertheless, organ transplantation remains the only viable option in a number of end-stage diseases.

THERAPEUTIC HIGHLIGHTS

A number of treatments have been developed to overcome rejection. The goal is to stop rejection without leaving the patient vulnerable to infections. One approach is to kill T lymphocytes by killing all rapidly dividing cells with drugs such as azathioprine, a purine antimetabolite, but this makes patients susceptible to infections and cancer. Another is to administer corticosteroids, which inhibit cytotoxic T cell proliferation by inhibiting production of IL-2, but these have side effects (see Chapter 20). More recently, immunosuppressive drugs such as **cyclosporine** or **tacrolimus (FK-506)** have found favor. Activation of the T cell receptor normally increases intracellular Ca^{2+}, which acts via calmodulin to activate calcineurin. Calcineurin dephosphorylates the transcription factor NF-AT, which moves to the nucleus and increases the activity of genes coding for IL-2 and stimulatory cytokines. Cyclosporine and tacrolimus prevent dephosphorylation of NF-AT. However, these drugs inhibit all T-cell–mediated immune responses, and cyclosporine causes kidney damage and cancer. A new and promising approach to transplant rejection is the production of T-cell unresponsiveness by using drugs that block the costimulation that is required for normal activation. Drugs that act in this fashion could be of great value to transplant surgeons.

Primary Immunodeficiencies

Mutations in regulators of acquired or innate immunity lead to primary immunodeficiencies. Typically, patients experience frequent infections or have an increased susceptibility to unusual infections, but they may also be subject to autoimmune problems, spontaneous inflammation, and malignancy. Mutations that prevent the development of many lymphoid lineages have the most serious consequences (Figure 3–3).

THERAPEUTIC HIGHLIGHTS

Mild immunodeficiencies may require only supportive therapies, but the most serious cause substantial morbidity and early mortality. Patients suffering from the latter conditions, therefore, are candidates for early and definitive therapy, and many have benefitted greatly from the transplant of allogeneic hematopoietic stem cells, provided they can tolerate the procedure and a suitable donor can be found. On the other hand, the monogenic nature of many serious primary immunodeficiencies has made them an attractive target for trials of gene therapy.

cytokine secreted by neutrophils and monocytes as well as platelets. It is an ether phospholipid produced from membrane lipids. It acts via a G-protein–coupled receptor to increase the production of arachidonic acid derivatives, including thromboxane A_2.

Platelet production is regulated by CSFs that control the production of the platelet precursors in the bone marrow, known as megakaryocytes, plus **thrombopoietin**, a circulating protein. This factor, which facilitates megakaryocyte maturation, is produced by the liver and kidneys, and there are thrombopoietin receptors on platelets. Consequently, when the number of platelets is low, less is bound and more is available to stimulate production of platelets. Conversely, when the number of platelets is high, more is bound and less is available, producing feedback control of platelet production.

clotting factors and **platelet-derived growth factor (PDGF)**. PDGF stimulates wound healing and is a potent mitogen for vascular smooth muscle. Blood vessel walls as well as platelets contain von Willebrand factor, which, in addition to its role in adhesion, regulates circulating levels of clotting factor VIII.

When a blood vessel wall is injured, platelets adhere to the exposed collagen and **von Willebrand factor** via membrane receptors, with platelet activation and release of granule contents. The released ADP acts on ADP receptors to produce further accumulation of platelets **(platelet aggregation)**. Aggregation is also fostered by **platelet-activating factor (PAF)**, an inflammatory

■ INFLAMMATION & WOUND HEALING

LOCAL INJURY

Inflammation is a localized response to foreign substances. It includes reactions initially involving cytokines, neutrophils, adhesion molecules, complement, and IgG. Later, monocytes and lymphocytes are involved. Arterioles in the inflamed area dilate, and capillary permeability is increased (see Chapters 32 and 33).

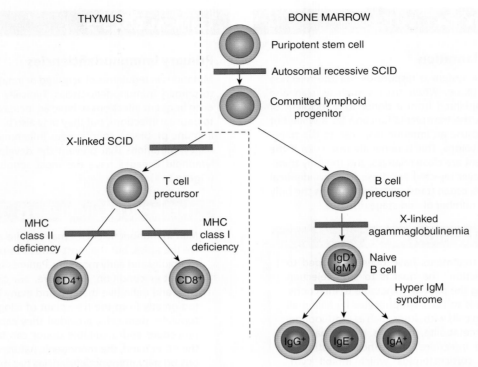

FIGURE 3–3 Sites of congenital blockade of B and T lymphocyte maturation in various primary immunodeficiency states.
SCID, severe combined immune deficiency.

The transcription factor **nuclear factor-κB** plays a key role in the inflammatory response. NF-κB is a heterodimer that normally exists in the cytoplasm of cells bound to IκBα, which renders it inactive. Stimuli induce signals that allow NF-κB to dissociate from IκBα, which is then degraded. NF-κB moves to the nucleus, where it binds to the DNA of genes for numerous inflammatory mediators. Corticosteroids inhibit the activation of NF-κB by increasing the production of IκBα, contributing to their anti-inflammatory action (see Chapter 20).

SYSTEMIC RESPONSE TO INJURY

Cytokines produced in response to injuries also produce systemic responses. These include alterations in plasma **acute phase proteins**, many of which are of hepatic origin. The changes in concentration are incompletely understood, but many make homeostatic sense. Thus, for example, an increase in C-reactive protein activates monocytes and causes further production of cytokines. Other changes that occur in response to injury include somnolence, negative nitrogen balance, and fever.

WOUND HEALING

When tissue is damaged, blood coagulation produces thrombin, which promotes platelet aggregation and granule release, generating an inflammatory response. Extravasated white blood cells and platelets release cytokines that upregulate integrins on macrophages,

which migrate to the area of injury, and on fibroblasts and epithelial cells, which mediate wound healing and scar formation. Plasmin aids healing by removing excess fibrin, aiding the migration of keratinocytes into the wound to restore the epithelium under the scab. Collagen synthesis is upregulated, producing the scar.

CHAPTER SUMMARY

- Immune and inflammatory responses are mediated by cells that arise predominantly from the bone marrow.
- Granulocytes mount phagocytic responses that engulf and destroy bacteria, accompanied by the release of reactive oxygen species and other mediators that may cause tissue injury.
- Mast cells and basophils underpin allergic reactions.
- Soluble mediators orchestrate the development of immunologic effector cells and their subsequent reactions.
- Innate immunity represents an evolutionarily conserved, primitive response to microbial components.
- Acquired immunity is slower to develop than innate immunity, but long-lasting and often more effective due to its greater specificity.
- Genetic rearrangements endow B and T lymphocytes with receptors capable of recognizing billions of antigens.
- Self-reactive lymphocytes are normally deleted; a failure of this process leads to autoimmune disease.
- Inflammatory responses occur in response to infection or injury. A number of chronic diseases reflect excessive inflammatory responses.

MULTIPLE-CHOICE QUESTIONS

For all questions, select the single best answer unless otherwise directed.

1. In an experiment, a scientist treats a group of mice with an antiserum that substantially depletes the number of circulating neutrophils. Compared with untreated control animals, the mice with reduced numbers of neutrophils were found to be significantly more susceptible to death induced by bacterial inoculation. The increased mortality can be ascribed to a relative deficit in which of the following?
   A. Acquired immunity
   B. Oxidants
   C. Platelets
   D. Granulocyte/macrophage colony stimulating factor (GM-CSF)
   E. Integrins

2. A 20-year-old college student comes to the student health center in April complaining of runny nose and congestion, itchy eyes, and wheezing. She reports that similar symptoms have occurred at the same time each year, and that she obtains some relief from over-the-counter antihistamine drugs, although they make her too drowsy to study. Her symptoms can most likely be attributed to inappropriate synthesis of which of the following antibodies specific for tree pollen?
   A. IgA
   B. IgD
   C. IgE
   D. IgG
   E. IgM

3. If a nasal biopsy were performed on the patient described in Question 2 while symptomatic, histologic examination of the tissue would most likely reveal degranulation of which of the following cell types?
   A. Dendritic cells
   B. Lymphocytes
   C. Neutrophils
   D. Monocytes
   E. Mast cells

4. A biotechnology company is working to design a new therapeutic strategy for cancer that involves triggering an enhanced immune response to cellular proteins that are mutated in the disease. Which of the following immune cells or processes will most likely **not** be required for a successful therapy?
   A. Cytotoxic T cells
   B. Antigen presentation in the context of MHC-II
   C. Proteasomal degradation
   D. Gene rearrangements producing T-cell receptors
   E. The immune synapse

5. A child is brought to her physician to be evaluated for repeated infections that are slow to resolve and poorly responsive to treatment. Laboratory investigations reveal a decreased number of circulating neutrophils and autoimmune production of antibodies to a specific cytokine. Her increased susceptibility to infection is most likely attributable to the resulting deficiency in
   A. interleukin-2 (IL-2)
   B. granulocyte colony-stimulating factor (G-CSF)
   C. erythropoietin
   D. interleukin-4 (IL-4)
   E. interleukin-5 (IL-5)

6. Another child evaluated for recurrent infections, similar to the patient in Question 5, has an increased number of circulating neutrophils but histologic examination of infected tissues shows a paucity of neutrophils at the site of infection; infections also result in little formation of pus. In this second child, symptoms are likely attributable to a defect in production of
   A. β_2 integrins
   B. granulocyte-monocyte colony stimulating factor (GM-CSF)
   C. stem cell factor (SCF)
   D. granulocyte colony stimulating factor (G-CSF)
   E. interleukin-3 (IL-3)

7. A keen amateur gardener injures his foot by stepping on a dirty nail while working in his yard. Later that night, his foot becomes red, painful, and swollen. This presumed initial response to an acute infection, mediated by cells responsible for innate immunity, is most likely to have been activated by
   A. glucocorticoids
   B. pollen
   C. carbohydrate sequences in bacterial cell walls
   D. immunoglobulin
   E. thrombopoietin

8. A patient suffering from an acute flare in his rheumatoid arthritis undergoes a procedure where fluid is removed from his swollen and inflamed knee joint. Biochemical analysis of the inflammatory cells recovered from the removed fluid would most likely reveal a decrease in which of the following proteins?
   A. Interleukin-1
   B. Tumor necrosis factor-α
   C. Nuclear factor-κB
   D. IκBα
   E. von Willebrand factor

9. A 6-year-old boy is brought to the pediatrician with complaints of progressive excessive thirst, increased urination, weight loss, and severe fatigue. A glucose tolerance test results in a diagnosis of type 1 diabetes mellitus, and the patient is treated effectively with injected insulin. The emergent symptoms in this patient reflect a failure of which immune process?
   A. Antibody synthesis
   B. Neutrophil chemotaxis
   C. Antigen presentation
   D. Tolerance
   E. Complement activation

10. A 40-year-old woman with kidney failure caused by an adverse reaction to a drug undergoes an autologous kidney transplant. After recovery from the surgery, she is administered tacrolimus in an effort to prevent rejection of the transplanted organ. This drug should be effective in preventing rejection by inhibiting an enzyme of which class in T cells?
    A. Protein kinase
    B. Protein phosphatase
    C. Glycogen synthase
    D. DNA polymerase
    E. ATPase

ANSWERS

1. The correct answer is **B.** Neutrophils are a critical source of oxidants, innate immune mediators that are involved in bacterial killing. While oxidants are also produced by macrophages, neutrophils are the primary source, making B the best answer. Acquired or adaptive immunity is mediated by lymphocytes, which should be unaffected by an experimental approach that targets neutrophils (excluding option **A**). Direct depletion of neutrophils also would not be expected to alter platelet numbers, and if anything would increase rather than decrease GM-CSF in an attempt to restore the neutrophil population (rules out options **C** and **D**, respectively). Finally, while integrins are involved in neutrophil diapedesis into tissues after infection, their expression also should not be reduced by a reduction in neutrophil numbers (excludes option **E**).

2. The correct answer is **C.** The symptoms described are typical for a seasonal allergy experienced when trees are in bloom. Allergic responses occur when allergens bind to and cross-link specific IgE molecules bound to the surface of mast cells located in mucosal sites, resulting in the release of histamine and other mediators. Mast cells do not express receptors for IgA, IgD, or IgM (rules out options **A**, **B**, and **E**). While there is some evidence that a specific subset of IgG molecules (IgG4) can contribute to allergic reactions, allergies are almost always attributable to synthesis of IgE specific for a substance that healthy subjects would find innocuous. This makes **C** the best answer and rules out option **D**.

3. The correct answer is **E.** Allergic reactions are produced by the actions of mast cell mediators on epithelial cells and airway smooth muscle, amongst other targets. Subsequent to mast cell activation, neutrophils may be attracted to mucosal sites and undergo a secondary wave of degranulation, but mast cells will be the primary effectors (rules out option **C** as the best completion). Finally, dendritic cells, lymphocytes and monocytes do not typically degranulate (rules out options **A**, **B**, and **D**).

4. The correct answer is **B.** Malignant cells are eliminated when cytotoxic T cells bearing receptors specific for tumor antigens (not synthesized by healthy cells) recognize fragments of these antigens produced by proteasomal degradation. The recognition of these diseased cells also requires presentation of the antigen fragment in the context of the immune synapse. Thus, because the question asks for factors **not** involved in a successful therapeutic strategy, options **A**, **C**, **D**, and **E** are ruled out. On the other hand, recognition of endogenous antigens, as opposed to those arising from bacterial or other exogenous sources, occurs in the context of MHC-I molecules on antigen-presenting cells, rather than MHC-II, making option **B** the best completion.

5. The correct answer is **B.** G-CSF is a key stimulus for the production of neutrophils and other granulocytes from bone marrow precursors. On the other hand, IL-2 is predominantly a growth factor for lymphocytes, IL-4 activates lymphocytes and monocytes and promotes IgE production, and IL-5 is required for the differentiation of eosinophils (rules out options **A**, **D**, and **E**, respectively). Erythropoietin stimulates the production of erythrocytes, and its deficiency would result in anemia but likely not infections (rules out option **C**).

6. The correct answer is **A.** Because neutrophils are present in the circulation, or even increased, this rules out a defect in the production of granulocytes from bone marrow precursors

(rules out option **B** and **D**). Similarly, SCF and IL-3 are required for the proliferation of pluripotent hematopoietic stem cells and their conversion to committed progenitors for downstream lineages, respectively (rules out options **C** and **E**). On the other hand, because neutrophils are absent from tissue sites of infection there is a defect in their chemotaxis and/or diapedesis in response to an infectious stimulus. The most likely cause of this outcome is a lack of β_2 integrins on neutrophils that are required for the tight adhesion of these cells to the endothelium and subsequent exit from the bloodstream (option **A**).

7. The correct answer is **C.** Innate immune mechanisms provide an immediate response to infection before adaptive or acquired immunity can be stimulated. Innate immunity relies on recognition of molecular patterns that are common amongst microbial species, but not found in eukaryotes. Glucocorticoids inhibit, rather than stimulating, inflammation and immunity (rules out **A**). Pollen is typically an innocuous antigen unless encountered by an allergic individual, and in any event enters the body predominantly through the nasal mucosa and airways (rules out **B**). Immunoglobulins are mediators of acquired immunity, and thrombopoietin is a growth factor for platelets (rules out **D** and **E**, respectively).

8. The correct answer is **D.** The patient is suffering from acute inflammation, a reaction that is orchestrated by the transcription factor nuclear factor-κB (NF-κB). In resting inflammatory cells, NF-κB is bound to IκBα and thereby held in an inactive form. When an inflammatory response is triggered (eg, by a rise in interleukin-1 or tumor necrosis factor-α, ruling out options **A** and **B**), IκBα is degraded by the proteasome, freeing NF-κB to activate gene expression. Von Willebrand factor is produced by endothelial cells and platelets, and involved in regulation of the clotting system rather than inflammation, ruling out option **E**.

9. The correct answer is **D.** Type 1 diabetes occurs secondary to an autoimmune attack on pancreatic beta cells, normally the source of insulin that is critical for glucose homeostasis. In susceptible individuals, there is a failure to delete lymphocyte precursors that are reactive with specific self-antigens (in this case, multiple components of the beta cell have been implicated). Presentation of these self-antigens to autoreactive T cells and synthesis of autoantibodies result (ruling out options **A** and **C**). It is unlikely that neutrophils or complement activation play a role in the disease, but in any event, these processes would if anything be activated in response to inflammation in the pancreas rather than deficient (rules out options **B** and **E**).

10. The correct answer is **B.** Tacrolimus is an immunosuppressive agent that inhibits calcineurin, a phosphatase that becomes active when ligation of the T-cell receptor causes an increase in intracellular calcium and associated calmodulin activation. The function of calcineurin is to dephosphorylate nuclear factor of activated T cells (NF-AT). In its unphosphorylated form, NF-AT can migrate to the nucleus and stimulate expression of IL-2, resulting in enhanced T cell numbers and activity. In theory, the impact of calcineurin inhibition on NF-AT could be mimicked by a drug that stimulated the activity of its kinase, but not by a kinase inhibitor (ruling out option **A**). The remaining enzymes listed are unrelated to the activity of tacrolimus (ruling out options **C**, **D**, and **E**).

Excitable Tissue: Nerve

OBJECTIVES

After studying this chapter, you should be able to:

- Name the various types of glia and their functions.
- Name the parts of a neuron and their functions.
- Describe the chemical nature of myelin, and summarize the differences in the ways in which unmyelinated and myelinated neurons conduct impulses.
- Describe orthograde and retrograde axonal transport.
- Describe the changes in ionic channels that underlie the action potential.
- List the various nerve fiber types found in the mammalian nervous system.
- Describe the function of neurotrophins.

INTRODUCTION

The human central nervous system (CNS) contains about 10^{11} (100 billion) **neurons** and 2–10 times this number of **glial cells.** It has been calculated that 40% of the human genes participate, at least to a degree, in the formation of the CNS. Neurons and glial cells along with brain capillaries form a functional unit that is required for normal brain function; their physiologic duties include synaptic activity, extracellular fluid homeostasis, energy metabolism, and neural protection. Disturbances in the interaction of these elements are the pathophysiological basis for many neurologic disorders. This chapter describes the cellular components of the CNS and the excitability of neurons, which involves the genesis of electrical signals that enable neurons to integrate and transmit impulses.

■ CELLULAR ELEMENTS IN THE CNS

GLIAL CELLS

For many years following their discovery, glial cells (or glia) were viewed as CNS connective tissue. In fact, the word *glia* is Greek for *glue*. However, today these cells are recognized for their role in communication within the CNS in partnership with neurons. Unlike neurons, glial cells continue to undergo cell division in adulthood and their ability to proliferate is particularly noticeable after brain injury (eg, stroke).

There are two major types of glial cells in the vertebrate nervous system: **microglia** and **macroglia.** Microglia are immune system cells; they are scavenger cells that resemble tissue macrophages and remove debris resulting from injury, infection, and disease (eg, multiple sclerosis [MS], AIDS-related dementia, Parkinson disease, and Alzheimer disease). Microglia arise from macrophages outside of the nervous system and are physiologically and embryologically unrelated to other neural cell types.

There are three types of macroglia: oligodendrocytes, Schwann cells, and astrocytes (**Figure 4–1**). **Oligodendrocytes** and **Schwann cells** are involved in myelin formation around axons in the CNS and peripheral nervous system, respectively. **Astrocytes**, which are found throughout the brain, are further subdivided into two groups. **Fibrous astrocytes**, which contain many intermediate filaments, are found primarily in white matter. **Protoplasmic astrocytes** are found in gray matter and

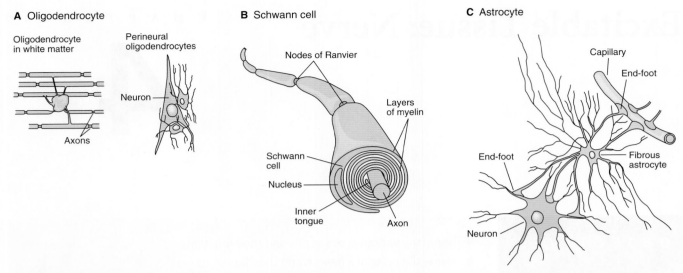

FIGURE 4–1 **The principal types of macroglia in the nervous system. (A)** Oligodendrocytes are small with relatively few processes. Those in the white matter provide myelin, and those in the gray matter support neurons. **(B)** Schwann cells provide myelin to the peripheral nervous system. Each cell forms a segment of myelin sheath about 1 mm long; the sheath assumes its form as the inner tongue of the Schwann cell turns around the axon several times, wrapping in concentric layers. Intervals between segments of myelin are the nodes of Ranvier. **(C)** Astrocytes are the most common glia in the CNS and are characterized by their starlike shape. They contact both capillaries and neurons and are thought to have a nutritive function. They are also involved in forming the blood–brain barrier. (Reproduced with permission from Kandel ER, Schwartz JH, Jessell TM, Siegelbaum SA, Hudspeth AJ (editors): *Principles of Neural Science*, 5th ed. New York, NY: McGraw-Hill; 2013.)

have a granular cytoplasm. Both types of astrocytes send processes to blood vessels, where they induce capillaries to form the tight junctions making up the **blood–brain barrier.** They also send processes that envelop synapses and the surface of nerve cells. Protoplasmic astrocytes have a membrane potential that varies with the external K⁺ concentration but do not generate propagated potentials. They produce substances that are tropic to neurons, and they help maintain the appropriate concentration of ions and neurotransmitters by taking up K⁺ and the neurotransmitters glutamate and γ-aminobutyrate (GABA).

NEURONS

Neurons in the mammalian CNS come in many different shapes and sizes. Most have the same parts as the typical spinal motor neuron illustrated in **Figure 4–2**. The cell body **(soma)** contains the nucleus and is the metabolic center of the neuron. Neurons have several processes called **dendrites** that extend outward from the cell body and arborize extensively. Particularly in the cerebral and cerebellar cortex, the dendrites have small knobby projections called **dendritic spines.** A typical neuron also has a long fibrous **axon** that originates from a somewhat thickened area of the cell

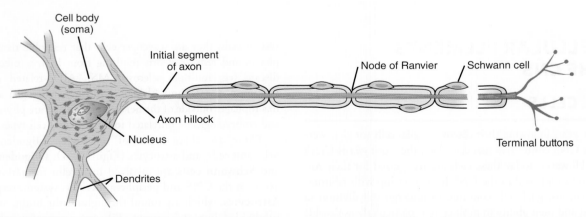

FIGURE 4–2 **Motor neuron with a myelinated axon.** A motor neuron is composed of a cell body (soma) with a nucleus, several processes called dendrites, and a long fibrous axon that originates from the axon hillock. The first portion of the axon is called the initial segment. A myelin sheath forms from Schwann cells and surrounds the axon except at its ending and at the nodes of Ranvier. Terminal buttons (boutons) are located at the terminal endings.

body, the **axon hillock.** The first portion of the axon is called the **initial segment.** The axon divides into **presynaptic terminals,** each ending in a number of **synaptic knobs** that are also called **terminal buttons** or **boutons.** They contain granules or vesicles in which the synaptic transmitters secreted by the nerves are stored. Based on the number of processes that emanate from their cell body, neurons can be classified as **unipolar, bipolar, pseudounipolar,** and **multipolar** (Figure 4–3).

The conventional terminology used for the parts of a neuron works well enough for spinal motor neurons and interneurons, but there are problems in terms of "dendrites" and "axons" when it is applied to other types of neurons found in the nervous system. From a functional point of view, neurons generally have four

important zones: (1) a receptor, or dendritic zone, where multiple local potential changes generated by synaptic connections are integrated; (2) a site where propagated action potentials are generated (the initial segment in spinal motor neurons, the initial node of Ranvier in cutaneous sensory neurons); (3) an axonal process that transmits propagated impulses to the nerve endings; and (4) the nerve endings, where action potentials cause the release of synaptic transmitters. The cell body is often located at the dendritic zone end of the axon, but it can be within the axon (eg, auditory neurons) or attached to the side of the axon (eg, cutaneous neurons). Its location makes no difference as far as the receptor function of the dendritic zone and the transmission function of the axon are concerned.

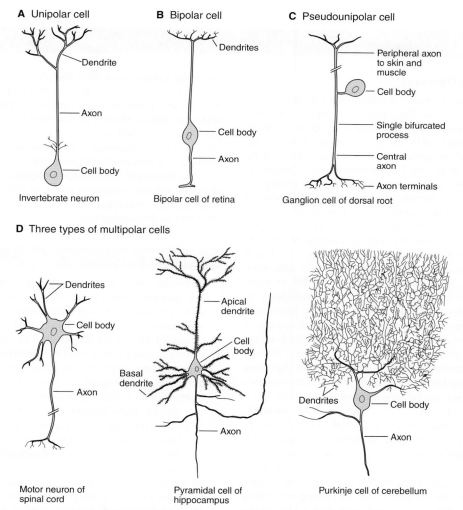

FIGURE 4–3 **Some of the types of neurons in the mammalian nervous system.** **(A)** Unipolar neurons have one process, with different segments serving as receptive surfaces and releasing terminals. **(B)** Bipolar neurons have two specialized processes: a dendrite that carries information to the cell and an axon that transmits information from the cell. **(C)** Some sensory neurons are in a subclass of bipolar cells called pseudounipolar cells. As the cell develops, a single process splits into two, both of which function as axons—one going to skin or muscle and another to the spinal cord. **(D)** Multipolar cells have one axon and many dendrites. Examples include motor neurons, hippocampal pyramidal cells with dendrites in the apex and base, and cerebellar Purkinje cells with an extensive dendritic tree in a single plane. (A, B, Reproduced with permission from Kandel ER, Schwartz JH, Jessell TM, Siegelbaum SA, Hudspeth AJ (editors): *Principles of Neural Science,* 5th ed. New York, NY: McGraw-Hill; 2013; C, Reproduced with permission from Ramón y Cajal S: *Histology,* 10th edition. Baltimore: Wood; 1933.)

The axons of many neurons are myelinated; that is, they acquire a sheath of **myelin**, a protein–lipid complex that is wrapped around the axon. In the peripheral nervous system, myelin forms when a Schwann cell wraps its membrane around an axon up to 100 times. The myelin is then compacted when the extracellular portions of a membrane protein called protein zero (P_0) lock to the extracellular portions of P_0 in the apposing membrane. Various mutations in the gene for P_0 cause peripheral neuropathies; 29 different mutations have been described that cause symptoms ranging from mild to severe. The myelin sheath envelops the axon except at its ending and at the **nodes of Ranvier**, periodic 1 μm constrictions that are about 1 mm apart (Figure 4–2).

Not all neurons are myelinated; **unmyelinated** neurons are surrounded by Schwann cells without the wrapping of the Schwann cell membrane that produces myelin around the axon.

In the CNS of mammals, most neurons are myelinated, but the cells that form the myelin are oligodendrocytes rather than Schwann cells. Unlike the Schwann cell, which forms the myelin between two nodes of Ranvier on a single neuron, oligodendrocytes emit multiple processes that form myelin on many neighboring axons. The loss of myelin is associated with delayed or blocked conduction in the demyelinated axons. In MS, patchy destruction of myelin occurs in the CNS (**Clinical Box 4–1**).

CLINICAL BOX 4–1

Demyelinating Diseases

Normal conduction of action potentials relies on the insulating properties of **myelin.** Thus, defects in myelin can have major adverse neurologic consequences. One example is **multiple sclerosis (MS)**, an autoimmune disease that affects over 3 million people worldwide, usually striking between the ages of 20 and 50 and affecting women about twice as often as men. The cause of MS appears to include both genetic and environmental factors. It is most common among whites living in countries with temperate climates including Europe, southern Canada, northern United States, and southeastern Australia. Environmental triggers include early exposure to viruses such as Epstein-Barr virus and those that cause measles, herpes, chickenpox, or influenza. In MS, antibodies and white blood cells in the immune system attack myelin, causing inflammation and injury to the sheath and eventually the nerves that it surrounds. Loss of myelin leads to leakage of K^+ through voltage-gated channels, hyperpolarization, and failure to conduct action potentials. Initial presentation commonly includes reports of **paraparesis** (weakness in lower extremities) that may be accompanied by mild spasticity and hyperreflexia; **paresthesia**; numbness; urinary incontinence; and heat intolerance. Clinical assessment often reports **optic neuritis**, characterized by blurred vision, a change in color perception, visual field defect (**central scotoma**), and pain with eye movements; **dysarthria**; and **dysphagia.** Symptoms are often exacerbated by increased body temperature or ambient temperature. Progression of the disease is quite variable. In the most common form called **relapsing-remitting MS**, transient episodes appear suddenly, last a few weeks or months, and then gradually disappear. Subsequent episodes can appear years later, and eventually full recovery does not occur. A steadily worsening course with only minor periods of remission (**secondary-progressive MS**) develops later in many individuals. Others have a progressive form of the disease in which there are no periods of remission (**primary-progressive MS**). Diagnosing MS is very difficult and generally is delayed until multiple episodes occur with deficits separated in time and space. **Nerve conduction tests** can detect slowed conduction in motor and sensory pathways. Cerebral spinal fluid analysis can detect the presence of **oligoclonal** bands indicative of an abnormal immune reaction against myelin. The most definitive assessment is **magnetic resonance imaging (MRI)** to visualize multiple scarred (sclerotic) areas or plaques in the brain. These plaques often appear in the periventricular regions of the cerebral hemispheres.

THERAPEUTIC HIGHLIGHTS

Although there is no cure for MS, **corticosteroids** (eg, **prednisone**) are the most common treatment used to reduce the inflammation that is accentuated during a relapse. Some drug treatments are designed to modify the course of the disease. For example, daily injections of β-**interferons** suppress the immune response to reduce the severity and slow the progression of the disease. **Glatiramer acetate** may block the immune system's attack on the myelin. **Natalizumab** interferes with the ability of potentially damaging immune cells to move from the bloodstream to the CNS. A clinical trial using B cell–depleting therapy with **rituximab**, an anti-CD20 monoclonal antibody, showed that the progression of the disease was slowed in patients younger than 51 years in whom the primary-progressive form of MS was diagnosed. Another clinical trial has shown that oral administration of **fingolimod** slowed the progression of the relapsing-remitting form of MS. This immunosuppressive drug acts by sequestering lymphocytes in the lymph nodes, thereby limiting their access to the CNS.

■ AXONAL TRANSPORT

Neurons are secretory cells, but they differ from other secretory cells in that the secretory zone is generally at the end of the axon, far removed from the cell body. The apparatus for protein synthesis is located for the most part in the cell body, with transport of proteins and polypeptides to the axonal ending by **axoplasmic flow.** Thus, the cell body maintains the functional and anatomic integrity of the axon; if the axon is cut, the part distal to the cut degenerates **(Wallerian degeneration).**

Orthograde transport occurs along microtubules that run along the length of the axon and requires two molecular motors, dynein and kinesin **(Figure 4–4)**. Orthograde transport moves from the cell body toward the axon terminals. It has both fast and slow components, **fast axonal transport** occurs at about 400 mm/day, and **slow axonal transport** occurs at 0.5–10 mm/day. **Retrograde transport**, which moves from the nerve ending to the cell body, occurs along microtubules at about 200 mm/day. Synaptic vesicles recycle in the membrane, but some used vesicles are carried back to the cell body and deposited in lysosomes. Some materials taken up at the ending by endocytosis, including **nerve growth factor (NGF)** and some viruses are also transported back to the cell body. A potentially important exception to these principles seems to occur in some dendrites. In them, single strands of mRNA transported from the cell body make contact with appropriate ribosomes, and protein synthesis appears to create local protein domains.

■ EXCITATION & CONDUCTION

A hallmark of nerve cells is their excitable membrane. Nerve cells respond to electrical, chemical, or mechanical stimuli. Two types of physicochemical disturbances are produced: local, nonpropagated potentials called, depending on their location, **synaptic, generator**, or **electrotonic potentials**; and propagated potentials, the **action potentials** (or **nerve impulses**). Action potentials are the primary electrical responses of neurons and other excitable tissues, and they are the main form of communication within the nervous system. They are due to changes in the conduction of ions across the cell membrane. The electrical events in neurons are rapid, being measured in milliseconds (ms); and the potential changes are small, being measured in millivolts (mV). The impulse is normally transmitted (conducted) along the axon to its termination. Conduction is an active, self-propagating process, and the impulse moves along the nerve at a constant amplitude and velocity.

IONIC CONTRIBUTIONS TO RESTING & ACTION POTENTIALS

When two electrodes are connected through a suitable amplifier and placed on the surface of a single axon, no potential difference is observed. However, if one electrode is inserted into the interior of the cell, a constant **potential difference** is observed, with the

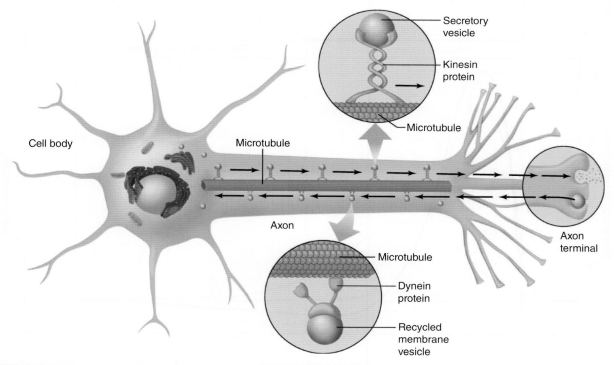

FIGURE 4–4 Axonal transport along microtubules by dynein and kinesin. Fast (400 mm/day) and slow (0.5–10 mm/day) axonal orthograde transport occurs along microtubules that run along the length of the axon from the cell body to the terminal. Retrograde transport (200 mm/day) occurs from the terminal to the cell body. (Reproduced with permission from Widmaier EP, Raff H, Strang KT: *Vander's Human Physiology*. New York, NY: McGraw-Hill; 2008.)

inside negative relative to the outside of the cell at rest. A membrane potential results from separation of positive and negative charges across the cell membrane. In order for a potential difference to be present across a membrane lipid bilayer, two conditions must be met. First, there must be an unequal distribution of ions of one or more species across the membrane (ie, a concentration gradient). Second, the membrane must be permeable to one or more of these ion species. The permeability is provided by the existence of channels or pores in the bilayer; these channels are usually permeable to a single species of ions. The resting membrane potential represents an equilibrium situation at which the driving force for the membrane-permeant ions down their concentration gradients across the membrane is equal and opposite to the driving force for these ions down their electrical gradients. In neurons, the concentration of K^+ is much higher inside than outside the cell, while the reverse is the case for Na^+. This concentration difference

is established by Na, K ATPase. The outward K^+ concentration gradient results in passive movement of K^+ out of the cell when K^+-selective channels are open. Similarly, the inward Na^+ concentration gradient results in passive movement of Na^+ into the cell when Na^+-selective channels are open.

In neurons, the **resting membrane potential** is usually about –70 mV, which is close to the equilibrium potential for K^+ (step 1 in Figure 4–5). Because there are more open K^+ channels than Na^+ channels at rest, the membrane permeability to K^+ is greater. Consequently, the intracellular and extracellular K^+ concentrations are the prime determinants of the resting membrane potential, which is therefore close to the equilibrium potential for K^+. Steady ion leaks cannot continue forever without eventually dissipating the ion gradients. This is prevented by the Na, K ATPase, which actively moves Na^+ and K^+ against their electrochemical gradients.

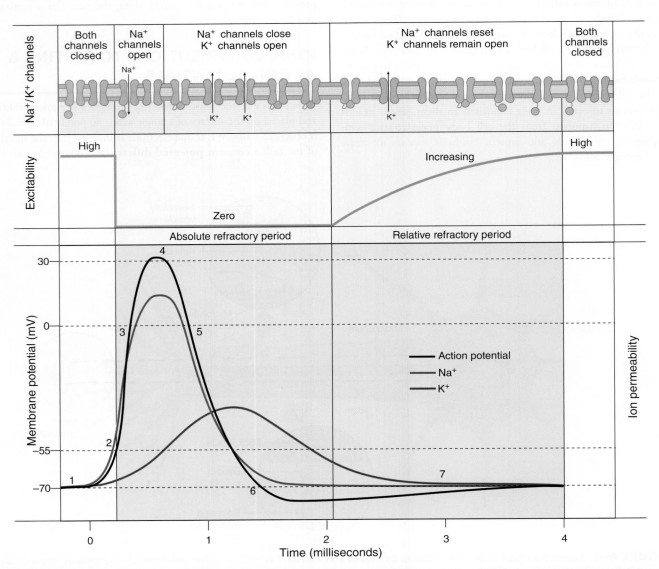

FIGURE 4–5 Changes in membrane potential and relative membrane permeability to Na+ and K+ during an action potential. Steps 1 through 7 are detailed in the text. These changes in threshold for activation (excitability) are correlated with the phases of the action potential. (Modified with permission from Silverthorn DU: *Human Physiology: An Integrated Approach*, 5th ed. New York: Pearson, 2010.)

The cell membranes of nerves, like those of other cells, contain many different types of ion channels. Some of these are voltage-gated and others are ligand-gated. It is the behavior of these channels, and particularly Na⁺ and K⁺ channels, that explains the electrical events in neurons. The changes in membrane conductance of Na⁺ and K⁺ that occur during the action potentials are shown by steps 1 through 7 in Figure 4–5. The conductance of an ion is the reciprocal of its electrical resistance in the membrane and is a measure of the membrane permeability to that ion. In response to a depolarizing stimulus, some of the voltage-gated Na⁺ channels open and Na⁺ enters the cell and the membrane is brought to its **threshold potential** (step 2) and the voltage-gated Na⁺ channels overwhelm the K⁺ and other channels. The entry of Na⁺ causes the opening of more voltage-gated Na⁺ channels and further depolarization, setting up a **positive feedback loop.** The rapid upstroke in the membrane potential ensues (step 3). The membrane potential moves toward the equilibrium potential for Na⁺ (+60 mV) but does not reach it during the action potential (step 4), primarily because the increase in Na⁺ conductance is short-lived. The Na⁺ channels rapidly enter a closed state called the **inactivated state** and remain in this state for a few milliseconds

before returning to the resting state, when they again can be activated. In addition, the direction of the electrical gradient for Na⁺ is reversed during the **overshoot** because the membrane potential is reversed, and this limits Na⁺ influx; also the voltage-gated K⁺ channels open. These factors contribute to **repolarization.** The opening of voltage-gated K⁺ channels is slower and more prolonged than the opening of the Na⁺ channels, and consequently, much of the increase in K⁺ conductance comes after the increase in Na⁺ conductance (step 5). The net movement of positive charge out of the cell due to K⁺ efflux at this time helps complete the process of repolarization. The slow return of the K⁺ channels to the closed state also explains the **after-hyperpolarization** (step 6), followed by a return to the resting membrane potential (step 7). Thus, voltage-gated K⁺ channels bring the action potential to an end and cause closure of their gates through a **negative feedback process.** Figure 4–6 shows the sequential feedback control in voltage-gated K⁺ and Na⁺ channels during the action potential.

Decreasing the external Na⁺ concentration reduces the size of the action potential but has little effect on the resting membrane potential. The lack of much effect on the resting membrane potential would be predicted, since the permeability of the

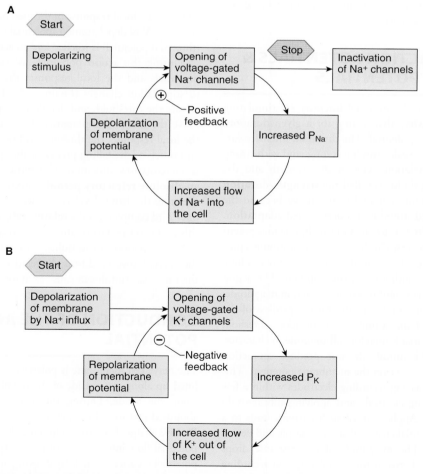

FIGURE 4–6 **Feedback control in voltage-gated ion channels in the membrane. (A)** Na⁺ channels exert positive feedback. **(B)** K⁺ channels exert negative feedback. P_{Na}, P_K is permeability to Na⁺ and K⁺, respectively. (Reproduced with permission from Widmaier EP, Raff H, Strang KT: *Vander's Human Physiology.* New York, NY: McGraw-Hill; 2008.)

membrane to Na^+ at rest is relatively low. In contrast, since the resting membrane potential is close to the equilibrium potential for K^+, changes in the external concentration of this ion can have major effects on the resting membrane potential. If the extracellular level of K^+ is increased (**hyperkalemia**), the resting potential moves closer to the threshold for eliciting an action potential, thus the neuron becomes more excitable. If the extracellular level of K^+ is decreased (**hypokalemia**), the membrane potential is reduced and the neuron is hyperpolarized.

Although Na^+ enters the nerve cell and K^+ leaves it during the action potential, very few ions actually move across the membrane. It has been estimated that only 1 in 100,000 K^+ ions cross the membrane to change the membrane potential from +30 mV (peak of the action potential) to –70 mV (resting potential). Significant differences in ion concentrations can be measured only after prolonged, repeated stimulation.

Other ions, notably Ca^{2+}, can affect the membrane potential through both channel movement and membrane interactions. A decrease in extracellular Ca^{2+} concentration increases the excitability of nerve and muscle cells by decreasing the amount of depolarization necessary to initiate the changes in the Na^+ and K^+ conductance that produce the action potential. Conversely, an increase in extracellular Ca^{2+} concentration can stabilize the membrane by decreasing excitability.

ALL-OR-NONE ACTION POTENTIALS & ELECTROTONIC POTENTIALS

It is possible to determine the minimal intensity of stimulating current (**threshold intensity**) that, acting for a given duration, will just produce an action potential. The threshold intensity varies with the duration; with weak stimuli it is long, and with strong stimuli it is short. The relation between the strength and the duration of a threshold stimulus is called the **strength–duration curve.** Slowly rising currents fail to fire the nerve because the nerve adapts to the applied stimulus, a process called **adaptation.**

Once threshold intensity is reached, a full-fledged action potential is produced. Further increases in the intensity of a stimulus produce no increment or other change in the action potential as long as the other experimental conditions remain constant. The action potential fails to occur if the stimulus is subthreshold in magnitude, and it occurs with constant amplitude and form regardless of the strength of the stimulus if the stimulus is at or above threshold intensity. The action potential is therefore **all-or-none** in character.

Although subthreshold stimuli do not produce an action potential, they do have an effect on the membrane potential. This can be demonstrated by placing recording electrodes within a few millimeters of a stimulating electrode and applying subthreshold stimuli of fixed duration. Application of such currents leads to a localized depolarizing potential change that rises sharply and decays exponentially with time. The magnitude of this response drops off rapidly as the distance between the stimulating and recording electrodes is increased. Conversely, an anodal current produces a hyperpolarizing potential change of similar duration. These potential changes are called **electrotonic potentials.** As the strength of the current is increased, the response is greater due to the increasing

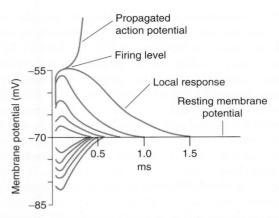

FIGURE 4–7 **Electrotonic potentials and local response.** The changes in the membrane potential of a neuron following application of stimuli of 0.2, 0.4, 0.6, 0.8, and 1.0 times threshold intensity are shown superimposed on the same time scale. The responses below the horizontal line are those recorded near the anode, and the responses above the line are those recorded near the cathode. The stimulus of threshold intensity was repeated twice. Once it caused a propagated action potential (top line), and once it did not.

addition of a **local response** of the membrane (**Figure 4–7**). Finally, at 7–15 mV of depolarization (potential of –55 mV), the **firing level** (threshold potential) is reached and an action potential occurs.

During the action potential, as well as during electrotonic potentials and the local response, the threshold of the neuron to stimulation changes (Figure 4–5). Hyperpolarizing responses elevate the threshold, and depolarizing potentials lower it as they move the membrane potential closer to the firing level. During the local response, the threshold is lowered, but during the rising and much of the falling phases of the spike potential, the neuron is refractory to stimulation. This **refractory period** is divided into an **absolute refractory period**, corresponding to the period from the time the firing level is reached until repolarization is about one-third complete, and a **relative refractory period**, lasting from this point to the start of after-depolarization. During the absolute refractory period, no stimulus, no matter how strong, will excite the nerve. However, during the relative refractory period, stronger than normal stimuli can cause excitation (Figure 4–5).

CONDUCTION OF THE ACTION POTENTIAL

The nerve cell membrane is polarized at rest, with positive charges lined up along the outside of the membrane and negative charges along the inside. During the action potential, this polarity is abolished and for a brief period is actually reversed (**Figure 4–8**). Positive charges from the membrane ahead of and behind the action potential flow into the area of negativity represented by the action potential ("current sink"). By drawing off positive charges, this flow decreases the polarity of the membrane ahead of the action potential. Such electrotonic depolarization initiates a local response, and when the firing level is reached, a propagated response occurs that in turn electrotonically depolarizes the membrane in front of it.

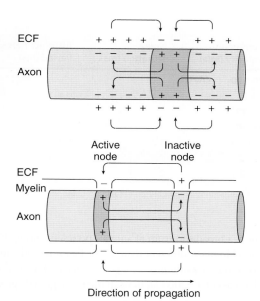

ECF

Axon

Active node   Inactive node

ECF

Myelin

Axon

Direction of propagation

FIGURE 4–8 **Local current flow (movement of positive charges) around an impulse in an axon. Top:** Unmyelinated axon. **Bottom:** Myelinated axon. Positive charges from the membrane ahead of and behind the action potential flow into the area of negativity represented by the action potential ("current sink"). In myelinated axons, depolarization appears to "jump" from one node of Ranvier to the next (saltatory conduction).

The spatial distribution of ion channels along the axon plays a key role in the initiation and regulation of the action potential. Voltage-gated Na⁺ channels are highly concentrated in the nodes of Ranvier and the initial segment in myelinated neurons. The number of Na⁺ channels per square micrometer of membrane in myelinated mammalian neurons has been estimated to be 50–75 in the cell body, 350–500 in the initial segment, less than 25 on the surface of the myelin, 2000–12,000 at the nodes of Ranvier, and 20–75 at the axon terminals. Along the axons of unmyelinated neurons, the number is about 110. In many myelinated neurons, the Na⁺ channels are flanked by K⁺ channels that are involved in repolarization.

Conduction in myelinated axons depends on a similar pattern of circular current flow as described above. However, myelin is an effective insulator, and current flow through it is negligible. Instead, depolarization in myelinated axons travels from one node of Ranvier to the next, with the current sink at the active node serving to electrotonically depolarize the node ahead of the action potential to the firing level (Figure 4–8). This "jumping" of depolarization from node to node is called **saltatory conduction.** It is a rapid process that allows myelinated axons to conduct up to 50 times faster than the fastest unmyelinated fibers.

An axon can conduct in either direction. When an action potential is initiated in the middle of the axon, two impulses traveling in opposite directions are set up by electrotonic depolarization on either side of the initial current sink. In the natural situation, impulses pass in one direction only, from synaptic junctions or receptors along axons to their termination. Such conduction is called **orthodromic.** Conduction in the opposite direction is called **antidromic.** Because synapses permit conduction in one direction only, an antidromic impulse will fail to pass the first synapse they encounter and die out at that point.

■ PROPERTIES OF MIXED NERVES

Peripheral nerves in mammals are made up of many axons bound together in a fibrous envelope called the **epineurium.** Potential changes recorded extracellularly from such nerves therefore represent an algebraic summation of the all-or-none action potentials of many axons. The thresholds of the individual axons in the nerve and their distance from the stimulating electrodes vary. With subthreshold stimuli, none of the axons are stimulated and no response occurs. When the stimuli are of threshold intensity, axons with low thresholds fire and a small potential change is observed. As the intensity of the stimulating current is increased, the axons with higher thresholds are also discharged. The electrical response increases proportionately until the stimulus is strong enough to excite all of the axons in the nerve. The stimulus that produces excitation of all the axons is the **maximal stimulus,** and application of greater, supramaximal stimuli produces no further increase in the size of the observed potential.

After a stimulus is applied to a nerve, there is a **latent period** before the start of the action potential. This interval corresponds to the time it takes the impulse to travel along the axon from the site of stimulation to the recording electrodes. Its duration is proportionate to the distance between the stimulating and recording electrodes and inversely proportionate to the speed of conduction. If the duration of the latent period and the distance between the stimulating and recording electrodes are known, **axonal conduction velocity** can be calculated.

■ NERVE FIBER TYPES & FUNCTION

Mammalian nerve fibers are divided into three major groups (A, B, and C); the A group is further subdivided into α, β, γ, and δ fibers (Table 4–1). By comparing the neurologic deficits produced by careful dorsal root section and other nerve-cutting experiments with the histologic changes in the nerves, the functions and histologic characteristics of each of the families of axons responsible for the various peaks of the compound action potential have been established. In general, the greater the diameter of a nerve fiber, the greater its speed of conduction. The large axons are concerned primarily with proprioceptive sensation, somatic motor function, conscious touch, and pressure, while the smaller axons subserve pain and temperature sensations and autonomic function. Further research has shown that not all the classically described lettered components are homogeneous, and a numerical system (Ia, Ib, II, III, and IV) has been used by some physiologists to classify sensory fibers. Unfortunately, this has led to confusion. A comparison of the number system and the letter system is shown in Table 4–2.

In addition to variations in speed of conduction and fiber diameter, the various classes of fibers in peripheral nerves differ in

TABLE 4–1 Types of mammalian nerve fibers.

Fiber Type	Function	Fiber Diameter (μm)	Conduction Velocity (m/s)	Spike Duration (ms)	Absolute Refractory Period (ms)
Aα	Proprioception; somatic motor	12–20	70–120		
Aβ	Touch, pressure	5–12	30–70	0.4–0.5	0.4–1
Aγ	Motor to muscle spindles	3–6	15–30		
Aδ	Pain, temperature	2–5	12–30		
B	Preganglionic autonomic	< 3	3–15	1.2	1.2
C, Dorsal root	Pain, temperature	0.4–1.2	0.5–2	2	2
C, Sympathetic	Postganglionic sympathetic	0.3–1.3	0.7–2.3	2	2

their sensitivity to hypoxia and anesthetics. This fact has clinical as well as physiologic significance. For example, local anesthetics depress transmission in the group C fibers before they affect group A touch fibers (Clinical Box 4–2). Conversely, pressure on a nerve can cause loss of conduction in large-diameter motor, touch, and pressure fibers while pain sensation remains relatively intact. Patterns of this type are sometimes seen in individuals who sleep with their arms under their heads for long periods, causing compression of the nerves in the arms.

■ NEUROTROPHINS: THEIR FUNCTION & RECEPTORS

Several proteins have been identified that are necessary for survival and growth of neurons. Some of these **neurotrophins** are products of the muscles or other structures that the neurons innervate, but many in the CNS are produced by astrocytes. These proteins bind to receptors at the endings of a neuron. They are internalized and then transported by retrograde transport to the neuronal cell body, where they foster the production of proteins associated with neuronal development, growth, and survival. Other neurotrophins are produced in neurons and transported in an anterograde fashion to the nerve ending, where they maintain the integrity of the postsynaptic neuron.

The first neurotrophin to be characterized was nerve growth factor (NGF), a protein found to be necessary for the growth and maintenance of sympathetic neurons and some sensory neurons. It

TABLE 4–2 Numerical classification of sensory nerve fibers.

Number	Origin	Fiber Type
Ia	Muscle spindle, annulospiral ending	Aα
Ib	Golgi tendon organ	Aα
II	Muscle spindle, flower-spray ending; touch, pressure	Aβ
III	Pain and cold receptors; some touch receptors	Aδ
IV	Pain, temperature, and other receptors	C

is present in a broad spectrum of animal species, including humans, and is found in many different tissues. The factor is made up of two α, two β, and two γ subunits. The β subunits, each of which has a molecular mass of 13,200 Da, have all the nerve growth-promoting

CLINICAL BOX 4–2

Local Anesthesia

Local or regional anesthesia is used to block the conduction of action potentials in sensory and motor nerve fibers. This usually occurs as a result of blockade of voltage-gated Na^+ channels on the nerve cell membrane. This causes a gradual increase in the threshold for electrical excitability of the nerve, a reduction in the rate of rise of the action potential, and a slowing of axonal conduction velocity. There are two major categories of local anesthetics: **ester-linked** (eg, **cocaine, procaine, tetracaine**) or **amide-linked** (eg, **lidocaine, bupivacaine**). In addition to either the ester or amide, all local anesthetics contain an aromatic and an amine group. The structure of the aromatic group determines the drug's hydrophobic characteristics, and the amine group determines its latency to onset of action and its potency. Application of these drugs into the vicinity of a central (eg, **epidural, spinal anesthesia**) or peripheral nerve can lead to rapid, temporary, and near complete interruption of neural traffic to allow a surgical or other potentially noxious procedure to be done without eliciting pain. Cocaine (from the coca shrub, *Erythroxylum coca*) was the first chemical to be identified as having local anesthetic properties and remains the only naturally occurring local anesthetic. In 1860, Albert Niemann isolated the chemical, tasted it, and reported a numbing effect on his tongue. The first clinical use of cocaine as a local anesthetic was in 1886 when Carl Koller used it as a topical ophthalmic anesthetic. Its addictive and toxic properties prompted the development of other local anesthetics. In 1905, procaine was synthesized as the first suitable substitute for cocaine. Nociceptive fibers (unmyelinated C fibers) are the most sensitive to the blocking effect of local anesthetics. This is followed by sequential loss of sensitivity to temperature, touch, and deep pressure. Motor nerve fibers are the most resistant to the actions of local anesthetics.

activity, the α subunits have trypsin-like activity, and the γ subunits are serine proteases. The function of the proteases is unknown. The structure of the β subunit of NGF resembles that of insulin. NGF is picked up by neurons and is transported in retrograde fashion from the endings of the neurons to their cell bodies. It is also present in the brain and appears to be responsible for the growth and maintenance of cholinergic neurons in the basal forebrain and the striatum. Injection of antiserum against NGF in newborn animals leads to almost total destruction of the sympathetic ganglia; it thus produces an **immunosympathectomy.** There is evidence that the NGF-mediated survival of neurons is actually due to suppression of apoptosis rather than promotion of cell metabolism.

In addition to NGF, there are several other neurotrophins, including **brain-derived neurotrophic factor (BDNF), neurotrophin 3 (NT-3)**, and **NT-4/5.** They each maintain a different pattern of neurons, although there is some overlap. NT-3 is important for proprioceptor neurons that innervate the muscle spindle and mechanoreceptors in the skin; NT-4/5 is important for neurons that innervate the hair follicle; NGF is important for skin nociceptive neurons. Sympathetic neurons depend on both NGF and NT-3. BDNF acts rapidly and can actually depolarize neurons. BDNF-deficient mice lose peripheral sensory neurons and have severe degenerative changes in their vestibular ganglia and blunted long-term potentiation.

These four established neurotrophins act through their three high-affinity **tyrosine kinase associated receptors (Trk A, B, C; Table 4–3).** All four neurotrophins can additionally bind a low-affinity NGF receptor, the **p75** receptor, with similar affinity. Interestingly, if a p75 receptor becomes activated in the absence of exposure to a neurotrophin, it causes apoptosis or cell death, an effect opposite to the usual growth-promoting and nurturing effects of neurotrophins.

The regulation of neuronal growth is a complex process and includes many other factors. Schwann cells and astrocytes produce **ciliary neurotrophic factor (CNTF).** This factor promotes the survival of damaged and embryonic spinal cord neurons and may prove to be of value in treating human diseases in which motor neurons degenerate. **Glial cell line–derived neurotrophic factor (GDNF)** maintains the survival of midbrain dopaminergic neurons and prevents the apoptosis of spinal motor neurons. Another factor that enhances the growth of neurons is **leukemia inhibitory factor (LIF).** In addition, neurons as well as other cells respond to **insulin-like growth factor I (IGF-I)** and the various forms of **transforming growth factor (TGF), fibroblast growth factor (FGF)**, and **platelet-derived growth factor (PDGF).** Clinical Box 4–3 compares the ability to regenerate neurons after central and peripheral nerve injury.

TABLE 4–3 Neurotrophins.

Neurotrophin	Receptor
Nerve growth factor (NGF)	Trk A
Brain-derived neurotrophic factor (BDNF)	Trk B
Neurotrophin 3 (NT-3)	Trk C, Trk B
Neurotrophin 4/5 (NT-4/5)	Trk B

CLINICAL BOX 4–3

Axonal Regeneration

Peripheral nerve damage is often reversible. Although the axon will degenerate distal to the damage, connective elements of the so-called **distal stump** often survive. **Axonal sprouting** occurs from the proximal stump, growing toward the nerve ending. This results from **growth-promoting factors** secreted by **Schwann cells** that attract axons toward the distal stump. Adhesion molecules of the immunoglobulin superfamily (eg, the neuron-glia cell adhesion molecule or NgCAM/L1) promote axon growth along cell membranes and extracellular matrices. Inhibitory molecules in the perineurium ensure that the regenerating axons grow in a correct trajectory. Denervated distal stumps are able to upregulate production of **neurotrophins** that promote growth. Once the regenerated axon reaches its target, a new functional connection (eg, neuromuscular junction) is formed, allowing for considerable, although not full, recovery. For example, fine motor control may be permanently impaired because some motor neurons are guided to an inappropriate motor fiber. Nonetheless, recovery of peripheral nerves from damage far surpasses that of central nerve pathways. The proximal stump of a damaged axon in the CNS will form short sprouts, but distant stump recovery is rare, and the damaged axons are unlikely to form new synapses. This is in part because CNS neurons do not have the growth-promoting chemicals needed for regeneration. In fact, CNS myelin is a potent inhibitor of axonal growth. In addition, after a CNS injury, **astrocytic proliferation, activation of microglia, scar formation, inflammation**, and **invasion of immune cells** create an inappropriate environment for regeneration. Thus, treatment of brain and spinal cord injuries focuses on rehabilitation rather than reversing the nerve damage. New research is aiming to identify ways to initiate and maintain axonal growth, to direct regenerating axons to reconnect with their target neurons, and to reconstitute original neuronal circuitry.

THERAPEUTIC HIGHLIGHTS

There is evidence showing that the use of **nonsteroidal anti-inflammatory drugs** (NSAIDs) such as ibuprofen can overcome the factors that inhibit axonal growth following injury. This effect is thought to be mediated by the ability of NSAIDs to inhibit RhoA, a small GTPase protein that normally prevents repair of neural pathways and axons. Growth cone collapse in response to myelin-associated inhibitors after nerve injury is prevented by drugs (such as **pertussis toxin**) that interfere with signal transduction via trimeric G-proteins. Experimental drugs that inhibit the **phosphoinositide 3-kinase (PI3K) pathway** or the **inositol triphosphate (IP3) receptor** have also been shown to promote regeneration after nerve injury.

CHAPTER SUMMARY

- There are two main types of glia: microglia and macroglia. Microglia are scavenger cells. Macroglia include oligodendrocytes, Schwann cells, and astrocytes. The first two are involved in myelin formation; astrocytes produce substances that are tropic to neurons, and they help maintain the appropriate concentration of ions and neurotransmitters.

- Neurons are composed of a cell body (soma) that is the metabolic center of the neuron, dendrites that extend outward from the cell body and arborize extensively, and a long fibrous axon that originates from a somewhat thickened area of the cell body, the axon hillock.

- The axons of many neurons acquire a sheath of myelin, a protein-lipid complex that is wrapped around the axon. Myelin is an effective insulator, and depolarization in myelinated axons travels from one node of Ranvier to the next, with the current sink at the active node serving to electrotonically depolarize to the firing level the node ahead of the action potential.

- Orthograde transport occurs along microtubules that run the length of the axon and requires two molecular motors: dynein and kinesin. It moves from the cell body toward the axon terminals and has both fast (400 mm/day) and slow (0.5–10 mm/day) components. Retrograde transport, which is in the opposite direction (from the nerve ending to the cell body), occurs along microtubules at about 200 mm/day.

- In response to a depolarizing stimulus, voltage-gated Na^+ channels become active, and when the threshold potential is reached, an action potential results. The membrane potential moves toward the equilibrium potential for Na^+. The Na^+ channels rapidly enter a closed state (inactivated state) before returning to the resting state. The direction of the electrical gradient for Na^+ is reversed during the overshoot because the membrane potential is reversed, and this limits Na^+ influx. Voltage-gated K^+ channels open and the net movement of positive charge out of the cell helps complete the process of repolarization. The slow return of the K^+ channels to the closed state explains after-hyperpolarization, followed by a return to the resting membrane potential.

- Nerve fibers are divided into different categories (A, B, and C) based on axonal diameter, conduction velocity, and function. A numerical classification (Ia, Ib, II, III, and IV) is also used for sensory afferent fibers.

- Neurotrophins such as NGF are carried by retrograde transport to the neuronal cell body, where they foster the production of proteins associated with neuronal development, growth, and survival and suppress neuronal apoptosis.

MULTIPLE-CHOICE QUESTIONS

For all questions, select the single best answer unless otherwise directed.

1. In an experiment, researchers engrafted human glia progenitor cells into neonatal mice and allowed them to mature. The mature mice demonstrated high numbers of human glial progenitors, mature human astrocytes and all types of mouse glial cells. The human and mice glial cells intercommunicated, with the human cells retaining larger structure. Interestingly, these human-grafted animals displayed increased neural network signaling and scored better in four independent learning tests when compared to vehicle- or mouse glial progenitor-engrafted mice. These data support the idea that glia contribute greatly to learning and cognition. When considering glia in the normal brain, which of the following statements is true?
   A. Microglia arise from macrophages outside of the nervous system and are physiologically and embryologically similar to other neural cell types.
   B. Glia do not undergo proliferation.
   C. Protoplasmic astrocytes produce substances that are tropic to neurons to help maintain the appropriate concentration of ions and neurotransmitters by taking up K^+ and the neurotransmitters glutamate and GABA.
   D. Oligodendrocytes and Schwann cells are involved in myelin formation around axons in the peripheral and central nervous systems, respectively.
   E. Macroglia are scavenger cells that resemble tissue macrophages and remove debris resulting from injury, infection, and disease.

2. Primary erythromelalgia, which may be due to a peripheral nerve sodium channelopathy, was diagnosed in a 13-year-old girl who was experiencing frequent episodes of red, painful, warm extremities. Which part of a neuron has the highest concentration of Na^+ channels per square micrometer of cell membrane?
   A. Dendrites
   B. Cell body near dendrites
   C. Initial segment
   D. Axonal membrane under myelin
   E. Node of Ranvier

3. A 45-year-old woman who works in an office had been experiencing tingling in her index and middle fingers and thumb of her right hand. Recently, her wrist and hand had become weak. Her physician ordered a nerve conduction test to evaluate her for carpal tunnel syndrome. Which one of the following nerves has the slowest conduction velocity?
   A. Aα fibers
   B. Aβ fibers
   C. Aγ fibers
   D. B fibers
   E. C fibers

4. While spending time in a neurophysiology laboratory, a summer research intern was able to monitor both electrical currents and vesicular transport in cultured neurons. As a way to remember basic fundamentals in neurophysiology, the intern commonly paired up specific features observed in vitro. Which of the following is *not* correctly paired?
   A. Synaptic transmission: antidromic conduction
   B. Molecular motors: dynein and kinesin
   C. Fast axonal transport: ~400 mm/day
   D. Slow axonal transport: 0.5–10 mm/day
   E. Nerve growth factor: retrograde transport

5. For a summer research project, a second-year medical student is introduced to the patch clamp technique in a neurophysiology laboratory. As part of her training, she learns to monitor both membrane potential and individual channel function. At the end for the summer, she is able to write up the specific techniques and findings from monitoring action potentials. Which of the following ionic changes is correctly matched with a component of the action potential?
   A. Opening of voltage-gated K^+ channels: after-hyperpolarization
   B. A decrease in extracellular Ca^{2+}: repolarization

C. Opening of voltage-gated Na⁺ channels: depolarization

D. Rapid closure of voltage-gated Na⁺ channels: resting membrane potential

E. Rapid closure of voltage-gated K⁺ channels: relative refractory period

6. A man falls into a deep sleep with one arm under his head. This arm is paralyzed when he awakens, but it tingles, and pain sensation in it is still intact. The reason for the loss of motor function without loss of pain sensation is
   A. A fibers are more susceptible to hypoxia than B fibers.
   B. A fibers are more sensitive to pressure than C fibers.
   C. C fibers are more sensitive to pressure than A fibers.
   D. Motor nerves are more affected by sleep than sensory nerves.
   E. Sensory nerves are nearer the bone than motor nerves and hence are less affected by pressure.

7. In classic experiments that covered many years, Dr. Rita Levi-Montalcini identified and isolated the first neurotrophin, nerve growth factor (NGF). She showed that NGF had specific actions on nerve cell differentiation. More specifically, she showed that NGF was expressed by peripheral cells, attracted spinal neurons and induced neurite formation. Later, other neurotrophins were identified and today neurotrophins are important factors used in the laboratory to differentiate neural stem cells into functional neurons. Which of the following statements about nerve growth factor is *not* true?
   A. It is made up of three polypeptide subunits.
   B. It is responsible for the growth and maintenance of adrenergic neurons in the basal forebrain and the striatum.
   C. It is necessary for the growth and development of the sympathetic nervous system.
   D. It is picked up by nerves from the organs they innervate.
   E. It can bind to both p75^NTR and Trk A receptors.

8. A 20-year-old female student awakens one morning with severe pain and blurry vision in her left eye; the symptoms abate over several days. About 6 months later, on a morning after playing volleyball with friends, she notices weakness but not pain in her right leg; the symptoms intensify while taking a hot shower. Which of the following is most consistent with her symptoms?
   A. The two episodes described are not likely to be related.
   B. She may have primary-progressive multiple sclerosis.
   C. She may have relapsing-remitting multiple sclerosis.
   D. She may have a lumbar disk rupture.
   E. She may have Guillain–Barrè syndrome.

9. A 60-year-old man visits his family physician after 3 days of abdominal pain, diarrhea, and fever. He is diagnosed with a gastrointestinal infection with *Campylobacter jejuni*. He recovers, but 3 weeks later, he develops weakness and tingling in his legs. The symptoms progress to paralysis in his legs and face within a few days and, he is admitted to a hospital where he is diagnosed with Guillain–Barrè syndrome. Which of the following is most likely the underlying cause of his muscle motor paralysis?
   A. Antibodies against nerve growth factor
   B. Antibodies against oligodendrocytes
   C. Demyelination of B fibers
   D. Demyelination of Aβ fibers
   E. Demyelination of C fibers

10. A family took a hike at Joshua Tree National Park to observe the beautiful desert scenery. During the hike, the 7-year-old son brushed into a Teddy Bear Cactus. Unfortunately for him, the interaction resulted in several pieces of cactus associated with his arm and hand. While the family was able to remove most of the cactus thorns, one needle in particular could not be removed. The family visited an urgent care facility where the boy was given a local injection of lidocaine to "numb" the area and the cactus needle was removed with minor surgical intervention. By which mechanism would lidocaine have acted to be helpful in this situation?
    A. Block of voltage-gated Ca²⁺ channels to limit excitability of sensory neurons
    B. Block of K⁺ channels to limit repolarization of the axon membrane potential
    C. Activation of voltage-gated Na⁺ channels to limit excitability of sensory neurons
    D. Block of voltage-gated Na⁺ channels to limit excitability of sensory neurons

ANSWERS

1. The correct answer is **C**. Astrocytes, one of the many glia phenotypes, play important roles in modulating extracellular neurotransmitters and ions. Microglia do arise from macrophages, but are physiologically and embryologically unrelated to other neural cell types, eliminating **A**. Glia do undergo proliferation, eliminating **B**. Oligodendrocytes are involved in myelin formation in the CNS and Schwann cells provide myelin formation around axons in the peripheral nervous system, eliminating **D**. The statement in **E** describes microglia, not macroglia.

2. The correct answer is **E**. The nodes of Ranvier along the axon are regions between the myelin sheaths that include high concentrations of Na⁺ channels to enhance propagation of the action potential. The dendrites **A** and cell body near the dendrites **B** function more as receptor areas, and do not have high concentrations of Na⁺ channels used in action potential propagation, so can be ruled out. While Na⁺ channel density can be high where action potentials initiate in the initial segment, densities are typically 1/5–1/20 that observed in the nodes of Ranvier, eliminating **C**. The insulated axonal membrane allows for propagation of the action potential with a limited density of Na⁺ channels, eliminating **D**.

3. The correct answer is **E**. The C type fibers associated with pain and temperature sensations in the Dorsal Root Ganglion tend to have small fiber diameters (~0.4–1.2 μm) and slow conductivity (~0.5–2 m/s). The various A fibers listed in **A**, **B**, and **C** have much larger fiber diameters (3–20 μm, depending on fiber type) with correspondingly higher conductivity (12–120 m/s). B fibers **D** are closer in size (< 3 μm) and conductivity (3 15 m/s) to the C fibers, but still are much faster and so can be eliminated.

4. The correct answer is **A**. Synapses permit conduction in one direction only; an antidromic impulse will fail to pass the first synapse they encounter and die out at that point. Molecular motors **B** that help to transport intracellular cargo in neurons include both dynein and kinesin and thus can be eliminated. These molecules help to transport intracellular cargo within neurons. Orthograde transport in neurons includes cargo

movement from the cell body toward the axon terminals. This transport has both fast **C** and slow **D** components with correctly listed distance measurements. Nerve growth factor can be taken up at the nerve ending by endocytosis are also transported back to the cell body (ie, retrograde transport), eliminating **E**.

5. The correct answer is **C**. A typical action potential begins with opening of Na^+ channels resulting in a large depolarization. The rapid closure of these Na^+ channels occurs during the depolarized state, eliminating **D**. It is also at this time that K^+ channels open to repolarize the cell, eliminating both **A** and **B**. K^+ channels do not undergo a rapid closure and can contribute to an after-hyperpolarization due to their extended opening time, further ruling out **A** and eliminating **E**.

6. The correct answer is **B**. The constant pressure on the arm has preferentially blocked conductance in the more sensitive to pressure, motor-sensing A fibers while allowing conduction in pain-sensing C fibers, ruling out **C**. Neither hypoxia **A**, sleep **D**, or neural placement **E** play significant roles in conduction changes related to the observed pressure-induced changes.

7. The correct answer is **B**. NGF is detected in the brain where it is thought to be responsible for cholinergic, not adrenergic, neurons. All of the other statements are accurate statements concerning NGF.

8. The correct answer is **C**. Diagnosing multiple sclerosis (MS) is very difficult and usually occurs only after multiple symptomatic presentations. While **A** is a possibility, the recurring symptoms require attention and it is ruled out as a best answer. Optic neuritis characterized by blurred vision and pain with eye movements is symptomatic of MS. Muscle weakness, especially without pain, and an increase in this weakness in response to heat are also symptomatic of MS. The transient nature of suddenly appearing symptoms is most consistent with relapsing-remitting MS; subsequent episodes can appear years later, and eventually full recovery does not occur. Primary-progressive MS **B** presents as a progressive form of the disease in which there are no periods of remission and thus, can be ruled out. Lumbar disk rupture **D** and Guillain–Barrè syndrome **E** can both present with muscle weakness; however, the initial symptoms of eye pain and blurry vision are not symptoms associated with either of these conditions.

9. The correct answer is **D**. Guillain–Barrè syndrome is an acute, rapidly inflammatory demyelinating neural disease that results in paralysis and sensory disturbance. It is the demyelination of Aβ fibers and subsequent conduction block that causes the paralysis. Up to 25% of Guillain–Barrè patients are diagnosed with *C. jejuni* infections. While Guillain–Barrè is an autoimmune disease, antibodies are not produced to nerve growth factor **A** or oligodendrocytes **B**, and these answers can be eliminated. Because B and C fibers are not associated with motor function, demyelination or conduction block in these neurons could not explain the paralysis, eliminating **C** and **E**.

10. The correct answer is **D**. Lidocaine can be used as a local anesthetic because it blocks voltage-gated Na^+ and thus prevents the development and/or propagation of an action potential. Without the action potential, local sensory fibers do not conduct pain signals. While voltage-gated Ca^{2+} channels are not a target for lidocaine, these channels also do not play a role in the initiation/propagation of the action potential in sensory neurons, and thus **A** can be eliminated. Lidocaine also does not interact with K^+ channels **B** nor cause activation of Na^+ channels **C**, eliminating these two answers.

Excitable Tissue: Muscle

- Differentiate the major classes of muscle in the body.
- Describe the molecular and electrical makeup of muscle cell excitation–contraction coupling.
- Define elements of the sarcomere that underlie striated muscle contraction.
- Differentiate the role(s) for Ca^{2+} in skeletal, cardiac, and smooth muscle contraction.
- Appreciate muscle cell diversity and function.

INTRODUCTION

Muscle cells can be excited chemically, electrically, and mechanically to produce an action potential that is transmitted along their cell membranes and leads to activation of a contractile mechanism. The contractile protein myosin and the cytoskeletal protein actin are abundant in muscle, where they are the primary structural components that bring about contraction. Muscle can be divided into three types: **skeletal, cardiac**, and **smooth**, although smooth muscle is not a homogeneous single category. The basic properties of these three groups of muscle cells will be discussed in this chapter.

■ SKELETAL MUSCLE MORPHOLOGY

ORGANIZATION

Skeletal muscle is made up of individual muscle fibers that are the "building blocks" of the muscular system. Most skeletal muscles begin and end in tendons, and the muscle fibers are arranged in parallel between the tendinous ends, so that the force of contraction of the units is additive. Each muscle fiber is a single cell that is multinucleated, long, cylindrical, and surrounded by a cell membrane, the **sarcolemma** (Figure 5–1). There are no syncytial bridges between cells. The muscle fibers are made up of myofibrils, which are divisible into individual filaments. These myofilaments contain several proteins that together make up the contractile machinery of the skeletal muscle.

The contractile mechanism in skeletal muscle largely depends on the proteins **myosin-II, actin, tropomyosin**, and **troponin.** Troponin is made up of three subunits: **troponin I, troponin T,** and **troponin C.** Other important proteins in muscle are involved in maintaining the proteins that participate in contraction in appropriate structural relation to one another and to the extracellular matrix.

STRIATIONS

Differences in the refractive indexes of the various parts of the muscle fiber are responsible for the characteristic cross-striations seen in skeletal muscle when viewed under the microscope. The parts of the cross-striations are frequently identified by letters (Figure 5–2). The light I band is divided by the dark Z line, and the dark A band has the lighter H band in its center. A transverse

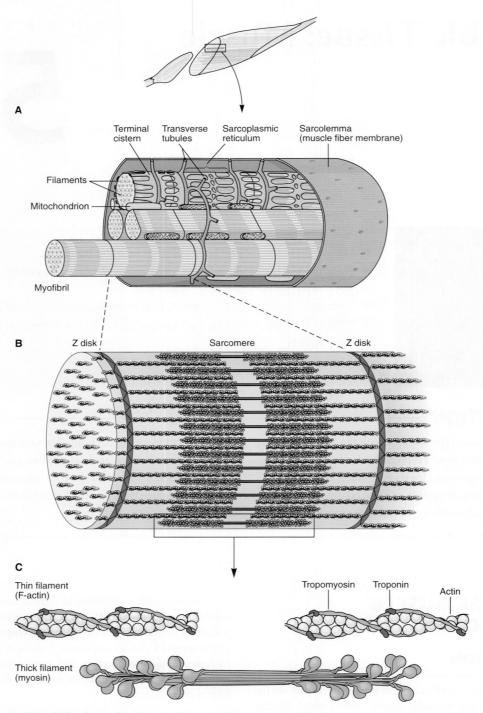

FIGURE 5–1 **Mammalian skeletal muscle. (A)** A single muscle fiber surrounded by its sarcolemma has been cut away to show individual myofibrils. The cut surface of the myofibrils shows the arrays of thick and thin filaments. The sarcoplasmic reticulum with its transverse (T) tubules and terminal cisterns surrounds each myofibril. The T tubules invaginate from the sarcolemma and contact the myofibrils twice in every sarcomere. Mitochondria are found between the myofibrils and a basal lamina surrounds the sarcolemma. **(B** and **C)** Structural elements of myofibril shown in detail (see also Figure 5–2).

M line is seen in the middle of the H band, and this line plus the narrow light areas on either side of it are sometimes called the pseudo-H zone. The area between two adjacent Z lines is called a **sarcomere.** The orderly arrangement of actin, myosin, and related proteins that produces this pattern can be seen in Figures 5–1 and 5–2. The thick filaments, which are about twice the diameter of the thin filaments, are made up of myosin; the thin filaments are made up of actin, tropomyosin, and troponin.

A

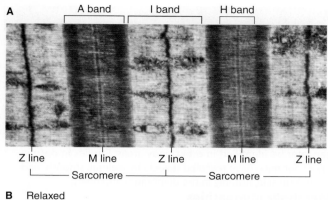

| A band | I band | H band |

Z line   M line   Z line   M line   Z line

└── Sarcomere ──┘ └── Sarcomere ──┘

B Relaxed

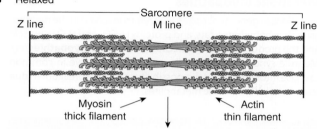

├────────── Sarcomere ──────────┤
Z line   M line   Z line

Myosin → ← Actin
thick filament   thin filament

C Contracted

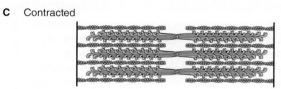

FIGURE 5–2 **Skeletal muscle sarcomere. (A)** Electron micrograph of human gastrocnemius muscle (× 13,500). The sarcomere, named bands, and lines are shown. (Used with permission from GM Walker and GR Schrodt.) **(B)** Arrangement of thin (actin) and thick (myosin) filaments and the Z line in a relaxed skeletal muscle. **(C)** Arrangement of thin and thick filaments and the Z line in a contracted skeletal muscle. Note that the Z lines come together as the thick and thin filaments slide next to each other during contraction. The thick and think filaments do not change in size.

The thick filaments are lined up to form the A bands, whereas the array of thin filaments extends out of the A band and into the less dense staining I bands. The lighter H bands in the center of the A bands are the regions where, when the muscle is relaxed, the thin filaments do not overlap the thick filaments. The Z lines allow for anchoring of the thin filaments. If a transverse section through the A band is examined under the electron microscope, each thick filament is seen to be surrounded by six thin filaments in a regular hexagonal pattern.

The form of myosin found in muscle is myosin-II, with two globular heads and a long tail. The heads of the myosin molecules form cross-bridges with actin. Myosin contains heavy chains and light chains, and its heads are made up of the light chains and the amino terminal portions of the heavy chains. These heads contain an actin-binding site and a catalytic site that hydrolyzes ATP. The myosin molecules are arranged symmetrically on either side of the center of the sarcomere, and it is this arrangement that creates the light areas in the pseudo-H zone. The M line is the

site of the reversal of polarity of the myosin molecules in each of the thick filaments. At these points, there are slender cross-connections that hold the thick filaments in proper array. Each thick filament contains several hundred myosin molecules.

The thin filaments are polymers made up of two chains of actin that form a long double helix. Tropomyosin molecules are long filaments located in the groove between the two chains in the actin. Each thin filament contains 300–400 actin molecules and 40–60 tropomyosin molecules. Troponin molecules are small globular units located at intervals along the tropomyosin molecules. Each of the three troponin subunits has a unique function: Troponin T binds the troponin components to tropomyosin, troponin I inhibits the interaction of myosin with actin, and troponin C contains the binding sites for the Ca^{2+} that helps initiate contraction.

Some additional structural proteins that are important in skeletal muscle function include **actinin, titin,** and **desmin.** Actinin binds actin to the Z lines. Titin connects the Z lines to the M lines and provides scaffolding for the sarcomere. It contains two kinds of folded domains that provide muscle with its elasticity. At first when the muscle is stretched there is relatively little resistance as the domains unfold, but with further stretch there is a rapid increase in resistance that protects the structure of the sarcomere. Desmin adds structure to the Z lines in part by binding the Z lines to the plasma membrane. Some muscle disorders associated with these structural components are described in **Clinical Box 5–1.** Although the described proteins are important in muscle structure/function, by no means do they represent an exhaustive list.

SARCOTUBULAR SYSTEM & DYSTROPHIN–GLYCOPROTEIN COMPLEX

The muscle fibrils are surrounded by structures made up of membranes that appear in electron micrographs as vesicles and tubules. These structures form the **sarcotubular system,** which is made up of a **T system** and a **sarcoplasmic reticulum.** The T system of transverse tubules, which is continuous with the sarcolemma of the muscle fiber, forms a grid perforated by the individual muscle fibrils (Figure 5–1). The space between the two layers of the T system is an extension of the extracellular space. The sarcoplasmic reticulum, which forms an irregular curtain around each of the fibrils, has enlarged **terminal cisterns** in close contact with the T system at the junctions between the A and I bands. At these points of contact, the arrangement of the central T system with a cistern of the sarcoplasmic reticulum on either side has led to the use of the term **triads** to describe the system. The T system, which is continuous with the sarcolemma, provides a path for the rapid transmission of the action potential from the cell membrane to all the fibrils in the muscle. The sarcoplasmic reticulum is an important store of Ca^{2+} and also participates in muscle metabolism. The large **dystrophin** protein forms a rod that connects the thin actin filaments to the transmembrane protein **β-dystroglycan** in the sarcolemma by smaller proteins in the cytoplasm, **syntrophins.** β-Dystroglycan is connected to **merosin** (merosin refers to laminins that contain the α2 subunit in their trimeric makeup)

Structural & Metabolic Disorders in Muscle Disease

The term **muscular dystrophy** is applied to diseases that cause progressive weakness of skeletal muscle. About 50 such diseases have been described, some of which include cardiac as well as skeletal muscle. They range from mild to severe and some are eventually fatal. They have multiple causes, but mutations in the genes for the various components of the dystrophin–glycoprotein complex are a prominent cause. The dystrophin gene is one of the largest in the body, and mutations can occur at many different sites in it. **Duchenne muscular dystrophy** is a serious form of dystrophy in which the dystrophin protein is absent from muscle. It is X-linked and usually fatal by the age of 30. In a milder form of the disease, **Becker muscular dystrophy**, dystrophin is present but altered or reduced in amount. Limb-girdle muscular dystrophies of various types are associated with mutations of the genes coding for the sarcoglycans or other components of the dystrophin–glycoprotein complex.

Due to its enormous size and structural role in the sarcomere, **titin** is a prominent target for mutations that give rise to muscle disease. Mutations that encode for shorter titin structure have been associated with dilated cardiomyopathy, while other mutations have been associated with hypertrophic cardiomyopathy. The skeletal muscle–associated tibialis muscular dystrophy is a genetic muscle disease of titin that is predicted to destabilize the folded state of the protein. Interestingly, many of the titin mutations identified thus far are in regions of titin that are expressed in all striated muscles, yet, not all muscles are affected in the same way. Such muscle type-specific phenotypes underscore the need to study titin's multiple functions in different muscles, under both normal and pathologic conditions.

Desmin-related myopathies are a very rare heterogeneous group of muscle disorders that typically result in cellular aggregates of desmin. Common symptoms of these diseases are failing and wasting in the distal muscles of the lower limbs that can later be identified in other body areas. Studies in desmin knockout mice have revealed defects in skeletal, smooth, and cardiac muscle, notably in the diaphragm and heart.

Metabolic Myopathies

Mutations in genes that code for enzymes involved in the metabolism of carbohydrates, fats, and proteins to CO_2 and H_2O in muscle and the production of ATP can cause **metabolic myopathies** (eg, McArdle syndrome). Metabolic myopathies all have in common exercise intolerance and the possibility of muscle breakdown due to accumulation of toxic metabolites.

THERAPEUTIC HIGHLIGHTS

Although acute muscle pain and soreness can be treated with anti-inflammatory drugs and rest, the genetic dysfunctions described above are not as easily addressed. The overall goals are to slow muscle function/structure loss and, when possible relieve symptoms associated with the disease. Extensive monitoring, physical therapy, and appropriate drugs including corticosteroids can aid to slow disease progression. Assistive devices and surgery are not uncommon as the diseases progress.

---

in the extracellular matrix by **α-dystroglycan** (Figure 5–3). The dystroglycans are in turn associated with a complex of four transmembrane glycoproteins: α-, β-, γ-, and **δ-sarcoglycan.** This **dystrophin–glycoprotein complex** adds strength to the muscle by providing a scaffolding for the fibrils and connecting them to the extracellular environment. Disruption of these important structural features can result in several different muscular dystrophies (see Clinical Box 5–1).

ELECTRICAL CHARACTERISTICS OF SKELETAL MUSCLE

The distribution of ions across the muscle fiber membrane is similar to that across the nerve cell membrane. Approximate values for the various ions and their equilibrium potentials are shown in Table 5–1. As in nerves, depolarization is largely a manifestation of Na^+ influx, and repolarization is largely a manifestation of K^+ efflux. The electrical events in skeletal muscle also share distinct similarities to those in nerve, with quantitative differences in timing and magnitude. The resting membrane potential of skeletal muscle is about –90 mV. The action potential lasts 2–4 ms and is conducted along the muscle fiber at about 5 m/s. The absolute refractory period is 1–3 ms long, and the after-polarizations, with their related changes in threshold to electrical stimulation, are relatively prolonged.

■ SKELETAL MUSCLE CONTRACTILE RESPONSES

It is important to distinguish between the electrical and mechanical events in skeletal muscle. Although one response does not normally occur without the other, their physiologic bases and characteristics are different. Muscle fiber membrane depolarization normally starts at the motor endplate, the specialized structure under the motor nerve ending. The action potential is transmitted along the muscle fiber and initiates the contractile response.

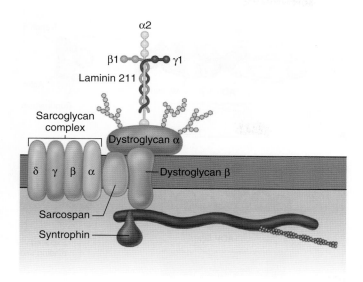

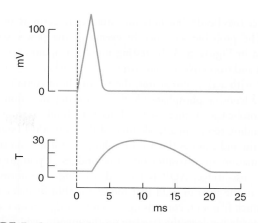

FIGURE 5–4 The electrical and mechanical responses of a mammalian skeletal muscle fiber to a single maximal stimulus. The electrical response (mV potential change) and the mechanical response (T, tension in arbitrary units) are plotted on the same abscissa (time). The mechanical response is relatively long-lived compared to the electrical response that initiates contraction.

FIGURE 5–3 The dystrophin–glycoprotein complex. Dystrophin connects F-actin to the two members of the dystroglycan (DG) complex, α- and β-dystroglycan, and these in turn connect to the merosin subunit of laminin 211 in the extracellular matrix. The sarcoglycan complex of four glycoproteins, α-, β-, γ-, and δ-sarcoglycan, sarcospan, and syntropins are all associated with the dystroglycan complex. There are muscle disorders associated with loss, abnormalities, or both of the sarcoglycans and merosin. (Used with permission from Justin Fallon and Kevin Campbell.)

A single action potential causes a brief contraction followed by relaxation. This response is called a **muscle twitch.** In **Figure 5–4**, the action potential and the twitch are plotted on the same time scale. The twitch starts about 2 ms after the start of depolarization of the membrane, before repolarization is complete. The duration of the twitch varies with the type of muscle being tested. "Fast" muscle fibers, primarily those concerned with fine, rapid, precise movement, have twitch durations as short as 7.5 ms. "Slow" muscle fibers, principally those involved in strong, gross, sustained movements, have twitch durations up to 100 ms.

MOLECULAR BASIS OF CONTRACTION

The process by which the contraction of muscle is brought about is a sliding of the thin filaments over the thick filaments. Note that this shortening is not due to changes in the actual lengths of the thick and thin filaments, rather, by their increased overlap within the muscle cell. The width of the A bands is constant, whereas the Z lines move closer together when the muscle contracts and farther apart when it relaxes (Figure 5–2).

The sliding during muscle contraction occurs when the myosin heads bind firmly to actin, bend at the junction of the head with the neck, and then detach. This "power stroke" depends on the simultaneous hydrolysis of ATP. Myosin-II molecules are dimers

TABLE 5–1 Steady-state distribution of ions in the intracellular and extracellular compartments of mammalian skeletal muscle, and the equilibrium potentials for these ions.

Ion[a]	Concentration (mmol/L)		Equilibrium Potential (mV)
	Intracellular Fluid	Extracellular Fluid	
Na^+	12	145	+65
K^+	155	4	–95
H^+	13×10^{-5}	3.8×10^{-5}	–32
Cl^-	3.8	120	–90
HCO_3^-	8	27	–32
A^-	155	0	…
Membrane potential = –90 mV			

[a]A^- represents organic anions. The value for intracellular Cl^- is calculated from the membrane potential, using the Nernst equation.

that have two heads, but only one attaches to actin at any given time. The probable sequence of events of the power stroke is outlined in Figure 5–5. In resting muscle, troponin I is bound to actin and tropomyosin and covers the sites where myosin heads interact with actin. Also at rest, the myosin head contains tightly bound adenosine phosphate (ADP). Following an action potential, cytosolic Ca^{2+} is increased and free Ca^{2+} binds to troponin C. This binding results in a weakening of the troponin I interaction with actin and exposes the actin binding site for myosin to allow for formation of myosin/actin cross-bridges. Upon formation of the cross-bridge, ADP is released, causing a conformational change in the myosin head that moves the thin filament relative to the thick filament, comprising the cross-bridge "power stroke." ATP quickly binds to the free site on the myosin, which leads to a detachment of the myosin head from the thin filament. ATP is hydrolyzed and inorganic phosphate (P_i) released, causing a "re-cocking" of the myosin head and completing the cycle. As long as Ca^{2+} remains elevated and sufficient ATP is available, this cycle repeats. Many myosin heads cycle at or near the same time, and they cycle repeatedly, producing gross muscle contraction. Each power stroke shortens the sarcomere about 10 nm. Each thick filament has about 500 myosin heads, and each head cycles about five times per second during a rapid contraction.

The process by which depolarization of the muscle fiber initiates contraction is called **excitation–contraction coupling.** The action potential is transmitted to all the fibrils in the fiber via the T tubule system (Figure 5–6). It triggers the release of Ca^{2+} from the terminal cisterns, the lateral sacs of the sarcoplasmic reticulum next to the T tubule system. Depolarization of the T tubule membrane activates the sarcoplasmic reticulum via **dihydropyridine receptors (DHPR;** Figure 5–7). DHPR are voltage-gated Ca^{2+} channels in the T tubule membrane. In skeletal muscle, the DHPR that serves as the voltage sensor unlocks release of Ca^{2+} from the nearby sarcoplasmic reticulum via physical interaction with the **ryanodine receptor (RyR)** on the sarcoplasmic reticulum. The RyR is a ligand-gated Ca^{2+} channel with Ca^{2+} as its natural ligand. The released Ca^{2+} is quickly amplified through calcium-induced calcium release. Ca^{2+} concentration is reduced in the muscle cell by the sarcoplasmic or endoplasmic reticulum Ca^{2+} ATPase (SERCA). The SERCA pump uses energy from ATP hydrolysis to remove Ca^{2+} from the cytosol back into the terminal cisterns, where it is stored until released by the next action potential. Once the Ca^{2+} concentration outside the sarcoplasmic reticulum has been lowered sufficiently, chemical interaction between myosin and actin ceases and the muscle relaxes. Note that ATP provides the energy for both contraction (at the myosin head) and relaxation (via SERCA). Alterations in the excitable response in muscle underscore a variety of pathologies (Clinical Box 5–2).

SUMMATION OF CONTRACTIONS

The electrical response of a muscle fiber to repeated stimulation is like that of nerve. The fiber is electrically refractory only during the rising phase and part of the falling phase of

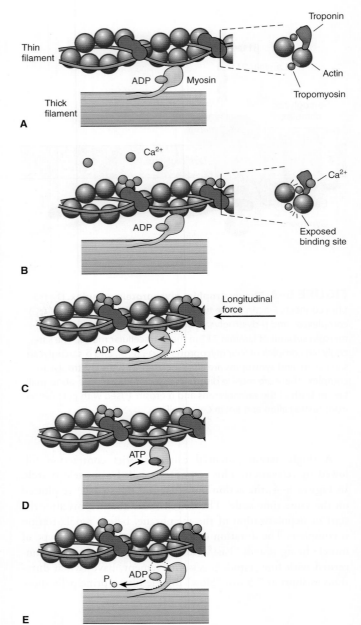

FIGURE 5–5　Power stroke of myosin in skeletal muscle.
(A) At rest, myosin heads are bound to adenosine diphosphate and are said to be in a "cocked" position in relation to the thin filament, which does not have Ca^{2+} bound to the troponin—tropomyosin complex. **(B)** Ca^{2+} bound to the troponin—tropomyosin complex induces a conformational change in the thin filament that allows for myosin heads to cross-bridge with thin filament actin. **(C)** Myosin heads rotate, move the attached actin and shorten the muscle fiber, forming the power stroke. **(D)** At the end of the power stroke, ATP binds to a now exposed site, and causes a detachment from the actin filament. **(E)** ATP is hydrolyzed into ADP and inorganic phosphate (P_i) and this chemical energy is used to "recock" the myosin head. (Data from Huxley AF, Simmons RM: Proposed mechanism of force generation in striated muscle. *Nature* Oct. 22;233(5321):533–538, 1971 and Squire JM: Molecular mechanisms in muscular contraction. *Trends Neurosci.* 6:409–413, 1093.)

Steps in contraction[a]

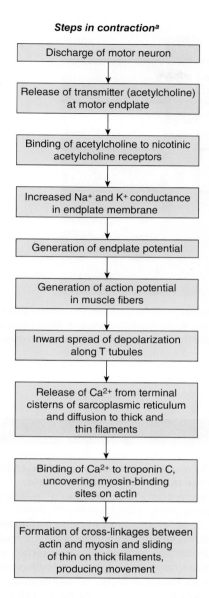

Discharge of motor neuron

Release of transmitter (acetylcholine) at motor endplate

Binding of acetylcholine to nicotinic acetylcholine receptors

Increased Na⁺ and K⁺ conductance in endplate membrane

Generation of endplate potential

Generation of action potential in muscle fibers

Inward spread of depolarization along T tubules

Release of Ca²⁺ from terminal cisterns of sarcoplasmic reticulum and diffusion to thick and thin filaments

Binding of Ca²⁺ to troponin C, uncovering myosin-binding sites on actin

Formation of cross-linkages between actin and myosin and sliding of thin on thick filaments, producing movement

Steps in relaxation

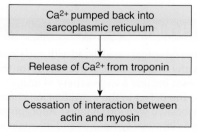

Ca²⁺ pumped back into sarcoplasmic reticulum

Release of Ca²⁺ from troponin

Cessation of interaction between actin and myosin

[a]The first six steps in contraction are discussed in Chapter 4.

FIGURE 5–6 **Flow of information that leads to muscle contraction.**

the spike potential. At this time, the contraction initiated by the first stimulus is just beginning. However, because the contractile mechanism does not have a refractory period, repeated stimulation before relaxation has occurred produces additional activation of the contractile elements and a response that is added to the contraction already present. This phenomenon is known as **summation of contractions.** The tension developed during summation is considerably greater than that during the single muscle twitch. With rapidly repeated stimulation, activation of the contractile mechanism occurs repeatedly before any relaxation has occurred, and the individual responses fuse into one continuous contraction. Such a response is called a **tetanus (tetanic contraction; Figure 5–8).** It is a **complete tetanus** when no relaxation occurs between stimuli and an **incomplete tetanus** when periods of incomplete relaxation take place between the summated stimuli. During a complete tetanus, the tension developed is about four times that developed by the individual twitch contractions. The stimulation frequency at which summation of contractions occurs is determined by the twitch duration of the particular muscle being studied. For example, if the twitch duration is 10 ms, frequencies less than 1/10 ms cause discrete responses interrupted by complete relaxation, and frequencies greater than 1/10 ms cause summation.

RELATION BETWEEN MUSCLE LENGTH, TENSION, & VELOCITY OF CONTRACTION

Both the tension that a muscle develops when stimulated to contract isometrically (the **total tension**) and the **passive tension** exerted by the unstimulated muscle vary with the length of the muscle fiber. This relationship can be studied in a whole skeletal muscle preparation. The length of the muscle can be varied by changing the distance between its two attachments. At each length, the passive tension is measured, the muscle is then stimulated electrically, and the total tension is measured. The difference between the two values at any length is the amount of tension actually generated by the contractile process, the **active tension**. The records obtained by plotting passive tension and total tension against muscle length are shown in **Figure 5–9.** The length of the muscle at which the active tension is maximal is usually called its **resting length.**

The observed length-tension relation in skeletal muscle can be explained by the sliding filament mechanism of muscle contraction. When the muscle fiber contracts isometrically (ie, contraction without change in length; think: "pushing against a hard wall"), the tension developed is proportional to the number of cross-bridges between the actin and the myosin molecules. When muscle is stretched, the overlap between actin and myosin is reduced and the number of cross-linkages is therefore reduced. Conversely, when the muscle is appreciably shorter than resting length, the distance the thin filaments can move is reduced. The velocity of muscle contraction varies inversely with the load on the muscle. At a given load, the velocity is maximal at the resting length and declines if the muscle is shorter or longer than this length.

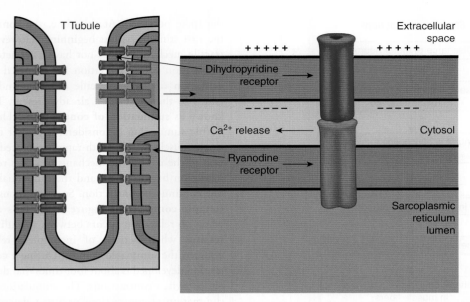

FIGURE 5-7   Relation of the T tubule to the sarcoplasmic reticulum in Ca²⁺ transport. In skeletal muscle, the voltage-gated dihydro-pyridine receptor in the T tubule triggers Ca²⁺ release from the sarcoplasmic reticulum (SR) via the ryanodine receptor (RyR). Upon sensing a voltage change, there is a physical interaction between the sarcolemmal-bound DHPR and the SR-bound RyR. This interaction gates the RyR and allows for Ca²⁺ release from the SR.

CLINICAL BOX 5-2

Muscle Channelopathies

Channelopathies are diseases that have as their underlying feature mutations or dysregulation of ion channels. Such diseases are frequently associated with excitable cells, including muscle. In the various forms of clinical **myotonia**, muscle relaxation is prolonged after voluntary contraction. The molecular bases of myotonias are due to dysfunction of channels that shape the action potential. Myotonia dystrophy is caused by an autosomal dominant mutation that leads to overexpression of a K⁺ channel (although the mutation is *not* at the K⁺ channel). A variety of myotonias are associated with mutations in Na⁺ channels (eg, hyperkalemic periodic paralysis, paramyotonia congenita, or Na⁺ channel congenita) or Cl⁻ channels (eg, dominant or recessive myotonia congenita). **Myasthenia,** defined as abnormal muscle weakness or disease, can also be related to loss of ion channel function in the muscle. In **congenital myasthenia**, the patient has an inheritable disorder of one of a group of ion channels necessary for the transmission of neuronal signaling to muscle response. Mutations in Ca²⁺ channels that allow for neuronal transmitter release or in the acetylcholine receptor nonspecific cation channels, important in recognition of neuronal transmitters, have both been shown to cause congenital myasthenia. Alterations of channel functions can also occur via autoimmune disease, such as that observed in **myasthenia gravis.** In this disease, antibodies to the nicotinic acetylcholine receptor can reduce its functional presence at the muscle membrane by up to 80%, and thus limit muscle response to neuronal transmitter release.

Channelopathies can also occur in the Ca²⁺ release channels in muscle (ryanodine receptors) that amplify the Ca²⁺ response within the cell. Such mutations can cause **malignant hyperthermia.** Patients with this condition display normal muscle function under normal conditions. However, certain anesthetic agents, or in rare cases exposure to high environmental heat or strenuous exercise, can trigger abnormal release of Ca²⁺ from the sarcoplasmic reticulum in the muscle cell, resulting in sustained muscle contraction and heat production. In severe cases, fatality can occur.

THERAPEUTIC HIGHLIGHTS

Although the symptoms associated with each individual channelopathy may be similar, treatments for the individual diseases include a wide variety of drugs that are targeted to the defect in the individual ion channel (or proteins associated with ion channel). Appropriate drug therapy helps improve symptoms and maintain acceptable muscle function. Further interventions related to individual diseases are to avoid muscle movements that exacerbate the disease.

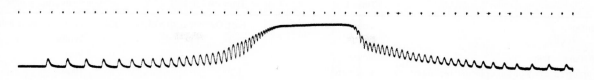

FIGURE 5–8 Tetanus. Isometric tension of a single muscle fiber during continuously increasing and decreasing stimulation frequency. Dots at the top are at intervals of 0.2 s. Note the development of incomplete and then complete tetanus as stimulation is increased, and the return of incomplete tetanus, then full response, as stimulation frequency is decreased.

FIBER TYPES

Although skeletal muscle fibers resemble one another in a general way, skeletal muscle is a heterogeneous tissue made up of fibers that vary in myosin ATPase activity, contractile speed, and other properties. Muscles are frequently classified into two types: "slow" and "fast." These muscles can contain a mixture of three fiber types: type I (or SO for slow oxidative), type IIA (FOG for fast oxidative glycolytic), or type IIB (FG for fast glycolytic). Some of the properties associated with type I, type IIA, and type IIB fibers are summarized in Table 5–2. Although these classification schemes are valid for muscles across many mammalian species, there are significant variations of fibers within and between muscles. For example, type I fibers in a given muscle can be larger than type IIA fibers from a different muscle in the same animal. Many of the differences in the fibers that make up muscles stem from differences in the proteins within them. Most of these are encoded by multigene families. There are different **isoforms** of the myosin heavy chains and each of the two types of light chains also have isoforms. There is only one known form of actin, but multiple isoforms of tropomyosin and all three components of troponin.

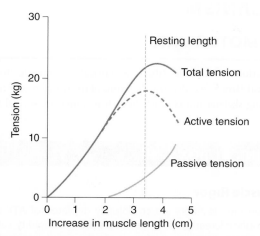

FIGURE 5–9 Length–tension relationship for the human triceps muscle. The passive tension curve measures the tension exerted by this skeletal muscle at each length when it is not stimulated. The total tension curve represents the tension developed when the muscle contracts isometrically in response to a maximal stimulus. The active tension is the difference between the two.

■ SKELETAL MUSCLE ENERGY SOURCES & METABOLISM

Muscle contraction requires energy, and muscle has been called "a machine for converting chemical energy into mechanical work." The immediate source of this energy is ATP, and this is formed by the metabolism of carbohydrates and lipids.

PHOSPHORYLCREATINE

ATP is resynthesized from ADP by the addition of a phosphate group. Some of the energy for this endothermic reaction is supplied by the breakdown of glucose to CO_2 and H_2O, but a second energy-rich phosphate compound, **phosphorylcreatine**, can supply this energy for short periods. Phosphorylcreatine is hydrolyzed to creatine and phosphate groups with the release of considerable energy. At rest, some ATP in the mitochondria transfers its phosphate to creatine, so that a phosphorylcreatine store is built up. During exercise, the phosphorylcreatine is hydrolyzed at the junction between the myosin heads and actin, forming ATP from ADP, and extending contraction.

CARBOHYDRATE & LIPID BREAKDOWN

At rest and during light exercise, muscles utilize lipids in the form of free fatty acids as their energy source. As the intensity of exercise increases, lipids alone cannot supply energy fast enough and so use of carbohydrate becomes the predominant component in the muscle fuel mixture. Thus, during exercise, much of the energy for phosphorylcreatine and ATP resynthesis comes from the breakdown of glucose to CO_2 and H_2O. Glucose in the bloodstream enters cells, where it is degraded through a series of chemical reactions to pyruvate. Another source of intracellular glucose, and consequently of pyruvate, is glycogen, the carbohydrate polymer that is especially abundant in liver and skeletal muscle. When adequate O_2 is present, pyruvate enters the citric acid cycle and is metabolized by **aerobic glycolysis.** The metabolism of glucose or glycogen to CO_2 and H_2O forms large quantities of ATP from ADP. If O_2 supplies are insufficient, the pyruvate formed from glucose does not enter the tricarboxylic acid cycle but is reduced to lactate. This process of **anaerobic glycolysis** is associated with the net production of much smaller quantities of energy-rich

TABLE 5–2 Classification of fiber types in skeletal muscles.

	Type 1	Type IIA	Type IIB
Other names	Slow, Oxidative (SO)	Fast, Oxidative, Glycolytic (FOG)	Fast, Glycolytic (FG)
Color	Red	Red	White
Myosin ATPase activity	Slow	Fast	Fast
Ca^{2+}-pumping capacity of sarcoplasmic reticulum	Moderate	High	High
Diameter	Small	Large	Large
Glycolytic capacity	Moderate	High	High
Oxidative capacity	High	Moderate	Low
Associated Motor Unit Type	Slow (S)	Fast Resistant to Fatigue (FR)	Fast Fatigable (FF)
Membrane potential = –90 mV			

phosphate bonds, but it does not require the presence of O_2. A brief overview of the various reactions involved in supplying energy to skeletal muscle is shown in Figure 5–10.

THE OXYGEN DEBT MECHANISM

During exercise, the muscle blood vessels dilate and blood flow is increased so that the available O_2 supply is increased. Up to a point, the increase in O_2 consumption is proportional to the energy expended, and all energy needs are met by aerobic processes. However, when muscular exertion is very great, aerobic resynthesis of energy stores cannot keep pace with their utilization. Under these conditions, phosphorylcreatine is still used to resynthesize ATP. In addition, some ATP synthesis is accomplished by using the energy released by the anaerobic breakdown of glucose to lactate. Use of the anaerobic pathway is self-limiting because in spite of rapid diffusion of lactate into the bloodstream, enough accumulates in the muscles to eventually exceed the capacity of the tissue buffers and produce an enzyme-inhibiting decline in pH. For short periods, the

presence of an anaerobic pathway for glucose breakdown permits muscular exertion of a far greater magnitude than would be possible without it. For example, in a 100-m dash that takes 10 s, 85% of the energy consumed is derived anaerobically; in a 2-mile race that takes 10 min, 20% of the energy is derived anaerobically; and in a long-distance race that takes 60 min, only 5% of the energy comes from anaerobic metabolism.

After a period of exertion is over, extra O_2 is consumed to remove the excess lactate, replenish the ATP and phosphorylcreatine stores, and replace the small amounts of O_2 that were released by myoglobin. Without replenishment of ATP, muscles enter a state of rigor (Clinical Box 5–3). The amount of extra O_2 consumed is proportional to the extent to which the energy demands during exertion exceeded the capacity for the aerobic synthesis of energy stores, that is, the extent to which an **oxygen debt** was incurred.

■ PROPERTIES OF SKELETAL MUSCLES IN THE INTACT ORGANISM

THE MOTOR UNIT

Innervation of muscle fibers is critical to muscle function (Clinical Box 5–4). Because the axons of the spinal motor neurons supplying skeletal muscle each branch to innervate several muscle

Energy in phosphate bond:
$$ATP + H_2O \rightarrow ADP + H_3PO_4 + 7.3 \text{ kcal}$$

ATP "storage" in muscle via creatine:
$$\text{Phosphorylcreatine} + ADP \rightleftharpoons \text{Creatine} + ATP$$

Anaerobic pathway:
$$\text{Glucose} + 2 ATP \longrightarrow 2 \text{ Lactic acid} + 4 ATP$$
$$(\text{or glycogen} + 1 ATP)$$

Aerobic pathway:
$$\text{Glucose} + 2 ATP \longrightarrow 6 CO_2 + 6 H_2O + 40 ATP$$
$$(\text{or glycogen} + 1 ATP)$$

$$FFA \longrightarrow CO_2 + H_2O + ATP$$

FIGURE 5–10   ATP turnover in muscle cells. Energy released by hydrolysis of 1 mol of ATP and reactions responsible for resynthesis of ATP. The amount of ATP formed per mole of free fatty acid (FFA) oxidized is large but varies with the size of the FFA. For example, complete oxidation of 1 mol of palmitic acid generates 140 mol of ATP.

CLINICAL BOX 5–3

Muscle Rigor

When muscle fibers are completely depleted of ATP and phosphorylcreatine, they develop a state of rigidity called rigor. When this occurs after death, the condition is called **rigor mortis.** In rigor, almost all of the myosin heads attach to actin but in an abnormal, fixed, and resistant way. The muscles effectively are locked into place and become quite stiff to the touch.

Denervation of Muscle

In the intact animal healthy skeletal muscle does not contract except in response to stimulation of its motor nerve supply. Destruction of this nerve supply causes muscle atrophy. It also leads to abnormal excitability of the muscle and increases its sensitivity to circulating acetylcholine (**denervation hypersensitivity**). Fine, irregular contraction of individual fibers (**fibrillations**) appears. This is the classic picture of a **lower motor neuron lesion.** If the motor nerve regenerates, the fibrillations disappear. Usually, the contractions are not visible grossly, and they should not be confused with **fasciculations**, which are jerky, visible contractions of groups of muscle fibers that occur as a result of pathologic discharge of spinal motor neurons.

fibers, the smallest possible amount of muscle that can contract in response to the excitation of a single motor neuron is all the muscle fibers supplied by the neuron. Each single motor neuron and the muscle fibers it innervates constitute a **motor unit.** The number of muscle fibers in a motor unit varies. In muscles concerned with fine, graded, precise movement (eg, in the fingers and eye), each motor unit innervates very few (on the order of three to six) muscle fibers. On the other hand, values of 600 muscle fibers per motor unit can occur in human leg muscles. The group of muscle fibers that contribute to a motor unit can be intermixed within a muscle. That is, although they contract as a unit, they are not necessarily "neighboring" fibers within the muscle.

Each spinal motor neuron innervates only one kind of muscle fiber, so that all the muscle fibers in a motor unit are of the same type. On the basis of the type of muscle fiber they innervate, and thus on the basis of the duration of their twitch contraction, motor units are divided into S (slow), FR (fast, resistant to fatigue), and FF (fast, fatigable) units. Interestingly, there is also a gradation of innervation of these fibers, with S fibers tending to have a low innervation ratio (ie, small units) and FF fibers tending to have a high innervation ratio (ie, large units). The recruitment of motor units during muscle contraction is not random; it follows a scheme called the **size principle.** In general, a specific muscle action is developed first by the recruitment of S muscle units that contract relatively slowly to produce controlled contraction. Next, FR muscle units are recruited, resulting in more powerful response over a shorter period of time. Lastly, FF muscle units are recruited for the most demanding tasks. For example, in muscles of the leg, the small, slow units are first recruited for standing. As walking motion is initiated, their recruitment of FR units increases. As this motion turns to running or jumping, the FF units are recruited. Of course, there is overlap in recruitment, but, in general, this principle holds true.

The differences between types of muscle units are not inherent but are determined by, among other things, their activity. When the nerve to a slow muscle is cut and the nerve to a fast muscle is spliced to the cut end, the fast nerve grows and innervates the previously slow muscle. However, the muscle becomes fast and corresponding changes take place in its muscle protein isoforms and myosin ATPase activity. This change is due to changes in the pattern of activity of the muscle; in stimulation experiments, changes in the expression of *MHC* genes and consequently of MHC isoforms can be produced by changes in the pattern of electrical activity used to stimulate the muscle. More commonly, muscle fibers can be altered by a change in activity initiated through exercise (or lack thereof). Increased activity can lead to muscle cell hypertrophy, which allows for increase in contractile strength. Type IIA and IIB fibers are most susceptible to these changes. Alternatively, inactivity can lead to muscle cell atrophy and a loss of contractile strength. Type I fibers—that is, the ones used most often—are most susceptible to these changes.

■ CARDIAC MUSCLE

The striations in cardiac muscle are similar to those in skeletal muscle, and Z lines are present. Large numbers of elongated mitochondria are in close contact with the muscle fibrils. The muscle fibers branch and interdigitate, but each is a complete unit surrounded by a cell membrane. Where the end of one muscle fiber abuts on another, the membranes of both fibers parallel each other through an extensive series of folds. These areas, which always occur at Z lines, are called **intercalated disks (Figure 5–11).** They provide a strong union between fibers, maintaining cell-to-cell cohesion, so that the pull of one contractile cell can be transmitted along its axis to the next. Along the sides of the muscle fibers next to the disks, the cell membranes of adjacent fibers fuse for considerable distances, forming gap junctions. These junctions provide low-resistance bridges for the spread of excitation from one fiber to another. They permit cardiac muscle to function as a syncytium. The T system in cardiac muscle is located at the Z lines rather than at the A–I junction, as seen in mammalian skeletal muscle.

RESTING MEMBRANE & ACTION POTENTIALS

The resting membrane potential of individual mammalian cardiac muscle cells is about –90 mV. Stimulation produces a propagated action potential that is responsible for initiating contraction. Although action potentials vary among the cardiomyocytes in different regions of the heart, the action potential of a typical ventricular cardiomyocyte can be used as an example (**Figure 5–12**). Depolarization proceeds rapidly and an overshoot of the zero potential is present, as in skeletal muscle and nerve, but this is followed by a plateau before the membrane potential returns to the baseline. In mammalian hearts, depolarization lasts about 2 ms, but the plateau phase and repolarization last 200 ms or more. Repolarization is therefore not complete until the contraction is half over.

As in other excitable tissues, changes in the external K$^+$ concentration affect the resting membrane potential of cardiac muscle, and changes in the external Na$^+$ concentration affect the

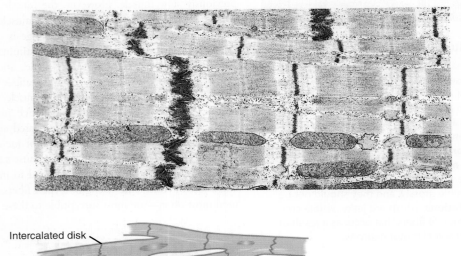

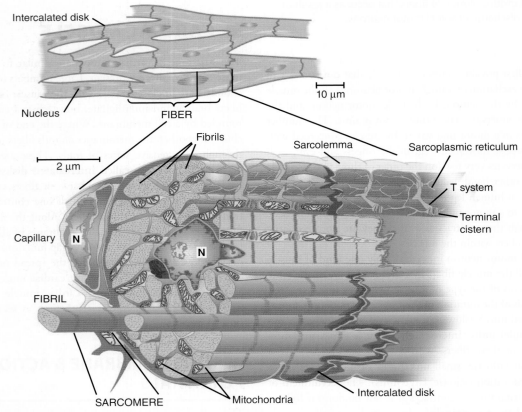

FIGURE 5–11 **Cardiac muscle. (A)** Electron micrograph of cardiac muscle. Note the similarity of the A-I regions seen in the skeletal muscle EM of Figure 5–2. The fuzzy thick lines are intercalated disks and function similarly to the Z lines but occur at cell membranes (×12,000). **(B)** Artist interpretation of cardiac muscle as seen under the light microscope (top) and the electron microscope (bottom). Again, note the similarity to skeletal muscle structure. N, nucleus. (A, Reproduced with permission from Bloom W, Fawcett DW: *A Textbook of Histology,* 10th ed. Saunders, 1975; B, Reproduced with permission from Braunwald E, Ross J, Sonnenblick EH: Mechanisms of contraction of the normal and failing heart. *N Engl J Med.* 1967 Oct 12; 277(15):794–800.)

magnitude of the action potential. The initial rapid depolarization and the overshoot (phase 0) are due to opening of voltage-gated Na^+ channels similar to that occurring in nerve and skeletal muscle **(Figure 5–13)**. The initial rapid repolarization (phase 1) is due to closure of Na^+ channels and opening of one type of K^+ channel. The subsequent prolonged plateau (phase 2) is due to a slower but prolonged opening of voltage-gated Ca^{2+} channels. Final repolarization

(phase 3) to the resting membrane potential (phase 4) is due to closure of the Ca^{2+} channels and a slow, delayed increase of K^+ efflux through various types of K^+ channels. Cardiac myocytes contain at least two types of Ca^{2+} channels (T- and L-types); the Ca^{2+} current is mostly due to opening of the slower L-type Ca^{2+} channels. Mutations or dysfunction in any of these channels lead to serious pathologies of the heart **(Clinical Box 5–5)**.

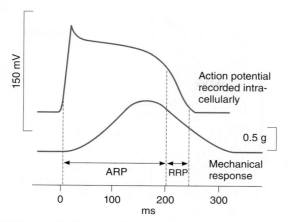

FIGURE 5–12 Comparison of action potentials and contractile response of a mammalian cardiac muscle fiber in a typical ventricular cell. In the top trace, the intracellular recording of the action potential shows the quick depolarization and extended recovery. In the bottom trace, the mechanical response is matched to the extracellular and intracellular electrical activities. Note that in the absolute refractory period (ARP), the cardiac myocyte cannot be excited, whereas in the relative refractory period (RRP) minimal excitation can occur.

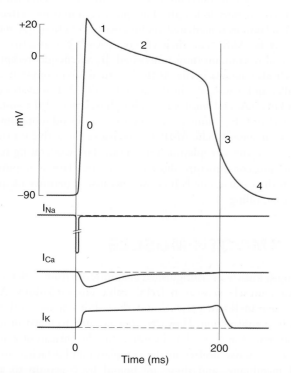

FIGURE 5–13 Dissection of the cardiac action potential. Top: The action potential of a cardiac muscle fiber can be broken down into several phases: 0, depolarization; 1, initial rapid repolarization; 2, plateau phase; 3, late rapid repolarization; 4, baseline. **Bottom:** Diagrammatic summary of Na+, Ca2+, and cumulative K+ currents during the action potential. As is convention, inward currents are downward, and outward currents are upward.

CONTRACTILE RESPONSE

The contractile response of cardiac muscle begins just after the start of depolarization and lasts about 1.5 times as long as the action potential (Figure 5–12). The role of Ca2+ in excitation–contraction coupling is similar to its role in skeletal muscle. However, it is the influx of extracellular Ca2+ through the voltage-sensitive DHPR in the T system that triggers calcium-induced calcium release through the RyR at the sarcoplasmic reticulum. Because there is a net influx of Ca2+ during activation, there is also a more prominent role for plasma membrane Ca2+ ATPases and the Na+/Ca2+ exchanger in recovery of intracellular Ca2+ concentrations. Specific effects of drugs that indirectly alter Ca2+ concentrations are discussed in **Clinical Box 5–6.**

During phases 0–2 and about half of phase 3 (until the membrane potential reaches approximately –50 mV during repolarization), cardiac muscle cannot be excited again; that is, it is in its **absolute refractory period.** It remains relatively refractory until phase 4. Therefore, tetanus of the type seen in skeletal muscle cannot occur.

Glycosidic Drugs & Cardiac Contractions

Ouabain and other digitalis glycosides are commonly used to treat failing hearts. These drugs have the effect of increasing the strength of cardiac contractions. Although there is discussion as to full mechanisms, a working hypothesis is based on the ability of these drugs to inhibit the Na, K ATPase in cell membranes of the cardiomyocytes. The block of the Na, K ATPase in cardiomyocytes would result in an increased intracellular Na^+ concentration. Such an increase would result in a decreased Na^+ influx and hence Ca^{2+} efflux via the Na^+-Ca^{2+} exchange antiport during the Ca^{2+} recovery period. The resulting increase in intracellular Ca^{2+} concentration in turn increases the strength of contraction of the cardiac muscle. With this mechanism in mind, these drugs can also be quite toxic. Overinhibition of the Na, K ATPase would result in a depolarized cell that could slow conduction, or even spontaneously activate. Alternatively, an overly increased Ca^{2+} concentration could also have ill effects on cardiomyocyte physiology.

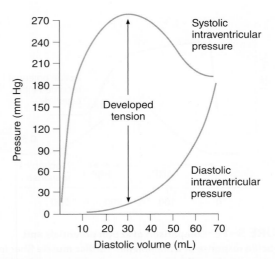

FIGURE 5–14 Length–tension relationship for cardiac muscle. Comparison of the systolic intraventricular pressure (top trace) and diastolic intraventricular pressure (bottom trace) display the developed tension in the cardiomyocyte. Values shown are for canine heart.

ISOFORMS

Cardiac muscle is generally slow and has relatively low ATPase activity. Its fibers are dependent on oxidative metabolism and hence on a continuous supply of O_2. The human heart contains both the α and β isoforms of myosin heavy chain (α MHC and β MHC). β MHC has lower myosin ATPase activity than α MHC. Both are present in the atria, with the α isoform predominating, whereas the β isoform predominates in the ventricle. The spatial differences in expression contribute to the well-coordinated contraction of the heart.

CORRELATION BETWEEN MUSCLE FIBER LENGTH & TENSION

The relation between initial fiber length and total tension in cardiac muscle is similar to that in skeletal muscle; there is a resting length at which the tension developed on stimulation is maximal. In the body, the initial length of the fibers is determined by the degree of diastolic filling of the heart, and the pressure developed in the ventricle is proportional to the volume of the ventricle at the end of the filling phase (**Starling law of the heart**). The developed tension (**Figure 5–14**) increases as the diastolic volume increases until it reaches a maximum and then tends to decrease. However, unlike skeletal muscle, the decrease in developed tension at high degrees of stretch is not due to a decrease in the number of cross-bridges between actin and myosin, because even severely dilated hearts are not stretched to this degree. The decrease is instead due to beginning disruption of the myocardial fibers.

The force of contraction of cardiac muscle can be also increased by catecholamines, and this increase occurs without a change in muscle length. This positive ionotropic effect of catecholamines is mediated via innervated β₁-adrenergic receptors, cyclic AMP, and their effects on Ca^{2+} homeostasis. The heart also contains non-innervated β₂-adrenergic receptors, which also act via cyclic AMP, but their ionotropic effect is smaller and is maximal in the atria. Cyclic AMP activates protein kinase A, and this leads to phosphorylation of the voltage-dependent Ca^{2+} channels, causing them to spend more time in the open state. Cyclic AMP also increases the active transport of Ca^{2+} to the sarcoplasmic reticulum, thus accelerating relaxation and consequently shortening systole. This is important when the cardiac rate is increased because it permits adequate diastolic filling.

■ SMOOTH MUSCLE

Smooth muscle is distinguished anatomically from skeletal and cardiac muscle because it lacks visible cross-striations. Actin and myosin-II are present, and they slide on each other to produce contraction. However, they are not arranged in regular arrays, as in skeletal and cardiac muscle. Instead of Z lines, there are **dense bodies** in the cytoplasm and attached to the cell membrane, and these are bound by α-actinin to actin filaments. Smooth muscle also contains tropomyosin, but troponin appears to be absent. The isoforms of actin and myosin differ from those in skeletal muscle. A sarcoplasmic reticulum is present, but it is less extensive than those observed in skeletal or cardiac muscle. In general, smooth muscles contain few mitochondria and depend, to a large extent, on glycolysis for their metabolic needs.

SMOOTH MUSCLE TYPES

There is considerable variation in the structure and function of smooth muscle in different parts of the body. In general, smooth muscle can be divided into **unitary** (or **visceral**) **smooth muscle** and **multiunit smooth muscle.** Unitary smooth muscle occurs in large sheets, has many low-resistance gap junctional connections between individual muscle cells, and functions in a syncytial fashion. Unitary smooth muscle is found primarily in the walls of hollow viscera such as the musculature of the intestine, the uterus, and the ureters. Multiunit smooth muscle is made up of individual units with few (or no) gap junctional bridges. It is found in structures such as the iris of the eye, in which fine, graded contractions occur. It is not under voluntary control, but it has many functional similarities to skeletal muscle. Each multiunit smooth muscle cell has en passant endings of nerve fibers, but in unitary smooth muscle there are en passant junctions on fewer cells, with excitation spreading to other cells by gap junctions. In addition, these cells respond to hormones and other circulating substances.

ELECTRICAL & MECHANICAL ACTIVITY

Unitary smooth muscle is characterized by the instability of its membrane potential and by the fact that it shows continuous, irregular contractions that are independent of its nerve supply. This maintained state of partial contraction is called **tonus**, or **tone.** The membrane potential has no true "resting" value, being relatively low when the tissue is active and higher when it is inhibited, but in periods of relative quiescence values for resting potential are on the order of –20 to –65 mV. Smooth muscle cells can display divergent electrical activity (**Figure 5–15**). There are slow sine wave-like fluctuations a few millivolts in magnitude and spikes that sometimes overshoot the zero potential line and sometimes do not. In many tissues, the spikes have durations of about 50 ms, whereas in some tissues the action potentials have a prolonged plateau during repolarization, like the action potentials in cardiac muscle. As in the other muscle types, there are significant contributions of K^+, Na^+, and Ca^{2+} channels and Na, K ATPase to this electrical activity. However, discussion of contributions to individual smooth muscle types is beyond the scope of this text.

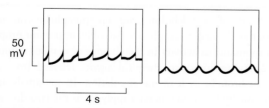

FIGURE 5–15 Electrical activity of individual smooth muscle cells in the guinea pig taenia coli. Left: Pacemaker-like activity with spikes firing at each peak. **Right:** Sinusoidal fluctuation of membrane potential with firing on the rising phase of each wave. In other fibers, spikes can occur on the falling phase of sinusoidal fluctuations and there can be mixtures of sinusoidal and pacemaker potentials in the same fiber.

Because of the continuous activity, it is difficult to study the relation between the electrical and mechanical events in unitary smooth muscle, but in some relatively inactive preparations, a single spike can be generated. In such preparations, the excitation–contraction coupling in unitary smooth muscle can occur with as much as a 500-ms delay. Thus, it is a very slow process compared with that in skeletal and cardiac muscle (< 10 ms). Because multiunit smooth muscle is nonsyncytial and contractions do not spread widely through it, the contractions of multiunit smooth muscle are more discrete, fine, and localized than those of unitary smooth muscle.

MOLECULAR BASIS OF CONTRACTION

As in skeletal and cardiac muscle, Ca^{2+} plays a prominent role in the initiation of contraction of smooth muscle. However, the source of Ca^{2+} increase can be quite different in unitary smooth muscle. Depending on the activating stimulus, Ca^{2+} increase can be due to influx through voltage- or ligand-gated plasma membrane channels, efflux from intracellular stores through the RyR, efflux from intracellular stores through the **inositol trisphosphate receptor (IP$_3$R)** Ca^{2+} channel, or via a combination of these channels. In addition, the lack of troponin in smooth muscle prevents Ca^{2+} activation via troponin binding. Rather, myosin in smooth muscle must be phosphorylated for activation of the myosin ATPase. Phosphorylation and dephosphorylation of myosin also occur in skeletal muscle, but phosphorylation is not necessary for activation of the ATPase. In smooth muscle, Ca^{2+} binds to calmodulin, and the resulting complex activates **calmodulin-dependent myosin light chain kinase.** This enzyme catalyzes the phosphorylation of the myosin light chain to increase its ATPase activity.

Myosin is dephosphorylated by **myosin light chain phosphatase** in the cell. However, dephosphorylation of myosin light chain kinase does not necessarily lead to relaxation of the smooth muscle. Various mechanisms are involved. One is a latch bridge mechanism by which myosin cross-bridges remain attached to actin for some time after the cytoplasmic Ca^{2+} concentration falls. This produces sustained contraction with little expenditure of energy, which is especially important in vascular smooth muscle. Relaxation of the muscle occurs when the Ca^{2+}-calmodulin complex finally dissociates or when some other mechanism comes into play. The events leading to contraction and relaxation of unitary smooth muscle are summarized in **Figure 5–16.** The events in multiunit smooth muscle are generally similar.

Unitary smooth muscle is unique in that, unlike other types of muscle, it contracts when stretched in the absence of any extrinsic innervation. Stretch is followed by a decline in membrane potential, an increase in the frequency of spikes, and a general increase in tone.

If epinephrine or norepinephrine is added to a preparation of intestinal smooth muscle arranged for recording of intracellular potentials in vitro, the membrane potential usually becomes larger, the spikes decrease in frequency, and the muscle relaxes

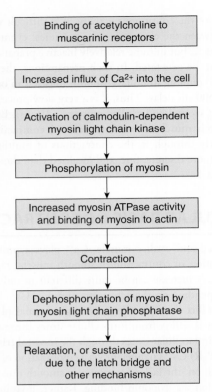

FIGURE 5–16 Sequence of events in contraction and relaxation of smooth muscle. Flow chart illustrates many of the molecular changes that occur from the initiation of contraction to its relaxation. Note the distinct differences from skeletal and cardiac muscle excitation.

(Figure 5–17). Norepinephrine is the chemical mediator released at noradrenergic nerve endings, and stimulation of the noradrenergic nerves to the preparation produces inhibitory potentials. Acetylcholine has an effect opposite to that of norepinephrine on the membrane potential and contractile activity of intestinal smooth muscle. If acetylcholine is added to the fluid bathing

a smooth muscle preparation in vitro, the membrane potential decreases and the spikes become more frequent. The muscle becomes more active, with an increase in tonic tension and the number of rhythmic contractions. The effect is mediated by phospholipase C, which produces IP_3 and allows for Ca^{2+} release through IP_3 receptors. In the intact animal, stimulation of cholinergic nerves causes release of acetylcholine, excitatory potentials, and increased intestinal contractions.

Like unitary smooth muscle, multiunit smooth muscle is very sensitive to circulating chemical substances and is normally activated by chemical mediators (acetylcholine and norepinephrine) released at the endings of its motor nerves. Norepinephrine in particular tends to persist in the muscle and to cause repeated firing of the muscle after a single stimulus rather than a single action potential. Therefore, the contractile response produced is usually an irregular tetanus rather than a single twitch. When a single twitch response is obtained, it resembles the twitch contraction of skeletal muscle except that its duration is 10 times longer.

RELAXATION

In addition to cellular mechanisms that increase contraction of smooth muscle, there are cellular mechanisms that lead to its relaxation (Clinical Box 5–7). This is especially important in smooth muscle that surrounds the blood vessels to increase blood flow. It was long known that endothelial cells that line the inside of blood cells could release a substance that relaxed smooth muscle, which was eventually identified as the gaseous second messenger molecule, **nitric oxide (NO).** NO produced in endothelial cells is free to diffuse into the smooth muscle to exert its effects. Once in muscle, NO directly activates a soluble guanylyl cyclase to produce another second messenger molecule, **cyclic guanosine monophosphate (cGMP).** This molecule can activate cGMP-specific protein kinases that affect ion channels, Ca^{2+} homeostasis, or phosphatases, or all of these, leading to smooth muscle relaxation.

FUNCTION OF THE NERVE SUPPLY TO SMOOTH MUSCLE

The effects of acetylcholine and norepinephrine on unitary smooth muscle serve to emphasize two of its important properties: (1) its spontaneous activity in the absence of nervous stimulation and (2) its sensitivity to chemical agents released from nerves locally or brought to it in the circulation. In mammals, unitary muscle usually has a dual nerve supply from the two divisions of the autonomic nervous system. The function of the nerve supply is not to initiate activity in the muscle but rather to modify it. Stimulation of one division of the autonomic nervous system usually increases smooth muscle activity, whereas stimulation of the other decreases it. In some organs, noradrenergic stimulation increases and cholinergic stimulation decreases smooth muscle activity; in others, the reverse is true.

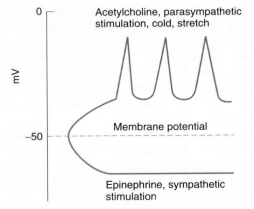

FIGURE 5–17 Effects of various agents on the membrane potential of intestinal smooth muscle. Drugs and hormones can alter firing of smooth muscle action potentials by raising (top trace) or lowering (bottom trace) resting membrane potential.

and no resting length can be assigned. In some ways, therefore, smooth muscle behaves more like a viscous mass than a rigidly structured tissue, and it is this property that is referred to as the **plasticity** of smooth muscle.

The consequences of plasticity can be demonstrated in humans. For example, the tension exerted by the smooth muscle walls of the bladder can be measured at different degrees of distension as fluid is infused into the bladder via a catheter. Initially, tension increases relatively little as volume is increased because of the plasticity of the bladder wall. However, a point is eventually reached at which the bladder contracts forcefully.

CHAPTER SUMMARY

- There are three main types of muscle cells: skeletal, cardiac, and smooth.
- Skeletal muscle is a true syncytium under voluntary control. Skeletal muscles receive electrical stimuli from neurons to elicit contraction: "excitation–contraction coupling." Action potentials in muscle cells are developed largely through coordination of Na^+ and K^+ channels. Contraction in skeletal muscle cells is coordinated through Ca^{2+} regulation of the actomyosin system that gives the muscle its classic striated pattern under the microscope.
- There are several different types of skeletal muscle fibers (I, IIA, IIB) that have distinct properties in terms of protein makeup and force generation. Skeletal muscle fibers are arranged into motor units of like fibers within a muscle. Skeletal motor units are recruited in a specific pattern as the need for force is increased.
- Cardiac muscle is a collection of individual cells (cardiomyocytes) that are linked as a syncytium by gap junctional communication. Cardiac muscle cells also undergo excitation–contraction coupling. Pacemaker cells in the heart can initiate propagated action potentials. Cardiac muscle cells also have a striated, actomyosin system that underlies contraction.
- Smooth muscle exists as individual cells and is frequently under control of the autonomic nervous system.
- There are two broad categories of smooth muscles: unitary and multiunit. Unitary smooth muscle contraction is synchronized by gap junctional communication to coordinate contraction among many cells. Multiunit smooth muscle contraction is coordinated by motor units, functionally similar to skeletal muscle.
- Smooth muscle cells contract through an actomyosin system, but do not have well-organized striations. Unlike skeletal and cardiac muscle, Ca^{2+} regulation of contraction is primarily through phosphorylation–dephosphorylation reactions.

MULTIPLE-CHOICE QUESTIONS

For all questions, select the single best answer unless otherwise directed.

1. A 22-year-old man is going in for surgery and requires intubation. He is put under a general anesthetic and prior to intubation given succinylcholine to temporarily "paralyze" muscles and allow for easier insertion of the endotracheal tube. Succinylcholine competes with the natural signal at

---

Common Drugs That Act on Smooth Muscle

Overexcitation of smooth muscle in the airways, such as that observed during an asthma attack, can lead to bronchoconstriction. Inhalers that deliver drugs to the conducting airway are commonly used to offset this smooth muscle bronchoconstriction, as well as other symptoms in the asthmatic airways. The rapid effects of drugs in inhalers are related to smooth muscle relaxation. Rapid response inhaler drugs (eg, ventolin, albuterol, salbutamol) frequently target β-adrenergic receptors in the airway smooth muscle to elicit a relaxation. Although these β-adrenergic receptor agonists targeting the smooth muscle do not treat all symptoms associated with asthma (eg, inflammation and increased mucus), they act rapidly and frequently allow for sufficient opening of the conducting airway to restore airflow, and thus allow for other treatments to reduce airway obstruction.

Smooth muscle is also a target for drugs developed to increase blood flow. As discussed in the text, NO is a natural signaling molecule that relaxes smooth muscle by raising cyclic guanosine monophosphate (cGMP). This signaling pathway is naturally downregulated by the action of **phosphodiesterase (PDE)**, which transforms cGMP into a nonsignaling form, GMP. The drugs sildenafil, tadalafil, and vardenafil are all specific inhibitors of PDE V, an isoform found mainly in the smooth muscle in the corpus cavernosum of the penis. Thus, oral administration of these drugs can block the action of PDE V, increasing blood flow in a very limited region in the body and offsetting erectile dysfunction.

FORCE GENERATION & PLASTICITY OF SMOOTH MUSCLE

Smooth muscle displays a unique economy when compared to skeletal muscle. Despite approximately 20% of the myosin content and a 100-fold difference in ATP use when compared with skeletal muscle, smooth muscle can generate similar force per cross-sectional area. One of the tradeoffs of obtaining force under these conditions is the noticeably slower contractions when compared to skeletal muscle. There are several known reasons for these noticeable changes, including unique isoforms of myosin and contractile-related proteins expressed in smooth muscle and their distinct regulation. The unique architecture of the smooth cell and its coordinated units also contribute.

Another special characteristic of smooth muscle is the variability of the tension it exerts at any given length. If a unitary smooth muscle is stretched, it first exerts increased tension. However, if the muscle is held at the greater length after stretching, the tension gradually decreases. Sometimes the tension falls to or below the level exerted before the muscle was stretched. It is consequently impossible to correlate length and developed tension accurately,

the neuromuscular junction (acetylcholine) and causes an extended depolarization that prevents muscles from initiating action potentials and contracting. The action potential of an unparalyzed skeletal muscle

A. has a prolonged plateau phase.
B. spreads inward to all parts of the muscle via the T tubules.
C. causes the immediate uptake of Ca^{2+} into the lateral sacs of the sarcoplasmic reticulum.
D. is longer than the action potential of cardiac muscle.
E. is not essential for contraction.

2. A physical therapy student recently joined a team at a hospital unit that specializes in evaluation, diagnosis and treatment plans for infants and children who have arthrogryposis. During his studies, a pre-adolescent patient with limited range of motion in the hands and feet is treated to improve range of motion. The physical therapist suspects that the patient could have Sheldon–Hall syndrome (arthrogryposis type 2B) and suggests genetic testing. Testing reveals a mutation in *TPM2*, a gene coding for tropomyosin, consistent with the Sheldon–Hall syndrome diagnosis. The patient's symptoms are attributable to the loss of which function of tropomyosin in skeletal muscle?

A. Sliding on actin to produce shortening
B. Releasing Ca^{2+} after initiation of contraction
C. Binding to myosin during contraction
D. Acting as a "relaxing protein" at rest by covering up the sites where myosin binds to actin
E. Generating ATP, which it passes to the contractile mechanism

3. Two students from a biophysical-based muscle laboratory have been testing a new drug that appears to hold muscle in a contracted state. They observe that application of their drug will cause muscle contraction that cannot be reversed by conventional means (eg, lowering $[Ca^+]$ or [ATP] in the preparation). They decide to obtain structural data on the sarcomere before and after drug application and attempts at relaxation. Fixed samples of the skinned skeletal muscle fibers showed shorter sarcomeres under the electron microscope, with thick filaments almost completely overlapping thin filaments between the Z lines. Which of the following proteins are in the thick filaments of the sarcomere?

A. Actin
B. Myosin
C. Troponin
D. Tropomyosin
E. Myelin

4. Two medical professors routinely meet each other at the gym for Monday, Wednesday, and Friday lunch breaks. While both professors consistently get through their 45 min workouts, they differ significantly in their choice of exercises. The older professor insists on limited stretching, followed by use of traditional weights with constant flexions and extensions. The younger professor prefers a series of stretches and isometric exercises, and then a short run on the treadmill. Both professors benefit greatly from their workouts, and fine-tune their abilities to argue by claiming they have the "best method" of addressing an exercise routine. When comparing the contractile response that each produces in their skeletal muscles, which of the following is a true statement?

A. Contraction starts only after completion of the skeletal muscle action potential.
B. Contraction is complete before the skeletal action potential is complete.
C. Isometric contractions produce more tension than isotonic contractions.
D. The contractile response produces more work when the muscle contracts isometrically than when the muscle contracts isotonically.
E. The contractile response decreases in magnitude with repeated stimulation.

5. A third-year MD/PhD student joined a laboratory interested in mechanisms underlying idiopathic atrial fibrillation. The laboratory group had access to cardiac tissue and blood samples from dozens of patients who had died following complications from stroke after a diagnosis of atrial fibrillation. In a subset of samples, the student found mutations in the gene for connexin 40 (*GJA5*), a protein known to contribute to gap junctions in the heart. It is also known that connexin 40, like other connexins, can form hemichannels that allow for transfer of select cytosolic and extracellular fluid components. Which of the following statements is true about gap junctions?

A. Gap junctions are absent in cardiac muscle.
B. Gap junctions are present but of little functional importance in cardiac muscle.
C. Gap junctions are present and provide the pathway for rapid spread of excitation from one cardiac muscle fiber to another.
D. Gap junctions are absent in smooth muscle.
E. Gap junctions connect the sarcotubular system to individual skeletal muscle cells.

6. A 30-year-old male is admitted to the hospital for surgery to repair a broken ankle. His medical history includes mild hypertension, acid reflux disease and a previous shoulder reconstruction with a risk for malignant hyperthermia (MH). The operating plan is for both general and regional anesthesia and precautions are taken to avoid the MH reaction (eg, the use of nontrigger anesthetics with no succinylcholine in the operating room). Other precautions include O_2 ventilator flow (> 10 L/min for 20 min), increased CO_2 absorbance, increased MH symptom monitoring and available dantrolene. MH can be caused by dysregulation of the ryanodine receptor (RyR) and result in sustained muscle contraction and heat generation. This is because the RyR is responsible for which of the following in skeletal muscle contraction?

A. ATP hydrolysis via myosin II
B. Voltage changes in the T tubule
C. Ca^{2+} release from intracellular stores
D. Reestablishment of skeletal muscle Ca^{2+} concentration following contraction
E. The prevention of myosin head/actin interaction

7. A youth soccer team has an early game on a brisk, autumn morning. One of the 12-year-olds involved has been diagnosed with mild asthma. As the game progresses, the child demonstrates increased wheezing and coughing to a point where breathing is strained. The child goes to the sideline, uses an asthma inhaler with a β-adrenergic agonist, and returns to the field. The child quickly resumes unobstructed breathing and has no more symptoms throughout the day.

The β-adrenergic agonist works to increase airflow by which of the following mechanisms?

A. Stimulation of β-adrenergic receptors on airway smooth muscle cells to induce contraction

B. Stimulation of β-adrenergic receptors on airway smooth muscle cells to induce relaxation

C. Stimulation of β-adrenergic receptors on vasculature smooth muscle cells to induce contraction

D. Stimulation of β-adrenergic receptors on vasculature smooth muscle cells to induce relaxation

E. Stimulation of β-adrenergic receptors on airway epithelial cells to increase the airway lumen

8. A family brings their 14-year-old child into a clinic. They explain to the attending physician that the child has been tiring more quickly than his peers in physical activities at school. They note that the child has always been clumsy, developed walking noticeably later than his siblings and demonstrated difficulty jumping and climbing when compared to his peers. A subsequent physical exam showed proximal muscle weakness and routine blood work showed an increase in creatine kinase. The physician ordered a genetic test and found a mutation in the dystrophin protein, and diagnosed Becker muscular dystrophy. How does the dystrophin protein contribute to muscle function?

A. Dystrophin is also known as the dihydropyridine receptor and responds to voltage changes by activating the ryanodine receptor.

B. Dystrophin is structural protein that connects actin to sarcolemma complex proteins.

C. Dystrophin is a myosin binding protein that helps regulate actin–myosin interactions.

D. Dystrophin is a gap junction protein that helps coordinate muscle fiber interactions.

E. Dystrophin is an intracellular Ca^{2+} channel that is activated following voltage changes at the sarcolemma.

9. On a recent road trip, a group of medical students were touring the Tennessee countryside when they came across a farm that advertised particularly meaty goats. The farm consisted of a population of goats with a genetic disorder that resulted in muscle stiffening, and the animals were prone to falling over after being startled. Further investigation of the goat breed uncovered that their genetic mutation delays relaxation in skeletal muscle fibers. Similar mutations can be observed in humans and result in myotonia congenita. Myotonia congenita is associated with mutations in skeletal muscle–expressed Cl^- channels. The action potential in skeletal muscle fibers includes which of the following?

A. Activation of the ryanodine receptor to release Ca^{2+} and depolarize the sarcoplasma membrane

B. Feedback from actin–myosin binding to depolarize the sarcoplasma membrane

C. An initial depolarization caused by the opening of ligand-gated K^+ channels

D. An initial depolarization caused by the opening of ligand-gated channels

E. An initial depolarization caused by the opening of voltage-gated Ca^{2+} channels

10. In a laboratory experiment on a mouse gastrocnemius muscle preparation, a student is able to directly perfuse and alternate Ca^{2+}-containing and Ca^{2+}-free balanced salt solutions supplemented with ATP to initiate contraction and relaxation sequences, respectively. Unfortunately, half way through the experiments, the student forgets to add ATP to the solutions while maintaining Ca^{2+} containing and Ca^{2+} free salt solution cycling. How would the preparation differ in the absence of supplemented ATP?

A. The muscle preparation would continue its contraction/relaxation cycle normally with the corresponding changes in Ca^{2+} concentration.

B. The muscle preparation would continue its contraction/relaxation cycle with reduced contraction size as long as changes in Ca^{2+} solution persisted.

C. The muscle preparation would stop its contraction/relaxation cycle and become flaccid.

D. The muscle preparation would stop its contraction/relaxation cycle and become rigid.

E. The muscle fibers would quickly lose their ability to hold together and the preparation would become dispersed.

ANSWERS

1. The correct answer is **B.** The initial signaling for muscle depolarization is quickly spread across the muscle plasma membrane via the T tubules. The repolarization phase of skeletal muscle varies by fiber type, however, in each case there is a limited plateau phase, especially when compared to a cardiomyocyte, ruling out **A** and **D.** Depolarization at the plasma membrane is followed by a quick release of Ca^{2+} from intracellular stores and not an uptake of Ca^{2+} as stated in **C.** Skeletal muscle cells are excitable cells and require electrical signaling (ie, action potential) for contraction, ruling out **E.**

2. The correct answer is **D.** Tropomyosin is a muscle protein found in thin filaments. At low $[Ca^{2+}]$, tropomyosin prevents myosin/actin binding. Increased $[Ca^{2+}]$ causes changes in troponin that can move tropomyosin to uncover myosin binding sites on actin and allow for the cross-bridge cycle. Tropomyosin does not slide on actin to produce shortening **A**, nor does it have Ca^{2+} **B** or myosin **C** binding sites. ATP is made in muscle via oxidative or anaerobic phosphorylation, or freed from phosphorylcreatine. Tropomyosin is not involved in any of these reactions, eliminating **E.**

3. The correct answer is **B.** In the sarcomere the thick filaments are made up of myosin molecules. Actin **A** is the primary structural molecule of thin filaments. Troponin **C** is the Ca^{2+} binding protein anchored to the thin filament that can interact with the thin filament protein tropomyosin **D** and expose myosin binding sites. Myelin **E** is not associated with skeletal muscle and refers to the cellular insulation that surrounds neuronal axons, and thus can be eliminated.

4. The correct answer is **C.** In an isometric exercise the muscle length does not change and tension continues to increase as more pressure is applied (eg, pushing against a wall). In contrast, there is no tension developed during actual muscle movement, or during isotonic contraction (iso = same; tonic = tension/force). In skeletal muscle, contraction begins as $[Ca^{2+}]$ levels rise. Since this occurs before the end of the action potential and continues after the end of the action potential, both **A** and **B** can be eliminated. There is no net movement during isometric exercise so there is no net work; this is not

the case for isotonic contractions where the muscle is moving and net work is recorded, eliminating **D** as a viable answer. In general, until tetanus is reached, increased stimulation will increase contractions in skeletal muscle, eliminating **E**.

5. The correct answer is **C**. Gap junctions formed by connexin 40 or connexin 43 proteins in the heart are essential in the establishment of cell-cell communication that allows for heart cells to communicate chemical and electrical signals, ruling out **A**. The coordination of the heart as an "electrical syncytium" is a key and necessary function of gap junctions, ruling out **B**. Unitary smooth muscle cells also contain gap junctions to help coordinate behavior, eliminating **D**. Gap junctions are not present in the sarcotubular system in individual skeletal muscles, ruling out **E**.

6. The correct answer is **C**. The RyR is the primary Ca^{2+} release channel on the sarcoplasmic reticulum of skeletal muscle, and thus is responsible for Ca^{2+} release from intracellular stores. The RyR is not involved in actin–myosin interactions nor electrical changes in the plasma membrane, eliminating **A**, **B**, and **D**. The reestablishment of $[Ca^{2+}]$ in the muscle cell is primarily due to the action of the SERCA pump that uses ATP to move Ca^{2+} from the cytosol of the muscle back into the sarcoplasmic reticulum, eliminating **E**.

7. The correct answer is **B**. The β-adrenergic agonist drugs in rapid inhalers target airway smooth muscle cell to cause relaxation, which then allows for opening of the lumen in the airways. Contraction of airway smooth muscle would result in lumen closing and further difficulty breathing, ruling out **A**. Vasculature smooth muscle cells are not a target of the β-adrenergic agonist inhaler delivery, and activation of the β-adrenergic receptor on these cells would not affect the airway, eliminating **C** and **D**. Finally, the caliber of the airways is controlled by the smooth muscle surrounding them, not by the epithelial cells that line them, ruling out **E**.

8. The correct answer is **B**. Dystrophin is an intracellular protein that binds specifically to F-actin in the cytosol and to dystroglycan in the sarcolemma. This tethering is essential for proper skeletal muscle contractions. The dihydropyridine receptor **A**, also known as DHPR, is a voltage sensitive receptor that translates voltage changes to the intracellular Ca^{2+} release channel **E**, also known as the ryanodine receptor, ruling out both of these answers. Dystrophin does not bind myosin, ruling out **C**. Skeletal muscles do not have gap junctions and do not express gap junction proteins (ie, connexins), ruling out **D**.

9. The correct answer is **D**. In myotonia congenita the lack of skeletal Cl^- channels causes hyperexcitability in skeletal muscles that can extend contraction because of the lack of a quick return to the resting potential. The normal action potential is initiated at the neuromuscular junction with release of acetylcholine and activation of ligand-gated cation channels that quickly depolarize the cell. Ryanodine receptors **A** are part of the intracellular machinery that releases Ca^{2+} from intracellular stores allowing for actin–myosin **B** interaction and contraction. Neither of these processes participates in action potential initiation and can be eliminated. While K^+ channels play an important role in the repolarization of the sarcolemma to allow for subsequent activation, voltage gated Ca^{2+} channels **E** and K^+ channels **C** are not activated by acetylcholine to initiate the skeletal muscle action potential and thus can be eliminated as answers.

10. The correct answer is **D**. The contraction/relaxation cycle is driven by Ca^{2+} concentration changes that allows for troponin to alter tropomyosin position and myosin/actin interaction. ATP hydrolysis in the myosin head, and more specifically, loss of ADP from the myosin head, is necessary for movement of myosin relative to actin. When ATP is depleted, the myosin heads cannot detach from actin and a state of rigor develops, ruling out **C**. Because ATP is required for the contraction/relaxation cycle, **A** and **B** are ruled out as answers. The muscle preparation can last for quite a while in balanced salt solutions, and thus, **E** is ruled out.

Synaptic & Junctional Transmission

O B J E C T I V E S

After studying this chapter, you should be able to:

- Describe the main morphologic features of synapses.
- Describe fast and slow excitatory and inhibitory postsynaptic potentials, outline the ionic fluxes that underlie them, and explain how the potentials interact to generate action potentials.
- Define and give examples of direct inhibition, indirect inhibition, presynaptic inhibition, and postsynaptic inhibition.
- Describe the neuromuscular junction, and explain how action potentials in the motor neuron at the junction lead to contraction of the skeletal muscle.
- Define denervation hypersensitivity.

INTRODUCTION

Impulses are transmitted over chemical or electrical synapses linking one neuron (presynaptic cell) with another neuron, muscle, or gland (postsynaptic cell). At chemical synapses, an impulse in the presynaptic axon causes secretion of a chemical that diffuses across the 30-nm-wide (approximately) synaptic cleft and binds to receptors on the surface of the postsynaptic cell. This triggers events that open or close channels in the membrane of the postsynaptic cell, mediating excitation or inhibition. At electrical synapses, the membranes of the presynaptic and postsynaptic neurons are close together, and gap junctions form low-resistance bridges through which ions pass with relative ease from one neuron to the next. Because most synaptic transmission is chemical, this chapter discusses chemical transmission.

STRUCTURE & FUNCTION OF SYNAPSES

A presynaptic axonal terminal can synapse on a cell body, dendrite, dendritic spine, or an axon to form axosomatic, axodendritic, and axoaxonic synapses, respectively (**Figure 6–1**). The thickening on the postsynaptic membrane is called a postsynaptic density. There are three kinds of membrane-enclosed vesicles in the presynaptic nerve terminal: small, clear synaptic vesicles that contain acetylcholine, glycine, GABA, or glutamate; small vesicles with a dense core that contain catecholamines; and large vesicles with a dense core that contain neuropeptides.

The vesicles and the chemicals they contain are synthesized in the neuronal cell body and transported along the axon to nerve terminals by fast axoplasmic transport. The large dense-core vesicles release their neuropeptide contents by exocytosis from all parts of the terminal. The small vesicles are located near the synaptic cleft and fuse to the membrane, discharging their contents very rapidly into the cleft at areas of membrane thickening called active zones (Figure 6–1).

In response to an action potential in the nerve terminal, Ca^{2+} enters and the transmitter is released close to the postsynaptic receptors. A response can occur in the postsynaptic neuron after

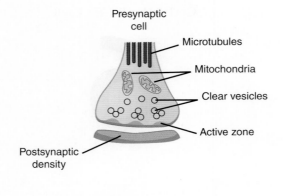

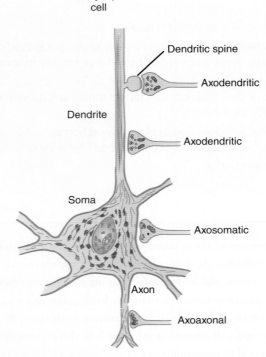

FIGURE 6–1 Axodendritic, axoaxonal, and axosomatic synapses. Many presynaptic neurons terminate on dendritic spines, as shown at the top, but some also end directly on the shafts of dendrites. Note the presence of clear and granulated synaptic vesicles in endings and clustering of clear vesicles at active zones.

EXCITATORY & INHIBITORY POSTSYNAPTIC POTENTIALS

Stimulation of a dorsal root afferent (sensory neuron) can be used to study excitatory and inhibitory transmission in an α-motor neuron (**Figure 6–2**). A single stimulus applied to the sensory nerve can produce either a transient depolarization or a transient hyperpolarization in a motor neuron. The initial depolarization produced by a single stimulus to the proper input begins about 0.5 ms after the afferent impulse enters the spinal cord; it reaches its peak 11.5 ms later and then declines exponentially. This potential is called an excitatory postsynaptic potential (EPSP). The excitatory transmitter (eg, glutamate) opens Na^+ or Ca^{2+} channels in the postsynaptic membrane, producing an inward current. The stimulus-induced hyperpolarization (inhibitory postsynaptic potential: IPSP) in the motor neuron involves an inhibitory interneuron and is mediated by an increase in Cl^- conductance.

In addition to the fast EPSPs and IPSPs, slow EPSPs and IPSPs occur in autonomic ganglia, cardiac and smooth muscle, and cortical neurons. These potentials have a latency of 100–500 ms and last several seconds. Slow EPSPs and IPSPs can result from decreases and increases in K^+ conductance, respectively.

ACTION POTENTIAL GENERATION IN A POSTSYNAPTIC NEURON

The interplay of excitatory and inhibitory activity produces a fluctuating membrane potential that is the algebraic sum of the hyperpolarizing and depolarizing activities. When the level of

a synaptic delay. The delay is due to the time it takes for the neurotransmitter to be released and to act on postsynaptic membrane receptors. The minimum time for transmission across a synapse is 0.5 ms, so one can determine if a given response is mediated by monosynaptic or polysynaptic (contains more than one synapse) pathway by measuring the synaptic delay.

The fusion of synaptic vesicles with the cell membrane involves the action of SNAP (soluble NSF attachment protein) and SNARE (SNAP receptors). **Clinical Box 6–1** describes how neurotoxins from the bacteria *Clostridium tetani* and *Clostridium botulinum* can disrupt neurotransmitter release in either the CNS or at the neuromuscular junction.

A Stretch reflex circuit for knee jerk

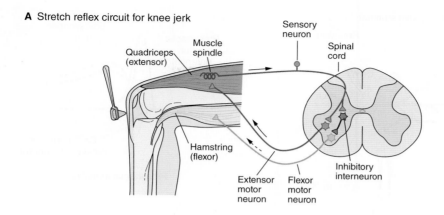

B Experimental setup for recording from cells in the circuit

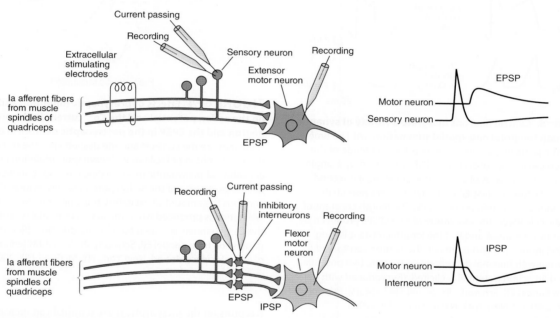

FIGURE 6–2 **Excitatory and inhibitory synaptic connections mediating the stretch reflex provide an example of typical circuits within the CNS. (A)** The stretch receptor sensory neuron of the quadriceps muscle makes an excitatory connection with the extensor motor neuron of the same muscle and an inhibitory interneuron projecting to flexor motor neurons supplying the antagonistic hamstring muscle. **(B)** Experimental setup to study excitation and inhibition of the extensor motor neuron. Top panel shows two approaches to elicit an excitatory (depolarizing) postsynaptic potential or EPSP in the extensor motor neuron–electrical stimulation of the whole Ia afferent nerve using extracellular electrodes and intracellular current passing through an electrode inserted into the cell body of a sensory neuron. Bottom panel shows that current passing through an inhibitory interneuron elicits an inhibitory (hyperpolarizing) postsynaptic potential or IPSP in the flexor motor neuron. (Reproduced with permission from Kandel ER, Schwartz JH, Jessell TM [editors]: *Principles of Neural Science*, 4th ed. New York, NY: McGraw-Hill; 2000.)

depolarization reaches the threshold voltage, a propagated action potential will occur. Two passive membrane properties of a neuron (time constant and length constant) affect the ability of postsynaptic potentials to summate to elicit an action potential (**Figure 6–3**). The time constant determines the time course of the synaptic potential; it can affect the amplitude of the depolarization caused by consecutive EPSPs produced by a single presynaptic neuron. The longer the time constant, the greater

is the chance for two potentials to summate to induce an action potential. If a second EPSP is elicited before the first EPSP decays, the two potentials summate to induce an action potential in the postsynaptic neuron (temporal summation). The length constant of a neuron determines the degree to which a depolarizing current is reduced as it spreads passively; it can affect the amplitude of the EPSPs produced by two presynaptic neurons in a process called spatial summation. If a neuron has a long length constant,

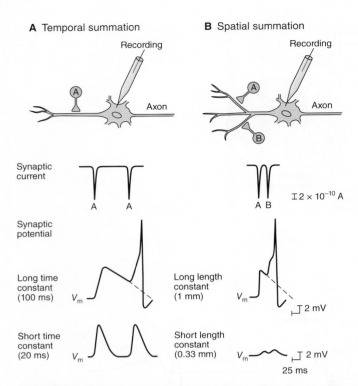

FIGURE 6–3 Central neurons integrate a variety of synaptic inputs through temporal and spatial summation. (A) The time constant of the postsynaptic neuron affects the amplitude of the depolarization caused by consecutive EPSPs produced by a single presynaptic neuron. In cases of a long time constant, if a second EPSP is elicited before the first EPSP decays, the two potentials summate to induce an action potential. **(B)** The length constant of a postsynaptic cell affects the amplitude of two EPSPs produced by two presynaptic neurons, A and B. If the length constant is long, the depolarization induced at two points on the neuron can spread to the trigger zone with minimal decrement so that the two potentials summate and an action potential is elicited. (Reproduced with permission from Kandel ER, Schwartz JH, Jessell TM [editors]: *Principles of Neural Science*, 4th ed. New York, NY: McGraw-Hill; 2000.)

the membrane depolarization induced by inputs arriving at two points on the neuron can spread to the trigger zone of the neuron with minimal decrement and summate to induce an action potential.

POSTSYNAPTIC & PRESYNAPTIC INHIBITION OR FACILITATION

Postsynaptic inhibition occurs when an inhibitory transmitter (eg, glycine or GABA) is released from a presynaptic nerve terminal to induce an IPSP in a postsynaptic neuron (Figure 6–2B). For example, there is an inhibitory interneuron interposed between the afferent fiber from the muscle spindle and the motor neurons supplying the antagonistic muscle. So stimulation of the afferent fiber produces an IPSP in that motor neuron. Presynaptic inhibition is mediated by an axoaxonal synapse on a neuron that releases an excitatory neurotransmitter **(Figure 6–4)**. Activation of GABA

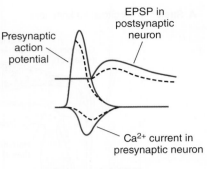

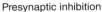

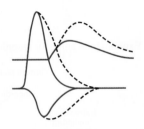

FIGURE 6–4 Effects of presynaptic inhibition and facilitation on the action potential and the Ca^{2+} current in the presynaptic neuron and the EPSP in the postsynaptic neuron. In each case, the solid lines are the controls and the dashed lines the records obtained during inhibition or facilitation. Presynaptic inhibition occurs when activation of presynaptic receptors increases Cl^- conductance, which decreases the size of the action potential. This reduces Ca^{2+} entry and thus the amount of excitatory transmitter released. Presynaptic facilitation is produced when the action potential is prolonged and the Ca^{2+} channels are open for a longer duration. (Reproduced with permission from Kandel ER, Schwartz JH, Jessell TM [editors]: *Principles of Neural Science*, 4th ed. New York, NY: McGraw-Hill; 2000.)

receptors on the presynaptic nerve terminal can increase Cl^- and/or K^+ conductance, which reduces Ca^{2+} entry and thus the amount of excitatory transmitter released. Conversely, presynaptic facilitation is produced when the action potential is prolonged and the Ca^{2+} channels are open for a longer period.

Both presynaptic and postsynaptic inhibitions are usually produced by stimulation of certain systems converging on a given postsynaptic neuron. Neurons may also inhibit themselves in a negative feedback manner (negative feedback inhibition). For instance, a spinal motor neuron emits a recurrent collateral that synapses with an inhibitory interneuron, which then terminates on the cell body of the spinal neuron and other spinal motor neurons.

NEUROMUSCULAR JUNCTION

Figure 6–5 shows the components of the neuromuscular junction. As the motor neuron approaches a skeletal muscle, it loses its myelin sheath and divides into a number of terminal boutons. The endings fit into depressions in the motor endplate (junctional folds) on the thickened portion of the muscle membrane

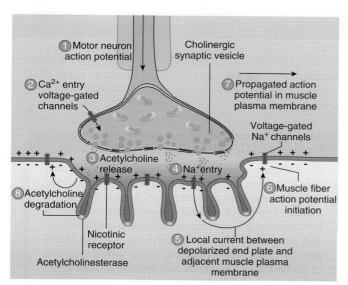

FIGURE 6–5 **Events at the neuromuscular junction that lead to an action potential in the muscle fiber plasma membrane.** The impulse arriving in the end of the motor neuron increases the permeability of its endings to Ca²⁺, which enters the endings and triggers exocytosis of the acetylcholine (ACh)-containing synaptic vesicles. ACh diffuses and binds to nicotinic cholinergic (N$_M$) receptors in the motor endplate, which increases Na⁺ and K⁺ conductance. The resultant influx of Na⁺ produces the endplate potential. The current sink created by this local potential depolarizes the adjacent muscle membrane to its firing level. Action potentials are generated on either side of the endplate and are conducted away from the endplate in both directions along the muscle fiber and the muscle contracts. ACh is then removed from the synaptic cleft by acetylcholinesterase. (Modified with permission from Widmaier EP, Raff H, Strang KT: *Vanders Human Physiology.* New York, NY: McGraw-Hill; 2008.)

at the junction. The space between the nerve and the thickened muscle membrane is comparable to the synaptic cleft at neuronal synapses. Only one nerve fiber ends on each endplate.

The events occurring during transmission of impulses from the motor nerve to the muscle are similar to those occurring at neuron-to-neuron synapses (Figure 6–5). The impulse arriving in the end of the motor neuron increases the permeability of its endings to Ca²⁺, which then causes exocytosis of acetylcholine from synaptic vesicles. The acetylcholine diffuses to nicotinic cholinergic receptors on the junctional folds. Binding of acetylcholine to these receptors increases the Na⁺ and K⁺ conductance; the influx of Na⁺ produces an endplate potential and subsequent depolarization of the adjacent muscle membrane. Action potentials are generated and conducted along the muscle fiber, leading in turn to muscle contraction. Acetylcholine is removed from the synaptic cleft by acetylcholinesterase, which is highly concentrated at the neuromuscular junction.

Small quanta (packets) of acetylcholine are released randomly from the nerve cell membrane at rest to induce a miniature endplate potential (~ 0.5 mV in amplitude). The size of the quanta released varies directly with the Ca²⁺ concentration and inversely with the Mg²⁺ concentration at the endplate. When a nerve impulse reaches the ending, the number of quanta released

increases by several orders of magnitude. Two diseases of the neuromuscular junction, myasthenia gravis and Lambert–Eaton myasthenic syndrome, are described in **Clinical Boxes 6–2** and **6–3**, respectively.

Myasthenia Gravis

Myasthenia gravis is sometimes a fatal disease characterized by muscle fatigue with sustained or repeated activity. It occurs in 25 to 125 of every 1 million people worldwide and can occur at any age, with peak occurrences in individuals in their 20s (mainly women) and 60s (mainly men). It is caused by the formation of circulating antibodies that destroy the muscle type of nicotinic receptors. In myasthenia gravis, neuromuscular transmission fails at low levels of quantal release of neurotransmitter with repetitive activation of the nerve. There are two major forms of the disease. In one form, the extraocular muscles are primarily affected. In the second form, there is a generalized skeletal muscle weakness. In severe cases, the diaphragm can become weak and respiratory failure and death can ensue. The major structural abnormality in myasthenia gravis is the appearance of sparse, shallow, and abnormally wide or absent synaptic clefts in the motor endplate. The postsynaptic membrane has a reduced response to acetylcholine and a 70–90% decrease in the number of receptors per endplate in affected muscles. Patients with myasthenia gravis have a greater than normal tendency to also have rheumatoid arthritis, systemic lupus erythematosus, or polymyositis. About 30% of patients with myasthenia gravis have a maternal relative with an autoimmune disorder. These associations suggest that individuals with myasthenia gravis share a genetic predisposition to autoimmune disease. The thymus may play a role in the pathogenesis of the disease by supplying helper T cells sensitized against thymic proteins that cross-react with acetylcholine receptors. In most patients, the thymus is hyperplastic; and 10–15% have a thymoma.

THERAPEUTIC HIGHLIGHTS

Muscle weakness due to myasthenia gravis improves after a period of rest or after administration of an acetylcholinesterase inhibitor such as neostigmine or pyridostigmine. Cholinesterase inhibitors prevent metabolism of acetylcholine, thus compensating for the normal decline in released neurotransmitters during repeated stimulation. Immunosuppressive drugs (eg, prednisone or cyclosporine) can suppress antibody production and can improve muscle strength in some cases. Thymectomy is indicated if a thymoma is suspected in the development of myasthenia gravis. Even in those without thymoma, thymectomy induces remission in 35% of patients.

CLINICAL BOX 6–3

Lambert–Eaton Syndrome

In a relatively rare condition called Lambert–Eaton myasthenic syndrome (LEMS), muscle weakness is caused by an autoimmune attack against one of the voltage-gated Ca^{2+} channels in the nerve endings at the neuromuscular junction. This decreases the Ca^{2+} influx needed for acetylcholine release. The incidence of LEMS in the United States is about 1 case per 100,000 people; it is usually an adult-onset disease. Proximal muscles of the lower extremities are primarily affected, producing a waddling gait and difficulty raising the arms. Repetitive stimulation of the motor nerve facilitates accumulation of Ca^{2+} in the nerve terminal and increases acetylcholine release, leading to an increase in muscle strength. About 40% of patients with LEMS also have cancer, especially small cell cancer of the lung. One theory is that antibodies that are produced to attack the cancer cells also attack Ca^{2+} channels, leading to LEMS. LEMS has also been associated with lymphosarcoma; malignant thymoma; and cancer of the breast, stomach, colon, prostate, bladder, kidney, or gallbladder. Clinical signs usually precede the diagnosis of cancer. A syndrome similar to LEMS can occur after the use of aminoglycoside antibiotics, which also impair Ca^{2+} channel function.

THERAPEUTIC HIGHLIGHTS

Since there is a high comorbidity with small cell lung cancer, the first treatment strategy is to determine if the individual also has cancer and, if so, to treat that appropriately. In patients without cancer, immunotherapy is initiated. Prednisone administration, plasmapheresis, and intravenous immunoglobulin are effective therapies for LEMS. Aminopyridines, which cause blockade of presynaptic K^+ channels and activate voltage-gated Ca^{2+} channels, can facilitate the release of acetylcholine in the neuromuscular junction and can improve muscle strength.

NERVE ENDINGS IN SMOOTH & CARDIAC MUSCLE

Postganglionic nerves branch extensively and come in close contact with smooth muscle cells which do not have endplates or postsynaptic specializations (**Figure 6–6**). The nerve fibers containing either clear vesicles (acetylcholine) or dense-core vesicles (norepinephrine) run along the membranes of the muscle cells and sometimes groove their surfaces. The multiple branches of postganglionic neurons are beaded with enlargements (varicosities) that contain synaptic vesicles. Transmitter is released at each varicosity at many locations along the axon, allowing one

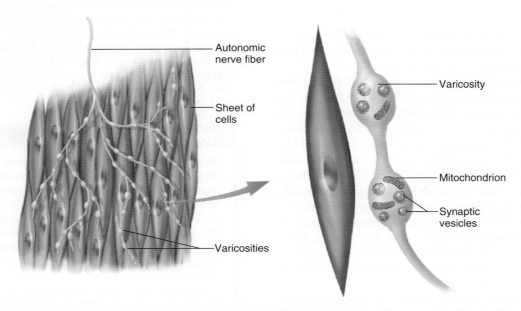

FIGURE 6–6 **Endings of postganglionic autonomic neurons on smooth muscle.** The nerve fibers run along the membranes of the smooth muscle cells and sometimes groove their surfaces. The multiple branches of postganglionic neurons are beaded with enlargements (varicosities) and contain synaptic vesicles. Neurotransmitter is released from the varicosities and diffuses to receptors on smooth muscle cell plasma membranes. (Reproduced with permission from Widmaier EP, Raff H, Strang KT: *Vanders Human Physiology.* New York, NY: McGraw-Hill; 2008.)

neuron to innervate many effector cells. This type of contact is called a *synapse en passant*. In the ventricle of the heart, the contacts between the sympathetic nerve and cardiac muscle fibers resemble those found in smooth muscle. In some smooth muscles, stimulation of the postganglionic nerves produces depolarizing excitatory junction potentials, which can summate with repeated stimuli. In other tissues, stimulation of the postganglionic nerves produces hyperpolarizing inhibitory junction potentials. Junctional potentials spread electrotonically.

AXONAL INJURY & DENERVATION SUPERSENSITIVITY

Reactions triggered by injury or section of an axon are shown in Figure 6–7. Orthograde degeneration (Wallerian degeneration) occurs from the point of injury to the nerve terminal, interrupting neural transmission. Distal to the injury, the membrane breaks down and the myelin sheath degenerates. The proximal axon may undergo retrograde degeneration and die. The cell body of the injured neuron swells, the nucleus moves to an eccentric position, and the rough endoplasmic reticulum gets fragmented (chromatolytic reaction).

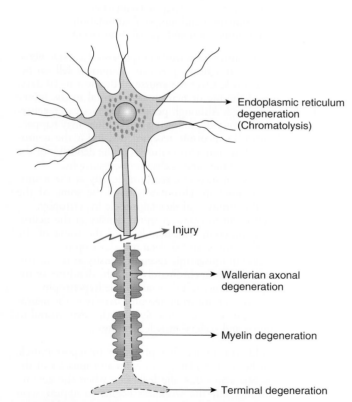

FIGURE 6–7 Changes occurring in a neuron when its axon is crushed or injured. The distal axon stump separates from the cell body, orthograde (Wallerian) degeneration occurs from the point of damage to the terminal, and the myelin sheath degenerates. The cell body of the injured neuron swells and the endoplasmic reticulum is fragmented as part of the chromatolytic reaction.

The nerve then starts to regrow, with multiple small branches projecting along the former path the axon (regenerative sprouting). Axons sometimes grow back to their original targets, especially in locations like the neuromuscular junction. However, nerve regeneration is generally limited because axons often become entangled in the area of tissue damage at the site where they were disrupted. Neurotrophins can facilitate nerve regeneration.

When the motor nerve to skeletal muscle is cut and allowed to degenerate, there is a marked proliferation of nicotinic receptors over a wide region of the neuromuscular junction and the muscle gradually becomes extremely sensitive to acetylcholine (denervation hypersensitivity or supersensitivity). Later, muscle atrophy occurs due to disuse. Although smooth muscle does not atrophy when denervated, it also becomes hyperresponsive to the neurotransmitter that activates it.

CHAPTER SUMMARY

- The presynaptic terminal is separated from the postsynaptic structure by a synaptic cleft. The postsynaptic membrane contains neurotransmitter receptors and usually a postsynaptic thickening called the postsynaptic density.
- An EPSP is produced by depolarization of the postsynaptic cell after a latency of 0.5 ms; the excitatory transmitter opens Na^+ or Ca^{2+} ion channels in the postsynaptic membrane, producing an inward current. An IPSP is produced by a hyperpolarization of the postsynaptic cell; it can be produced by a localized increase in Cl^- transport.
- Postsynaptic inhibition during the course of an IPSP is called direct inhibition. Indirect inhibition is due to the effects of previous postsynaptic neuron discharge; an example is the change in excitability during the refractory period. Presynaptic inhibition is mediated by an axoaxonal synapse on a neuron that releases an excitatory neurotransmitter; a series of events leads to reduced release of the excitatory neurotransmitter.
- A neuromuscular junction is formed by the axon terminal of motor neurons that synapses on the motor endplate on the skeletal muscle membrane. Acetylcholine released from the motor neuron diffuses and binds to nicotinic cholinergic receptors on the motor endplate, causing an increase in Na^+ and K^+ conductance; the influx of Na^+ induces the endplate potential and subsequent depolarization of the adjacent muscle membrane. Action potentials are generated and conducted along the muscle fiber to mediate muscle contraction.
- When a nerve is damaged and degenerates, the postsynaptic structure gradually becomes extremely sensitive to the transmitter released by the nerve to cause denervation hypersensitivity.

MULTIPLE-CHOICE QUESTIONS

For all questions, select the single best answer unless otherwise directed.

Scenario for Questions 1–3: A neurology resident was conducting research in an electrophysiology laboratory. He was recording from the soma of two motor neurons while electrically stimulating the dorsal root afferent fiber very close to its entry into the spinal cord. In motor neuron A he recorded an inward current that had an onset latency of 0.75 ms after the stimulus. In motor neuron B, the same stimulus induced an outward current whose onset latency was 1.45 ms.

1. Which of the following could explain the response recorded from motor neuron A?
    A. The stimulus caused the release of GABA that led to the opening of Cl⁻ channels and a fast inhibitory postsynaptic potential (IPSP).
    B. The stimulus caused the release of glycine that led to the closing of Cl⁻ channels and a fast IPSP.
    C. The stimulus caused the release of glutamate that led to opening of Na⁺ channels and a fast excitatory postsynaptic potential (EPSP).
    D. The stimulus caused the release of glutamate that led to an increase in Na⁺ conductance and an endplate potential in the postsynaptic neuron.
    E. The stimulus caused the release of glycine that led the closure of K⁺ channels and a fast IPSP.

2. Which of the following could explain the response recorded from motor neuron B?
    A. The stimulus caused the release of GABA that led to the opening of Cl⁻ channels and a fast inhibitory postsynaptic potential (IPSP).
    B. The stimulus caused the release of glycine that led to the closing of Cl⁻ channels and a fast IPSP.
    C. The stimulus caused the release of glutamate that led to opening of Na⁺ channels and a fast excitatory postsynaptic potential (EPSP).
    D. The stimulus caused the release of glutamate that led to an increase in Na⁺ conductance and an endplate potential in the postsynaptic neuron.
    E. The stimulus caused the release of glycine that led the closure of K⁺ channels and a fast IPSP.

3. On the basis of the information provided, how many synapses can there be between the afferent fiber and motor neuron A and between the afferent fiber and motor neuron B?
    A. There can be at least two synapses between the afferent and motor neuron A, and there can be at least three synapses between the afferent and motor neuron B.
    B. There can be at most one synapse between the afferent and motor neuron A, and there can be at most two synapses between the afferent and motor neuron B.
    C. There can be at least two synapses between the afferent and both motor neuron A and B.
    D. There can be only one synapse between the afferent and motor neuron A, and there can be three synapses between the afferent and motor neuron B.
    E. There is not enough information to estimate the number of synapses.

Scenario for Questions 4–6. A medical student was studying the passive membrane properties of neurons and their ability to affect the amplitude of an EPSP recorded from the neuron. She compared the responses of two different neurons to electrical stimulation of either one or two of their presynaptic inputs.

4. In the first experiment the student found that in one neuron, applying two stimuli separated by 25 ms to one presynaptic input induced two EPSPs of identical amplitude. In a second neuron, the same type of stimulation induced an EPSP followed an action potential? What can she conclude from this experiment?

A. The second neuron had a longer time constant than the first neuron.
B. The second neuron had a shorter time constant than the first neuron.
C. The second neuron had a longer length constant than the first neuron.
D. The second neuron had a shorter length constant than the first neuron.

5. The student recorded an EPSP followed by an action potential in one neuron when a stimulus was applied to one presynaptic input and 25 ms later a stimulus was applied to a second presynaptic input. When recording from a second neuron, the same stimulus protocol induced two EPSPs. What can she conclude from this experiment?
    A. The second neuron had a longer time constant than the first neuron.
    B. The second neuron had a shorter time constant than the first neuron.
    C. The second neuron had a longer length constant than the first neuron.
    D. The second neuron had a shorter length constant than the first neuron.

6. Experiments 1 and 2, respectively, demonstrated the following properties of synaptic transmission.
    A. Presynaptic facilitation and postsynaptic facilitation
    B. Both demonstrate presynaptic inhibition
    C. Both demonstrate presynaptic facilitation
    D. Spatial summation and temporal summation
    E. Temporal summation and spatial summation

7. A 27-year-old construction worker experienced a severe nerve compression when a heavy piece of equipment fell on his wrist while at work. Over the course of the next 6–10 days, the portion of the motor neuron axons distal to the injury slowly degenerated. Although peripheral nerves can regenerate, prior to recovery the following three things may happen.
    A. A decrease in nicotinic receptor density at the neuromuscular junction, chromatolysis of the dendrites of the damaged neurons, and skeletal muscle atrophy.
    B. An increase in nicotinic receptor density at the neuromuscular junction, chromatolysis of the soma of the damaged neurons, and skeletal muscle hypertrophy.
    C. An increase in nicotinic receptor density at the neuromuscular junction, chromatolysis of the soma of the damaged neurons, and skeletal muscle atrophy.
    D. A decrease in muscarinic receptor density at the neuromuscular junction, chromatolysis of the dendrites of the damaged neurons, and skeletal muscle hypertrophy.
    E. An increase in muscarinic receptor density at the neuromuscular junction, chromatolysis of the axon rostral to the injury, and skeletal muscle atrophy.

8. A 35-year-old woman sees her physician to report muscle weakness in her extraocular eye muscles and muscles of the extremities. She states that she feels fine when she gets up in the morning, but the weakness begins to appear soon after she becomes active. The weakness is improved by rest. Sensation appears normal. The physician treats her with an acetylcholinesterase inhibitor, and she notes almost immediate return of muscle strength. These signs and symptoms are consistent with a diagnosis of
    A. Lambert–Eaton syndrome.
    B. myasthenia gravis.

C. multiple sclerosis.
D. Parkinson disease.
E. muscular dystrophy.

9. A 50-year-old man visits his physician for his annual physical, 2 years after the diagnosis of small cell lung cancer. The patient mentions to his physician that he has noted muscle weakness in his legs and arms. Also, he sometimes finds it difficult to raise his left arm; and he has begun to experience difficulty walking. Upon questioning, he says that the greater the effort he exerts in trying to raise his arm, the easier it becomes to move it. These signs and symptoms are consistent with a diagnosis of
A. Lambert–Eaton syndrome.
B. myasthenia gravis.
C. multiple sclerosis.
D. Parkinson disease.
E. muscular dystrophy.

10. A 55-year-old woman had an autonomic neuropathy that disrupted the sympathetic nerve supply to the pupillary dilator muscle of her right eye. While having her eyes examined, the ophthalmologist placed phenylephrine in her eyes. The right eye became much more dilated than the left eye. This suggests that
A. the sympathetic nerve to the right eye had regenerated.
B. the parasympathetic nerve supply to the right eye remained intact and compensated for the loss of the sympathetic nerve.
C. phenylephrine blocked the pupillary constrictor muscle of the right eye.
D. denervation supersensitivity had developed in her right eye.
E. the left eye also had nerve damage and so was not responding as expected.

11. A 47-year-old woman was admitted to the hospital after experiencing nausea and vomiting for about 2 days followed by severe muscle weakness and neurologic symptoms, including ptosis and dysphagia. She indicated she had eaten meat that seemed to be undercooked at a restaurant the evening before the symptoms began. Laboratory tests were positive for *Clostridium botulinum*. The mechanism of action of this neurotoxin to cause these effects is
A. blockade of the reuptake of acetylcholine into presynaptic terminals.
B. irreversible binding to the receptor on the postsynaptic membrane at the neuromuscular junction.
C. blockade of the synthesis of acetylcholine in the cholinergic neuron.
D. a direct action on skeletal muscle fibers to prevent its ability to contract.
E. prevention of the docking of synaptic vesicles to the membrane of the nerve terminal that is needed for the release of acetylcholine.

12. A 54-year-old man came to the emergency department of his local hospital after a few days of worsening jaw discomfort. Today he was having difficulty opening his mouth. He said he has not had a physical exam since his physician retired more than 15 years ago, and this episode is the first time he has felt the need to get professional help for any health concern. The medical student doing his clerkship in the ED noticed a puncture wound on the man's hand and queried him about it. The man said about 10 days ago he was cleaning out an old shed when a rusty nail punctured his hand. Upon further questioning, he said he did not recall the last time he had a tetanus booster but certainly more than 15 years ago. Assuming his jaw problems are due to tetanus toxin, what is the mechanism of action of this neurotoxin to cause these effects?
A. Blockade of acetylcholinesterase in the neuromuscular junction
B. Excessive activation of α-motor neurons to the masseter muscle due to dysfunction of spinal inhibitory interneurons
C. Reduced activity in inhibitory α-motor neurons that normally relax the mandibular muscle
D. Excessive activation of Ia spindle afferents that increases the activity in α-motor neurons
E. Loss of function of Ib afferent fibers from the Golgi tendon organ causing excessive tension in skeletal muscle

ANSWERS

1. The best answer is **C.** An inward current denotes depolarization (fast EPSP) which would occur due to an action of an excitatory neurotransmitter such as glutamate to increase Na^+ conductance. Options **A, B,** and **E** can be ruled out since the release of an inhibitory neurotransmitter such as GABA or glycine induces hyperpolarization (outward current, fast IPSP) due to either an increase in Cl^- or K^+ conductance. Option **D** can be ruled out since an endplate potentials are recorded at the neuromuscular junction and result from release of acetylcholine by a motor neuron.

2. The best answer is **A.** An outward current denotes depolarization (fast IPSP) which would occur due to an action of an inhibitory neurotransmitter such as GABA to an increase in Cl^- conductance. Glycine also increases Cl^- or K^+ conductance (rules out options **B** and **E**). The appearance of an outward current is inconsistent with a fast EPSP (rules out option **C**). Option **D** can be ruled out since an endplate potentials are recorded at the neuromuscular junction and is an excitatory potential due to release of acetylcholine by a motor neuron.

3. The best answer is **B.** The minimum latency at a synapse is 0.5 ms so a latency of 0.75 ms is consistent with a single synapse and a latency of 1.45 ms can be no more than two synapses. A latency of 0.75 ms between the afferent fiber and motor neuron A rules out options **A** and **C**; a latency of 1.45 ms between the afferent fiber and motor neuron B rules out **A** and **D**. Option **E** can be ruled out because their is sufficient information to determine the number of synapses.

4. The best answer is **A.** The time constant of a neuron can affect the amplitude of the depolarization caused by consecutive EPSPs produced by a single presynaptic neuron. The longer the time constant, the greater is the chance for two potentials to summate to induce an action potential (temporal summation) as occurred here for the second neuron. This rules out option **B.** The length constant is determined by activating two separate presynaptic inputs which rules out options **C** and **D**.

5. The best answer is **D.** The length constant of a neuron determines the degree to which a depolarizing current is reduced as it spreads passively. If a neuron has a long length constant, the depolarization induced by inputs arriving at two points can spread to the trigger zone of the neuron with minimal decrement and summate to induce an action potential (spatial summation) as occurred in the first neuron but

not the second. So the first neuron has a longer time constant than the first neuron (rules out option **C**). The time constant is determined by repetitive stimulation of a single presynaptic input which rules out options **A** and **B**.

6. The best answer is **E**. See the answers to Questions 4 and 5 above for definitions of temporal and spatial summation which also rule out option **D**. Presynaptic inhibition occurs when activation of presynaptic receptors increases Cl^- conductance, which decreases the size of the action potential (rules out option **B**). With presynaptic facilitation, the duration of the action potential is prolonged (rules out options **A** and **C**).

7. The best answer is **C**. When the motor nerve to skeletal muscle is cut and undergoes degeneration, there is a marked proliferation of nicotinic receptors over a wide region of the neuromuscular junction and the muscle gradually becomes extremely sensitive to acetylcholine. Also, the soma of the injured neuron swells, the nucleus moves to an eccentric position, and the rough endoplasmic reticulum gets fragmented (chromatolytic reaction). Later, muscle atrophy occurs due to disuse. Thus all other options (**A, B, D,** and **E**) can be ruled out.

8. The best answer is **B**. Myasthenia gravis is caused by the formation of circulating antibodies that destroy skeletal muscle nicotinic receptors. Normally, the number of quanta released from the motor nerve terminal declines with successive repetitive stimuli. In myasthenia gravis, neuromuscular transmission fails at these low levels of quantal release. This leads to the major clinical feature of the disease, muscle fatigue with sustained or repeated activity. The muscle weakness improves after a period of rest or after administration of an acetylcholinesterase inhibitor, which prevents metabolism of the released acetylcholine. The muscle weakness due to Lambert–Eaton syndrome is actually reduced (not enhanced) with repetitive stimulation, which rules out option **A**. As described in Chapter 4, multiple sclerosis is a demyelinating disease which presents with various combinations of muscle weakness, spasticity, hyperreflexia, paresthesia, numbness, and visual problems (rules out option **C**). As described in Chapter 12, Parkinson disease leads to both hypokinetic (akinesia and bradykinesia) and hyperkinetic (cogwheel rigidity and tremor at rest) characteristics which rules out option **D**. As described in Chapter 5, muscular dystrophy refers to diseases that cause progressive muscle weakness, which is not reduced by rest or corrected by cholinesterase inhibitors (rules out option **E**).

9. The best answer is **A**. The muscle weakness due to Lambert–Eaton syndrome is caused by an autoimmune attack against voltage-gated Ca^{2+} channels in the nerve endings at the neuromuscular junction, which leads to reduced acetylcholine release. Proximal muscles of the lower extremities are primarily affected, producing a waddling gait and difficulty raising the arms. Repetitive stimulation of the motor nerve facilitates accumulation of Ca^{2+} in the nerve terminal and increases acetylcholine release, leading to an increase in muscle strength. About 40% of patients with LEMS also have cancer, especially small cell cancer of the lung. See the response to Question 8 to rule out the other options (**B, C, D,** and **E**).

10. The best answer is **D**. Phenylephrine is an agonist of the adrenergic receptors on the pupillary dilator muscle. After the nerve supply to smooth muscle such as the pupillary dilator muscle is damaged and degenerates, the receptors on the muscle become hyperresponsive to both endogenous and exogenous agonists (denervation hypersensitivity or supersensitivity). If the nerve had regenerated, it would resume normal function and receptors on the smooth muscle would respond normally to an agonist such as phenylephrine (rules out option **A**). There is no parasympathetic innervation of the pupillary dilator muscle; parasympathetic control of pupillary diameter is mediated by contraction of the pupillary constrictor muscle (rules out option **B**). The pupillary constrictor muscle contraction is dependent on activation of cholinergic receptors, and phenylephrine does not bind to these receptors (rules out option **C**). If the sympathetic nerve to the pupillary dilator muscle of the left eye was also damaged, that eye would also have an exaggerated response to phenylephrine (rules out option **E**).

11. The best answer is **E**. Botulinum toxins A and E cleave synaptosome-associated protein-25 (SNAP-25), a presynaptic membrane protein needed for fusion of synaptic vesicles containing acetylcholine to the terminal membrane, an important step in neurotransmitter release. By blocking acetylcholine release at the neuromuscular junction, these toxins cause flaccid paralysis. Symptoms can include ptosis, diplopia, dysarthria, dysphonia, and dysphagia. There is not an acetylcholine reuptake mechanism; rather, acetylcholine is rapidly hydrolyzed to acetate and choline after its release. The choline is transported into the nerve terminal via a choline transporter that can be blocked by hemicholinium (rules out option **A**). Irreversible binding of acetylcholine to postsynaptic receptors is caused by acetylcholinesterase inhibitors not neurotoxins (rules out option **B**). Synthesis of acetylcholine is slowed by hemicholinium since it prevents the transport of choline into the nerve terminal, a step needed for synthesis of acetylcholine (rules out option **C**). As their name implies, neurotoxins do not act directly on the skeletal muscle (rules out option **D**).

12. The best answer is **B**. Tetanus toxin from the gram-negative bacteria *Clostridium tetani* binds irreversibly to the presynaptic membrane of the neuromuscular junction and travels via retrograde axonal transport to the cell body of motor neurons. From there it is picked up by the terminals of presynaptic inhibitory interneurons and attaches to gangliosides to block the release of glycine and GABA, thereby increasing the activity of motor neurons. Clinically, tetanus toxin causes spasms of the masseter muscle (lockjaw). The widespread use of tetanus toxoid vaccine in the United States beginning in the mid-1940s has led to a marked decline in the incidence of tetanus toxicity. Cholinesterase inhibitors (including organophosphates) prevent the breakdown of acetylcholine and therefore prolong its actions and causes skeletal muscle twitching and the excessive activation of cholinergic symptoms in autonomic targets is associated with miosis, salivation, sweating, bronchial constriction, vomiting, and diarrhea (rules out option **A**). There are no inhibitory α-motor neurons; skeletal muscle relaxation occurs when α-motor neurons are silenced (rules out **C**). Excessive activation of Ia muscle spindle afferents would increase the activity of α-motor neurons, but neurotoxins are not associated with a direct effect on these afferents (rules out option **D**). Neurotoxins are also not known to specifically target Ib tendon afferent fibers (rules out option **E**).

Neurotransmitters & Neuromodulators

- List the major types of neurotransmitters.
- Summarize the steps involved in the biosynthesis, release, action, and removal from the synaptic cleft of the major neurotransmitters.
- Describe the various types of receptors for amino acids, acetylcholine, monoamines, neuropeptides, and opioids.

INTRODUCTION

The dominant form of neuron-to-neuron or neuron-to-effector organ communication within the mammalian nervous system is mediated by the release of a chemical neurotransmitter that induces excitation or inhibition of the postsynaptic target. Neuromodulators are chemicals released by neurons that have little or no direct effects on their own but can modify the effects of neurotransmitters. This chapter provides a summary of the major properties of some of the most common chemical neurotransmitters, including excitatory and inhibitory amino acids, acetylcholine,

catecholamines, and neuropeptides. For many of these chemicals, there are some common steps involved in the process of neurotransmission (**Figure 7–1**). These steps include uptake of a neurotransmitter precursor, biosynthesis of the neurotransmitter, its storage within synaptic vesicles, its release into the synaptic cleft in response to nerve impulses, binding of the neurotransmitter to receptors on the membrane of the postsynaptic target, and finally termination of its actions via diffusion away from the synapse, reuptake into the nerve terminal, or enzymatic degradation.

■ CHEMICAL NEUROTRANSMISSION

Figure 7–2 shows the steps involved in the biosynthesis of some of the common neurotransmitters in the central nervous system (CNS) or peripheral nervous system. **Table 7–1** summarizes properties of major neurotransmitters, including their receptors, second messengers, ion channel effects, and examples of receptor agonists and antagonists.

Several factors contribute to the types of responses that result from release of a neurotransmitter. One, each chemical mediator has the potential to act on many different subtypes of receptors. Two, binding of a neurotransmitter on the autoreceptors and heteroreceptors on presynaptic nerve terminals can inhibit or

facilitate further neurotransmitter release. Three, with prolonged exposure to their ligands, most receptors undergo homologous desensitization (loss of responsiveness to a specific ligand) or heterologous desensitization (loss of responsiveness to more than one ligand).

Receptors are either ligand-gated ion channels (ionotropic receptors) or 7-transmembrane G-protein–coupled receptors (GPCR; metabotropic receptors). In the case of ionotropic receptors, a membrane channel is opened when a ligand binds to it; its activation can elicit a brief (few to tens of milliseconds) increase in ionic conductance to mediate fast synaptic transmission. In the case of GPCRs, binding of a neurotransmitter initiates the production of a second messenger that modulates the voltage-gated channels on cell membranes.

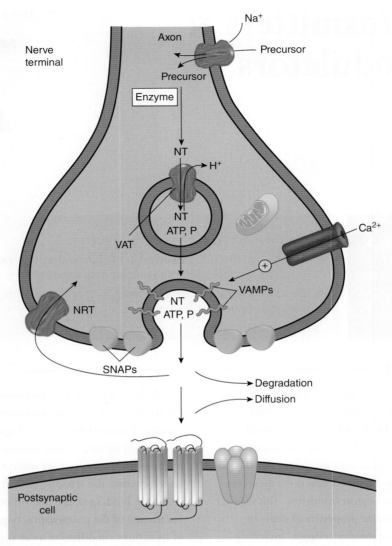

FIGURE 7–1 Biochemical events at a neuronal synapse. The drawing shows the common steps involved in neurotransmission. Step 1: Transport of a neurotransmitter precursor into a nerve terminal. Step 2: Synthesis of the neurotransmitter. Step 3: Transport of the neurotransmitter into a synaptic vesicle via a vesicle transporter. Step 4: An action potential induced influx of Ca^{2+}, which leads to fusion of vesicles with the surface membrane and expulsion of the neurotransmitter and co-transmitters into the synaptic cleft. This step can involve synaptosome-associated proteins (SNAPs) and vesicle-associated membrane proteins (VAMPs). Step 5: The neurotransmitter acts on G-protein–coupled receptors or ionotropic receptors on the membrane of the postsynaptic target (a neuron, smooth muscle, skeletal muscle, or gland). Step 6: The action of the neurotransmitter is terminated by diffusion away from the synapse, reuptake into the nerve terminal, or enzymatic degradation. Specifics regarding each of these steps involved in transmission at cholinergic, adrenergic, and serotonergic synapses is detailed in the text.

After their release, many neurotransmitters are rapidly transported back into the cytoplasm of the nerve terminal (reuptake), which involves a high-affinity, Na^+-dependent membrane transporter. Reuptake is a major mechanism to terminate the action of neurotransmitters; if inhibited, the prolonged action of the neurotransmitter can have clinical or pathological consequences. For example, some antidepressant drugs are inhibitors of the reuptake of amine transmitters. If glutamate reuptake into neurons and glia is prevented (eg, during ischemia or anoxia), cell death can occur because glutamate is an excitotoxin that can kill cells by overstimulation (**Clinical Box 7–1**).

■ COMMON NEUROTRANSMITTERS

Glutamate

Glutamate is the main excitatory neurotransmitter within the CNS. The glutamate released from a nerve terminal into the synaptic cleft can be transported via a glutamate reuptake transporter into glia, where it is converted to glutamine by glutamine synthetase (**Figure 7–3**). Glutamine then diffuses back into the nerve terminal where glutaminase hydrolyzes it back to glutamate.

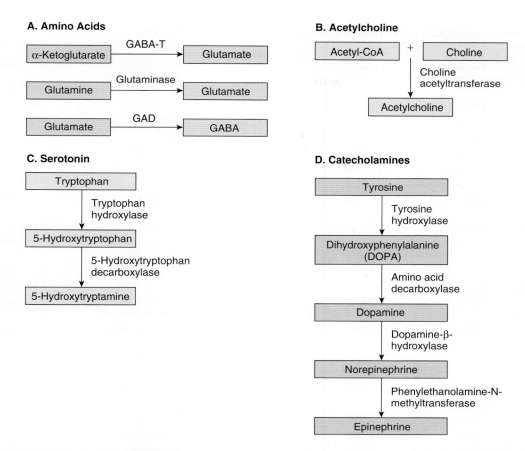

A. Amino Acids

B. Acetylcholine

C. Serotonin

D. Catecholamines

FIGURE 7–2 **Biosynthesis of some common small-molecule neurotransmitters. (A)** Glutamate is synthesized in the Krebs cycle by the conversion of α-ketoglutarate to the amino acid via the enzyme γ-aminobutyric acid transferase (GABA-T) or in nerve terminals by the hydrolysis of glutamine by the enzyme glutaminase. GABA is synthesized by the conversion of glutamate by the enzyme glutamic acid decarboxylase (GAD). **(B)** Acetylcholine is synthesized in the cytoplasm of a nerve terminal from acetyl-Co-A and choline by the enzyme choline acetyltransferase. **(C)** Serotonin is synthesized from the amino acid tryptophan in a two-step process: the enzymatic hydroxylation of tryptophan to 5-hydroxytryptophan and the enzymatic decarboxylation of this intermediate to form 5-hydroxytryptamine (also called serotonin). **(D)** Catecholamines are synthesized from the amino acid tyrosine by a multi-step process. Tyrosine is oxidized to dihydroxyphenylalanine (DOPA) by the enzyme tyrosine hydroxylase in the cytoplasm of the neuron; DOPA is then decarboxylated to dopamine. In dopaminergic neurons, the process stops there. In noradrenergic neurons, the dopamine is transported into synaptic vesicles where it is converted to norepinephrine by dopamine-β-hydroxylase. In neurons that also contain the enzyme phenylethanolamine-N-methyltransferase, norepinephrine is converted to epinephrine.

The transporter also returns glutamate into the nerve terminal. Within neurons, glutamate is concentrated in synaptic vesicles by a vesicular glutamate transporter.

There are three types of ionotropic glutamate receptors and seven types of metabotropic receptors (mGluR). Kainate and AMPA receptors are on glia and neurons; NMDA receptors are only on neurons. Table 7–1 shows the second messengers and ionic changes induced by activation of these receptors as well as some common agonists and antagonists. Binding of glutamate to AMPA or kainate receptors leads to fast excitatory postsynaptic potentials (EPSP); activation of the NMDA receptor leads to a slow EPSP. The mGluRs are involved in synaptic plasticity in the hippocampus and the cerebellum. The clinical application of drugs that modulate glutamatergic transmission is in its infancy because glutamate was not identified as a neurotransmitter until

the 1970s, more than 50 years after the discovery of chemical neurotransmission.

GABA & Glycine

GABA is the major inhibitory neurotransmitter throughout the brain; glycine is another inhibitory mediator, primarily in the brainstem and spinal cord. A vesicular GABA transporter moves GABA and glycine into synaptic vesicles. Following release of these inhibitory neurotransmitters, there is an active reuptake mechanism.

Table 7–1 shows the ionic changes induced by activation of GABA and glycine ionotropic receptors and some of their common agonists and antagonists. Activation of GABA$_A$ receptors mediates fast inhibitory postsynaptic potentials (IPSP); activation

TABLE 7-1 Pharmacological properties of some common neurotransmitters.

Neurotransmitter	Receptor	Second Messenger	Net Channel Effects	Agonists	Antagonists
Glutamate	AMPA		$\uparrow Na^+, K^+$	AMPA	CNQX, DNQX
	Kainate		$\uparrow Na^+, K^+$	Kainate	CNQX, DNQX
	NMDA		$\uparrow Na^+, K^+, Ca^{2+}$	NMDA	AP5, AP7
	$mGluR_1$	$\uparrow cAMP, IP_3, DAG$	$\downarrow K^+, \uparrow Ca^{2+}$	DHPG	
	$mGluR_5$	$\uparrow IP_3, DAG$	$\downarrow K^+, \downarrow Ca^{2+}$	Quisqualate	
	$mGluR_2, mGluR_3$	$\downarrow cAMP$	$\downarrow K^+, Ca^{2+}$	DCG-IV	
	$mGluR_4, mGluR_{6-7}$	$\downarrow cAMP$	$\downarrow Ca^{2+}$	L-AP4	
GABA	$GABA_A$		$\uparrow Cl^-$	Muscimol	Bicuculline, Gabazine, Picrotoxin
	$GABA_B$	$\uparrow IP_3, DAG$	$\uparrow K^+, \downarrow Ca^{2+}$	Baclofen	Saclofen
Glycine	Glycine		$\uparrow Cl^-$	Taurine, β-alanine	Strychnine
Acetylcholine	N_M		$\uparrow Na^+, K^+$	Nicotine	Tubocurarine, Gallamine triethiodide
	N_N		$\uparrow Na^+, K^+$	Nicotine, lobeline	Trimethaphan
	M_1, M_3, M_5	$\uparrow IP_3, DAG$	$\uparrow Ca^{2+}$	Muscarine, Bethanechol, Oxotremorine (M_1)	Atropine, Pirenzepine (M_1)
	M_2, M_4	$\downarrow cAMP$	$\uparrow K^+$	Muscarine, Bethanechol (M_2)	Atropine, Tropicamide (M_4)
Norepinephrine	α_1	$\uparrow IP_3, DAG$	$\downarrow K^+$	Phenylephrine	Prazosin, Tamsulosin
	α_2	$\downarrow cAMP$	$\uparrow K^+, \downarrow Ca^{2+}$	Clonidine	Yohimbine
	β_1	$\uparrow cAMP$	$\downarrow K^+$	Isoproterenol, Dobutamine	Atenolol, Esmolol
	β_2	$\uparrow cAMP$		Albuterol	Butoxamine
Serotonin	$5HT_{1A}$	$\downarrow cAMP$	$\uparrow K^+$	8-OH-DPAT	Metergoline, Spiperone
	$5HT_{1B}$	$\downarrow cAMP$		Sumatriptan	
	$5HT_{1D}$	$\downarrow cAMP$	$\downarrow K^+$	Sumatriptan	
	$5HT_{2A}$	$\uparrow IP_3, DAG$	$\downarrow K^+$	Dobutamine	Ketanserin
	$5HT_{2C}$	$\uparrow IP_3, DAG$		α-Methyl-5-HT	
	$5HT_3$		$\uparrow Na^+$	α-Methyl-5-HT	Ondansetron
	$5HT_4$	$\uparrow cAMP$	$\downarrow K^+$	5-Methoxytryptamine	

8-OH-DPAT, 8-hydroxy-N, N-dipropyl-2-aminotetralin; AMPA, α-amino-3-hydroxyl-5-methyl-4-isoxazole-propionate; DAG, diacylglycerol; DCG-IV, 2-(2, 3-dicarboxycyclopropyl) glycine; DHPG, 3-5 dihydroxyphenylglycine; IP_3, inositol triphosphate; L-AP4, 2-amino-4-phosphonobutyrate; NMDA, N-methyl-D-aspartate.

CLINICAL BOX 7-1

Excitotoxins

Glutamate is usually cleared from the brain's extracellular fluid by a Na^+-dependent uptake system in neurons and glia to maintain micromolar levels of the chemical in the extracellular fluid despite millimolar levels within neurons. Ischemia, anoxia, hypoglycemia, or trauma leads to an increase in extracellular levels of glutamate. Glutamate is an excitotoxin that can induce enough Ca^{2+} influx that the neuron dies. When a cerebral artery is occluded (stroke), the cells in the severely ischemic area die. The surrounding partially ischemic neurons may survive but lose their ability to maintain the transmembrane Na^+ gradient. The elevated levels of intracellular Na^+ prevent the reuptake of glutamate into glia and neurons; thus, glutamate accumulates and acts on NMDA receptors to cause excitotoxic damage and cell death in the penumbra, the region around the completely infarcted area. Excessive glutamate receptor activation may also contribute to the pathophysiology of neurodegenerative diseases such as amyotrophic lateral sclerosis (ALS), Parkinson disease, and Alzheimer disease.

THERAPEUTIC HIGHLIGHTS

Riluzole is a voltage-gated channel blocker that antagonizes NMDA receptors. It can slow the progression of impairment and modestly improve the life expectancy of patients with ALS. Another NMDA receptor antagonist memantine slows the progressive decline in patients with Alzheimer disease. Another NMDA receptor antagonist, amantadine, in conjunction with levodopa, improves function in patients with Parkinson disease.

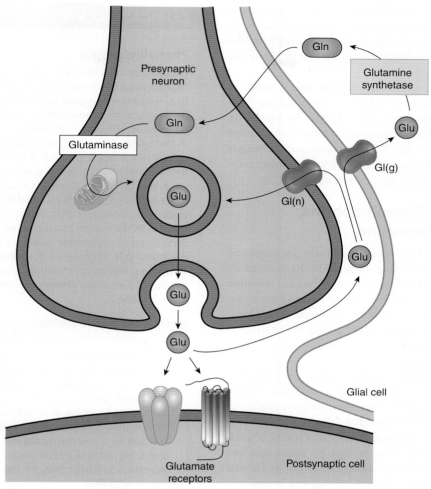

FIGURE 7–3 Biochemical events at a glutamatergic synapse. Glutamate (Glu) released into the synaptic cleft by Ca^{2+}-dependent exocytosis. Released Glu can act on ionotropic and G-protein–coupled receptors on the postsynaptic neuron. Synaptic transmission is terminated by the active transport of Glu via by a Na^+-dependent glutamate transporters located on membranes of the presynaptic terminal [Gt(n)] and glia [Gt(g)]. In glia, Glu is converted to glutamine (Gln) by the enzyme glutamine synthetase; Gln then diffuses into the nerve terminal where it is hydrolyzed back to Glu by the enzyme glutaminase. In the nerve terminal, Glu is highly concentrated in synaptic vesicles by a vesicular glutamate transporter.

of $GABA_B$ mediates both presynaptic (decreased Cl^- conductance) and slow postsynaptic inhibition (increased K^+ conductance). Glycine induces an IPSP and modulates excitatory neurotransmission by potentiating the action of glutamate on NMDA receptors.

The effects of activation of $GABA_A$ receptors are potentiated by benzodiazepines (eg, diazepam), which are effective as muscle relaxants, anticonvulsants, and sedatives. Barbiturates such as phenobarbital are effective anticonvulsants because they enhance $GABA_A$ receptor–mediated inhibition and suppress AMPA receptor–mediated excitation. The anesthetic actions of barbiturates (thiopental, pentobarbital, and methohexital) result from their actions as agonists at $GABA_A$ receptors and as neuromodulators of GABA transmission. In contrast, inhaled anesthetics act by inhibiting NMDA and AMPA receptors. Glycine's actions are antagonized by strychnine. The clinical picture of convulsions and muscular hyperactivity produced by strychnine emphasizes the importance of postsynaptic inhibition in normal neural function.

Acetylcholine

Acetylcholine is the neurotransmitter at the neuromuscular junction, in autonomic ganglia, and in all postganglionic parasympathetic and some postganglionic sympathetic nerve-target organ junctions. It is also found in the basal forebrain complex (septal nuclei and nucleus basalis), which projects to the hippocampus and neocortex, and the pontomesencephalic cholinergic complex, which projects to the dorsal thalamus and forebrain. These systems are involved in regulation of sleep-wake states, learning, and memory.

Acetylcholine is stored in small, clear synaptic vesicles in high concentration in the terminals of cholinergic neurons. It is synthesized there from choline and acetyl-CoA by choline acetyltransferase (Figures 7–1 and 7–2). The choline is transported from the extracellular space into the nerve terminal via a Na^+-dependent choline transporter. It is then transported from the cytoplasm into vesicles by a vesicle-associated transporter and is released when a nerve impulse triggers the influx of Ca^{2+} into the nerve terminal. Acetylcholinesterase in the synaptic cleft rapidly hydrolyzes acetylcholine to choline and acetate to terminate the actions of acetylcholine.

Nicotinic ionotropic receptors are found in skeletal muscle at the neuromuscular junction (N_M) and on autonomic ganglia (N_N). There are five types of muscarinic (M_1–M_5) GPCRs located on glands and smooth muscle. Both nicotinic and muscarinic receptors are also found in the CNS. Table 7–1 shows the second messengers and ionic changes induced by activation of these cholinergic receptors and some of their common agonists and antagonists.

Catecholamines: Norepinephrine, Epinephrine, & Dopamine

Norepinephrine is released by most sympathetic postganglionic neurons; both norepinephrine and epinephrine are secreted by the adrenal medulla. Noradrenergic neurons in the locus coeruleus innervate the spinal cord, cerebellum, several nuclei of the hypothalamus, thalamus, basal telencephalon, and neocortex. Dopaminergic neurons in the substantia nigra project to the striatum in the basal ganglia; those in the midbrain ventral tegmental area project to the prefrontal cortex.

Norepinephrine, epinephrine, and dopamine are formed by hydroxylation and decarboxylation of the amino acid tyrosine (Figures 7–1 and 7–2). Most of the tyrosine is of dietary origin, but some is formed from phenylalanine. Phenylalanine hydroxylase is found primarily in the liver (**Clinical Box 7–2**). Tyrosine is transported into catecholaminergic neurons via a Na^+-dependent carrier. Its conversion to dihydroxy-phenylalanine (dopa) by tyrosine hydroxylase in the cytoplasm is the rate-limiting step in catecholamine synthesis. Dopa decarboxylase converts dopa to dopamine in the cytoplasm. Dopamine is then transported into the vesicle by vesicular monoamine transporters where it is converted to norepinephrine by dopamine β-hydroxylase. An action potential triggers the expulsion of norepinephrine and co-transmitters like ATP and peptides.

Norepinephrine and other amines can also be carried by vesicular monoamine transporters. Some CNS neurons and adrenal medullary cells contain the cytoplasmic enzyme phenylethanolamine-N-methyltransferase, which catalyzes the conversion of norepinephrine to epinephrine. In these cells, norepinephrine leaves the vesicles, is converted to epinephrine in the cytoplasm, and then enters other vesicles for storage until it is released by exocytosis.

Epinephrine and norepinephrine act on various subtypes of α- and β-adrenergic receptors (adrenoceptors); dopaminergic receptors are divided into D_1-like (D_1 and D_5) and D_2-like (D_2, D_3, and D_4) receptors. All catecholaminergic receptors are GPCR. Table 7–1 shows the second messengers and ionic changes induced by activation of adrenoceptors and some of their common agonists and antagonists. At many synapses, activation of α_1-adrenoceptors is excitatory to the postsynaptic target. In contrast, at many synapses, activation of α_2-adrenoceptors inhibits the postsynaptic target. Overstimulation of D_2 receptors and D_4

CLINICAL BOX 7–2

Phenylketonuria

Phenylketonuria (PKU) is an inborn error of metabolism and characterized by severe intellectual disability; it is often due to a mutation of the gene for phenylalanine hydroxylase on the long arm of chromosome 12. The cognitive impairment is due to accumulation of phenylalanine and its derivatives in the blood. PKU can also be caused by tetrahydrobiopterin (BH4) deficiency. BH4 is a cofactor for phenylalanine hydroxylase, tyrosine hydroxylase, and tryptophan hydroxylase. BH4 deficiency also leads to catecholamine and serotonin deficiencies. BH4 is essential for the synthesis of nitric oxide (NO), so severe BH4 deficiency can lead to impairment of NO formation and increased oxidative stress in the CNS. Blood phenylalanine levels are usually determined in newborns in North America, Australia, and Europe; if PKU is diagnosed, dietary interventions should be started before the age of 3 weeks to prevent the development of an intellectual disability.

THERAPEUTIC HIGHLIGHTS

PKU can usually be treated successfully by markedly reducing the amount of phenylalanine in the diet. This means restricting the intake of high-protein foods such as milk, eggs, cheese, meats, and nuts. In individuals with a BH4 deficiency, treatment can include BH4, levodopa, and 5-hydroxytryptophan in addition to a low-phenylalanine diet. The US Food and Drug Administration approved the drug sapropterin, a synthetic BH4, for the treatment of some people with PKU.

receptors may contribute to the pathophysiology of schizophrenia (**Clinical Box 7–3**).

Reuptake of norepinephrine via a norepinephrine transporter (NET) is a major mechanism to terminate its actions. Active reuptake of dopamine occurs via a Na^+- and Cl^--dependent dopamine transporter. Catecholamines are metabolized to biologically inactive products by oxidation and methylation via monoamine oxidase (MAO) and catechol-O-methyltransferase (COMT). Vanillylmandelic acid is the major catecholamine metabolite found in the urine of humans.

Serotonin

Tryptophan is transported into the serotonergic nerve terminal by a Na^+-dependent aromatic L-amino acid transporter (Figure 7–1). The rate-limiting step in the synthesis of serotonin (5-hydroxytryptamine; 5-HT) is the conversion of tryptophan to 5-hydroxytryptophan by tryptophan hydroxylase (Figure 7–2). This is then converted to serotonin by the aromatic L-amino acid decarboxylase. Serotonin is transported into the vesicles by vesicular monoamine transporters. After its release, serotonin

CLINICAL BOX 7–3

Schizophrenia

Schizophrenia is associated with deficits of multiple brain systems that alter an individual's inner thoughts and their interactions with others. Individuals with schizophrenia experience hallucinations, delusions, and racing thoughts (positive symptoms) as well as apathy, difficulty dealing with novel situations, and little spontaneity or motivation (negative symptoms). Worldwide, 1–2% of the population lives with schizophrenia. A combination of genetic, biologic, cultural, and psychologic factors contributes to the illness. A defect in the mesocortical system (eg, overstimulation of limbic D_2 dopamine receptors), contributes to the development of some of the symptoms of schizophrenia. Brain levels of D_2 receptors are elevated in individuals with schizophrenia; there is a positive correlation between the antischizophrenic activity of many drugs and their ability to block D_2 receptors. Several recently developed antipsychotic agents are weak antagonists of D_2 receptors, but they bind to D_4 receptors. Ongoing research is assessing whether these receptors are abnormal in individuals with schizophrenia.

THERAPEUTIC HIGHLIGHTS

Since the mid-1950s antipsychotic drugs (eg, chlorpromazine and haloperidol) have been used to treat schizophrenia. In the 1990s, new "atypical" antipsychotics (eg, clozapine) were developed; they reduce psychotic symptoms, hallucinations, suicidal behavior, and breaks with reality. Clozapine has greater affinity for D_4 receptors than the other dopamine receptors. A potential adverse side effect is agranulocytosis (a loss of the white blood cells) that impairs the ability to fight infections. Other atypical antipsychotics do not cause agranulocytosis (eg, risperidone, olanzapine, quetiapine, ziprasidone, and aripiprazole).

---

reuptake occurs via the relatively selective serotonin transporter (SERT). Once serotonin is returned to the nerve terminal, it is either taken back into the vesicles or is inactivated by MAO to form 5-hydroxyindoleacetic acid (5-HIAA). This substance is the principal urinary metabolite of serotonin; urinary output of 5-HIAA is an index of the rate of serotonin metabolism in the body.

Serotonin is in highest concentration in blood platelets and in the gastrointestinal tract. It is also found within the brainstem in the raphe nuclei, which project to a wide portion of the CNS (eg, hypothalamus, limbic system, neocortex, cerebellum, and spinal cord).

Serotonin acts on various subtypes of 5-HT receptors (5-HT$_1$–5-HT$_7$); all except 5-HT$_3$ are GPCR and affect adenylyl cyclase or phospholipase C (Table 7–1). Serotonin receptors are found at both presynaptic and postsynaptic sites. Tricyclic antidepressants inhibit the reuptake of serotonin by blocking SERT. Selective serotonin uptake inhibitors (SSRIs) such as fluoxetine are widely used in the treatment of depression (Clinical Box 7–4).

Large Molecule Neurotransmitters

Substance P is a polypeptide containing 11 amino acid residues that is found in the intestine, some peripheral nerves, and many parts of the CNS. It is one of a family of polypeptides called tachykinins that includes neurokinin A and neurokinin B. There are three neurokinin receptors (NK$_1$–NK$_3$); all are GPCR. Substance P is the preferred ligand for NK$_1$ receptors in the CNS, and activation of this receptor increases the formation of IP$_3$ and DAG. Substance P is highly concentrated in the endings of primary afferent neurons in the spinal cord, and it is the mediator at the first synapse in the pathways for pain transmission in the dorsal horn. In the intestine, it is involved in peristalsis. Some centrally active NK$_1$ receptor antagonists have antidepressant activity, and they are used as antiemetics in patients undergoing chemotherapy.

The brain and the gastrointestinal tract contain receptors that bind morphine. The endogenous ligands for these receptors include two closely related opioid peptides (enkephalins): met-enkephalin and leu-enkephalin. Enkephalins are found in the substantia gelatinosa and have analgesic activity when injected into the brainstem; they also decrease intestinal motility. There are three classes of opioid receptors (μ, κ, and δ) which differ in physiologic effects and affinity for various opioid peptides (Table 7–2).

Neuropeptide Y is a polypeptide that is abundant throughout the brain and the autonomic nervous system; it acts on Y$_1$–Y$_8$ receptors; except for Y$_3$, these are GPCR. Activation of the GPCR mobilizes Ca^{2+} and inhibits adenylyl cyclase. Neuropeptide Y acts within the CNS to increase food intake; Y$_1$ and Y$_5$ receptor antagonists may be used to treat obesity. It also acts in the periphery to cause vasoconstriction and on heteroreceptors on postganglionic sympathetic nerve terminals to reduce the release of norepinephrine.

CHAPTER SUMMARY

- Major neurotransmitters include glutamate, GABA, glycine, acetylcholine, norepinephrine, serotonin, and opioids.
- The amino acid glutamate is the main excitatory transmitter in the CNS. There are two major types of glutamate receptors: metabotropic (GPCR) and ionotropic (ligand-gated ion channels receptors, including kainate, AMPA, and NMDA).
- GABA is the major inhibitory mediator in the brain. There are three subtypes of GABA receptors: GABAA and GABAC (ligand-gated ion channel) and GABAB (G-protein–coupled).

CLINICAL BOX 7–4

Major Depression

According to the National Institutes of Mental Health, nearly 21 million Americans over the age of 18 have a mood disorder that includes major depressive disorder, dysthymia, and bipolar disease. The largest group is those with major depression. Major depression has a median age of onset of 32 years and is more prevalent in women than men. Symptoms of major depression include depressed mood, anhedonia, loss of appetite, insomnia or hypersomnia, restlessness, fatigue, feelings of worthlessness, diminished ability to think or concentrate, and recurrent thoughts of suicide. Typical depression is characterized by feelings of sadness, early-morning awakenings, decreased appetite, restlessness, and anhedonia. Symptoms of atypical depression include pleasure-seeking behavior and hypersomnia.

The precise cause of depression is unknown, but genetic factors likely contribute as well as a role of central monoamines (norepinephrine, serotonin, and dopamine). The hallucinogenic agent lysergic acid diethylamide (LSD) is a central 5-HT$_2$ receptor agonist. The transient hallucinations produced by this drug were discovered when the chemist who synthesized it inhaled some by accident. Its discovery drew attention to the correlation between behavior and variations in brain serotonin content. 3,4-Methylenedioxymethamphetamine (MDMA or Ecstasy) is a drug of abuse that produces euphoria followed by difficulty in concentrating and depression. The drug causes release of serotonin followed by serotonin depletion; the euphoria may be due to the release and the later symptoms to the depletion.

THERAPEUTIC HIGHLIGHTS

In cases of typical depression, drugs such as fluoxetine (Prozac), which are selective serotonin reuptake inhibitors (SSRIs), are effective as antidepressants. SSRIs are also used to treat anxiety disorders. In atypical depression, SSRIs are often ineffective. Instead, monoamine oxidase inhibitors (MAOIs) such as phenelzine and selegiline are effective as antidepressants. However, they have adverse consequences including hypertensive crisis if the patient ingests large quantities of products high in tyramine, which include aged cheese, processed meats, avocados, dried fruits, and red wines (especially Chianti). Since atypical depression may result from a decrease in both serotonin and dopamine, drugs acting more generally on monoamines have been developed. These drugs, called atypical antidepressants, include bupropion, which resembles amphetamine and increases both serotonin and dopamine levels in the brain. Bupropion is also used as smoking cessation therapy.

The GABAA and GABAB receptors are widely distributed in the CNS.

- Acetylcholine is found at the neuromuscular junction, in autonomic ganglia, and in postganglionic parasympathetic nerve-target organ junctions and a few postganglionic sympathetic nerve-target junctions. It is also found in the CNS. There are two types of cholinergic receptors: muscarinic (GPCR) and nicotinic (ligand-gated ion channel receptors).

- Catecholamines (norepinephrine, epinephrine, and dopamine) are found in the brain; norepinephrine is also the major neuurotransmitter released by sympathetic postganglionic neurons. Norepinephrine and epinephrine act on α- and β-adrenoceptors; they are GPCR, and each has multiple forms. Dopamine acts on dopaminergic receptors; all are GPCRs.

TABLE 7–2 Physiologic effects produced by stimulation of opioid receptors.

Receptor	Endogenous Opioid Peptide Affinity	Effect
μ	Endorphins > Enkephalins > Dynorphins	Supraspinal and spinal analgesia Respiratory depression Constipation Euphoria Sedation Increased secretion of growth hormone and prolactin Miosis
κ	Enkephalins > Endorphins and Dynorphins	Supraspinal and spinal analgesia Diuresis Sedation Miosis Dysphoria
γ	Dynorphins > > Endorphins and Enkephalins	Supraspinal and spinal analgesia

MULTIPLE-CHOICE QUESTIONS

For all questions, select the single best answer unless otherwise directed.

1. A medical student is doing a research project in a neurophysiology laboratory that is studying the neuromuscular junction. As a first experiment, he tested the effects of three different drugs on the potential recorded from the skeletal muscle during stimulation of the nerve to the skeletal muscle. Drug A enhanced the response, drug B blocked the response, and drug C did not alter the potential in the skeletal muscle. Drugs A, B, and C might be the following types of drugs, respectively.
   A. An acetylcholinesterase inhibitor, a muscarinic receptor antagonist, and a nicotinic receptor agonist
   B. A nicotinic receptor agonist, a GPCR antagonist, and a muscarinic receptor agonist

C. A glycine receptor antagonist, a GABA receptor agonist, and a glutamate receptor agonist

D. A glutamate receptor agonist, a glutamate receptor antagonist, and a GABA reuptake inhibitor

E. An acetylcholinesterase inhibitor, a nicotinic receptor antagonist, and a muscarinic receptor antagonist

2. A medical student is studying transmission through autonomic ganglia. She studied the effects of two different drugs on the activity of a postganglionic neuron. Drug A induced an EPSP in the postganglionic neuron, and drug B blocked the EPSP produced by electrical stimulation of a preganglionic nerve. Drugs A and B might be the following drugs, respectively.
   A. Glutamate and glycine
   B. Nicotine and atropine
   C. Strychnine and atenolol
   D. Nicotine and trimethaphan
   E. Acetylcholine and phenylephrine

3. An MD/PhD candidate was planning to study patients diagnosed with schizophrenia for her doctoral research. In preparation for writing her thesis proposal, she was reviewing the literature to determine which brain pathways or neurons might be defective in these patients, which types of neurotransmitters and receptors contribute to the symptoms of the disease, and what drugs are used to treat schizophrenia. Her search of the literature would lead to the following information:
   A. The nigrostriatal pathway is defective, increased release of dopamine acting on metabotropic D_2 receptors might lead to symptoms of schizophrenia, and dopamine receptor antagonists are effective in treatment of the disease.
   B. The mesocortical pathway is defective, increased release of dopamine acting on metabotropic D_4 receptors might lead to symptoms of schizophrenia, and atypical antipsychotic drugs are effective in the treatment of the disease.
   C. The mesocortical pathway is defective, decreased release of GABA preventing the activation of $GABA_A$ ionotropic receptors might lead to symptoms of schizophrenia, and benzodiazepines are effective in the treatment of the disease.
   D. Midbrain raphe neurons are defective, decreased release of serotonin preventing the activation of $5-HT_2$ metabotropic receptors might lead to symptoms of schizophrenia, and selective serotonin reuptake inhibitors are effective in the treatment of the disease.
   E. Locus coeruleus neurons are defective, increased norepinephrine release acting on α_2-adrenoceptors might lead to symptoms of schizophrenia, and MAO inhibitors are effective in the treatment of the disease.

4. A 27-year-old man was brought to the emergency department by a friend who suspected he had overdosed on a drug. Upon arrival at the emergency department, he had depressed respiration, miosis, and reduced consciousness. Based on these symptoms, what drug did the individual likely take and what is its mechanism of action?
   A. Haloperidol acting as a D_2 receptor agonist
   B. Lysergic acid diethylamide (LSD) acting as a $5-HT_2$ receptor antagonist
   C. An opioid acting on as a δ and κ receptor agonist
   D. Ecstasy acting as a serotonin reuptake inhibitor
   E. An opioid acting as a μ-opioid receptor agonist

5. A 38-year-old woman was referred to a psychiatrist after telling her primary care physician that she had difficulty sleeping (awakening at 4 AM frequently for the past few months) and a lack of appetite causing a weight loss of over 20 lb. She also said she no longer enjoyed going out with her friends or doing volunteer service for underprivileged children. What type of drug is her doctor most likely to suggest as an initial step in her therapy?
   A. A serotonergic receptor antagonist
   B. A selective serotonin reuptake inhibitor
   C. An inhibitor of monoamine oxidase (MAO)
   D. An amphetamine-like drug
   E. A drug that causes an increase in both serotonin and dopamine

6. A 55-year-old woman had been receiving long-term treatment with phenelzine for her atypical depression. After she consumed Chianti wine, aged cheddar cheese, processed meats, and dried fruits one night at a party, the following symptoms developed: a severe headache, chest pain, rapid heartbeat, enlarged pupils, increased sensitivity to light, and nausea. What is the most likely cause of these symptoms?
   A. The foods were contaminated with botulinum toxin.
   B. She had a myocardial infarction.
   C. She experienced a migraine headache.
   D. She had an adverse reaction to the mixture of alcohol with her antidepressant.
   E. She had a hypertensive crisis from eating foods high in tyramine while taking a monoamine oxidase inhibitor for her depression.

7. A 72-year-old man was admitted to intensive care after having a stroke in his primary motor cortex. There was evidence for cell death in the brain region surrounding the stroke. A potential contributing factor for this is
   A. reduced levels of intracellular Na^+ in these neurons prevented the release of glutamate.
   B. an NMDA receptor-induced influx of large amounts of Ca^{2+} into neurons caused by excessive amounts of glutamate in the synaptic cleft.
   C. glycine released by neurons damaged by the stroke acts as an excitotoxin on the NMDA receptors on surrounding neurons.
   D. these neurons lost their normal excitatory drive when the stroke destroyed their presynaptic input.
   E. excessive levels of GABA in the region led to sustained postsynaptic inhibition.

8. A full-term infant boy is delivered without complications and has normal APGAR scores. Routine newborn screening tests reveal elevated levels of phenylalanine in his blood, leading to a diagnosis of phenylketonuria (PKU). What is the likely outcome if a dietary intervention with restricted intake of high-protein foods is not initiated by the age of three weeks?
   A. Development of cholestasis
   B. Development of neonatal seizures
   C. Malformation of the enteric nervous system
   D. Autism
   E. Profound intellectual disability

9. A medical student was doing research on drug that produces euphoria (possibly due to release of serotonin) followed by

depression (possibly due to depletion of serotonin). What drug has these characteristics?

A. 3,4-Methylenedioxymethamphetamine
B. Lysergic acid diethylamide
C. N,N-dimethyltryptamine
D. Haloperidol
E. Amphetamine

10. For the past several years, an unemployed 29-year-old had been experiencing a mix of hallucinations, delusions, racing thoughts, apathy, and a lack of spontaneity or motivation. His partner has been very concerned and insisted that he go to a local clinic to be examined. What is a likely diagnosis and what is a potential therapeutic strategy?

A. Adverse side effects of using LSD, central 5-HT$_2$ receptor agonist
B. Anxiety disorder, selective serotonin reuptake inhibitor
C. Adverse side effects of using amphetamine, norepinephrine reuptake inhibitor
D. Adverse reaction to his haloperidol therapy, terminate use of haloperidol immediately
E. Schizophrenia, clozapine

ANSWERS

1. The best answer is **E.** The motor neuron releases acetylcholine that binds to a nicotinic receptor on the skeletal muscle end plate to increase N$^+$ and K$^+$ conductance to generate an end plate potential followed by an action potential in the skeletal muscle fiber and eventual muscle contraction. The duration of action of acetylcholine is very short but can be prolonged by the administration of an acetylcholinesterase inhibitor to prevent the hydrolysis of acetylcholine to choline and acetate. A nicotinic receptor antagonist will prevent the binding of the acetylcholine released by nerve stimulation to the nicotinic receptor, thus preventing a response in the skeletal muscle. There are no muscarinic receptors in the neuromuscular junction, thus a muscarinic receptor agonist will not alter the response to electrical stimulation. This also rules out option **A** as the best answer; this option is also incorrect because administration of a nicotinic receptor agonist would activate the muscle. Option **B** can be ruled out because the receptors at the neuromuscular junction are ionotropic receptors not GPCR. Options **C** and **D** are ruled out because the neuromuscular junction does not contain excitatory or inhibitory amino acid receptors.

2. The best answer is **D.** Preganglionic neurons release acetylcholine on nicotinic receptors on postganglionic neurons in sympathetic and parasympathetic ganglia. Nicotine (or acetylcholine) is an example of a nicotinic receptor agonist and trimethaphan is a nicotinic receptor antagonist. Autonomic ganglia do not have excitatory and inhibitory amino acid receptors thus it would not be activated by glutamate or strychnine or inhibited by glycine (rules out options **A** and **C**). Since atropine is a muscarinic receptor antagonist, it would not prevent the EPSP in the postganglionic neuron (rules out option **B**). Preganglionic nerve terminals contain adrenoceptors that modulate neurotransmitter release, but neither a β-adrenoceptor antagonist (atenolol) nor a α$_1$-adrenoceptor agonist (phenylephrine) would block the response to stimulation of the preganglionic neuron (rules out options **C** and **E**).

3. The best answer is **B.** A defect in the dopaminergic mesocortical system is responsible for the development of at least some of the symptoms of schizophrenia which includes hallucinations, delusions, and racing thoughts (positive symptoms) as well as apathy, difficulty dealing with novel situations, and little spontaneity or motivation (negative symptoms). Although brain levels of D$_2$ receptors are elevated in individuals with schizophrenia; several recently developed drugs atypical antipsychotic drugs (eg, clozapine) bind to D$_2$ receptors to only a limited degree. Since they bind to D$_4$ receptors, current research is addressing the possibility that D$_4$ receptors are abnormal in individuals with schizophrenia. A reduction in the levels of dopamine within the nigrostriatal pathway is the basis for Parkinson disease (rules out option **A**). Decreased release of GABA would increase excitability within the CNS and can contribute to seizure activity but not the symptoms of schizophrenia (rules out option **C**). There are many serotonergic receptors throughout the limbic system; these receptors receive input from the midbrain raphe nuclei. In contrast to drugs used to treat schizophrenia, many drugs that are effective in the treatment of depression or anxiety alter serotonergic neurotransmission (rules out option **D**). Noradrenergic neurons in the locus coeruleus innervate the spinal cord, cerebellum, hypothalamus, and neocortex; changes in noradrenergic pathways are not linked to the symptoms of schizophrenia (rules out option **E**).

4. The best answer is **E.** Depressed respiration, miosis, and reduced consciousness are classic signs of opioid intoxication. There are three types of opioid receptors: μ, δ, and κ. Activation of κ-opioid receptors causes miosis and sedation but not respiratory depression; activation of δ-opioid receptors leads to analgesia. Thus, the symptoms noted are most indicative of activation of the μ-opioid receptor (rules out option **C**). Haloperidol is D$_2$ receptor antagonist (not an agonist) that is used to reduce the positive symptoms of schizophrenia (see Question 3 above); although some symptoms of overdose are similar to that of opioids (sedation, respiratory depression), a major symptom is muscle rigidity and tremor (rules out option **A**). LSD binds to a variety of receptors (dopaminergic, serotonergic, and adrenergic) and acts as an agonist; it causes excessive wakefulness and hallucinations (rules out option **B**). Ecstasy causes the release of serotonin and euphoria followed by serotonin depletion and depression (rules out option **E**).

5. The best answer is **B.** The signs listed are characteristic of typical depression which is commonly treated with a selective serotonin reuptake inhibitor (SSRI) such as fluoxetine (Prozac). Since depression may be linked with reduced levels of serotonin, a serotonergic receptor antagonist would not be an effective therapy (rules out option **A**). MAO inhibitors as well as drugs that increase both serotonin and dopamine levels (eg, bupropion) are used to treat atypical depression which presents with pleasure-seeking behavior and hypersomnia (rules out options **C** and **E**). Amphetamine-like drugs are a substrate for NET block the reuptake of norepinephrine; they are CNS stimulants that have restricted therapeutic use in the US (rules out option **D**).

6. The best answer is **E.** Phenelzine is an MAO inhibitor that has been associated with adverse consequences including "hypertensive crisis" and the responses noted above if the patient ingests large quantities of products high in tyramine (eg, aged cheese, processed meats, avocados, dried fruits, and

red wines). The exact mechanism of this adverse event is not known, but it may be related to the displacement of norepinephrine from synaptic vesicles. Some of the symptoms could be due to myocardial infarction, but headache and sensitivity to light are not (rules out option **B**). Botulinum is a toxin that prevents release of GABA and glycine in the CNS and acetylcholine in the neuromuscular junction; it causes spastic paralysis (rules out option **A**). A migraine headache is not typically associated with chest pain and tachycardia (rules out option **C**). Symptoms of mixing alcohol and antidepressants include drowsiness, dizziness, and suicidal thoughts (rules out option **D**).

7. The best answer is **B**. When a cerebral artery is occluded (stroke), the cells in the severely ischemic area die. The surrounding partially ischemic neurons may survive but lose their ability to maintain the transmembrane Na^+ gradient. The elevated levels of intracellular Na^+ (rules out option **A**) prevent the reuptake of glutamate into glia and neurons. Glutamate is an excitotoxin so when high levels of it are present in the synaptic cleft, it kills cells by overstimulation of NMDA receptors and an influx of Ca^{2+} into neurons. Glycine is an inhibitory neurotransmitter not an excitotoxin (rules out option **C**). Loss of excitatory drive or sustained inhibitory input would make the neurons quiescent but would not kill them (rules out options **D** and **E**).

8. The best answer is **E**. PKU is an inborn error of metabolism and characterized by severe intellectual disability. Causes include a mutation of the gene for phenylalanine hydroxylase or tetrahydrobiopterin (BH4) deficiency; the cognitive impairment is due to accumulation of phenylalanine and its derivatives in the blood. Neonatal cholestasis is due to the accumulation of bile in the bloodstream (rules out option **A**). There are various causes of neonatal seizures including metabolic disorders and intracranial infections (rules out option **B**). Malformations of the enteric nervous result from congenital disorders and are diagnosed by histopathology or rectal biopsies (rules out option **C**). The causes of autism are unknown but may include genetic and environmental factors; no simple blood test can be used to diagnose it (rules out option **D**).

9. The best answer is **A**. 3,4-Methylenedioxymethamphetamine (MDMA or Ecstasy) is a drug of abuse that produces euphoria followed by difficulty in concentrating and depression. It causes the release of serotonin followed by serotonin depletion; the euphoria may be due to the release and the later symptoms to the depletion. Lysergic acid diethylamide (LSD) is a hallucinogenic agent that is a central 5-HT_2 receptor agonist (rules out **B**). N,N-dimethyltryptamine (DMT) is a serotonergic hallucinogenic drug that is a derivative of tryptamine and may act as an agonist at 5-HT_{2A} and 5-HT_{2C} receptors (rules out option **C**). Haloperidol is an antipsychotic drug that is an antagonist at dopaminergic receptors (rules out option **D**). Amphetamine causes release of dopamine as well as norepinephrine in the brain, and it causes a schizophrenia-like psychosis (rules out option **E**).

10. The best answer is **E**. Individuals with schizophrenia experience hallucinations, delusions, and racing thoughts (positive symptoms) as well as apathy, difficulty dealing with novel situations, and little spontaneity or motivation (negative symptoms). Since the 1990s, new "atypical" antipsychotics have been used (eg, clozapine) which reduces psychotic symptoms, hallucinations, suicidal behavior, and breaks with reality. LSD is a potent mood-altering drug and often leads to loss of appetite, sleeplessness, dry mouth, tremors, delusions and visual hallucinations. Since LSD is a 5-HT2 receptor agonist, one would not use another agonist for therapy (rules out option **A**). Symptoms of anxiety disorder include feelings of panic and fear, inability to relax, sweaty hands, and palpitations; anxiety does not cause hallucinations and delusions (rules out option **B**). Amphetamine causes release of dopamine as well as norepinephrine in the brain, and it causes a schizophrenia-like psychosis; but a norepinephrine reuptake inhibitor would magnify the effects of the drug (rules out option **C**). Common adverse side effects of haloperidol (an antipsychotic drug) include difficulty speaking, trembling, restlessness, and uncontrolled movements of the arms and legs, twitches in the eye, lips, and tongue (rules out option **D**).

SECTION II CENTRAL & PERIPHERAL NEUROPHYSIOLOGY

INTRODUCTION TO NEUROPHYSIOLOGY

The central nervous system (CNS) can be likened to a computer processor that is the command center for the functions of the body. The peripheral nervous system is like a set of cables that transfers critical data from the CNS to the body and then feeds back information from the body to the CNS. This sophisticated "computer system" continually makes appropriate adjustments to its inputs and outputs to allow us to react and adapt to changes in the external and internal environments (sensory systems), to maintain posture, permit locomotion, and use the fine motor control in our hands to create pieces of art (somatomotor system), to maintain homeostasis (autonomic nervous system), to regulate the transitions between sleep and wakefulness (consciousness), and to allow us to recall past events and to communicate with the outside world (higher cortical functions). This section on neurophysiology will describe the fundamental properties and integrative capabilities of neural systems that allow for the exquisite control of this vast array of physiologic functions. Medical fields such as neurology, neurosurgery, and clinical psychology build on the foundation of neurophysiology.

There are over 600 known neurologic disorders. Nearly 50 million people in the United States and a 1 billion people worldwide have experienced damage to the central or peripheral nervous system. Each year, nearly 7 million people die of a neurologic disorder or its complications. Neurologic disorders include genetic disorders (eg, Huntington disease), demyelinating diseases (eg, multiple sclerosis), developmental disorders (eg, cerebral palsy), degenerative diseases (eg, Parkinson disease and Alzheimer disease), an imbalance of neurotransmitters (eg, depression, anxiety, and eating disorders), trauma (eg, spinal cord and head injury), and convulsive disorders (eg, epilepsy). There are also neurologic complications associated with cerebrovascular problems (eg, stroke) and exposure to neurotoxic chemicals (eg, nerve gases, mushroom poisoning, and pesticides).

Advances in stem cell biology and brain imaging techniques, a greater understanding of the basis for synaptic plasticity of the brain, a wealth of new knowledge about the regulation of receptors and the release of neurotransmitters, and the detection of genetic and molecular defects that lead to neurologic problems have advanced our understanding of the pathophysiologic basis for neurologic disorders. They have also led to better therapies to prevent or reverse the physiologic deficits resulting from neurologic disorders.

Somatosensory Neurotransmission: Touch, Pain, & Temperature

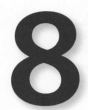

O B J E C T I V E S

After studying this chapter, you should be able to:

- Describe the cutaneous receptors that mediate the sensations of touch, pressure, pain, and temperature.
- Explain the four attributes of a stimulus to sensory receptors.
- Explain acute and chronic pain, hyperalgesia, and allodynia.
- Describe referred pain.
- Compare the pathway that mediates sensory input from touch, proprioceptive, and vibratory senses to that mediating information from nociceptors and thermoreceptors.
- Describe processes involved in modulation of transmission in pain pathways.
- Identify drugs used for relief of pain, their mechanism of action, and the rationale for their use.

INTRODUCTION

Sensory receptors are transducers that change a particular form of energy in the environment into electrical signals, which are then relayed to the central nervous system (CNS) which can then interpret the information received. Table 8–1 is a list of different types of receptors in the skin, muscles, and specialized organs like the eye and ear and the specific energy (stimulus) to which they

respond. The emphasis in this chapter is on the characteristics of cutaneous mechanoreceptors, thermoreceptors, and nociceptors; the way they generate impulses in afferent neurons; and the central pathways that mediate or modulate information from these receptors. Subsequent chapters cover sensory receptors in the eye, ear, tongue and nose, and skeletal muscles and joints.

■ TOUCH, PRESSURE, PAIN, & TEMPERATURE RECEPTORS

Touch and pressure are sensed by four types of mechanoreceptors that are specialized dendritic endings of Aα and Aβ afferent nerve fibers (Figure 8–1). Meissner corpuscles respond to changes in texture and slow vibrations; Merkel cells respond to sustained pressure and touch; Ruffini corpuscles respond to sustained pressure; and Pacinian corpuscles respond to deep pressure and fast vibration.

Pain and temperature sensations arise from thinly myelinated Aδ fibers or unmyelinated C fibers in skin and deep tissue.

Mechanical nociceptors respond to strong pressure (eg, from a sharp object). Thermal nociceptors are activated by skin temperatures above 42°C or by severe cold. Chemically sensitive nociceptors respond to various chemicals such as bradykinin, histamine, high acidity, and environmental irritants. Polymodal nociceptors respond to combinations of these stimuli.

Activation of Aδ fibers releases glutamate to elicit a rapid response (first or fast pain) responsible for the discriminative aspect of pain (ability to localize the site and intensity of the stimulus). Activation of C fibers releases both glutamate and substance P to elicit a delayed second or slow pain; this is the

TABLE 8–1 **Principle sensory modalities.**

Sensory Receptor	Receptor Class	Modality	Stimulus
Meissner corpuscles	Cutaneous mechanoreceptor	Touch	Tap, flutter 5–40 Hz
Hair follicle receptors	Cutaneous mechanoreceptor	Touch	Motion
Pacinian corpuscles	Cutaneous mechanoreceptor	Touch	Deep pressure, vibration 60–300 Hz
Merkel cells	Cutaneous mechanoreceptor	Touch	Touch, pressure
Ruffini corpuscles	Cutaneous mechanoreceptor	Touch	Sustained pressure
Muscle spindles	Mechanoreceptor	Proprioception	Stretch
Golgi tendon organ	Mechanoreceptor	Proprioception	Tension
Cold and warmth receptors	Thermoreceptor	Temperature	Thermal
Chemical, thermal, and mechanical nociceptors (or polymodal)	Chemoreceptor, thermoreceptor, and mechanoreceptor	Pain	Chemical, thermal, and mechanical
Rods, cones	Photoreceptor	Vision	Light
Hair cells (cochlea)	Mechanoreceptor	Hearing	Sound
Hair cells (semicircular canals)	Mechanoreceptor	Balance	Angular acceleration
Hair cells (otolith organs)	Mechanoreceptor	Balance	Linear acceleration, gravity
Olfactory sensory neuron	Chemoreceptor	Smell	Chemical
Taste buds	Chemoreceptor	Taste	Chemical

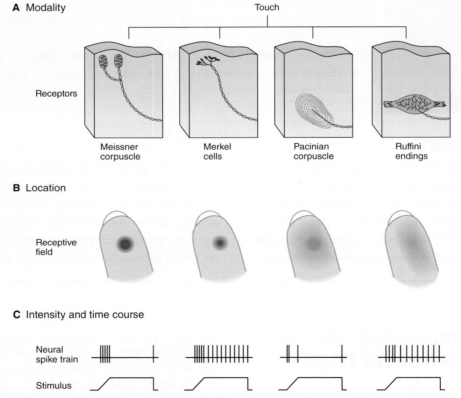

FIGURE 8–1 **Sensory systems encode four elementary attributes of stimuli: modality, location (receptive field), intensity, and duration (timing). (A)** The human hand has four types of mechanoreceptors; their combined activation produces the sensation of contact with an object. Selective activation of Merkel cells and Ruffini endings causes sensation of steady pressure; selective activation of Meissner and Pacinian corpuscles causes tingling and vibratory sensation. **(B)** Location of a stimulus is encoded by spatial distribution of the population of receptors activated. A receptor fires only when the skin close to its sensory terminals is touched. These receptive fields of mechanoreceptors (shown as red areas on fingertips) differ in size and response to touch. Merkel cells and Meissner corpuscles provide the most precise localization as they have the smallest receptive fields and are most sensitive to pressure applied by a small probe. **(C)** Stimulus intensity is signaled by firing rates of individual receptors; duration of stimulus is signaled by time course of firing. The spike trains indicate action potentials elicited by pressure from a small probe at the center of each receptive field. Meissner and Pacinian corpuscles adapt rapidly, the others adapt slowly. (Modified with permission from Kandel ER, Schwartz JH, Jessell TM [editors]: *Principles of Neural Science*, 4th ed. New York, NY: McGraw-Hill; 2000.)

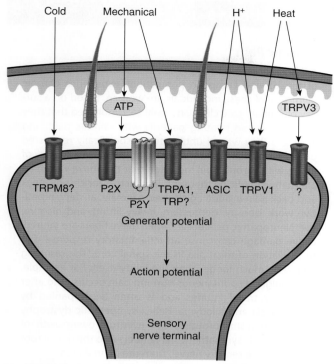

FIGURE 8–2 Receptors on nociceptive unmyelinated nerve terminals in the skin. Nociceptive stimuli (eg, heat) can activate some receptors directly due to transduction of the stimulus energy by receptors (eg, transient receptor potential (TRP) channel TRPV1) or indirectly by activation of TRP channels on keratinocytes (eg, TRPV3). Nociceptors (eg, mechanoreceptors) can also be activated by the release of intermediate molecules (eg, ATP). ASIC, acid-sensitive ion channel; P2X, ionotropic purinoceptor; P2Y, G-protein–coupled purinergic receptor.

dull, intense, diffuse, and unpleasant feeling associated with a noxious stimulus.

Noxious thermal, mechanical, or chemical stimuli activate ionotropic or G-protein–coupled receptors (GPCR) on nociceptive nerve terminals (**Figure 8–2**). Transient receptor potential (TRPV1) receptors are activated by intense heat, acids, and chemicals (eg, capsaicin). Noxious mechanical, cold, and chemical stimuli activate TRPA1 receptors. Acid-sensing ion channel (ASIC) receptors are activated by pH changes within a physiologic range. Some stimuli release intermediate molecules that activate receptors on the nerve ending; stimulation of nociceptive mechanical receptors releases adenosine triphosphate (ATP) that acts on purinergic (P2X, P2Y) receptors. Tyrosine receptor kinase A (TrkA) is activated by nerve growth factor (NGF) released with tissue damage. Nerve endings have receptors that respond to immune mediators released due to tissue injury (inflammatory pain); these include B_1 and B_2 receptors (bradykinin), prostanoid receptors (prostaglandins), and cytokine receptors (interleukins).

Innocuous cold receptors are on Aδ and C nerve endings, and innocuous warmth receptors are on C fibers. The threshold for activation of warmth receptors is 30°C; their firing rate increases as the skin temperature rises to 46°C. Cold receptors are inactive at 40°C, but

steadily increase their firing rate as skin temperature fall to 24°C. The firing rate of cold receptors decreases until the temperature reaches 10°C; below that temperature, they are inactive and cold becomes an effective local anesthetic. Moderate cold activates TRPM8 receptors; TRPV4 receptors are activated by warm temperatures up to 34°C; TRPV3 receptors respond to temperatures of 35–39°C.

■ MODALITY, LOCATION, INTENSITY, & DURATION

All sensory systems code for four elementary attributes of a stimulus: modality, location, intensity, and duration (Figure 8–1). Modality is the type of energy (mechanical, thermal, electromagnetic, or chemical) transmitted by a stimulus. Location is the site of origin of the stimulus on the body or space. Intensity is signaled by the response amplitude or frequency of action potentials generated. Duration is the time from start to end of a response in the receptor. The sensory component of a neurologic exam includes an assessment of sensory modalities for touch, proprioception, vibratory sense, and pain (**Clinical Box 8–1**).

Lateral inhibition enables localization of a stimulus. Sensory neurons whose receptors are at the periphery of the stimulus send less information to the CNS than the sensory neurons at the center of the stimulus. Lateral inhibition enhances the contrast between the center and periphery of a stimulated area so the brain can localize a sensory input; it underlies two-point discrimination (see Clinical Box 8–1). As a greater pressure is applied to the skin, the frequency of the action potentials in a single axon transmitting information to the CNS is increased. As the strength of a stimulus is increased, it can spread over a large area and activates the sense organs immediately in contact and those in the surrounding area (recruitment).

If a stimulus of constant strength is maintained on a sensory receptor, the firing rate of the sensory nerve declines over time (receptor adaptation or desensitization). Meissner and Pacinian corpuscles are rapidly adapting (phasic) receptors; Merkel cells and Ruffini endings (also muscle spindles and nociceptors) are slowly adapting (tonic) receptors.

■ PAIN

One of the main reasons an individual seeks medical advice is because he or she is in pain. Painful stimuli generally initiate potent withdrawal and avoidance responses. Pain differs from other sensations in that it sounds a warning that something is wrong, preempts other signals, and is associated with an unpleasant affect. It is very complex because when tissue is damaged, central nociceptive pathways are sensitized and reorganized, which leads to persistent or chronic pain (**Clinical Box 8–2**).

CLASSIFICATION OF PAIN

Pain is defined by the International Association for the Study of Pain (IASP) as, "an unpleasant sensory and emotional experience associated with actual or potential tissue damage, or described

CLINICAL BOX 8–1

Neurologic Exam

The size of the receptive fields for light touch can be measured by the two-point threshold test. In this procedure, the two points on a pair of calipers are simultaneously positioned on the skin to determine the minimum distance between the two caliper points that can be perceived as separate points of stimulation (two-point discrimination threshold). If the distance is very small, each caliper point is touching the receptive field of only one sensory neuron. If the distance between stimulation points is less than this threshold, only one point of stimulation can be felt. Thus, this is a measure of tactile acuity. The magnitude of two-point discrimination thresholds is smallest where touch receptors are most abundant. Stimulus points on the back, for instance, must be separated by at least 65 mm before they can be distinguished as separate, whereas on the fingertips two stimuli are recognized if they are separated by as little as 2 mm. Two-point discrimination is used to test the integrity of the dorsal column (medial lemniscus) system, the central pathway for touch and proprioception.

Vibratory sensibility is tested by applying a vibrating (128-Hz) tuning fork to the skin on the fingertip, tip of the toe, or bony prominences of the toes. The normal response is a "buzzing" sensation, most marked over bones; this sensation is mediated via touch receptors (Pacinian corpuscles) and dorsal column pathway. Degeneration of the spinal cord dorsal columns occurs in poorly controlled diabetes, pernicious anemia, vitamin B_{12} deficiencies, or early tabes dorsalis. An increased threshold for vibratory stimuli is an early symptom of this degeneration. Vibratory sensation and proprioception are closely related; when one is diminished, so is the other.

Stereognosis is the perception of the form and nature of an object without looking at it and depends on intact touch and pressure sensation; it is compromised with damage to the dorsal column pathway. Tactile agnosia is the inability to identify an object by touch. Stereognosia can be due to the failure to identify an object by sight (visual agnosia), sounds or words (auditory agnosia), color (color agnosia), or position of an extremity (position agnosia).

CLINICAL BOX 8–2

Chronic Pain

A 2009 report in *Scientific American* indicated that 10–20% of the US and European populations experience chronic pain; 59% of these individuals are women. Based on a survey of primary care clinicians, only 15% indicated that they felt comfortable treating patients with chronic pain; and 41% said they waited until patients specifically requested opioid pain killers before prescribing them. Nearly 20% of adults with chronic pain indicated that they have visited an alternative medicine therapist. Risk factors for chronic neck and back pain include aging, being female, anxiety, repetitive work, obesity, depression, heavy lifting, and nicotine use. Neuropathic pain occurs when nerve fibers are injured. Nerve damage can cause an inflammatory response due to activation of microglia in the spinal cord. The resulting pain lasts much longer than the injury itself. For example, in causalgia, a spontaneous burning pain occurs long after seemingly trivial injuries and is often accompanied by hyperalgesia and allodynia. Reflex sympathetic dystrophy may result from sprouting and eventual overgrowth of noradrenergic sympathetic nerve fibers into the dorsal root ganglia of the sensory nerves from the injured area.

THERAPEUTIC HIGHLIGHTS

Some current chronic pain therapies act directly on nociceptors or on sensory transduction. Capsaicin transdermal patches or creams reduce pain by exhausting the supply of substance P in nerves and by acting on TRPV1 receptors in the skin. Voltage-gated N-type Ca^{2+} channels on presynaptic terminals of sensory neurons are a target of some drugs used to treat pain, particularly neuropathic pain. Ziconotide, a voltage-gated N-type Ca^{2+} channel blocker, is used for intrathecal analgesia in patients with refractory chronic pain. Gabapentin is used to treat neuropathic and inflammatory pain and acts on voltage-gated Ca^{2+} channels. Topiramate and valproate, voltage-gated Na^+ channel blockers, are used to treat migraines. Another Na^+ channel blocker, carbamazepine, is the gold standard for treating trigeminal neuralgia. The last four drugs are anticonvulsants.

in terms of such damage." Nociception is defined as the unconscious activity induced by a harmful stimulus applied to sense receptors.

Pain can be classified as physiologic or acute pain and pathologic or chronic pain including inflammatory and neuropathic pain. Acute pain has a sudden onset and recedes during the healing process; it serves a protective mechanism as demonstrated by the withdrawal reflex. Chronic pain persists long after recovery from an injury and is often refractory to common analgesic agents, including nonsteroidal anti-inflammatory drugs (NSAIDs) and opioids. Chronic pain can result from nerve injury (neuropathic pain) including diabetic neuropathy, toxin-induced nerve damage, and ischemia.

HYPERALGESIA & ALLODYNIA

Hyperalgesia is an exaggerated response to a noxious stimulus, and allodynia is a sensation of pain in response to a normally innocuous stimulus. Both signify increased sensitivity of nociceptive fibers. Injured cells release chemicals such as K⁺ that directly depolarize nerve terminals, making nociceptors more responsive (sensitization). Injured cells also release bradykinin and substance P to further sensitize nociceptive terminals. The release of histamine from mast cells, serotonin (5-HT) from platelets, and prostaglandins from cell membranes contribute to the inflammatory process; they activate or sensitize nociceptors. Some released substances act by releasing another one (eg, bradykinin activates Aδ and C nerve endings and increases prostaglandin synthesis and release). Prostaglandin E$_2$ (a cyclooxygenase metabolite of arachidonic acid) is released from damaged cells to produce hyperalgesia; this is why NSAIDs (nonselective inhibitors of cyclooxygenase) alleviate pain.

Changes in the periphery and CNS contribute to chronic pain. NGF released by tissue damage is picked up by nerve terminals and transported retrogradely via activation of TrkA receptors to cell bodies in dorsal root ganglia. There NGF increases production of substance P and converts non-nociceptive neurons to nociceptive neurons (a phenotypic change). NGF also increases the expression of a tetrodotoxin-resistant voltage-gated sodium channel (Nav1.8) that is unique to dorsal root ganglia cells of nociceptive fibers.

Damaged nerve fibers undergo sprouting, so fibers from touch receptors synapse on dorsal horn neurons that normally receive only nociceptive input, contributing to allodynia. Substance P and glutamate release from nociceptive afferents causes excessive activation of NMDA (N-methyl-D-aspartate) receptors on spinal neurons ("wind-up") to increase activity in pain transmitting pathways. Microglia near afferent nerve terminals in the spinal cord are activated by the release of transmitters from sensory afferents; this leads to the release of proinflammatory cytokines and chemokines that modulate pain processing by increasing presynaptic release of neurotransmitters and postsynaptic excitability.

VISCERAL PAIN

Visceral pain is poorly localized, unpleasant, and associated with nausea and autonomic symptoms. Afferent fibers from visceral structures reach the CNS via sympathetic and parasympathetic nerves. Their cell bodies are located in the dorsal root and cranial nerve ganglia. The nociceptors in the walls of the viscera are sensitive to distension of the organ; the pain waxes and wanes (intestinal colic) as the intestine contracts and relaxes. When a visceral organ is inflamed or hyperemic, relatively minor stimuli cause severe pain, a form of hyperalgesia.

Irritation of a visceral organ can produce pain that is felt in a somatic structure some distance away (referred pain). Knowledge of the common sites of pain referral from visceral organs is of importance to a clinician. For example, cardiac pain is often referred to the inner aspect of the left arm, pain in the tip of the shoulder is caused by irritation of the central portion of the diaphragm, and pain in the testicle is due to distension of the ureter. Sites of reference are not stereotyped (eg, cardiac pain may be

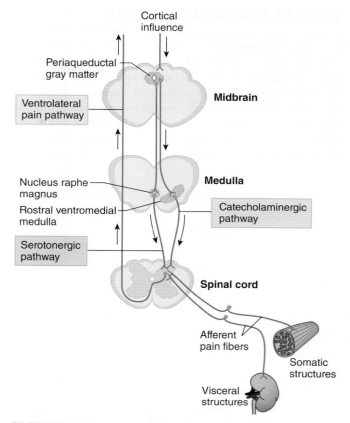

FIGURE 8–3 **Schematic illustration of the convergence-projection theory for referred pain and descending pathways involved in pain control.** The basis for referred pain may be convergence of somatic and visceral pain fibers on the same second-order neurons in the dorsal horn of the spinal cord that project higher brain regions. The periaqueductal gray is a part of a descending pathway that includes serotonergic neurons in the nucleus raphe magnus and catecholaminergic neurons in the rostral ventromedial medulla to modulate pain transmission by inhibition of primary afferent transmission in the dorsal horn.

referred to the right arm, abdominal region, back, neck, or jaw). The basis for referred pain may be convergence of somatic and visceral pain fibers on the same neurons in the dorsal horn that project to the thalamus and then to the somatosensory cortex (**Figure 8–3**).

■ SOMATOSENSORY PATHWAYS

The sensation evoked by impulses from a sensory receptor depends in part on the specific part of the brain it activates. The ascending sensory pathway that mediates touch, vibratory sense, and proprioception is the dorsal column (or medial lemniscal) pathway; that which mediates pain and temperature is the ventrolateral spinothalamic pathway.

DORSAL COLUMN PATHWAY

The dorsal column pathway mediates the sensations of touch, vibratory sense, and proprioception (**Figure 8–4A**). Fibers ascend ipsilaterally in the spinal dorsal columns and synapse in the medullary gracilis and cuneate nuclei. From here, fibers cross the midline and ascend in the medial lemniscus to end in the contralateral ventral posterior lateral (VPL) nucleus and related specific sensory thalamic relay nuclei. Fibers within this pathway are joined in the brainstem by fibers mediating sensation from

the head via the main sensory and mesencephalic nuclei of the trigeminal nerve.

The pathway is somatotopically organized throughout its extent; fibers from the sacral cord are the most medial and those from the cervical cord are the most lateral. Lower and upper body representation continues in the gracilis nucleus and cuneate nucleus, respectively; the medial lemniscus is organized dorsal to ventral representing neck to foot. VPL neurons relay sensory information in a highly specific way to the primary somatosensory cortex in the postcentral gyrus

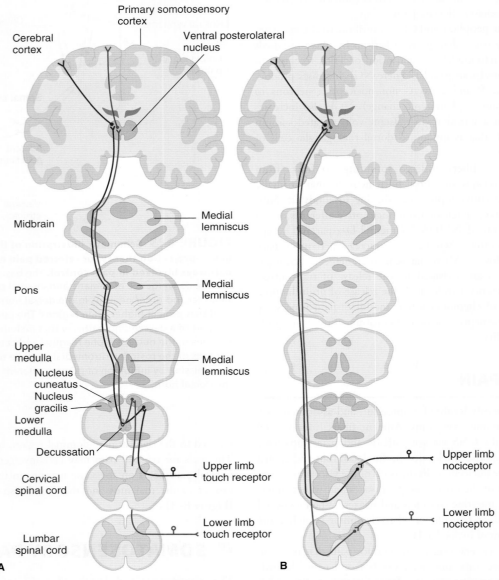

FIGURE 8–4 **Ascending tracts carrying sensory information from peripheral receptors to the cerebral cortex. (A)** Dorsal column pathway mediates touch, vibratory sense, and proprioception. Sensory fibers ascend ipsilaterally via the spinal dorsal columns to medullary gracilis and cuneate nuclei; from there the fibers cross the midline and ascend in the medial lemniscus to the contralateral thalamic ventral posterior lateral (VPL) and then to the primary somatosensory cortex. **(B)** Ventrolateral spinothalamic tract mediates pain and temperature. These sensory fibers terminate in the dorsal horn and projections from there cross the midline and ascend in the ventrolateral quadrant of the spinal cord to the VPL and then to the primary somatosensory cortex.

of the parietal lobe. The size of the cortical receiving area for impulses from a body part is proportional to the use of the part. The sensory association area (parietal cortex) and the secondary somatosensory cortex (lateral or sylvian fissure) help integrate sensory information and receive input from the primary somatosensory cortex.

VENTROLATERAL SPINOTHALAMIC TRACT

Fibers from nociceptors and thermoreceptors synapse on neurons in the dorsal horn of the spinal cord. The axons from these neurons cross the midline and ascend in the ventrolateral quadrant of the spinal cord to begin the ventrolateral spinothalamic pathway (Figure 8–4B). Fibers within this tract synapse in the VPL which projects to the primary somatosensory cortex; this pathway is responsible for the discriminative aspect of pain. The motivational-affective component of pain is relayed via dorsal horn neurons that synapse in the reticular formation of the brainstem (spinoreticular pathway) with projections to the centrolateral nucleus of the thalamus and then to the frontal lobe, limbic system, and insular cortex.

CORTICAL PLASTICITY & EFFECTS OF CNS LESIONS

Cortical plasticity occurs because connections of sensory units to the cortex have extensive convergence and divergence, with connections that can become weak with disuse and strong with use. PET scans document plastic changes, sometimes from one sensory modality to another. For example, tactile and auditory stimuli increase metabolic activity in the visual cortex in blind individuals; and deaf individuals respond faster and more accurately than normal individuals to moving stimuli in the visual periphery.

Clinical Box 8–1 describes some of the deficits noted after damage within the somatosensory pathways. Damage to the dorsal columns leads to ipsilateral loss of discriminative touch, vibration, and proprioception below the level of the lesion. Damage to the ventrolateral spinothalamic pathway leads to contralateral loss of pain and temperature sensation below the level of the lesion. An infarct in the thalamus can lead to a loss of sensation. Thalamic pain syndrome is sometimes seen during recovery from a thalamic infarct and is characterized by chronic pain on the side of the body contralateral to the stroke.

Lesions of the primary somatosensory cortex do not abolish somatic sensation. Irritation of this region causes paresthesia or an abnormal sensation of numbness and tingling on the contralateral side of the body. Lesions impair the ability to localize noxious stimuli in time, space, and intensity. Damage to the cingulate cortex impairs the recognition of the aversive nature of a noxious stimulus.

■ MODULATION OF PAIN TRANSMISSION

ROLES OF SPINAL CORD, BRAINSTEM, & PERIAQUEDUCTAL GRAY

Transmission in nociceptive pathways can be interrupted by actions within the dorsal horn of the spinal cord at the site of sensory afferent termination. Rubbing or shaking an injured area decreases the pain due to an injury. The activation of cutaneous mechanosensitive afferents may reduce the responsiveness of dorsal horn neurons to their input from nociceptive afferent terminals. This may explain why transcutaneous electrical nerve stimulation (TENS) can be effective for pain relief; this method uses electrodes to activate $A\alpha$ and $A\beta$ fibers in the vicinity of the injury.

Opioids exert their analgesic effects at various places in the CNS, including the spinal cord and dorsal root ganglia (Figure 8–5). Endogenous opioid peptides (eg, enkephalin, dynorphin) are released from interneurons to act on the terminals of nociceptive fibers and on dendrites of dorsal horn neurons. Activation of the postsynaptic opioid receptors hyperpolarizes the dorsal horn interneuron by causing an increase in K^+ conductance. Activation of the presynaptic opioid receptors decreases Ca^{2+} influx, resulting in a decrease in release of glutamate and substance P. Together these actions reduce the duration of the EPSP in the dorsal horn neuron. Activation of opioid receptors on dorsal root ganglia cell bodies also contributes to reduced transmission from nociceptive afferents.

Patients who receive long-term pain management with morphine may become resistant to the drug, requiring progressively higher doses for pain relief. This acquired tolerance is different from addiction, which refers to a psychological craving. Psychological addiction rarely occurs when morphine is used to treat chronic pain, provided the patient does not have a history of drug abuse. Clinical Box 8–3 describes mechanisms involved in motivation and addiction.

Morphine and endogenous opioid peptides also act in the midbrain periaqueductal gray (PAG) to induce analgesia. The PAG is a part of a descending pathway that modulates pain transmission by inhibition of primary afferent transmission in the dorsal horn (Figure 8–3). These PAG neurons activate neurons in the nucleus raphe magnus and rostral ventromedial medulla that project to the spinal cord where they release serotonin and norepinephrine, respectively, to inhibit the activity of dorsal horn neurons that receive input from nociceptive afferent fibers. This inhibition involves the activation of the dorsal horn enkephalin-containing interneurons.

STRESS-INDUCED ANALGESIA

Soldiers wounded in battle often feel no pain until the battle is over; this is an example of stress-induced analgesia. The release of endogenous cannabinoids such as 2-arachidonoylglycerol and anandamide may contribute to stress-induced analgesia. These chemicals can act on at least two types of GPCRs (CB_1 and CB_2). CB_1 receptors are

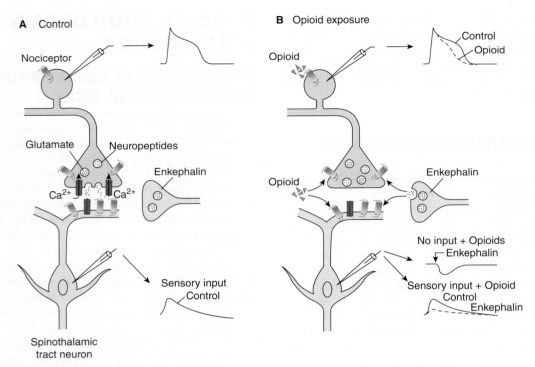

FIGURE 8–5 **Actions of opioids to reduce sensory transmission in pain pathways at the level of the dorsal root ganglion (DRG) and spinal cord dorsal horn region. (A)** Activation of a nociceptor leads to the release of glutamate and neuropeptides from its nerve terminals that synapse on spinothalamic tract projection neurons. This leads to the depolarization (activation) of spinothalamic tract projection neurons. Enkephalin-containing (ENK) interneurons mediate their effects via opioid receptors on the terminals of nociceptive afferent fibers and on dendrites of dorsal horn neurons to exert both presynaptic and postsynaptic inhibition. **(B)** The action of an opioid (eg, morphine) within the DRG is to decrease Ca^{2+} influx leading to a decrease in the duration of the invoked action potential in the nociceptive neuron and a reduction in transmitter release from the nociceptive neuron onto a neuron in the dorsal horn. Opioids also hyperpolarize the membrane of dorsal horn neuron by activation of a K^+ conductance; opioids also decrease the amplitude of the excitatory postsynaptic potential (EPSP) produced by stimulation of nociceptors.

CLINICAL BOX 8–3

Motivation & Addiction

Addiction, defined as the repeated compulsive use of a substance despite negative health consequences, can be produced by various drugs. According to the World Health Organization, over 76 million people worldwide suffer from alcohol abuse and over 15 million suffer from drug abuse. Addictive drugs include opioids (eg, morphine and heroin), cocaine, amphetamine, alcohol, cannabinoids, and nicotine. Each of these drugs increase the amount of dopamine available to act on D_3 receptors in the nucleus accumbens to stimulate the brain's reward system, which is comprised of the main dopamine pathways of the brain (mesolimbic pathway), the ventral tegmental area, and nucleus accumbens. Long-term addiction involves the development of tolerance or the need for increasing amounts of a drug to produce a high. Withdrawal produces psychological and physical symptoms. For opioid addicts, the relapse rate in the first year is about 80%. Relapse often occurs on exposure to sights, sounds, and situations that were previously associated with drug use. Even a single dose of an addictive drug facilitates release of excitatory neurotransmitters in brain areas concerned with memory. The medial frontal cortex, hippocampus, and amygdala are concerned with memory, and they all project via excitatory glutamatergic pathways to the nucleus accumbens. Absence of

β-arrestin-2 blocks tolerance but has no effect on dependence; β-arrestin-2 is a member of a family of proteins that inhibit heterotrimeric G-proteins by phosphorylating them.

THERAPEUTIC HIGHLIGHTS

Withdrawal symptoms and cravings associated with addiction to opioids can be reversed by treatment with various drugs that act on the same CNS receptors as morphine and heroin (eg, methadone and buprenorphine). The US Federal Drug Administration has approved the use of three drugs for treatment of alcohol abuse: naltrexone, acamprosate, and disulfiram. Naltrexone is an opioid receptor antagonist that blocks the reward system and the craving for alcohol. Acamprosate may reduce the withdrawal effects associated with alcohol abuse. Disulfiram causes an accumulation of acetaldehyde by preventing the full degradation of alcohol. This leads to an unpleasant reaction to alcohol ingestion (eg, flushing, nausea, and palpitations). Topiramate, a Na^+ channel blocker, is showing promise in clinical trials of alcohol addiction.

located in many brain regions, and activation of these receptors accounts for the euphoric actions of cannabinoids. CB_2 receptors are expressed in activated microglia under various pathologies that are associated with chronic neuropathic pain. Binding of an agonist to CB_2 receptors on microglia reduces the inflammatory response and has an analgesic effect.

CHAPTER SUMMARY

- Touch and pressure are sensed by mechanoreceptors that are innervated by $A\alpha$ and $A\beta$ sensory afferents. They include Meissner corpuscles (respond to changes in texture and slow vibrations), Merkel cells (respond to sustained pressure and touch), Ruffini corpuscles (respond to sustained pressure), and Pacinian corpuscles (respond to deep pressure and fast vibrations).

- Nociceptors and thermoreceptors are free nerve endings on C fibers or $A\delta$ fibers in skin and deep tissues. These nerve endings have various types of receptors that are activated by noxious chemical (eg, TRPV1 and ASIC), mechanical (eg, P2X, P2Y and TRPA1), and thermal (eg, TRPV1) stimuli. Chemical mediators (eg, bradykinin, prostaglandin, serotonin, and histamine) released in response to tissue injury directly activate or sensitize nociceptors.

- Converting a receptor stimulus to a recognizable sensation is termed "sensory coding." All sensory systems code for four elementary attributes of a stimulus: modality, location, intensity, and duration.

- Acute pain has a sudden onset, recedes during the healing process, and serves as an important protective mechanism. Chronic pain is persistent and caused by nerve damage; it is often associated with hyperalgesia (an exaggerated response to a noxious stimulus) and allodynia (a sensation of pain in response to an innocuous stimulus).

- Visceral pain is poorly localized, unpleasant, and associated with nausea and autonomic symptoms. It often radiates (or is referred) to other somatic structures perhaps due to convergence of somatic and visceral nociceptive afferent fibers on the same spinothalamic tract neurons.

- Discriminative touch, proprioception, and vibratory sensations are relayed via the dorsal column (medial lemniscus) pathway to the VPL in the thalamus and primary somatosensory cortex. Pain and temperature sensations are mediated via the ventrolateral spinothalamic tract, which projects to the VPL and cortex. The discriminative aspect of pain results from activation of the primary somatosensory cortex; the motivational-affective component of pain is from activation of the frontal lobe, limbic system, and insular cortex.

- Transmission in pain pathways is modulated by endogenous opioids that act in the PAG, brainstem, spinal cord, and dorsal root ganglia. Descending pain modulating pathways include neurons in the PAG, nucleus raphe magnus, rostral ventromedial medulla, and locus coeruleus.

- New pain therapies focus on synaptic transmission in nociception and peripheral sensory transduction. Capsaicin transdermal patches or creams acts on TRPV1 receptors; lidocaine blocks Nav1.8, which is uniquely associated with nociceptive neurons in dorsal root ganglia; ziconotide blocks voltage-gated N-type Ca^{2+} channels; gabapentin blocks voltage-gated Ca^{2+} channels; topiramate blocks a Na^+ channel blocker; NMDA

receptor antagonists can be coadministered with an opioid to reduce tolerance to an opioid.

MULTIPLE-CHOICE QUESTIONS

For all questions, select the single best answer unless otherwise directed.

1. A 28-year-old man was seen by a neurologist because he had experienced prolonged episodes of tingling and numbness in his right arm. He underwent a neurologic exam to evaluate the integrity of his sensory nervous system, including a measure of the ability to discern that two pointed objects touching the skin are indeed two distinct points. What does this two-point discrimination test measure and what central nervous system pathway is being evaluated?
   A. Nociceptive sensitivity and the spinothalamic pathway
   B. Stereognosis and medial lemniscal pathway
   C. Stereognosis and spinoreticular pathway
   D. Tactile acuity and the dorsal column pathway
   E. Tactile acuity and the spinothalamic pathway

2. A 62-year-old man had a gunshot wound to the left side of his head that damaged the top portion of the lateral postcentral gyrus very close to the midline of the brain (posterior portion of the paracentral lobule). What sensory modalities will likely be compromised by his injury?
   A. He will lose the sense of touch and the discriminative aspect of pain over his left hand and wrist.
   B. He will lose the sense of touch, pressure, and vibration over his right forearm.
   C. He will lose the sense of touch and the discriminative aspect of pain over his right leg and hip.
   D. He will lose the sense of touch over his left leg and the discriminative aspect of pain over his right leg.
   E. He will lose the sense of touch, pressure, and vibration but maintain the discriminative aspect of pain over his right leg.

3. A 27-year-old woman experienced pain in her jaw, especially when chewing that had increased in severity and frequency over the past 6 months and was not controlled by over-the-counter analgesics. Her physician prescribed a mixture of codeine and acetaminophen which initially provided considerable pain relief, but within a few weeks the severity and frequency of the pain increased. The doctor increased the dose of codeine. What is the most likely explanation for why the original dose of codeine no longer provided pain relief?
   A. She had acquired tolerance to the codeine.
   B. She had developed psychological addiction to codeine.
   C. She had developed physical dependence to codeine.
   D. Nociceptors in her facial nerve had developed sensitization to the codeine.

4. A 27-year-old woman experienced pain in her jaw, especially when chewing that had increased in severity and frequency over the past 6 months and was not controlled by over-the-counter analgesics. She was prescribed a mixture of codeine and acetaminophen; and although a social drinker, she decided to refrain from alcohol while taking the medication. After nearly 2 months of treatment and little if any relief, she decided to stop taking the medication. She drank two glasses of wine when out with friends that evening. Soon after that she developed abdominal cramping, nausea, vomiting, and

diarrhea. Which of the following is the most likely explanation for the appearance of these symptoms?
A. She had coincidentally developed the flu when she stopped taking her medication.
B. She had developed gastrointestinal toxicity from the acetaminophen.
C. She had developed physical dependence to codeine.
D. She had developed psychological dependence to codeine.
E. These are symptoms of an overdose of acetaminophen and codeine.

5. A resident in internal medicine is asked to give a presentation on referred pain to second year medical students. What is the definition of referred pain and what is a potential basis for it?
A. Referred pain is pain that originates within a visceral organ but is sensed as pain arising from a somatic structure. It may be due to the convergence of somatic and visceral nociceptive fibers on the same neurons in the dorsal horn that project to the thalamus and then to the somatosensory cortex.
B. Referred pain is pain that is referred to a body part that has been removed. It may result from the reorganization of the somatosensory cortex after the sensory input is cut off.
C. Referred pain is poorly localized pain from a visceral structure that is relayed to the central nervous system by branches of sensory neurons from the nearby skin or skeletal muscle. It may occur because the same nociceptive fiber transmits information from visceral and somatic structures to the spinal cord dorsal horn.
D. Referred pain resembles "fast pain" produced by noxious stimulation of the skin since it also originates from unmyelinated C fibers. It may result from the activation of sympathetic nerves to the visceral organ causing the release of chemicals into the circulation that sensitize nociceptors in the skin and skeletal muscle.

6. A resident in internal medicine is asked to give a presentation on referred pain to second year medical students. He explains the importance of recognizing the common sites of pain referral from each of the visceral organs. What might be the actual origin of the pain if it was referred to the left arm and jaw, the tip of the left shoulder, and in the testicle, respectively?
A. Appendicitis, myocardial infarction, and kidney stone
B. Myocardial infarction, pancreatitis, and irritation of the central portion of the diaphragm
C. Stomach ulcer, distension of the ureter, and hepatitis
D. Myocardial infarction, irritation of the central portion of the diaphragm, and distension of the ureter
E. Appendicitis, kidney stone, gastric cancer

7. A 64-year-old man had been experiencing severe pain in his right leg as a result of inoperable bone cancer. The pain is not controlled by opioids or other pain therapies. After trying many alternative therapies without success, a neurosurgeon performed a ventrolateral cordotomy which relieved the pain. This surgery was effective because it interrupted the
A. left dorsal column.
B. left ventrolateral spinothalamic tract.
C. right ventrolateral spinothalamic tract.
D. right medial lemniscal pathway.
E. a direct projection to the primary somatosensory cortex.

8. A 29-year-old woman had a spinal cord injury that resulted in a loss of touch, pressure, and vibration from his left leg and left arm. Pain and temperature sensitivity in all limbs was unchanged. Which part of the spinal cord was most likely damaged as a result of the injury?
A. Left gracilis fasciculus in the thoracic spinal cord
B. Right cuneate fasciculus in the upper lower cervical spinal cord
C. Upper cervical dorsal horn
D. Left dorsal column in the mid-cervical spinal cord
E. Right medial lemniscal pathway in the lower cervical spinal cord

9. A 50-year-old woman with uncontrolled diabetes was undergoing vibratory sensibility testing by applying a vibrating (128-Hz) tuning fork to the skin on the fingertip, tip of the toe, and bony prominences of the toes. What kind of receptors are activated by this stimulus?
A. Meissner corpuscles
B. Merkel cells
C. Pacinian corpuscles
D. Ruffini corpuscles
E. Mechanical nociceptors

10. Long after his arm had healed from third degree burns, a 47-year-old man experienced frequent episodes of pain that was not relieved by his current pain medications. He was entered into a clinical trial for a drug that acted on an ion channel receptor that is located exclusively on dorsal root ganglia of unmyelinated, small-diameter sensory fibers. What ion channel is this?
A. TRPVI
B. ASIC
C. Voltage-gated N-type Ca^{2+} channel
D. TrkA
E. Nav1.8

11. A 40-year-old man loses his right hand in a farm accident. Four years later, he has episodes of severe pain in the missing hand (phantom limb pain). A detailed PET scan study of his cerebral cortex might be expected to show
A. expansion of the right-hand area in his right primary somatosensory cortex.
B. expansion of the right-hand area in his left primary somatosensory cortex.
C. a metabolically inactive spot where his hand area in his left primary somatosensory cortex would normally be.
D. projection of fibers from neighboring sensory areas into the right-hand area of his right primary somatosensory cortex.
E. projection of fibers from neighboring sensory areas into the right-hand area of his left primary somatosensory cortex.

12. A 50-year-old man undergoes a neurologic exam that indicates loss of pain and temperature sensitivity, vibratory sense, and proprioception and weakness in the left arm. These symptoms could be explained by
A. a tumor on the right medial lemniscal pathway in the cervical spinal cord.
B. a peripheral neuropathy.
C. a tumor on the left medial lemniscal pathway in the sacral spinal cord.
D. a tumor affecting the left posterior paracentral gyrus.
E. a large tumor in the right lumbar ventrolateral spinal cord.

13. A medical student was doing research in a sensory neurophysiology laboratory. In preparation for his research, the principal investigator of the laboratory asked him to compare

the four basic attributes of a stimulus to sensory receptors. The four attributes of sensory coding are

A. modality, location, intensity, and duration.
B. adequate threshold, receptive field, adaptation, and projection.
C. adequate threshold, energy, sensation, and duration.
D. sensitization, discrimination, energy, and projection.
E. modality, adequate threshold, sensitivity, and location.

14. A 29-year-old man fell off of his bicycle and scraped the skin off of his elbow, enough to cause bleeding and pain. Over the next week he was careful not to bend his elbow a lot as each time he did so, it hurt. As the abrasion healed, he was able to regain full use of his arm. The type of pain he experienced after the fall and until the injury healed is best described as

A. neuropathic pain.
B. nociceptive pain.
C. chronic pain.
D. pathologic pain.

15. A 13-month-old boy, who had just recently learned to walk, stepped on hot coals left from a backyard cook-out at his family home. He did not cry and after standing there for several seconds he stepped off the coals and playfully walked away. His mother quickly picked him up and found severe burns on his feet. Which of the following is the most likely explanation of the child's behavior following stepping on the coals?

A. He does not have a functional withdrawal reflex.
B. He has a selective absence of TRPM8 receptors on the bottom of his feet.
C. He has a selective absence of TRPA1 receptors on the bottom of his feet.
D. He has congenital insensitivity to pain.
E. He has a high tolerance for pain.

16. A 23-year-old woman fell asleep on the beach while sunbathing. She awoke a few hours later and to find that she had a very bad sunburn. That evening while taking a shower, the lukewarm water (40°C) touching her back caused her to feel pain. What types of receptors were activated by the lukewarm water and why did she experience pain?

A. Thermal nociceptors and nociceptive pain
B. Thermal nociceptors and allodynia
C. Thermal nociceptors and hyperalgesia
D. Innocuous thermal receptors and hyperalgesia
E. Innocuous thermal receptors and allodynia

17. A medical student is working in a laboratory that studies modulation of transmission in nociceptive pathways. She is particularly interested in studying neurons in the brainstem that project to the spinal cord and release neurotransmitters that inhibit nociceptive transmission in the dorsal horn. What medullary regions is she likely to study and what neurotransmitters do they release in the dorsal horn?

A. Periaqueductal gray (endorphin) and rostral ventromedial medulla (serotonin)
B. Nucleus raphe magnus (serotonin) and rostral ventromedial medulla (norepinephrine)
C. Periaqueductal gray (enkephalin) and nucleus raphe magnus (serotonin)
D. Locus coeruleus (endorphin) and rostral ventromedial medulla (serotonin)
E. Periaqueductal gray (dynorphin) and rostral ventromedial medulla (norepinephrine)

ANSWERS

1. The best answer is **D.** The two-point threshold test measures the size of the receptive field for light touch which is a measure of tactile acuity. It is used to test the integrity of the dorsal column (medial lemniscus) system, the central pathway for touch and proprioception (rules out option **E**). Stereognosis is the perception of the form and nature of an object without looking at it (rules out options **B** and **C**) and also requires an intact dorsal column. Option **A** is ruled out since pain sensitivity, which requires an intact spinothalamic tract, is measured by asking a patient, with their eyes closed, if a stimulus to the skin is sharp (needle) or dull (brush).

2. The best answer is **C.** The lateral postcentral gyrus within the parietal lobe is the location of the primary somatosensory cortex, the sensory receptive area for the sense of touch and discriminative aspect of pain. This region is somatotopically organized with the lower part of the body (foot, leg, hip) represented in the posterior paracentral lobule and the upper body (chest, arm, and hand) represented in the upper postcentral gyrus (rules out **A** and **B**). The pathway for touch and pain are both crossed, so the primary somatosensory cortex on the left side of the brain represents the right side of the body (rules out **D** and **E**).

3. The best answer is **A.** There is a gradual reduction in the effectiveness of a narcotic analgesic (tolerance) with chronic administration of a therapeutic dose. Thus, to get an equivalent analgesic effect, a larger dose or increased frequency of administration is needed. Tolerance is different from addiction, which refers to a psychological craving and behavioral pattern characterized by compulsive use and overwhelming involvement in its procurement and use (rules out **B**). Physical dependence is a set of changes that cause a disturbance in the homeostatic set point if a drug is suddenly stopped (rules out **C**). Codeine would not increase sensitivity of nociceptor afferent fibers; in fact via its binding to μ-opioid receptors on the terminals of nociceptive fibers leads to a decrease in Ca^{2+} influx, resulting in a decrease in release of glutamate and substance P (rules out **D**).

4. The best answer is **C.** Although it is possible that she coincidentally developed the flu (option **A**), there is a physiological basis for the appearance of these symptoms. Physical dependence occurs when a narcotic analgesic is suddenly stopped, leading to signs of withdrawal which can include diarrhea, vomiting, tremors, abdominal cramps, irritability and insomnia, and drug craving and seeking behavior. Although not likely to occur after a single episode of moderate drinking, hepatotoxicity is associated with the use of acetaminophen in combination with alcohol (rules out option **B**). See the answer to Question 3 to rule out option **D**. Symptom of an overdose of acetaminophen and codeine include shallow breathing, drowsiness, miosis, and coma (rules out **E**).

5. The best answer is **A.** A general definition of referred pain is "pain in a part other than that in which the cause that produced it is situated." But it is commonly used with reference to pain that originates in a visceral organ and is "sensed" at a remote site (see Question 6 for examples). One explanation for the referral is the convergence of somatic and visceral nociceptive fibers on the same dorsal horn neurons. Option **B** is a definition of "phantom pain." Between 50% and 80% of amputees experience phantom sensations, usually pain, in the region of their amputated

limb. Phantom sensations may also occur after the removal of other body parts (eg, phantom tooth pain after extraction of a tooth). It may be due to reorganization of the brain after the sensory input is cut off. In patients who have had their leg amputated, the ventral posterior thalamic nucleus that once received input from the leg and foot now respond to stimulation of the stump (thigh). Pain of visceral origin is commonly poorly localized, but unlike the statement in option **C**, visceral organs have their own sensory fibers that travel with the sympathetic or parasympathetic nerves to that organ. Option **D** is ruled out because fast pain is mediated by lightly myelinated Aδ fibers; visceral referred pain is typically mediated via activation of unmyelinated C fibers. Also chemicals released from visceral organs mediate some cases of referred pain, but the chemicals can act locally to sensitize or activate the sensory fibers in the visceral organ not remote sites to induce the pain.

6. The best answer is **D.** Pain due to myocardial infarction commonly is referred to the left chest wall, left neck or jaw, left shoulder, or left arm. Pain due to irritation of the central portion of the diaphragm (eg, due to ruptured spleen, gallbladder, hepatitis which are organs that can push against the diaphragm) is referred to the tip of the left or right shoulder. Pain due to distension of the ureter (or a kidney stone) is referred to the testicle or flank radiating the groin. Appendicitis is referred to periumbilical area (rules out options **A** and **E**); pancreatitis is referred to the upper abdominal region (rules out option **B**); pain due to stomach ulcer or gastric cancer is referred to the epigastrium or mid-back between the scapulae (rules out **C** and **E**).

7. The best answer is **B.** Fibers in the ventrolateral spinothalamic tract (from the spinal dorsal horn to the thalamus) cross soon after entry of the afferent into the spinal cord; thus it relays nociceptive information from the opposite side of the body to the primary somatosensory cortex. Thus a ventrolateral cordotomy would need to be completed on the left side to interrupt nociceptive information from the right leg (rules out option **C**). Surgical section of the left or right dorsal column (medial lemniscal pathway) would interrupt transmission of touch, pressure, vibration, and proprioception from the left or side of the body, respectively (rules out options **A** and **D**). There is no pathway that projects directly (ie, monosynaptically) from the spinal cord to the primary somatosensory cortex (rules out option **E**).

8. The best answer is **D.** For a single site of injury to cause loss of sensation from both the upper and lower body, the lesion must be at a cervical level (entry of sensory information in the arm is C5-T2). Sensations of touch, pressure, and vibration from the left side are relayed ipsilaterally via the dorsal column (rules out **E**). A lesion of the left gracilis fasciculus in the thoracic spinal cord would interrupt information from the left leg but not the arm (rules out **A**); a lesion of the right cuneate fasciculus would interrupt transmission from the right arm but not the leg (rules out option **B**). The upper cervical dorsal horn would interrupt all sensory information (including nociception) mediated by sensory fibers entering at that level (rules out option **C**).

9. The best answer is **C.** Pacinian corpuscles respond to deep pressure and fast vibration. Other options are ruled out since Meissner corpuscles respond to changes in texture and slow vibrations (5–40 Hz); Merkel cells respond to sustained pressure and touch; Ruffini corpuscles respond to sustained pressure; and mechanical nociceptors respond to strong pressure (eg, from a sharp object).

10. The best answer is **E.** A tetrodotoxin-resistant voltage-gated sodium channel (Nav1.8) is uniquely associated with dorsal root ganglia cells from nociceptive afferents; these could be an excellent target for new pain therapies. TRPV1 and ASIC are located on sensory nerve endings in the periphery and respond to noxious stimuli such as heat and acids (rules out **A** and **B**). Voltage-gated N-type Ca²⁺ channels are located on presynaptic nerve terminals in the dorsal horn; the anticonvulsant (and analgesic) drug Ziconotide blocks these channels (rules out **C**). TrkA receptors are located on nerve fibers and may be activated to transport nerve growth factor from the site of nerve injury to the dorsal root ganglia where it can convert a non-nociceptive to a nociceptive neuron (rules out **D**).

11. The best answer is **E.** If a body part is amputated, the cortical representation of the neighboring body parts spreads into the cortical area that was formerly occupied by the representation of the amputated body part. Since representation in one side of the cortex is for body parts on the opposite side, all responses to changes on the right side can be ruled out (**A** and **D**). Since the afferent fibers from the limb are no longer intact, there is no ability for them to increase their projection area (rules out option **B**). A decrease in metabolic activity implies reduced activity which is the opposite of what would be expected by the description of this patient's presentation (rules out option **C**).

12. The best answer is **B.** The patient reports loss of both motor (weakness) and sensory loss from the same limb. This could be explained by damage to a peripheral nerve. Damage to the lumbar or sacral cord would not impact sensation or motor control of the arm (rules out **A** and **E**). Damage to the medial lemniscus would interrupt sensory but not motor control of the left arm (rules out **C**). Since both sensory (ascending) and motor (descending) pathways cross below the cortex, any cortical damage would have to be on the right side (rules out option **D**).

13. The best answer is **A.** All sensory systems code for four elementary attributes of a stimulus: modality, location, intensity, and duration. Modality is the type of energy or stimulus (mechanical, thermal, electromagnetic, or chemical) to which the receptor responds; location is the site on the body or space where the stimulus originated; intensity is the magnitude of the stimulus; and duration is the time from start to end of a stimulus. Options **B** through **E** can be ruled out although they all provide some information about activation of sensory receptors. The adequate stimulus is the form of energy (modality) to which a receptor is most sensitive. The receptive field of an individual sensory neuron is the extent of the region (location) from which a stimulus will activate the neuron. Adaptation refers to changes in the sensitivity or responsiveness of receptors during a sustained stimulus; receptors can be divided into rapidly and slowly adapting types, depending on the rate of decay of the generator potential. Projection refers to the pathway that transmits information from the receptor to the central nervous system. Sensation is the conscious awareness of a stimulus. Sensitization is a process in which repeated stimulation of a receptor results in the progressive amplification of a response; this contributes to the development of chronic pain.

14. The best answer is **B.** Nociceptive pain (also called physiological or acute pain) has a sudden onset due to tissue injury

and recedes during the healing process; it serves an important protective mechanism. Neuropathic pain is due to damage to a peripheral or central nerve; there is no indication of nerve damage in this scenario (rules out **A**). Chronic pain (also called pathologic pain) persists long after recovery from an injury (rules out C and D).

15. The best answer is **D**. Congenital insensitivity to pain is a rare condition in which an individual does not feel pain; it is due to mutations in the *SCN9A* gene. Options **A** can be ruled out since it is more than simply a lack of this spinal reflex that protects the body from damaging stimuli; this child had no reaction to a noxious stimulus. Options **B** and **C** can be ruled out as these deficiencies reflect an absence of sensitivity to moderate cold and noxious mechanical, cold, and chemical stimuli, respectively. Option **E** can be ruled out because he did not even have an automatic withdrawal reflex.

16. The best answer is **E**. A temperature of 40°C activates innocuous thermal receptors; sensing pain in response to an innocuous stimulus is called allodynia. The threshold for activation of thermal nociceptors is above 42°C (rules out options **A**, **B**, and **C**). Hyperalgesia is an exaggerated response to a noxious stimulus (rules out option **D**).

17. The best answer is **B**. Neurons in the nucleus raphe magnus and rostral ventromedial medulla project to the spinal cord where they release serotonin and norepinephrine, respectively (rules out option **A**), to inhibit the activity of dorsal horn neurons that receive input from nociceptive afferent fibers. The periaqueductal gray is in the midbrain not the medulla (rules out options **C** and **E**) and is also involved in pain modulation; neurons in this region release enkephalin to activate neurons in the nucleus raphe magnus and rostral ventromedial medulla. Pontine locus coeruleus neurons also release norepinephrine to modulate pain transmission (rules out option **D**).

Vision

- Describe the various parts of the eye and list the functions of each.
- Describe the organization of the retina.
- Explain how light rays in the environment are brought to a focus on the retina and the role of accommodation in this process.
- Define hyperopia, myopia, astigmatism, presbyopia, and strabismus.
- Describe the electrical responses produced by rods and cones, and explain how these responses are produced.
- Describe the electrical responses and function of bipolar, horizontal, amacrine, and ganglion cells.
- Trace the neural pathways that transmit visual information from the rods and cones to the visual cortex.
- Define and explain dark adaptation and visual acuity.
- Describe the neural pathways involved in color vision.
- Identify the muscles involved in eye movements.

INTRODUCTION

The eye is often compared to a camera, with the cornea acting as the lens, the pupillary diameter functioning like the aperture of the camera, and the retina serving as the film. However, the eye, especially the retina, is far more sophisticated than even the most expensive camera. Within its protective casing, each eye has a layer of photoreceptors that respond to light, a lens system that focuses the light on these receptors, and a system of nerves that conducts impulses from the receptors to the brain. This chapter reviews the way the components of the visual system operate to set up conscious visual images.

■ ANATOMY OF THE EYE

The major parts of the eye are the sclera (protective covering), cornea (transfer light rays), choroid (nourishment), retina (photoreceptor cells), crystalline lens, and a pigmented iris containing circular and radial muscle fibers that constrict and dilate the pupil, respectively, to control the amount of light reaching the retina (**Figure 9–1**). The iris, ciliary body, and choroid are collectively called the uvea. The lens is held in place by the suspensory ligament (zonule) attached to the ciliary body. The eye is well protected from injury by the bony walls of the orbit. The cornea is moistened and kept clear by tears from the lacrimal gland that empty via the lacrimal duct into the nose. Blinking helps keep the cornea moist.

The aqueous humor, which flows through the pupil and fills the anterior chamber, is produced in the ciliary body by diffusion and active transport from plasma. It is reabsorbed through a network of trabeculae into the canal of Schlemm (filtration angle). Obstruction of this outlet leads to increased intraocular pressure, a risk factor for

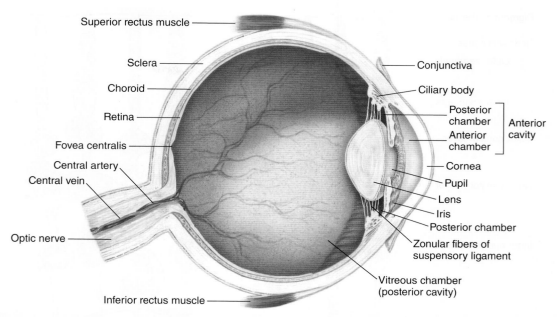

FIGURE 9–1 **A schematic of the anatomy of the eye.** (Reproduced with permission from Fox SI. *Human Physiology*, 10th ed. New York, NY: McGraw-Hill; 2008.)

glaucoma (**Clinical Box 9–1**). The posterior chamber is a narrow aqueous-containing space between the iris, zonule, and the lens. The vitreous chamber is the space between the lens and the retina that is filled with a clear gelatinous material (vitreous humor).

RETINA & PHOTORECEPTORS

The outer nuclear layer of the retina contains photoreceptors (rods and cones) and the inner nuclear layer contains bipolar cells, horizontal cells, and amacrine cells (**Figure 9–2**). The optic nerve is formed by the axons of the only output neuron of the retina, the ganglion cells. The outer plexiform layer is between the outer and inner nuclear layers; the inner plexiform layer is between the inner nuclear and ganglion cell layers. The neural elements of the retina are bound together by Müller cells, which form the inner limiting membrane. The outer limiting membrane separates the inner segment portion of the rods and cones from their cell bodies. The rods and cones synapse with bipolar cells, and bipolar cells synapse with ganglion cells. Horizontal cells interconnect photoreceptor cells in the outer plexiform layer. Amacrine cells interconnect

---

CLINICAL BOX 9–1

Glaucoma

Increased intraocular pressure (IOP) is a critical risk factor for the development of glaucoma, a degenerative disease in which there is loss of retinal ganglia cells. In 20–50% of the patients with this disease, IOP is normal (10–20 mm Hg); however, increased IOP makes glaucoma worse, and treatment is aimed at lowering the pressure. Elevations in IOP due to injury or surgery can cause glaucoma. Glaucoma is caused by poor drainage of the aqueous humor through the filtration angle formed between the iris and the cornea. Open-angle glaucoma, a chronic disease, is caused by decreased permeability through the trabeculae into the canal of Schlemm, which leads to an increase in IOP. In some cases, this type of glaucoma is due to a genetic defect. Closed-angle glaucoma results from a forward ballooning of the iris so that it reaches the back of the cornea and obliterates the filtration angle, thus reducing the outflow of aqueous humor. If left untreated, glaucoma can lead to blindness.

THERAPEUTIC HIGHLIGHTS

Glaucoma can be treated with agents that decrease the secretion or production of aqueous humor or with drugs that increase outflow of the aqueous humor. β-Adrenergic antagonists (eg, timolol) and carbonic anhydrase inhibitors (eg, dorzolamide, acetazolamide) decrease the secretion of aqueous humor. Glaucoma can also be treated with cholinergic agonists (eg, pilocarpine, carbachol, physostigmine) that increase aqueous outflow by causing ciliary muscle contraction. Aqueous outflow is also increased by prostaglandins.

Pigment epithelium

Rods and cones

Outer segments

Inner segments

Outer nuclear layer

Outer plexiform layer

Inner nuclear layer

Inner plexiform layer

Ganglion cell layer

Optic nerve fibers

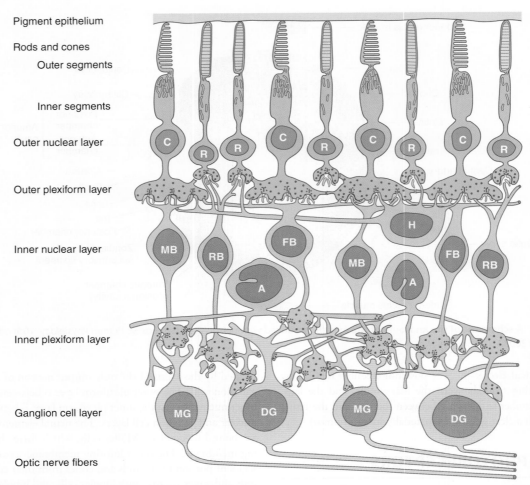

FIGURE 9–2   Neural components of the extrafoveal portion of the retina. A, amacrine cells; C, cone; DG and MG, diffuse and midget ganglion cells; H, horizontal cells; MB, RB, and FB, midget, rod, and flat bipolar cells; R, rod. (Modified with permission from Dowling JE, Boycott BB: Organization of the primate retina: Electron microscopy, Proc R Soc Lond Ser B [Biol] 1966 Nov 15; 166(1002):80–111.)

ganglion cells in the inner plexiform layer and make connections on the terminals of bipolar cells. The receptor layer of the retina rests on the pigment epithelium next to the choroid.

Each rod and cone photoreceptor is divided into an outer segment, an inner segment that includes a nuclear region, and a synaptic terminal zone (Figure 9–2). The outer segment is modified cilia composed of regular stacks of flattened saccules or membranous disks. The inner segment, rich in mitochondria, and is the region that synthesizes the photosensitive compounds. The inner and outer segments are connected by a ciliary stalk through which photosensitive compounds reach the rods and cones. Rods are extremely sensitive to light and are the receptors for night vision; cones have a much greater acuity and are responsible for vision in bright light and for color vision.

An ophthalmoscope is used to view the fundus or interior surface of the eye that includes the retina, optic disk, macula and fovea (Figure 9–3). The optic disk is the region where the optic nerve leaves the eye. Since there are no photoreceptors over the disk, this area does not respond to light (blind spot). The macula, a yellowish pigmented spot, is near the posterior pole of the eye.

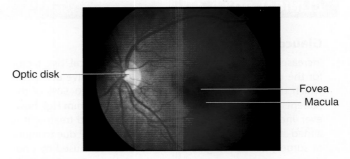

Optic disk

Fovea
Macula

FIGURE 9–3   The fundus of the eye in a healthy human as seen through the ophthalmoscope. The fundus of the eye is the interior surface of the eye, opposite the lens, and includes the retina, optic disk, macula and fovea, and posterior pole. Optic nerve fibers leave the eyeball at the optic disk to form the optic nerve. The arteries, arterioles, and veins in the superficial layers of the retina near its vitreous surface can be seen through the ophthalmoscope. (Used with permission from Dr AJ Weber, Michigan State University.)

CLINICAL BOX 9–2

Visual Acuity & Age-Related Macular Degeneration

Visual acuity is the degree to which the details and contours of objects are perceived, and it is usually defined in terms of the shortest distance by which two lines can be separated and still be perceived as two lines. Clinically, visual acuity is often determined by the use of Snellen letter charts viewed at a distance of 20 ft (6 m). The individual being tested reads aloud the smallest line distinguishable. Normal visual acuity is 20/20; a 20/15 score is better than normal visual acuity; and a 20/100 score is subnormal visual acuity (ie, this individual can read at a distance of 20 ft what a person with normal visual acuity can read at a distance of 100 ft). Visual acuity is influenced by many factors, including optical factors (eg, the state of the image-forming mechanisms of the eye), retinal factors (eg, the state of the cones), and stimulus factors (eg, illumination, brightness of the stimulus, contrast between the stimulus and the background, length of time the subject is exposed to the stimulus). Some drugs can have adverse side effects on visual acuity. The antiarrhythmic drug amiodarone can cause blurred vision, glare and halos around lights, or light sensitivity. Aspirin and other anticoagulants can cause conjunctival or retinal hemorrhaging. Maculopathy is a risk factor for those treated with tamoxifen for breast cancer.

There are over 20 million individuals in the United States and Europe with age-related macular degeneration (AMD),

a deterioration of central visual acuity. Nearly 30% of those aged 75 or older have this disorder; it is the most common cause of visual loss in those aged 50 or older. Women are at greater risk than men for AMD; whites have a greater risk than blacks. There are two types: wet and dry. Wet AMD occurs when fragile blood vessels begin to form under the macula. Blood and fluid leak from these vessels and rapidly damage the macula. Vascular endothelial growth factors (VEGF) may contribute to the growth of these blood vessels. Dry AMD occurs when the cones in the macula slowly break down, causing a gradual loss of central vision.

THERAPEUTIC HIGHLIGHTS

The US Food and Drug Administration approved ranibizumab which acts by inhibiting VEGF and pegaptanib sodium which attacks VEGF for the treatment of wet AMD. Photodynamic therapy uses an injection of verteporfin into the vein in an arm; it is activated by a laser light to produce a chemical reaction that destroys abnormal blood vessels. Laser surgery can be done to repair damaged blood vessels if they are at a distance from the fovea. However, new vessels may form after the surgery, and vision loss may progress.

The fovea (center of the macula) is a thin, rod-free portion of the retina where cones are densely packed. Each cone synapses on a single bipolar cell, which, in turn, synapses on a single ganglion cell, providing a direct pathway to the brain. Since there are few overlying cells and no blood vessels, the fovea is the point where visual acuity is greatest. Age-related macular degeneration is a disease in which sharp, central vision is gradually destroyed (Clinical Box 9–2).

The fundus is the one place in the body where arterioles are readily visible, making ophthalmoscopy of great value in the diagnosis and evaluation of diabetes mellitus, hypertension, and other diseases that affect blood vessels. A characteristic of glaucomatous optic neuropathy is that the disk becomes pale, especially in the center (Clinical Box 9–1). The retinal blood vessels are distorted, especially at the disk margin, due to a lack of support tissue; and there is increased "cupping" of the disk.

■ THE PHOTORECEPTOR MECHANISM

The receptor potentials of the photoreceptors and the electrical responses of most of the other neural elements in the retina are local, graded potentials. Action potentials are only

generated in the ganglion cells. In response to light, the rods, cones, and horizontal cells are hyperpolarized; bipolar cells are either hyperpolarized or depolarized; and amacrine cells are depolarized and develop spikes that may act as generator potentials for the propagated spikes produced in the ganglion cells.

Rod responses are proportional to stimulus intensity at levels of illumination that are below the threshold for cones. Cone responses are proportional to stimulus intensity at high levels of illumination when the rod responses are maximal. Thus, cones generate good responses to changes in light intensity above background but do not represent absolute illumination well, and rods detect absolute illumination.

IONIC BASIS OF PHOTORECEPTOR POTENTIALS

Rhodopsin (visual purple) is the photosensitive pigment in the rods; it is composed of retinal, an aldehyde of vitamin A, and the protein opsin. Vitamin A deficiency produces visual abnormalities (Clinical Box 9–3). The sequence of events in photoreceptors by which incident light leads to production of a signal in the next neural unit in the retina is summarized in Figure 9–4.

CLINICAL BOX 9–3

Vitamin A Deficiency

Vitamin A is composed of a family of compounds called retinoids. Deficiency is rare in the United States but is a major public health problem in the developing world. Annually, about 80,000 individuals worldwide lose their sight from severe vitamin A deficiency due to inadequate intake of foods high in vitamin A (liver, kidney, whole eggs, milk, cream, and cheese) or β-carotene, a precursor of vitamin A, found in dark green leafy vegetables and yellow or orange fruits and vegetables. One of the earliest visual defects to appear with vitamin A deficiency is night blindness (nyctalopia). It also contributes to blindness by causing the eye to become very dry, which damages the cornea (xerophthalmia) and retina. Vitamin A first alters rod function, but concomitant cone degeneration occurs as vitamin A deficiency develops. Prolonged deficiency is associated with anatomic changes in the rods and cones followed by degeneration of the neural layers of the retina. Treatment with vitamin A can restore retinal function if given before the receptors are destroyed. Vitamin A–rich foods include liver, chicken, beef, eggs, whole milk, yams, carrots, spinach, kale, and other green vegetables. Other vitamins, especially those of the B complex, are also necessary for the normal functioning of the retina and other neural tissues.

In the dark, the retinal in rhodopsin is in the 11-*cis* configuration. Light changes the shape of the retinal, converting it to the all-*trans* isomer which alters the configuration of the opsin; the opsin change activates its associated heterotrimeric G-protein transducin. After 11-*cis* retinal is converted to the all-*trans* configuration, it separates from the opsin in a process called bleaching. This changes the color from the rosy red of rhodopsin to the pale yellow of opsin.

Some of the all-*trans* retinal is converted back to the 11-*cis* retinal by retinal isomerase to replenish the rhodopsin supply. Some 11-*cis* retinal is also synthesized from vitamin A. All of these reactions, except the formation of the all-*trans* isomer of retinal, are independent of the light intensity. Thus, the amount of rhodopsin in the receptors varies inversely with the incident light level. The transducin exchanges GDP for GTP, and the α-subunit separates and remains active until its intrinsic GTPase activity hydrolyzes the GTP. Termination of the activity of transducin is accelerated by its binding of β-arrestin. The α-subunit activates cGMP phosphodiesterase, which converts cGMP to 5′-GMP.

In darkness, when phosphodiesterase activity is low, cGMP-gated Na⁺ channels in the outer segment are maintained in an open state; Na⁺ and Ca²⁺ enter the photoreceptor, the cell is depolarized, and glutamate is released (**Figure 9–5**). The light-induced decline in the cytoplasmic cGMP concentration causes some cGMP-gated Na⁺ channels to close, reducing the entry of Na⁺ and Ca²⁺. This hyperpolarizes the synaptic terminal of the photoreceptor, reducing the release of glutamate. This generates a signal in the bipolar cells that ultimately leads to action potentials in ganglion cells that are transmitted to the brain.

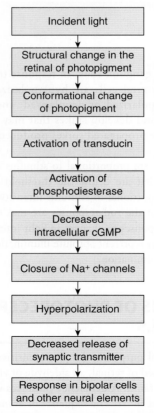

FIGURE 9–4 **Sequence of events involved in phototransduction in rods and cones.**

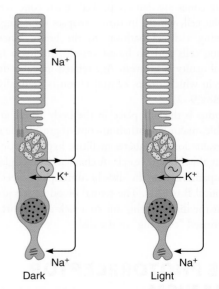

FIGURE 9–5 **Effect of light on current flow in visual receptors.** In the dark, Na⁺ channels in the outer segment are held open by cGMP. Light leads to increased conversion of cGMP to 5′-GMP, and some of the channels close. This produces hyperpolarization of the synaptic terminal of the photoreceptor.

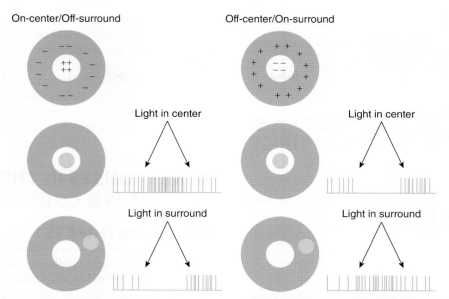

FIGURE 9–6 **Responses of two types of retinal ganglion cells to light (yellow circle) focused on a portion of their receptive field.**
Left side: An *on-center/off-surround* cell responds with an increase in firing rate when the light is placed in the center of the receptive field and with a decrease in firing rate when the light is placed in the surround portion of the receptive field. **Right side:** An *off-center/on-surround* cell responds with a decrease in firing rate when the light is placed in the center and with an increase in firing rate when the light is placed in the surround.

PROCESSING OF VISUAL INFORMATION IN THE RETINA

A characteristic of the retinal bipolar and retinal ganglion cells (as well as the lateral geniculate neurons and the neurons in layer 4 of the visual cortex) is that they respond best to a small, circular stimulus and that, within their receptive field, an annulus of light around the center (surround illumination) antagonizes the response to the central spot (**Figure 9–6**). The center can be excitatory with an inhibitory surround (an on-center/off-surround cell) or inhibitory with an excitatory surround (an off-center/on-surround cell). The inhibition of the center response by the surround is probably due to inhibitory feedback from one photoreceptor to another mediated via horizontal cells. Thus, activation of nearby photoreceptors by addition of the annulus triggers horizontal cell hyperpolarization, which in turn inhibits the response of the centrally activated photoreceptors. The inhibition of the response to central illumination by an increase in surrounding illumination is an example of lateral inhibition.

■ THE IMAGE-FORMING MECHANISM

The bending of light rays (refraction) allows one to focus an accurate image onto the retina. In the eye, light is refracted at the anterior surface of the cornea and at the anterior and posterior surfaces of the lens. The retinal image is inverted but the connections of the retinal receptors from birth view any inverted image on the retina as being right side up and project to the visual field on the side opposite to the area stimulated.

COMMON DEFECTS OF THE IMAGE-FORMING MECHANISM

In hyperopia (farsightedness), the eyeball is too short and light rays are focused behind the retina (**Figure 9–7**). Sustained accommodation partially compensates for the defect, but prolonged convergence of the visual axes may lead to strabismus, a misalignment of the eyes (**Clinical Box 9–4**). Hyperopia can be corrected by using glasses with convex lenses, which aid the refractive power of the eye in shortening the focal distance. In myopia (nearsightedness), the anteroposterior diameter of the eyeball is too long. This defect can be corrected by glasses with biconcave lenses, which make parallel light rays diverge slightly before they strike the eye. Astigmatism is a common condition in which the curvature of the cornea is not uniform. When the curvature in one meridian is different from that in others, light rays in that meridian are refracted to a different focus, so that part of the retinal image is blurred. Astigmatism can usually be corrected with cylindrical lenses placed in such a way that they equalize the refraction in all meridians.

ACCOMMODATION

To bring diverging rays from close objects to a focus on the retina, the curvature of the lens is increased, a process called accommodation. At rest, the lens is held under tension by the lens ligaments. Because the lens substance is malleable and the lens capsule has considerable

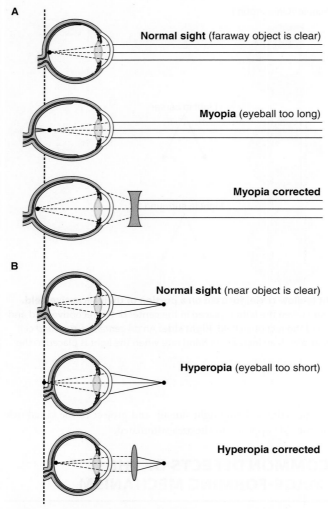

FIGURE 9–7 Common defects of the optical system of the eye. (A) In myopia (nearsightedness), the eyeball is too long and light rays focus in front of the retina. Placing a biconcave lens in front of the eye causes the light rays to diverge slightly before striking the eye, so that they are brought to a focus on the retina. **(B)** In hyperopia (farsightedness), the eyeball is too short and light rays come to a focus behind the retina. A biconvex lens corrects this by adding to the refractive power of the lens of the eye. (Reproduced with permission from Widmaier EP, Raff H, Strang KT: *Vander's Human Physiology*, 11th ed. New York, NY: McGraw-Hill; 2008.)

elasticity, the lens is pulled into a flattened shape. If the gaze is directed at a near object, the ciliary muscle contracts. This decreases the distance between the edges of the ciliary body and relaxes the lens ligaments, so that the lens springs into a more convex shape. Changes in accommodation with age are described in Clinical Box 9–5.

PUPILLARY LIGHT REFLEXES

When light is directed into one eye, the pupil constricts (direct light response). The pupil of the other eye also constricts (consensual light response). The optic nerve fibers that carry the impulses initiating this pupillary reflex leave the optic tract near the lateral geniculate bodies. On each side, they enter the midbrain via the brachium of the superior colliculus and terminate in the pretectal nucleus. From this nucleus, nerve fibers project to the ipsilateral and contralateral Edinger–Westphal nuclei that contain preganglionic parasympathetic neurons within the oculomotor nerve. These neurons terminate in the ciliary ganglion from which postganglionic nerves project to the ciliary muscle.

■ RESPONSES IN THE VISUAL PATHWAYS & CORTEX

NEURAL PATHWAYS

The axons of the ganglion cells pass caudally in the optic nerve and optic tract to end in the lateral geniculate body in the thalamus (Figure 9–8). The fibers from each nasal hemiretina decussate in the optic chiasm. In the geniculate body, the fibers from the nasal half of one retina and the temporal half of the other synapse on the cells whose axons form the geniculocalcarine tract. This tract passes to the occipital lobe of the cerebral cortex.

The axons of retinal ganglion cells project a precise point-for-point representation of the retina on the 6-layered lateral geniculate body (Figure 9–9). Layers 3–6 are called parvocellular (small cells); layers 1 and 2 are called magnocellular (large cells). Layers 1, 4, and 6 receive input from the contralateral eye and layers 2, 3, and 5 from the ipsilateral eye. All six layers are in register so that along a line perpendicular to the layers, receptive fields of the cells in each layer are almost identical. Only 10–20% of the input to the lateral geniculate nucleus (LGN) comes from the retina; input from the visual cortex is involved in visual processing related to the perception of orientation and motion.

Large retinal ganglion cells (magno, or M cells) add responses from different kinds of cones and are concerned with movement and stereopsis. Small ganglion cells (parvo, or P cells) subtract input from one type of cone from input from another and are concerned with color, texture, and shape. The M and P ganglion cells project to the magnocellular and parvocellular portions of the lateral geniculate, respectively. From the LGN, a magnocellular pathway and a parvocellular pathway project to the visual cortex. The magnocellular pathway carries signals for detection of movement, depth, and flicker. The parvocellular pathway carries signals for color vision, texture, shape, and fine detail.

EFFECT OF LESIONS IN THE OPTIC PATHWAYS

A lesion that interrupts one optic nerve causes blindness in that eye, but a lesion in one optic tract causes blindness in half of the visual field (Figure 9–9). This defect is classified as a homonymous (same side of both visual fields) hemianopia (half-blindness).

CLINICAL BOX 9–4

Strabismus & Amblyopia

Strabismus is a misalignment of the eyes and one of the most common eye problems in children, affecting about 4% of children under 6 years of age. It is characterized by one or both eyes turning inward (esotropia), outward (exotropia), upward, or downward. Strabismus is also commonly called "wandering eye" or "crossed-eyes." It results in visual images that do not fall on corresponding retinal points. When visual images chronically fall on noncorresponding points in the two retinas in young children, one is eventually suppressed (suppression scotoma). This suppression is a cortical phenomenon, and it usually does not develop in adults. It is important to institute treatment before age 6 in affected children, because if the suppression persists, the loss of visual acuity in the eye generating the suppressed image is permanent. A similar suppression with subsequent permanent loss of visual acuity can occur in children in whom vision in one eye is blurred or distorted owing to a refractive error. The loss of vision in these cases is called amblyopia ex anopsia, a term that refers to uncorrectable loss of visual acuity not directly due to organic disease of the eye. Typically, an affected child has one weak eye with poor vision and one strong eye with normal vision. It affects about 3% of the general population. Amblyopia is also referred to as "lazy eye," and it often coexists with strabismus.

THERAPEUTIC HIGHLIGHTS

Atropine (muscarinic receptor antagonist) and miotics (eg, echothiophate iodide) can be administered in the eye to correct strabismus and amblyopia. Atropine will blur the vision in the good eye to force the individual to use the weaker eye. Eye muscle training through optometric vision therapy has also been proven to be useful, even in patients older than 17 years. Some types of strabismus can be corrected by surgical shortening of some of the eye muscles, by eye muscle training exercises, and by the use of glasses with prisms that bend the light rays sufficiently to compensate for the abnormal position of the eyeball. However, subtle defects in depth perception persist. Congenital abnormalities of the visual tracking mechanisms may cause both strabismus and the defective depth perception.

Lesions affecting the optic chiasm (eg, pituitary tumors) destroy fibers from both nasal hemiretinas and produce a heteronymous (opposite sides) hemianopia. Selective visual field defects are further classified as bitemporal, binasal, and right or left.

CLINICAL BOX 9–5

Accommodation & Aging

Accommodation is an active process, requiring muscular effort, and can therefore be tiring. The ciliary muscle is one of the most used muscles in the body. The degree to which the lens curvature can be increased is limited, and light rays from an object very near the individual cannot be brought to a focus on the retina, even with the greatest of effort. The nearest point to the eye at which an object can be brought into clear focus by accommodation is called the near point of vision. The near point recedes throughout life, slowly at first and then rapidly with advancing age, from approximately 9 cm at age 10 to approximately 83 cm at age 60. This recession is due principally to increasing hardness of the lens, with a resulting loss of accommodation due to the steady decrease in the degree to which the curvature of the lens can be increased. By the time a healthy individual reaches age 40–45 years, the loss of accommodation is usually sufficient to make reading and close work difficult. This condition (presbyopia) can be corrected by wearing glasses with convex lenses.

The optic nerve fibers from the upper retinal quadrants (lower half of the visual field) terminate in the medial half of the lateral geniculate body; the fibers from the lower retinal quadrants terminate in the lateral half. The geniculocalcarine fibers from the medial half of the lateral geniculate terminate on the superior lip of the calcarine fissure; those from the lateral half terminate on the inferior lip. The fibers from the lateral geniculate body that mediate macular vision separate from those that mediate peripheral vision and end more posteriorly on the lips of the calcarine fissure. As a result, occipital lobe lesions may produce discrete quadrantic visual field defects (upper and lower quadrants of each half visual field).

Macular sparing (loss of peripheral vision with intact macular vision) is common with occipital lesions because the macular representation is separate from that of the peripheral fields and very large relative to that of the peripheral fields. Therefore, occipital lesions must extend considerable distances to destroy macular as well as peripheral vision. Bilateral destruction of the occipital cortex causes subjective blindness. The fibers to the pretectal region that mediate the pupillary reflex leave the optic tracts near the geniculate bodies. Therefore, blindness with preservation of the pupillary light reflex is usually due to bilateral lesions caudal to the optic tract.

PRIMARY VISUAL CORTEX

The primary visual cortex is located on the sides of the calcarine fissure. The lateral geniculate body projects a similar point-for-point representation on the primary visual cortex. The axons from

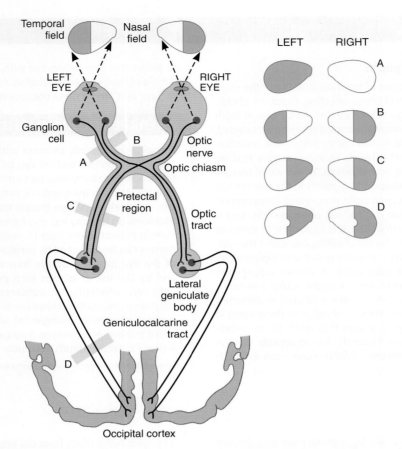

FIGURE 9–8   Visual pathways. Transection of the pathways at the locations indicated by the letters causes the visual field defects shown in the diagrams on the right. The fibers from the nasal half of each retina decussate in the optic chiasm, so that the fibers in the optic tracts are those from the temporal half of one retina and the nasal half of the other. A lesion that interrupts one optic nerve causes blindness in that eye **(A)**. A lesion in one optic tract causes blindness in half of the visual field **(C)** and is called homonymous (same side of both visual fields) hemianopia (half-blindness). Lesions affecting the optic chiasm destroy fibers from both nasal hemiretinas and produce a heteronymous (opposite sides of the visual fields) hemianopia **(B)**. Occipital lesions may spare the fibers from the macula (as in **D**) because of the separation in the brain of these fibers from the others subserving vision.

the LGN that form the magnocellular pathway end in layer 4, specifically in its deepest part, layer 4C. Many of the axons that form the parvocellular pathway also end in layer 4C. The axons from the interlaminar region end in layers 2 and 3 which contain clusters of cells (blobs) that contain a high concentration of the mitochondrial enzyme cytochrome oxidase. They are arranged in a mosaic in the visual cortex and are concerned with color vision. The parvocellular pathway also carries color opponent data to the deep part of layer 4.

Simple cells respond to bars of light, lines, or edges, but only when they have a particular orientation. Complex cells have a preferred orientation of a linear stimulus but are less dependent on the location of a stimulus in the visual field than the simple cells and the cells in layer 4. They often respond maximally when a linear stimulus is moved laterally without a change in its orientation. The simple and complex cells are called feature detectors because they respond to and analyze certain features of the stimulus.

The visual cortex is arranged in vertical columns that are concerned with orientation (orientation columns). For each ganglion cell receptive field in the visual field, there is a collection of

columns in a small area of visual cortex, representing the possible preferred orientations at small intervals throughout the full 360°. Another feature of the visual cortex is the presence of ocular dominance columns; the cells in layer 4 receive input from only one eye and alternate with cells receiving input from the other eye.

■ COLOR VISION

Color vision relies on three kinds of cones, each containing a different photopigment and that are maximally sensitive to one of the three primary colors, with the sensation of any given color being determined by the relative frequency of the impulses from each of these cone systems. The blue, green, and red cones are also called S (short), M (medium), and L (long) because they respond maximally to wavelengths of light centered at 440, 535, and 565 nm, respectively.

Color is mediated by ganglion cells that subtract or add input from one type of cone to input from another type. Processing in the ganglion cells and the LGN produces impulses that pass

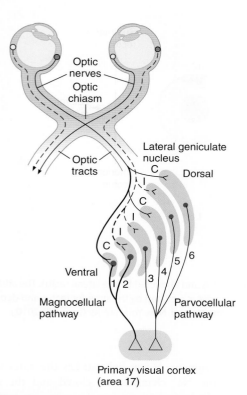

FIGURE 9–9 Ganglion cell projections from the right hemiretina of each eye to the right lateral geniculate body and from this nucleus to the right primary visual cortex. Note the six layers of the geniculate body. P ganglion cells project to layers 3–6, and M ganglion cells project to layers 1 and 2. The ipsilateral (I) and contralateral (C) eyes project to alternate layers. Not shown are the interlaminar area cells, which project via a separate component of the P pathway to blobs in the visual cortex. (Modified with permission from Kandel ER, Schwartz JH, Jessell TM [editors]: *Principles of Neural Science*, 4th ed. New York, NY: McGraw-Hill; 2000.)

along three types of neural pathways that project to the primary visual cortex: a red-green pathway that signals differences between L- and M-cone responses, a blue-yellow pathway that signals differences between S-cone and the sum of L- and M-cone responses, and a luminance pathway that signals the sum of L- and M-cone responses. These pathways project to the blobs and the deep portion of layer 4C. From the blobs and layer 4, color information is projected to the visual cortex.

■ OTHER ASPECTS OF VISUAL FUNCTION

DARK ADAPTATION

If a person spends a considerable length of time in brightly lighted surroundings and then moves to a dimly lighted environment, the retinas slowly (over a period of about 20 min) become more sensitive to light (dark adaptation). The time required for dark adaptation is determined in part by the time required to build up

the rhodopsin stores. When one passes suddenly from a dim to a brightly lighted environment, the light seems intensely and even uncomfortably bright until the eyes adapt to the increased illumination and the visual threshold rises. This light adaptation occurs over a period of about 5 min.

The dark adaptation response has two components. The first drop in visual threshold, rapid but small in magnitude, is due to dark adaptation of the cones because when only the foveal, rod-free portion of the retina is tested, the decline proceeds no further. In the peripheral portions of the retina, a further drop occurs as a result of adaptation of the rods.

VISUAL FIELDS & BINOCULAR VISION

The visual field of each eye is the portion of the external world visible out of that eye. Mapping the visual fields is important in neurologic diagnosis. The peripheral portions of the visual fields are mapped with an instrument called a perimeter, and the process is referred to as perimetry. One eye is covered while the other is fixed on a central point. A small target is moved toward this central point along selected meridians, and, along each, the location where the target first becomes visible is plotted in degrees of arc away from the central point. The central visual fields are mapped with a tangent screen, a black felt screen across which a white target is moved. By noting the locations where the target disappears and reappears, the blind spot and any objective scotomas (blind spots due to disease) can be outlined.

The central parts of the visual fields of the two eyes coincide; therefore, anything in this portion of the field is viewed with binocular vision. The impulses set up in the two retinas by light rays from an object are fused at the cortical level into a single image. The term corresponding points is used to describe the points on the retina on which the image of an object must fall if it is to be seen binocularly as a single object. If one eye is gently pushed out of alignment while staring fixedly at an object in the center of the visual field, double vision (diplopia) results; the image on the retina of the eye that is displaced no longer falls on the corresponding point. When visual images no longer fall on corresponding retinal points, strabismus occurs (Clinical Box 9–4).

EYE MOVEMENTS

Eye movement is controlled by six ocular muscles innervated by the oculomotor, trochlear, and abducens nerves (Figure 9–10). The inferior oblique muscle turns the eye upward and outward; the superior oblique turns it downward and outward. The superior rectus muscle turns the eye upward and inward; the inferior rectus turns it downward and inward. The medial rectus muscle turns the eye inward; the lateral rectus turns it outward.

There are four types of eye movements, each controlled by a different neural system. Saccades (sudden jerky movements) occur as the gaze shifts from one object to another; they reduce adaptation in the visual pathway that would occur if gaze were fixed on a single object for long periods. Smooth pursuit

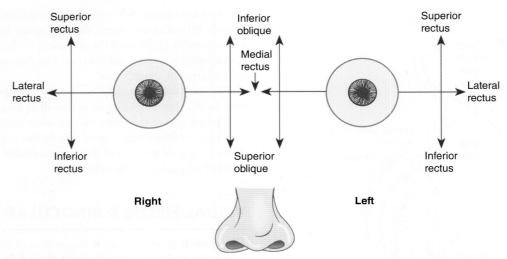

FIGURE 9–10 Diagram of eye muscle actions. The eye is adducted by the medial rectus and abducted by the lateral rectus. The adducted eye is elevated by the inferior oblique and depressed by the superior oblique; the abducted eye is elevated by the superior rectus and depressed by the inferior rectus. (Reproduced with permission from Waxman SG: *Clinical Neuroanatomy*, 26th ed. New York, NY: McGraw-Hill; 2010.)

movements are tracking movements of the eyes as they follow moving objects. Vestibular movements occur in response to stimuli in the semicircular canals to maintain visual fixation as the head moves. Convergence movements bring the visual axes toward each other as attention is focused on objects near the observer.

CHAPTER SUMMARY

- The major parts of the eye are the sclera (protective covering), cornea (transfer light rays), choroid (nourishment), retina (receptor cells), lens, and iris.

- The retina is organized into several layers: the outer nuclear layer contains the photoreceptors (rods and cones); the inner nuclear layer contains bipolar cells, horizontal cells, and amacrine cells; and the ganglion cell layer contains the only output neuron of the retina.

- The bending of light rays (refraction) allows one to focus an accurate image onto the retina. Light is refracted at the anterior surface of the cornea and at the anterior and posterior surfaces of the lens. To bring diverging rays from close objects to a focus on the retina, the curvature of the lens is increased, a process called accommodation.

- In hyperopia (farsightedness), the eyeball is too short and light rays come to a focus behind the retina. In myopia (nearsightedness), the anteroposterior diameter of the eyeball is too long. Astigmatism is a common condition in which the curvature of the cornea is not uniform. Presbyopia is the loss of accommodation for near vision. Strabismus is a misalignment of the eyes; it is also known as "crossed eyes." Eyes can be deviated outward (exotropia) or inward (esotropia).

- Na^+ channels in the outer segments of the rods and cones are open in the dark, so current flows from the inner to the outer segment. When light strikes the outer segment, some of the Na^+ channels are closed and the cells are hyperpolarized.

- In response to light, horizontal cells are hyperpolarized; bipolar cells are either hyperpolarized or depolarized; and amacrine cells are depolarized and develop spikes that may act as generator potentials for the propagated spikes produced in the ganglion cells.

- The visual pathway is from the rods and cones to bipolar cells to ganglion cells then via the optic tract to the thalamic lateral geniculate body to the occipital lobe of the cerebral cortex. The fibers from each nasal hemiretina decussate in the optic chiasm; the fibers from the nasal half of one retina and the temporal half of the other synapse on the cells whose axons form the geniculocalcarine tract.

- The decline in visual threshold after spending long periods of time in a dimly lit room is called dark adaptation. The fovea in the center of the retina is the point where visual acuity is greatest.

- The Young–Helmholtz theory of color vision postulates the existence of three kinds of cones, each containing a different photopigment and that are maximally sensitive to one of the three primary colors, with the sensation of any given color being determined by the relative frequency of the impulses from each of these cone systems.

- Eye movement is controlled by six ocular muscles innervated by the oculomotor, trochlear, and abducens nerves. The inferior oblique muscle turns the eye upward and outward; the superior oblique turns it downward and outward. The superior rectus muscle turns the eye upward and inward; the inferior rectus turns it downward and inward. The medial rectus muscle turns the eye inward; the lateral rectus turns it outward.

MULTIPLE-CHOICE QUESTIONS

For all questions, select the single best answer unless otherwise directed.

1. A visual exam in an 80-year-old man shows he has loss of vision in the temporal visual field of the left eye and the nasal visual field of the right eye but some vision remains in the central area of the visual field. The diagnosis is
   A. central scotoma.
   B. heteronymous hemianopia with macular sparing.
   C. lesion of the optic chiasm.
   D. homonymous hemianopia with macular sparing.
   E. retinopathy.

2. A visual exam in a 70-year-old woman shows blindness in the temporal visual field of the right eye and the nasal visual field of the left eye. This visual defect could result from a lesion of the
   A. the left optic nerve.
   B. right optic tract.
   C. left lateral geniculate nucleus.
   D. optic chiasm.
   E. right occipital cortex.

3. A 45-year-old woman who had never needed to wear glasses experienced difficulty reading a menu in a dimly lit restaurant. She then recalled that as of late she needed to hold the newspaper further away in order to read it. Her scientist friend recommended she purchase reading glasses and explained that she was experiencing a loss in accommodation for near vision that is common at her age (presbyopia) and is due to
   A. the inability to increase the tension on the lens ligaments.
   B. the inability to increase the curvature of the lens.
   C. relaxation of the sphincter muscle of the iris.
   D. contraction of the ciliary muscle.
   E. increased softness of the lens.

4. A 28-year-old man with severe myopia made an appointment to see his ophthalmologist when he began to notice flashing lights and floaters in his visual field. He was diagnosed with a retinal detachment and underwent laser surgery to correct the problem. The inner nuclear layer of the retina
   A. is also called the pigment epithelial layer.
   B. contains the photoreceptors (rods and cones).
   C. contains bipolar cells, horizontal cells, and amacrine cells.
   D. contains ganglion cells whose axons form the optic nerve.
   E. is formed by glia called Müller cells.

5. A 62-year-old man went to his ophthalmologist for his routine eye exam. It included ophthalmoscopy to visualize the interior surface of his eye, opposite to the lens. This portion of the eye is called
   A. the optic disk.
   B. the macula.
   C. the sclera.
   D. the conjunctiva.
   E. the fundus.

6. A 72-year-old white woman experienced a rapid onset of blurry vision along with loss of central vision. A comprehensive eye exam showed that she had wet age-related macular degeneration. Two important features of the fovea of the eye are that
   A. it has the highest concentration of rods and has the lowest light threshold.
   B. it is a rod-free portion of the retina and is the region of highest visual acuity.
   C. it contains no visual receptors (blind spot) and it is the one place in the body where arterioles are readily visible.
   D. it contains rods and cones and is located within the center of the fovea.
   E. it has the lowest light threshold and is the region with the highest visual acuity.

7. A medical student was interested in learning more about visual acuity, especially the reason that center of the macula (the fovea) is the region of highest visual acuity. She understood that it had to do with the connections between the cones and the visual cortex. Which of the following explains the connections from the cone receptor to the visual cortex?
   A. Each cone synapses on a single bipolar cell, which, in turn, synapses on a single ganglion cell, providing a direct pathway from the retina to the primary visual cortex.
   B. Each cone synapses on a single ganglion cell, which in turn synapses on a horizontal cell that projects direct pathway from the retina to the primary visual cortex.
   C. Each cone synapses on a single bipolar cell, which, in turn, synapses on a single ganglion cell that terminates in the lateral geniculate body.
   D. Each cone synapses on a single horizontal cell, which, in turn, synapses on a single ganglion cell, providing a direct pathway from the retina to the lateral geniculate body.
   E. Each cone synapses on a single bipolar cell and a horizontal cell, which, in turn, synapse directly in the lateral geniculate neuron which then projects to the primary visual cortex.

8. A medical student was working in a laboratory that studied the steps involved in phototransduction in rods and cones. The correct sequence of events involved in phototransduction in rods after activation by light is
   A. activation of transducin, decreased release of glutamate, structural changes in rhodopsin, closure of Na^+ channels, and decrease in intracellular cGMP.
   B. decreased release of glutamate, activation of transducin, closure of Na^+ channels, decrease in intracellular cGMP, and structural changes in rhodopsin.
   C. structural changes in rhodopsin, decrease in intracellular cGMP, decreased release of glutamate, closure of Na^+ channels, and activation of transducin.
   D. structural changes in rhodopsin, activation of transducin, decrease in intracellular cGMP, closure of Na^+ channels, and decreased release of glutamate.
   E. activation of transducin, structural changes in rhodopsin, closure of Na^+ channels, decrease in intracellular cGMP, and decreased release of glutamate.

9. A 25-year-old medical student spent a summer volunteering in the sub-Saharan region of Africa. There he noted a high incidence of people reporting difficulty with night vision due to a lack of vitamin A in their diet. Why does a lack of vitamin A lead to difficulty with night vision?
   A. A lack of vitamin A prevents the synthesis of the opsin protein in both rod and cone photoreceptors which are critical for night vision.

B. A lack of vitamin A prevents the synthesis of β-carotene that is a precursor for retinal and rhodopsin in rod photoreceptors which is critical for night vision.

C. A lack of vitamin A prevents the synthesis of retinal and consequently rhodopsin in rod photoreceptors which is critical for night vision.

D. A lack of vitamin A prevents the synthesis of cone transducin which is critical for night vision.

10. An 11-year-old boy was having difficulty reading the graphs that his teacher was showing at the front of the classroom. Not only was he asked to look at a Snellen letter chart for visual acuity but he was also asked to identify numbers in an Ishihara chart. He responded that he merely saw a bunch of dots. Abnormal color vision is 20 times more common in males than females because most cases are caused by an abnormal

A. dominant gene on the Y chromosome.

B. recessive gene on the Y chromosome.

C. dominant gene on the X chromosome.

D. recessive gene on the X chromosome.

E. recessive gene on chromosome 22.

11. At the age of 11, a girl learned that she was red-green color blind. Ten years later when she was taking a college course in physiology, she learned that this is an inherited abnormality and is very rare in women, only occurring in 0.4% of white females. She began to read more about how color vision was processed and learned that there are only three types of cones that process color. They are S (short), M (medium), and L (long) cones that respond maximally to wavelengths of light centered at 440, 535, and 565 nm, respectively. Thus, S, M, and L cones relay information about these three primary colors, respectively.

A. Red, blue, and yellow

B. Blue, green, and red

C. Green, blue, and red

D. Blue, yellow, and red

E. Yellow, blue, and red

12. A tumor was diagnosed near the base of the skull in a 56-year-old woman, impinging on her right optic tract. Which parts of the visual field of each eye are relayed through the right optic tract?

A. The fibers from each temporal hemiretina decussate in the optic chiasm, so that the fibers in the right optic tract are those from the temporal half of left retina and the nasal half of the right retina.

B. The fibers from each nasal hemiretina decussate in the optic chiasm, so that the fibers in the right optic tract are those from the nasal half of left retina and the temporal half of the right retina.

C. The fibers from each temporal hemiretina decussate in the optic chiasm, so that the fibers in the right optic tract are those from the temporal half of right retina and the nasal half of the left retina.

D. The fibers from each nasal hemiretina decussate in the optic chiasm, so that the fibers in the right optic tract are those from the nasal half of right retina and the temporal half of the left retina.

E. The fibers from both halves of the retina decussate in the optic chiasm, so that the fibers in the right optic tract are those from both the temporal and nasal halves of the left retina.

13. A 32-year-old man was brought to the emergency department after being found comatose by his wife. The resident in the emergency department assessed his pupillary light reflex as a useful gauge of his brainstem function. He found that when the light was shone into his left eye, neither pupil constricted; but when the light was shone in his right eye, both pupils constricted. The physician determined that damage was within

A. the left optic nerve.

B. the left oculomotor nerve.

C. the right optic nerve.

D. the right oculomotor nerve.

E. the sphincter muscle of the left eye.

14. A 32-year-old man was brought to the emergency department after being found comatose by his wife. The resident in the emergency department assessed his pupillary light reflex as a useful gauge of his brainstem function. He found that when the light was shone into either his right or left eye, only his left pupil constricted. The physician determined that damage was within

A. the left optic nerve.

B. the left oculomotor nerve.

C. the right optic nerve.

D. the right oculomotor nerve.

15. A 63-year-old woman began having difficulty moving her right eye sideways, toward her right temporal visual field. She also reported double vision. She had an appointment with her primary care physician who did further testing and revealed that she had damage to one of her cranial nerves that innervated one of the muscles controlling eye movement. Which nerve and muscle allow the eye to move sideways?

A. The oculomotor nerve and the inferior oblique muscle

B. The trochlear nerve and the medial rectus muscle

C. The abducens nerve and the lateral rectus muscle

D. The oculomotor nerve and the superior oblique muscle

E. The trochlear nerve and the inferior rectus muscle

16. A 70-year-old man presented with the ptosis and outward and downward deviation of the left eye and dilation of the pupil in the same eye. He was diagnosed with oculomotor nerve palsy. Which eye muscles were directly impacted by the loss of function of this cranial nerve?

A. Levator palpebrae superioris, superior rectus, medial rectus, inferior rectus, inferior oblique, sphincter, and ciliary muscles

B. Levator palpebrae superioris, inferior rectus, medial rectus, superior oblique, sphincter, and ciliary muscles

C. Superior rectus, medial rectus, inferior rectus, superior oblique, radial, and ciliary muscles

D. Levator palpebrae superioris, lateral rectus, superior rectus, inferior rectus, superior oblique, radial, and ciliary muscles

E. Lateral rectus, superior rectus, inferior rectus, lateral rectus, superior oblique, sphincter, and ciliary muscles

17. A 55-year-old African–American farsighted woman had experienced a loss of peripheral vision that had progressed over time. Recently she also noticed loss of visual acuity. She decided that she should go to her ophthalmologist for the first time in several years. An ophthalmoscopic exam revealed that her disk had become pale, especially in the center; the retinal blood vessels were distorted and there is increased "cupping" of the disk. Her intraocular pressure was elevated. What is the likely diagnosis and what type of treatment should be initiated?

A. She has open angle glaucoma and drug treatment should be directed at increasing aqueous humor outflow and reducing aqueous humor production.

B. She has open angle glaucoma and surgery should be done immediately to lower intraocular pressure.

C. She has closed angle glaucoma and drug treatment should be directed at increasing aqueous humor outflow and reducing aqueous humor production.

D. She has closed angle glaucoma and surgery should be done immediately to lower intraocular pressure.

ANSWERS

1. The best answer is **D**. Blindness in the left half of both visual fields (temporal field in the left eye and nasal field in the right eye) is classified as a homonymous hemianopia; maintained vision within the central portion of the visual field indicates that there has been macular sparing. All other options can be ruled out for the following reasons. Central scotoma is impaired vision in the center of the visual field. A heteronymous hemianopia is the loss of the temporal visual field in both eyes and is caused by a lesion of the optic chiasm. Retinopathy would cause loss of vision only in the eye with the pathology.

2. The best answer is **C**. The left lateral geniculate nucleus receives information from the nasal field of the left eye and the temporal field of the right eye. All other options can be ruled out for the following reasons. A lesion of the left optic nerve would cause blindness in the left eye. A lesion of the right optic tract would cause blindness in the nasal field of the right eye and the temporal field of the left eye. A lesion of the optic chiasm causes blindness in the nasal field of both eyes. A lesion of the right occipital cortex is likely to cause visual defects in portions of the nasal field of the right eye and portions of the temporal field of the left eye with maintained vision in the central visual field because of the fibers from the foveal (central) region are spread over a large region of the primary sensory cortex.

3. The best answer is **B**. Presbyopia is to due increasing hardness of the lens (rules out **E**), with a resulting loss of accommodation due to a reduction in the degree to which the curvature of the lens can be increased. Increased tension in the lens ligaments flattens the lens (rules out option **A**). Relaxation of the sphincter muscle dilates the pupil and does not affect accommodation (rules out **C**). Contraction of the ciliary muscle allows for accommodation (rules out **D**).

4. The best answer is **C**. The inner nuclear layer of the retina contains the cell bodies of the various types of excitatory and inhibitory interneurons including bipolar cells, horizontal cells, and amacrine cells. The pigment epithelium layer is next to the choroid and absorbs light rays, preventing the reflection of rays back through the retina to prevent blurring of the visual images (rules out **A**). The outer nuclear layer contains the photoreceptors (rules out **B**). The ganglion cell layer contains ganglion cells whose axons form the optic nerve (rules out **D**). The inner limiting membrane is formed by glia called Müller cells (rules out **E**).

5. The best answer is **E**. Ophthalmoscopy (also called fundoscopy) visualizes the fundus of the eye that includes the retina, optic disk, macula and fovea, and posterior pole. The optic disk and macula are just part of the region viewed by the ophthalmoscope (rules out **A** and **B**). The sclera is the outer protective layer of the eyeball (rules out **C**), and the conjunctiva is a clear mucous membrane that covers the sclera (rules out **D**).

6. The best answer is **B**. The fovea is a thinned-out, rod-free portion of the retina in which cones are densely packed; the region contains very few overlying cells and no blood vessels, so it is the point where visual acuity is greatest. Rods are in highest concentration in the parafoveal region, and they have the lowest threshold to light (rules out option **A** and **E**). Since the fovea contains cones but not rods, options **C** and **D** can be ruled out.

7. The best answer is **C**. The synaptic terminal of each cone photoreceptor synapses on a single bipolar cell that then synapses on a single ganglion cell, the only output neuron of the retina and their axons form the optic nerve which terminates in the lateral geniculate body in the thalamus. This in turn projects to the primary visual cortex (rules out option **A**). Cones do not make direct contact with the output ganglion cell (rules out **B**), and horizontal cells do not project to ganglion cells (rules out **D**). Option **E** is ruled out because neither bipolar nor horizontal cells project directly to the lateral geniculate body.

8. The best answer is **D**. The full sequence of events is structural changes in the retinal component of rhodopsin, conformational change in the opsin component of rhodopsin, activation of transducin, activation of phosphodiesterase, decrease in intracellular cGMP, closure of Na^+ channels, hyperpolarization, and decreased release of glutamate.

9. The best answer is **C**. The photosensitive pigment in the rods (rhodopsin) is composed of retinal, an aldehyde of vitamin A, and a protein called opsin. Because of the importance of vitamin A in the synthesis of retinal and because rods are critical for night vision, one of the earliest visual defects to result from a deficiency in vitamin A is night blindness. Vitamin A is not responsible for the synthesis of opsin or transducin (rules out options **A** and **D**. β-Carotene is actually a precursor to vitamin A (rules out option **B**).

10. The best answer is **D**. The most common test for color blindness uses the Ishihara charts, which are plates containing figures made up of colored spots on a background of similarly shaped colored spots. The figures are intentionally made up of colors that are liable to look the same as the background to an individual who is color blind. Color blindness is inherited as a recessive and X-linked characteristic. It is present in males if the X chromosome has the abnormal gene; females show a defect only when both X chromosomes contain the abnormal gene. However, female children of a man with X-linked color blindness are carriers and pass the defect on to half of their sons. Therefore, X-linked color blindness skips generations, appearing in males of every second generation. Color blindness can also be due to a lesions of area V8 of the visual cortex, a region concerned with color vision in humans.

11. The best answer is **B**. The blue, green, and red cones respond maximally to wavelengths of light centered at 440, 535, and 565 nm, respectively; thus blue, green, and red are called primary colors or colors that can be combined to make other colors.

12. The best answer is **A.** The fibers from temporal visual field but not the nasal visual field decussate in the optic chiasm (rules out options **B, D,** and **E**), so that the fibers in the right optic tract are those from the temporal half of contralateral retina and the nasal half of the ipsilateral retina (rules out option **C**). The trajectory from the nasal fields of both eyes is uncrossed all the way to the cortex.

13. The best answer is **A.** Left optic nerve damage prevents the ability of light shone into the left eye to signal the brain to initiate a reflex, so neither eye responds. Since the pupil of the left eye was able to constrict when light was shone into the right eye, the left oculomotor nerve and left sphincter muscles were intact (rules out **B** and **E**). Also, since the pupil of the right eye constricted when the light was shone into that eye, both its afferent (optic) and motor (oculomotor) nerves were intact (rules out **C** and **D**).

14. The best answer is **D.** Right oculomotor nerve damage would prevent a stimulus to either eye from being able to elicit contraction of the sphincter muscle in the right eye. Since the pupil of the left eye constricted when light was shone into either eye, both its afferent (optic) and motor (oculomotor) nerves were intact (rules out **A** and **B**) and the afferent fiber from the right eye was also intact (rules out **C**).

15. The best answer is **C.** Movement of the eye toward the temporal visual field is called abduction and is mediated via the abducens nerve controlling the lateral rectus muscle. The oculomotor nerve innervates the inferior oblique muscle to elevate the eye (rules out option **A**); it does not innervate the superior oblique muscle (rules out option **D**). The trochlear nerve innervates the superior oblique muscle to depress the eye (rules out options **B** and **E**).

16. The best answer is **A.** The somatomotor division of the oculomotor nerve innervates the levator palpebrae superioris, superior rectus, medial rectus, inferior rectus, and inferior oblique muscles; the visceromotor component innervates the sphincter and ciliary muscles. The trochlear nerve supplies the superior oblique muscle (rules out options **B, D,** and **E**); sympathetic nerves innervate the radial muscle (rules out options **C** and **D**); the abducens nerve supplies the lateral rectus (rules out **D** and **E**).

17. The best answer is **A.** Women over 40 years of age are particularly susceptible to open angle glaucoma; and it is more common in African–American than Caucasian individuals. Farsightedness is a risk factor for development of open angle glaucoma. Open-angle glaucoma progresses slowly and can be treated with agents that decrease the secretion or production of aqueous humor or with drugs that increase outflow of the aqueous humor (rules out option **B**). Closed angle glaucoma is caused by a rapid or sudden increase in intraocular pressure, causing eye pain, headaches, loss of vision, nausea, and vomiting (rules out options **C** and **D**). It is a medical emergency and requires surgery.

Hearing & Equilibrium

- Describe the components and functions of the external, middle, and inner ear.
- Describe the way that movements of molecules in the air are converted into impulses generated in hair cells in the cochlea.
- Explain the roles of the tympanic membrane, the auditory ossicles (malleus, incus, and stapes), and scala vestibule in sound transmission.
- Explain how auditory impulses travel from the cochlear hair cells to the auditory cortex.
- Explain how pitch, loudness, and timbre are coded in the auditory pathways.
- Describe the various forms of deafness and the tests used to distinguish between them.
- Explain how the receptors in the semicircular canals detect rotational acceleration and how the receptors in the saccule and utricle detect linear acceleration.
- List the major sensory inputs that provide the information that is synthesized in the brain into the sense of position in space.

INTRODUCTION

Specialized receptors (hair cells) for two sensory modalities (hearing and equilibrium) are housed in the ear. The external ear, middle ear, and cochlea of the inner ear are involved with hearing. The semicircular canals, utricle, and saccule of the inner ear are involved with equilibrium. There are six groups of hair cells in each inner ear: one in each of the three semicircular canals, the utricle, the saccule, and the cochlea. Receptors in the semicircular canals detect rotational acceleration, those in the utricle detect linear acceleration in the horizontal direction, and those in the saccule detect linear acceleration in the vertical direction.

■ STRUCTURE & FUNCTION OF THE EAR

EXTERNAL, MIDDLE, & INNER EAR

Sound travels inward from the external auditory meatus to the tympanic membrane of the external ear or pinna (Figure 10–1). Auditory ossicles (malleus, incus, and stapes) and two small muscles (tensor tympani and stapedius) are located in the middle ear (Figure 10–2). The inner ear (or labyrinth) has three components: the cochlea, three semicircular canals, and the otolith organs with hair cells that respond to sound, head rotation, and changes in gravity and head tilt, respectively (Figure 10–3).

The basilar membrane and Reissner membrane divide the cochlea into the upper scala vestibuli and lower scala tympani, which contain perilymph and communicate with each other, and the scala media which is continuous with the membranous

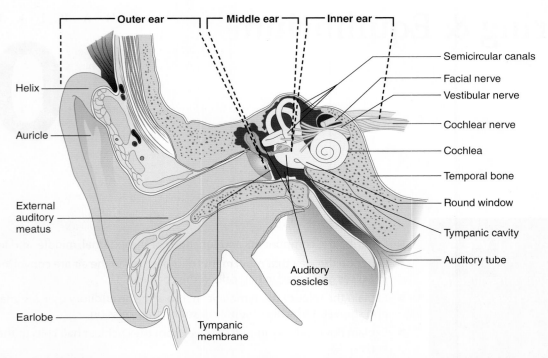

FIGURE 10–1   The structures of the external, middle, and inner portions of the human ear. Sound waves travel from the external ear to the tympanic membrane via the external auditory meatus. The middle ear is an air-filled cavity in the temporal bone; it contains the auditory ossicles. The inner ear is composed of the bony and membranous labyrinths. To make the relationships clear, the cochlea has been turned slightly and the middle ear muscles have been omitted. (Reproduced with permission from Fox SI. *Human Physiology*, 10th ed. New York, NY: McGraw-Hill; 2008.)

labyrinth and does not communicate with the other two scalae (**Figure 10–4**). Endolymph is formed in the scala media by the stria vascularis and has an unusually high concentration of K⁺. The difference in K⁺ concentration in the perilymph and endolymph creates a potential difference across the Reissner membrane of about +80 mV in the endolymph.

The organ of Corti contains the hair cells whose processes pierce the reticular lamina that is supported by the pillar cells or rods of Corti (Figure 10–4). Three rows of outer hair cells are lateral to the tunnel formed by the rods of Corti, and one row of inner hair cells is medial to the tunnel. The tips of the hairs of the outer (not inner) hair cells are embedded in the viscous, elastic tectorial membrane. The cell bodies of the sensory neurons are in the spiral ganglion; 90–95% of them innervate the inner hair cells, and 5–10% innervate the outer hair cells. The axons of the sensory neurons form the cochlear division of the eighth cranial nerve.

The semicircular canals are perpendicular to each other with a receptor structure (crista) in the ampulla (Figure 10–3). The crista consists of the hair cells and supporting cells embedded in a gelatinous mass (cupula). The otolith organs (saccule and utricle) are near the center of the membranous labyrinth; their sensory epithelium (macula) contains supporting cells and hair cells, surrounded by a membrane in which crystals of calcium carbonate (otoliths, otoconia, or ear dust) are embedded. The nerve fibers from the hair cells of the semicircular canals and otolith organs form the vestibular division of the eighth cranial nerve.

HAIR CELLS

The specialized sensory mechanoreceptors in the ear consist of six patches of hair cells in the membranous labyrinth (**Figure 10–5**). The hair cells in the organ of Corti signal hearing; those in the utricle and saccule signal horizontal and vertical acceleration, respectively, and those in the semicircular canals signal rotational acceleration. A single kinocilium (a nonmotile cilium) is found in all except the cochlea; stereocilia are found in all hair cells. Along an axis toward the kinocilium, the stereocilia increase progressively in height; along the perpendicular axis, all the stereocilia are of the same height.

Tip links are fine processes that tie each stereocilium to the side of its higher neighbor; they are mechanically sensitive cation channels in the taller process (**Figure 10–6**). When shorter stereocilia are pushed toward taller ones, the channels open and K⁺ and Ca²⁺ enter and produce depolarization. The influx of K⁺ results from the high concentration of K⁺ in the endolymph and the positive endoplasmic membrane potential. A myosin-based molecular motor in the taller neighbor then moves the channel toward the base, releasing tension in the tip link; the channel closes to restore the resting state. Depolarization of hair cells causes the release of a neurotransmitter to initiate depolarization of afferent neurons. The changes in membrane potential in the cilia are proportional to the direction and distance the hair cell moves.

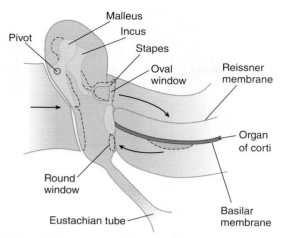

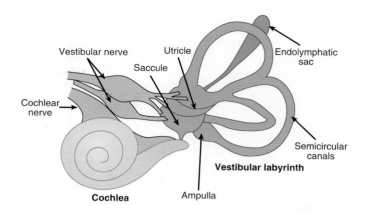

FIGURE 10–2 Schematic representation of the auditory ossicles and the way their movement translates movements of the tympanic membrane into a wave in the fluid of the inner ear. The wave is dissipated at the round window. The movements of the ossicles, the membranous labyrinth, and the round window are indicated by dashed lines. The waves are transformed by the eardrum and auditory ossicles into movements of the footplate of the stapes. These movements set up waves in the fluid of the inner ear. In response to the pressure changes produced by sound waves on its external surface, the tympanic membrane moves in and out to function as a resonator that reproduces the vibrations of the sound source. The motions of the tympanic membrane are imparted to the manubrium of the malleus, which rocks on an axis through the junction of its long and short processes, so that the short process transmits the vibrations of the manubrium to the incus. The incus moves so that the vibrations are transmitted to the head of the stapes. Movements of the head of the stapes swing its footplate.

■ HEARING

SOUND WAVES & SOUND TRANSMISSION

Sound is the sensation produced when vibrations of molecules in the external environment strike the tympanic membrane. These movements, expressed as changes in pressure per unit of time, are a series of sound waves that travel through air at a speed of ~344 m/s (770 mph) at 20°C at sea level. The speed of sound increases with temperature and altitude, but the speed of sound is 1450 m/s at 20°C in freshwater and is even greater in saltwater.

The loudness and pitch of a sound is directly correlated to the amplitude (expressed on a decibel scale) and frequency of the sound wave, respectively. Prolonged or frequent exposure to sounds above 85 dB can cause hearing loss. The sound frequencies audible to humans range from ~20 to 20,000 Hz. The threshold varies with the pitch of the sound, the greatest sensitivity being in the 1000- to 4000-Hz range. The pitch of the average male conversational voice is ~120 Hz; that of the average female voice is ~250 Hz.

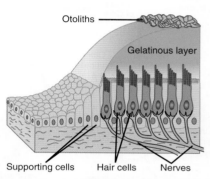

FIGURE 10–3 The membranous labyrinth of the inner ear has three components: semicircular canals, cochlea, and otolith organs. Hair cells in the semicircular canals are sensitive to angular accelerations that deflect the gelatinous cupula. Cochlea hair cells spiral along the basilar membrane within the organ of Corti. Airborne sounds set the eardrum in motion, which is conveyed to the cochlea by bones of the middle ear, and the membrane flexes up and down. Hair cells in the organ of Corti are stimulated by shearing motion. The otolithic organs (saccule and utricle) are sensitive to linear acceleration in vertical and horizontal planes. Hair cells are attached to the otolithic membrane. Information from the cochlear hair cells is carried by the cochlear division of the auditory (VIII cranial) nerve. Information from the hair cells in the semicircular canals and otolith organs is carried by the vestibular divisions of the auditory nerve.

In response to the pressure changes produced by sound waves on its external surface, the tympanic membrane resonates to reproduce the vibrations of the sound source (Figure 10–2). The ossicles function as a lever system that converts the resonant vibrations of the tympanic membrane into movements of the stapes against the perilymph-filled scala vestibuli of the cochlea. The action of the waves on the organ of Corti generates action potentials in the nerve fibers.

Outer hair cells amplify sound vibrations entering the inner ear. These changes occur in parallel with changes in prestin, the motor protein of outer hair cells. The olivocochlear bundle is the efferent fibers in the auditory nerve that arise from the superior olivary complex and end primarily around the bases of the outer hair cells of the organ of Corti. The activity in this nerve modulates the sensitivity

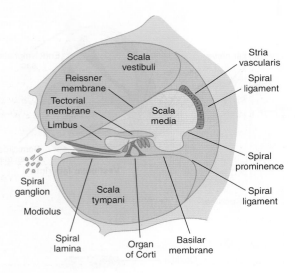

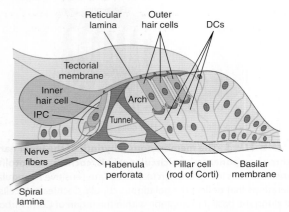

FIGURE 10–4 Schematic of the cochlea and organ of Corti in the membranous labyrinth of the inner ear. Top: A cross section of the cochlea showing the organ of Corti and the three scalae of the cochlea. **Bottom:** The structure of the organ of Corti as it appears in the basal turn of the cochlea. DC, Deiters cells supporting outer hair cells; IPC, inner phalangeal cells supporting inner hair cell.

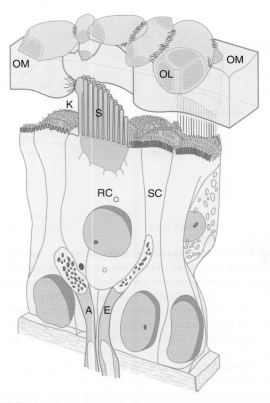

FIGURE 10–5 Structure of hair cell in the saccule. Hair cells in the membranous labyrinth of the ear have a common structure, and each is within an epithelium of supporting cells (SC) surmounted by an otolithic membrane (OM) embedded with crystals of calcium carbonate, the otoliths (OL). Projecting from the apical end are rod-shaped processes, or hair cells (RC), in contact with afferent (A) and efferent (E) nerve fibers. Except in the cochlea, one of these, kinocilium (K), is a nonmotile cilium with nine pairs of microtubules around its circumference and a central pair of microtubules. The stereocilia (S) are found in all hair cells; they have cores of actin filaments coated with isoforms of myosin. Within the clump of processes on each cell there is an orderly structure. Along an axis toward the kinocilium, the stereocilia increase progressively in height; along the perpendicular axis, all the stereocilia are the same height.

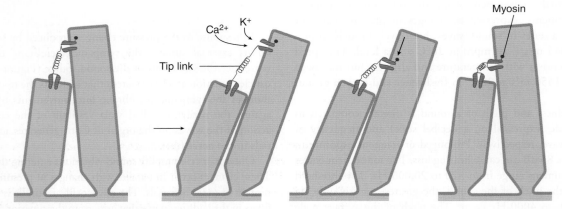

FIGURE 10–6 Schematic representation of the role of tip links in the responses of hair cells. When a stereocilium is pushed toward a taller stereocilium, the tip link is stretched and opens an ion channel in its taller neighbor. The channel next is presumably moved down the taller stereocilium by a molecular motor, so the tension on the tip link is released. When the hairs return to the resting position, the motor moves back up the stereocilium.

of hair cells via the release of acetylcholine. The effect is inhibitory and may function to block background noise.

Determining the direction from which a sound emanates depends on detecting the difference in the arrival time of the stimulus in the two ears and the difference in phase of the sound waves on the two sides. Also, sound is louder on the side closest to the source. Sounds coming from directly in front of an individual differ in quality from those coming from behind because each pinna is turned slightly forward. Lesions of the auditory cortex disrupt sound localization.

CENTRAL AUDITORY PATHWAY

The afferent fibers in the auditory division of the eighth cranial nerve end in dorsal and ventral cochlear nuclei (Figure 10–7). From there, impulses travel to the inferior colliculi, the centers for auditory reflexes, and the thalamic medial geniculate body to the auditory cortex on the superior temporal gyrus of the temporal lobe. Information from both ears converges on each superior olive; from there most

of the neurons respond to inputs from both sides. The responses of second-order neurons in the cochlear nuclei to sound stimuli are like those of the auditory nerve fibers. The frequency at which sounds of the lowest intensity evoke a response varies from unit to unit; with increased sound intensities, the band of frequencies to which a response occurs becomes wider. However, there is a sharper "cutoff" on the low-frequency side in the medullary neurons that is probably due to an inhibitory process in the brainstem. The auditory pathways are modified by experience; for example, in individuals who become deaf before language skills are fully developed, sign language activates auditory association areas. Conversely, individuals who become blind early in life are demonstrably better at localizing sound than individuals with normal eyesight.

DEAFNESS

Deafness is due to conductive or sensorineural hearing loss. Conductive deafness refers to impaired sound transmission in the external or middle ear and impacts all sound frequencies. It

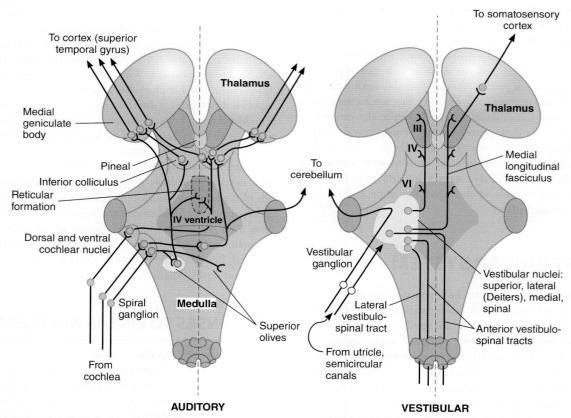

FIGURE 10–7 **Simplified diagram of main auditory (left) and vestibular (right) pathways superimposed on a dorsal view of the brainstem.** Cerebellum and cerebral cortex have been removed. For the auditory pathway, eighth cranial nerve afferent fibers form the cochlea end in dorsal and ventral cochlear nuclei. From there, most fibers cross the midline and terminate in the contralateral inferior colliculus. From there, fibers project to the medial geniculate body in the thalamus and then to the auditory cortex located on the superior temporal gyrus of the temporal lobe. For the vestibular pathway, the vestibular nerve terminates in the ipsilateral vestibular nucleus. Most fibers from the semicircular canals terminate in the superior and medial divisions of the vestibular nucleus and project to nuclei controlling eye movement. Most fibers from the utricle and saccule terminate in the lateral division, which then projects to the spinal cord. They also terminate on neurons that project to the cerebellum and the reticular formation. The vestibular nuclei also project to the thalamus and from there to the primary somatosensory cortex. The ascending connections to cranial nerve nuclei are concerned with eye movements.

TABLE 10–1 Common tests with a tuning fork to distinguish between sensorineural and conduction deafness.

	Weber	Rinne	Schwabach
Method	Base of vibrating tuning fork placed on vertex of skull	Base of vibrating tuning fork placed on mastoid process until subject no longer hears it, then held in air next to ear	Bone conduction of patient compared with that of healthy subject
Normal	Hears equally on both sides	Hears vibration in air after bone conduction is over	
Conduction deafness (one ear)	Sound louder in diseased ear because masking effect of environmental noise is absent on diseased side	Vibrations in air not heard after bone conduction is over	Bone conduction better than normal (conduction defect excludes masking noise)
Sensorineural deafness (one ear)	Sound louder in normal ear	Vibration heard in air after bone conduction is over, as long as nerve deafness is partial	Bone conduction worse than normal

can result from plugging of the external auditory canals with wax or foreign bodies, otitis externa (inflammation of the outer ear, "swimmer's ear") and otitis media (inflammation of the middle ear), perforation of the eardrum, and otosclerosis (an abnormal growth of bone in the middle ear). Conduction and sensorineural deafness can be differentiated by simple tests with a tuning fork (Table 10–1).

Sensorineural deafness is often the result of loss of cochlear hair cells but can be due to problems with the eighth cranial nerve or within central auditory pathways. It can impair the ability to hear certain pitches. Aminoglycoside antibiotics (eg, streptomycin and gentamicin) obstruct the mechanosensitive channels in the stereocilia of hair cells (especially outer hair cells) and the cells degenerate, causing sensorineural hearing loss and abnormal vestibular function. Damage to the hair cells by prolonged exposure to noise can result in hearing loss (Clinical Box 10–1). Other causes include tumors of the eighth cranial nerve and cerebellopontine angle and vascular damage in the medulla.

■ VESTIBULAR SYSTEM

The vestibular apparatus within the inner ear detects head motion and position and transduces this information to a neural signal (Figure 10–3). The cell bodies of the vestibular sensory neurons are in the vestibular ganglion; the vestibular nerve terminates in the ipsilateral vestibular nuclei that are primarily concerned with maintaining the position of the head in space; the tracts that descend from these nuclei mediate head-on-neck and head-on-body adjustments (Figure 10–7). Fibers from the semicircular canals terminate primarily in the superior and medial divisions of the nucleus; from here neurons project to nuclei controlling eye movement. Fibers from the utricle and saccule project to Deiters nucleus which then projects to the spinal cord (lateral vestibulospinal tract). Fibers from the utricle and saccule also terminate on neurons that project to the cerebellum and reticular formation. The vestibular nuclei project to the primary somatosensory cortex via the thalamus.

RESPONSES TO ROTATIONAL ACCELERATION

Rotational acceleration in the plane of a given semicircular canal stimulates its crista; the endolymph is displaced in a direction opposite to that of the rotation. The fluid pushes on the cupula, deforming it and bending the processes of the hair cells (Figure 10–3). When a constant speed of rotation is reached, the fluid spins at the same rate as the body and the cupula swings back into the upright position. When rotation is stopped, deceleration displaces the endolymph in the direction of the rotation, and the cupula is deformed in a direction opposite to that during acceleration. Movement of the cupula in one direction increases the firing rate of nerve fibers from the crista, and movement in the opposite direction inhibits neural activity.

Rotation causes maximal stimulation of the semicircular canals most nearly in the plane of rotation. Because the canals on one side of the head are a mirror image of those on the other side, the endolymph is displaced toward the ampulla on one side and away from it on the other. Thus, the pattern of stimulation reaching the brain varies with both the direction and plane of rotation. Clinical Box 10–2 describes the characteristic eye movements that occur during rotation.

RESPONSES TO LINEAR ACCELERATION

The utricular and saccular maculae respond to horizontal and vertical acceleration, respectively. The otoliths in the surrounding membrane are denser than the endolymph, and acceleration in any direction causes them to be displaced in the opposite direction, distorting the hair cell processes and generating activity in the nerve fibers. The maculae also discharge tonically in the absence of head movement due to the pull of gravity on the otoliths.

The impulses generated from these receptors mediate in part the labyrinth righting reflex in which tilting of the head stimulates the otolithic organs; the response is compensatory contraction of the neck muscles to keep the head level. Visual cues can initiate

CLINICAL BOX 10-1

Hearing Loss

Hearing loss is the most common sensory defect in humans. According to the World Health Organization, over 270 million people worldwide have moderate to profound hearing loss, with one-fourth of these cases beginning in childhood. According to the National Institutes of Health, ~15% of Americans between 20 and 69 years of age have high-frequency hearing loss due to exposure to loud sounds (noise-induced hearing loss). Outer hair cells are particularly vulnerable to damage by excessive noise. Hearing loss can result from the use of some antibiotics (streptomycin), loop diuretics (furosemide), and platinum-based chemotherapy agents (cisplatin). These ototoxic agents damage the outer hair cells or the stria vascularis. Presbycusis, gradual hearing loss associated with aging, affects more than one-third of those over age 75 and is due to gradual cumulative loss of hair cells and neurons. In most cases, hearing loss is a multifactorial disorder caused by both genetic and environmental factors. Single-gene mutations can cause hearing loss that is a monogenic disorder with an autosomal dominant, autosomal recessive, X-linked, or mitochondrial mode of inheritance. Monogenic forms can be syndromic (hearing loss associated with other abnormalities) or nonsyndromic (only hearing loss). About 0.1% of newborns have genetic mutations leading to deafness. Nonsyndromic deafness due to genetic mutations can first appear in adults and may account for many of the 16% of all adults who have significant hearing impairment. The products of 100 or more genes are essential for normal hearing, and deafness loci have been described in all but 5 of the 24 human chromosomes. The most common mutation leading to congenital hearing loss is that of the protein connexin 26. This defect prevents the normal recycling of K^+ through the sustentacular cells. Mutations in three nonmuscle myosins also cause deafness: myosin-VIIa (associated with the actin in the hair cell processes), myosin-Ib (part of the "adaptation motor" that adjusts tension on the tip links), and myosin-VI (essential for the formation of cilia). Deafness is also associated with mutant forms of α-tectin, a protein in the tectorial membrane. In Pendred syndrome a mutant multifunctional anion exchanger causes deafness and goiter. A mutation of the K^+ channel protein KVLQT1 is linked to deafness. In the stria vascularis, the normal form of this protein maintains the high K^+ concentration in endolymph, and in the heart it helps maintain a normal QT interval. Individuals who are homozygous for mutant KVLQT1 are deaf and predisposed to ventricular arrhythmias and sudden death that characterize long QT syndrome. The membrane protein barttin is mutated in a form of Bartter syndrome associated with congenital deafness and renal failure.

THERAPEUTIC HIGHLIGHTS

Cochlear implants are used to treat children and adults with severe hearing loss. According to the US Food and Drug Administration in 2012, ~324,000 people worldwide have received cochlear implants. These devices consist of a microphone (picks up environmental sounds), speech processor (selects and arranges sounds), transmitter and receiver/stimulator (converts sounds into electrical impulses), and an electrode array (sends impulses to the auditory nerve). Although the implant cannot restore normal hearing, it provides a useful representation of sounds to a deaf person. Those with adult-onset deafness can learn to associate the signals the implant provides with sounds they remember. Children who receive cochlear implants in conjunction with intensive therapy have been able to acquire speech and language skills. Research is ongoing to develop cells that can replace the hair cells in the inner ear.

CLINICAL BOX 10-2

Nystagmus

Nystagmus, the jerky movement of the eye seen at the start and end of a period of rotation, is a vestibuloocular reflex that maintains visual fixation on stationary points while the body rotates. When rotation starts, the eyes move slowly in a direction opposite to that of rotation. When the limit of this movement is reached, the eyes quickly snap back to a new fixation point and then again move slowly in the other direction. The slow component is initiated by impulses from the vestibular labyrinths; the quick component is triggered by neurons in the brainstem. Nystagmus is often horizontal (ie, eyes move in a horizontal plane), but it can be vertical if the head is tipped sideways during rotation or rotatory if the head is tipped forward. The direction of eye movement is identified by the direction of the quick component. The direction of the quick component during rotation is the same as that of the rotation, but the postrotatory nystagmus that occurs with displacement of the cupula is in the opposite direction. Nystagmus at rest is a sign of a pathology. Acquired nystagmus can be seen after acute temporal bone fracture affecting semicircular canals, after damage to the flocculonodular lobe or midline structures (eg, fastigial nucleus), and as a result of stroke, multiple sclerosis, head injury, and brain tumors. Nystagmus can be used as a diagnostic indicator of the integrity of the vestibular system. In the case of a unilateral lesion in the vestibular pathway, nystagmus is reduced or absent on the side of the lesion.

CLINICAL BOX 10–3

Vestibular Disorders

Vestibular balance disorders are one of the most common reasons elderly people seek medical advice. Neither lightheadedness nor dizziness is necessarily a symptom of vestibular problems, but vertigo is a prominent symptom of a disorder of the inner ear or vestibular system, especially when a labyrinth is inflamed. Benign paroxysmal positional vertigo is the most common vestibular disorder; it is characterized by episodes of vertigo during changes in body position. It can occur if otoconia separate from the otolith membrane and become lodged in the semicircular canal. Ménière disease is an abnormality of the inner ear causing vertigo or severe dizziness, tinnitus, fluctuating hearing loss, and the sensation of pressure or pain in the affected ear lasting several hours. Symptoms can occur suddenly and recur daily or very rarely. The hearing loss is initially transient but can become permanent. The pathophysiology may involve an immune reaction. An inflammatory response can increase fluid volume within the membranous labyrinth, causing it to rupture and allowing the endolymph and perilymph to intermix. The worldwide prevalence for Ménière disease is ~12 per 1000 individuals. It is diagnosed most often between the ages of 30 and 60 and affects both sexes similarly. The nausea, blood pressure changes, sweating, pallor, and vomiting that are common symptoms of motion sickness are produced by excessive vestibular stimulation and occur when conflicting information is fed into the vestibular and other sensory systems. The symptoms may be due to reflexes mediated via vestibular connections in the brainstem and the flocculonodular lobe of the cerebellum.

THERAPEUTIC HIGHLIGHTS

Symptoms of benign paroxysmal positional vertigo often subside over weeks or months; if treatment is needed, one option is canalith repositioning which consists of simple and slow maneuvers to position the head to move the otoconia from the semicircular canals back into the vestibule that houses the utricle. There is no cure for Ménière disease, but the symptoms can be controlled by reducing the fluid retention through dietary changes (low-salt diet, no caffeine, no alcohol), diuretics, or vestibulosuppressants (eg, antihistamines) that decrease the excitability of the middle ear labyrinth and block conduction in the vestibular-cerebellar pathway. Motion sickness can be prevented with the use of antihistamines or scopolamine, a muscarinic receptor antagonist.

the optical righting reflex which maintains the head in a stable position and the eyes fixed on visual targets despite movements of the body.

Although most of the responses to stimulation of the maculae are reflex in nature, vestibular impulses reach the cerebral cortex and are responsible for conscious perception of motion and provide information necessary for orientation in space. Vertigo is the sensation of rotation in the absence of actual rotation and is a prominent symptom when one labyrinth is inflamed. Visual cues are also important for orientation in space. Other information comes from proprioceptors in joint capsules and cutaneous touch and pressure receptors. These inputs are synthesized at a cortical level into a continuous picture of the individual's orientation in space. Clinical Box 10–3 describes some common vestibular disorders.

CHAPTER SUMMARY

- Sound waves travel from the external ear, to the external auditory meatus and tympanic membrane, and then pass through three auditory ossicles (malleus, incus, and stapes) in the middle ear. The inner ear contains the cochlea and organ of Corti.
- The organ of Corti hair cells signal hearing. The stereocilia provide a mechanism for generating changes in membrane potential proportional to the direction and distance the hair moves. Sound is the sensation produced when longitudinal vibrations of air molecules strike the tympanic membrane.
- The pressure changes produced by sound waves cause the tympanic membrane to move in and out, acting as a resonator to reproduce the vibrations of the sound source. Auditory ossicles serve as a lever system to convert these vibrations into movements of the stapes against the perilymph-filled scala vestibuli of the cochlea.
- The auditory pathway includes the eighth cranial nerve afferent fibers, dorsal and ventral cochlear nuclei, inferior colliculi, thalamic medial geniculate body, and the auditory cortex.
- Loudness is correlated with the amplitude of a sound wave, pitch with the frequency, and timbre with harmonic vibrations.
- Conductive deafness is due to impaired sound transmission in the external or middle ear and impacts all sound frequencies. Sensorineural deafness is usually due to loss of cochlear hair cells but can result from damage to the eighth cranial nerve or central auditory pathway. Conduction and sensorineural deafness can be differentiated by simple tests with a tuning fork.
- Rotational acceleration stimulates the crista in the semicircular canals, displacing the endolymph in a direction opposite to the direction of rotation, deforming the cupula and bending the hair cell. The utricle responds to horizontal acceleration and the saccule to vertical acceleration. Acceleration in any direction displaces the otoliths, distorting the hair cell processes and generating neural activity.
- Spatial orientation is dependent on input from vestibular receptors, visual cues, proprioceptors in joint capsules, and cutaneous touch and pressure receptors.

MULTIPLE-CHOICE QUESTIONS

For all questions, select the single best answer unless otherwise directed.

1. A 40-year-old woman made an appointment with her primary care physician after she experienced sudden onset of vertigo, tinnitus and hearing loss in her left ear, nausea, and vomiting. This was the second episode in the past few months. She was referred to an otolaryngologist to rule out Ménière disease. Which of the following is a possible cause of Ménière disease?
   A. Ménière disease is autosomal dominant genetic disorder that weakens the membranous labyrinth of the inner ear.
   B. The hair cells of the cochlea are altered to give the sensation of motion even at rest.
   C. The otoliths dislodge, enter the semicircular canal, and stimulate the hair cells.
   D. An inflammatory response increases fluid volume within the membranous labyrinth, causing it to rupture and allowing the endolymph and perilymph to intermix.
   E. The membranous labyrinth on one side has become inflamed.

2. A 45-year-old man with testicular cancer underwent chemotherapy treatment with cisplatin. He reported several adverse side effects including changes in taste, numbness and tingling in his fingertips, and reduced sound clarity. What is a likely basis for the reduced sound clarity in this individual?
   A. The cancer had metastasized to the spiral ganglion.
   B. Cisplatin preferentially damaged the inner versus outer hair cells in the cochlea.
   C. Cisplatin preferentially damaged the outer versus inner hair cells in the organ of Corti.
   D. The cancer had metastasized to the auditory cortex.
   E. Cisplatin damaged the auditory (cochlear) division of the eighth cranial nerve.

3. After playing the violin for the Boston Symphony Orchestra for 18 years, a 40-year-old man was given the opportunity to follow the dream he had as a child to be a physician like his father. Compared to other students in his medical school class, what distinctive features might be expressed in his auditory system?
   A. The pitch of his conversational voice will be about 120 Hz compared to his younger male classmates whose voices are likely to have a pitch of about 250 Hz.
   B. He will be able to distinguish about 2000 pitches; in contrast, his younger classmates will be able to distinguish only about 1000 pitches.
   C. As a musician, he will be better able to localize sound than his nonmusician classmates.
   D. The Wernicke area on the right side of his brain is more concerned with melody, pitch, and sound; in contrast, Wernicke area on the left side of the brain of his nonmusician classmates is more concerned with these sound qualities.
   E. When presented with musical tones, a larger area of his auditory cortex will be activated compared to the area activated in the cortex of his nonmusician classmates.

4. A 40-year-old man, employed as a road construction worker for over 20 years, went to his clinician to report that he recently began to notice difficulty hearing during normal conversations. A Weber test indicated that sound from a vibrating tuning fork was localized to the right ear. A Schwabach test showed that bone conduction was below normal. A Rinne test showed that both air and bone conduction were abnormal, but air conduction lasted longer than bone conduction. The diagnosis was
   A. sensorineural deafness in both ears.
   B. conduction deafness in the right ear.
   C. sensorineural deafness in the right ear.
   D. conduction deafness in the left ear.
   E. sensorineural deafness in the left ear.

5. What would the diagnosis be if a patient had the following test results? Weber test showed that sound from a vibrating tuning fork was louder than normal; Schwabach test showed that bone conduction was better than normal; and Rinne test showed that air conduction did not outlast bone conduction.
   A. Sensorineural deafness in both ears
   B. Conduction deafness in both ears
   C. Normal hearing
   D. Both sensorineural and conduction deafness
   E. A possible tumor on the left eighth cranial nerve

6. A faculty member that is a neurophysiologist agreed to participate in a Grand Rounds at a local teaching hospital. She was paired with an otolaryngologist who was presenting the medical problems and treatment of a 21-year-old woman who had progressive hearing loss. The neurophysiologist was asked to describe the central pathway that transmits the sensation of sound to the cortex. She would have told the audience in attendance that the auditory pathway is composed of
   A. sensory fibers in the eighth cranial nerve that synapse in the spiral ganglia and from there the nerve projects to the ipsilateral lateral cochlear nucleus which connects with the superior colliculi bilaterally and then the auditory cortex.
   B. afferent fibers of the eighth cranial nerve that synapse bilaterally in the dorsal and ventral cochlear nuclei, which in turn synapses in the inferior colliculi which connects to the lateral geniculate body, and then the auditory cortex.
   C. sensory fibers of the eighth cranial nerve that synapse in the ipsilateral dorsal and ventral cochlear nuclei, which in turn synapses in the contralateral superior colliculi which connects to the lateral geniculate body, and then the auditory cortex.
   D. sensory fibers of the eighth cranial nerve that synapse in the ipsilateral dorsal and ventral cochlear nuclei, which in turn project bilaterally to the inferior colliculi which connects with the medial geniculate body, and then the auditory cortex.
   E. afferent fibers of the eighth cranial nerve that synapse in the ipsilateral medial and lateral cochlear nuclei, which in turn project bilaterally to the inferior colliculi which connects with the medial geniculate body, and then the auditory cortex.

7. A healthy male medical student volunteered to undergo evaluation of the function of his vestibular system for a class demonstration. The direction of his nystagmus is expected to be vertical when he is rotated
   A. after warm water is put in one of his ears.
   B. with his head tipped backward.
   C. after cold water is put in both of his ears.
   D. with his head tipped sideways.
   E. with his head tipped forward.

8. A healthy male medical student volunteered to undergo evaluation of the function of his vestibular system for a class demonstration. After a period of spinning, the chair was suddenly stopped and the fast phase of his eye movement was noted to be in the opposite direction of the rotation, known as the "postrotatory nystagmus." Postrotatory nystagmus is caused by continued movement of
   A. aqueous humor over the ciliary body in the eye.
   B. cerebrospinal fluid over the parts of the brainstem that contain the vestibular nuclei.
   C. endolymph in the semicircular canals, with consequent bending of the cupula and stimulation of hair cells.
   D. endolymph toward the helicotrema.
   E. perilymph over hair cells that have their processes embedded in the tectorial membrane.

9. An MD/PhD candidate was doing her research in a laboratory that studied the vestibular system. Her research involved an assessment of the specialized mechanoreceptors in the utricle. In the utricle, tip links in hair cells are involved in
   A. formation of perilymph.
   B. depolarization of the stria vascularis.
   C. movements of the tympanic membrane.
   D. perception of sound.
   E. regulation of mechanically sensitive cation channels.

10. At the age of 10 months, a boy was diagnosed with sensorineural deafness. Upon further examination, it was evident that the child also experienced polydipsia and polyuria. These symptoms persisted as he grew to a young adult. At that time he was found to have a normal blood pressure but elevated renin levels. This clinical profile could be due to a mutation in the gene encoding
   A. the membrane protein barttin.
   B. a multifunctional anion exchanger.
   C. the protein connexin 26.
   D. the protein α-tectin.
   E. myosin-VIIa.

11. A 78-year-old man noticed that he needed to increase the volume on his television in order to listen to the nightly news. Also, he frequently noticed that when he would answer the phone, the person on the other end seemed to be mumbling. One day he decided to call the phone number on a mailing that he received from a company that sold hearing aids. He was told that he likely had presbycusis. What is presbycusis and what is its most common cause?
    A. Presbycusis is an age-related gradual loss in hearing commonly due to a progressive loss of hair cells in the cochlea.
    B. Presbycusis is a sudden loss in hearing due to a defect in calcium metabolism that causes a progressive accumulation of otoconia in the ear canal.
    C. Presbycusis is a combination of hearing loss and an enlarged thyroid gland due to a mutant multifunctional anion exchanger.
    D. Presbycusis is a gradual hearing loss due to a progressive buildup of cerumen in the external auditory canal.
    E. Presbycusis is a gradual hearing loss associated with aging and is most often due to thickening of the tympanic membrane.

12. A 2-year-old girl was diagnosed with a type of sensorineural deafness. After being evaluated by an audiologist, she was determined to be a good candidate for a cochlear implant. The child's mother asked the audiologist about the causes of sensorineural deafness and she learned that it includes
    A. otitis externa, otitis media, and excessive accumulation of endolymph.
    B. lack of development or damage to saccule hair cells, damage of the eighth cranial nerve, and a lesion of the lateral geniculate nucleus.
    C. thickening of the tympanic membrane, dysfunction of the malleus, incus, and stapes in the middle ear, and a mutation of a K⁺ channel protein KVLQT1.
    D. lack of development or damage to hair cells in the organ of Corti, damage of the eighth cranial nerve, and obstruction of the mechanosensitive channels in the stereocilia of outer hair cells.
    E. damage to the tensor tympani or stapedius muscles in the middle ear and vascular damage in the medulla.

13. A 48-year-old man was diagnosed with conductive deafness and learned that he was not a candidate for a cochlear implant. He asked his otolaryngologist about the causes of this type of deafness and he learned that it includes
    A. otitis externa, otitis media, and a buildup of cerumen in the ear canal.
    B. loss of outer hair cells in the cochlea, a lesion of the medial geniculate nucleus, and obstruction of the mechanosensitive channels in the stereocilia of hair cells.
    C. the use of streptomycin, furosemide, and cisplatin.
    D. loss of cochlear hair cells, a lesion in Deiters nucleus, and tumor in the auditory cortex.
    E. damage to the otolith organ and Ménière disease.

14. A 36-year-old man made an appointment with his primary care physician after he had experienced several episodes of vertigo when he was bending over. He was diagnosed with benign paroxysmal positional vertigo which is often caused by
    A. the use of streptomycin or furosemide.
    B. otoconia lodged in the cupula of the semicircular canal.
    C. a fracture of the temporal bone affecting semicircular canals or damage to the flocculonodular lobe of the cerebellum.
    D. loss of saccular hair cells and a rupture of the membranous labyrinth.
    E. inflammation of the otolith organ and damage to the ossicles in the middle ear.

15. A 9-year-old girl complained of ear pain which was found to be due to an inflammation and build-up of fluids in the middle ear. She was diagnosed with a middle ear infection, acute otitis media of bacterial origin, and she was treated with an antibiotic. The middle ear contains
    A. hair cells that mediate linear acceleration.
    B. the membranous labyrinth containing endolymph.
    C. the bony labyrinth containing perilymph fluid.
    D. hair cells that mediate hearing.
    E. the auditory ossicles and skeletal muscles.

ANSWERS

1. The best answer is **D**. The pathophysiology of Ménière disease likely involves an immune reaction. An inflammatory response can increase fluid volume within the membranous labyrinth, causing it to rupture and allowing the endolymph and perilymph to mix together. It is not a genetic disorder; an example an autosomal dominant pattern of genetic disorder that leads to hearing loss is some cases of nonsyndromic deafness (rules out option **A**). Damage to the cochlear hair cells would be most apt to cause hearing loss but not the symptoms of damage to the vestibular system described by this subject (rules out **B**). Option **C** is ruled out as this is a description of the cause of benign paroxysmal positional vertigo, which is the most common vestibular disorder and is characterized by episodes of vertigo during changes in body position (eg, turning over in bed, bending over). Vertigo can occur if one labyrinth is inflamed, but it does not account for the other symptoms described here (rules out option **E**).

2. The best answer is **C**. The platinum-based chemotherapy agents like cisplatin are ototoxins that damage the outer hair cells in the cochlea (organ of Corti) or the stria vascularis; activation of outer hair cells improves sound clarity by amplifying sound vibrations entering the inner ear. Very few outer hair cells (5–10%) are connected to the sensory fibers. Cisplatin is less likely to damage inner hair cells (which are innervated by sensory fibers in the eighth cranial nerve); it is a neurotoxin and primarily affects sensory fibers in the limbs rather than cranial nerves (rules out options **B** and **E**). Testicular cancer has not been shown to metastasize commonly to the cranial nerves and auditory cortex, thus options **A** and **D** are not the best answer.

3. The best answer is **E**. Musicians provide an example of cortical plasticity. In these individuals, the size of the auditory areas activated by musical tones is increased. The pitch of the average adult male voice in conversation is about 120 Hz and that of the average adult female voice about 250 Hz (rules out option **A**). The number of pitches that can be distinguished by an average individual is about 2000, but trained musicians can improve on this figure considerably (rules out option **B**). Being a musician does not impact sound localization (rules out option **C**). Wernicke area on the right side is more concerned with melody, pitch, and sound intensity in all individuals (rules out option **D**).

4. The best answer is **E**. Prolonged or frequent exposure to sounds above 85 dB can cause hearing loss. The results of each of these tests indicates that he has sensorineural hearing loss in one ear, since the Weber test showed that sound was localized to the right ear, it means the left ear is the one with hearing loss (rules out options **A** and **C**). Options **B** and **D** can be ruled out because conduction deafness would show that sound is louder in diseased ear because masking effect of environmental noise is absent on diseased side (Weber test), vibrations in air not heard after bone conduction is over (Rinne test), and bone conduction better than normal because a conduction defect excludes masking noise (Schwabach test).

5. The best answer is **B**. As described above in Question 4, these results are indicative of conduction deafness in both ears. Also see the comments for Question 4 to explain why these results are not indicative of sensorineural deafness (rules out options **A** and **D**). Option **C** is ruled out because normal hearing would show equal sound from both ears (Weber test) and

vibrations heard in air after bone conduction is over (Rinne test). A tumor on the left eighth cranial nerve would not cause bilateral hearing loss (rules out option **E**).

6. The best answer is option **D**. The auditory pathway goes from the eighth cranial nerve to the ipsilateral dorsal and ventral cochlear nuclei and bilaterally to the inferior colliculi to the medial geniculate body to the auditory cortex. Information from both ears converges on each superior olive, and beyond this, most of the neurons respond to inputs from both sides. The spiral ganglion is the location of cell bodies of the eighth cranial nerve, not a synaptic site (rules out option **A**). The eighth cranial nerve terminates ipsilaterally not bilaterally in the cochlear nuclei (rules out option **B**). The cochlear nuclei project to the inferior not superior colliculi (rules out option **C**). The eighth cranial nerve synapses in the dorsal and ventral (not medial and lateral) cochlear nuclei (rules out option **E**).

7. The best answer is **D**. Nystagmus can be vertical when the head is tipped sideways during rotation. By convention, the direction of eye movement is identified by the direction of the quick component. The direction of the quick component during rotation is the same as that of the rotation, but the postrotatory nystagmus that occurs with displacement of the cupula is in the opposite direction. The semicircular canals are stimulated by instilling warm (40°C) or cold (30°C) water into the external auditory meatus. The temperature difference sets up convection currents in the endolymph and motion of the cupula. Options **A** and **C** can be ruled out because in healthy persons, the test follows the mnemonic COWS (Cold water nystagmus is opposite sides; Warm water nystagmus is same side). To avoid nystagmus, vertigo, and nausea when irrigating the ear canals in the treatment of ear infections, it is important that the fluid used is at body temperature. Nystagmus is rotatory when the head is tipped backward or forward (rules out options **B** and **E**).

8. The best answer is **C**. When rotation is suddenly stopped, the deceleration displaces the endolymph in the direction of the rotation, and the cupula is deformed which activates the hair cells. Aqueous humor and cerebrospinal fluid are not involved in nystagmus (rules out options **A** and **B**). The helicotrema is a small opening in the cochlea and it contains perilymph not endolymph (rules out option **D**). The tectorial membrane is in the cochlea (hearing), not semicircular canals which are involved in nystagmus (rules out option **E**).

9. The best answer is **E**. Tip links connect the tip of each stereocilium to the side of its higher neighbor to regulate mechanically sensitive cation channels in the taller process. Perilymp is extracellular fluid in the scala vestibule and scala tympani in the cochlea not utricle (rules out option **A**). The stria vascularis is capillary loops and small blood vessels that produce endolymph in the scala media of the cochlea (rules out option **B**). The tympanic membrane is part of the external ear (rules out option **C**). The utricle is not involved in the perception of sound (rules out **D**).

10. The best answer is **A**. The combination of hearing loss and renal dysfunction is indicative of infantile Bartter syndrome with sensorineural deafness that is caused by a mutation of the gene that encodes barttin protein. A mutation in the gene encoding a multifunctional anion exchanger is associated with Pendred syndrome (rules out **B**). A mutation in the gene encoding the protein connexin 26 is associated with some forms of congenital deafness, and mutation in the gene encoding the protein α-tectin and myosin-VIIa also are associated with forms of deafness but not combined with renal dysfunction (rules out options **C, D**, and **E**).

11. The best answer is **A.** Presbycusis is the gradual hearing loss associated with aging; it affects more than one-third of those over age 75 and is most often due to a gradual and cumulative loss of cochlear hair cells in the inner ear. Less frequently, presbycusis can be due to abnormalities of the tympanic membrane or dysfunction of the ossicles in the middle ear (rules out option **E**). Presbycusis does not have a sudden onset and is not due to a defect in calcium metabolism; when otoconia separate from the otolith membrane, they become lodged in the semicircular canal and cause vertigo not hearing impairment (rules out option **B**). A combination of hearing loss and an enlarged thyroid is indicative of Pendred syndrome (rules out option **C**). Accumulation of cerumen (ear wax) is an example of conductive deafness and is not age-related (rules out option **D**).

12. The best answer is **D.** Sensorineural deafness is most commonly the result of loss of cochlear (organ of Corti) hair cells due to a variety of causes including ototoxins, excessive hearing, and genetic factors; it can also be due to damage (eg, tumors) to the eighth cranial nerve or within central auditory pathways, and vascular damage to the medullary regions involved in hearing. Options **A, C**, and **E** all include problems in non-neural components which do not account for sensorineural deafness. Option **B** can be ruled out because the saccule hair cells and lateral geniculate nucleus are not involved in hearing.

13. The best answer is **A.** Conductive deafness refers to impaired sound transmission in the external or middle ear and the causes include plugging of the external auditory canals with wax (cerumen) or foreign bodies, otitis externa (inflammation of the outer ear, "swimmer's ear") and otitis media (inflammation of the middle ear) causing fluid accumulation, perforation of the eardrum, and osteosclerosis. Options **B, C**, and **D** can be ruled out as they include causes of sensorineural deafness. Damage to the otolith and Ménière disease are examples of vestibular disorders (rules out option **E**).

14. The best answer is **B.** Benign paroxysmal positional vertigo is the most common vestibular disorder characterized by episodes of vertigo that occur with particular changes in body position (eg, turning over in bed and bending over). It can occur if otoconia from the utricle separate from the otolith membrane and become lodged in the semicircular canal, causing abnormal deflections when the head changes position relative to gravity. The use of streptomycin or furosemide can lead to sensorineural hearing loss (rules out option **A**). Acquired nystagmus is due to acute temporal bone fracture affecting semicircular canals or damage to the flocculonodular lobe or midline structures such as the fastigial nucleus (rules out option **C**). A rupture of the membranous labyrinth can occur in Ménière disease and can contribute to vertigo and hearing loss (rules out **D**). Damage to the auditory ossicles would cause conductive hearing loss (rules out option **E**).

15. The best answer is **E.** The middle ear is an air-filled cavity in the temporal bone and contains the three auditory ossicles (malleus, incus, and stapes) and two small skeletal muscles (tensor tympani and stapedius). Hair cells that detect linear acceleration are located in the utricle of the inner ear; hair cells that mediate hearing are located in the cochlea of the inner ear (rules out options **A** and **D**). The membranous labyrinth containing endolymph and the bony labyrinth containing perilymph are located within the inner ear (rules out options **B** and **C**). Infections of the inner ear are typically of viral rather than bacterial origin. Symptoms of an inner ear infection include vertigo, dizziness, and difficulties with balance, vision, or hearing may result.

Smell & Taste

OBJECTIVES

After studying this chapter, you should be able to:

- Describe the basic features of the neural elements in the olfactory epithelium and olfactory bulb.
- Describe signal transduction in odorant receptors.
- Outline the pathway by which impulses generated in the olfactory epithelium reach the olfactory cortex.
- Describe the location and cellular composition of taste buds.
- Name the five major taste receptors and signal transduction mechanisms in these receptors.
- Outline the pathways by which impulses generated in taste receptors reach the insular cortex.

INTRODUCTION

Smell (olfaction) and taste (gustation) receptors are chemoreceptors that are stimulated by molecules in a solution within the nasal mucus and saliva in the mouth. The sensations of smell and taste allow individuals to distinguish between estimates of up to 30 million compounds that are present in food, predators, and mates and to convert the information received into appropriate behaviors. Odors from food enter our nasal passages at the same time that the taste receptors in our mouth are stimulated by the food. Smell and taste are separate senses but interact with each other to account for the flavor we experience when we eat and drink. Flavor refers to the overall perception that results from a combination of taste and smell.

■ SMELL

OLFACTORY EPITHELIUM & OLFACTORY BULBS

Olfactory sensory neurons are located in the yellowish pigmented olfactory epithelium of the nasal mucosa (**Figure 11–1A**). These sensory neurons are interspersed with glia-like supporting (sustentacular) cells and basal stem cells. New olfactory sensory neurons are generated by basal stem cells to replace those damaged by exposure to the environment. The olfactory epithelium is covered by a thin layer of mucus secreted by the supporting cells and Bowman glands, which lie beneath the epithelium.

Each olfactory sensory neuron has a short, thick dendrite that projects into the nasal cavity where it terminates in a knob containing 6–12 cilia (Figure 11–1). The cilia are unmyelinated processes that protrude into the mucus overlying the epithelium. Odorant molecules (chemicals) dissolve in the mucus and bind to odorant receptors on the cilia of olfactory sensory neurons. The mucus provides the appropriate molecular and ionic environment for odor detection.

The axons of the olfactory sensory neurons (first cranial nerve) enter the olfactory bulbs where they contact the primary dendrites of the mitral cells and tufted cells to form anatomically discrete synaptic units called olfactory glomeruli (**Figure 11–2**). The olfactory bulbs also contain periglomerular cells, which are inhibitory neurons connecting one glomerulus to another, and granule cells, which have no axons and make reciprocal synapses with the dendrites of the mitral and tufted cells. At these synapses, the mitral or tufted cells excite granule cells by releasing glutamate, and the granule cells inhibit the mitral or tufted cell by releasing GABA.

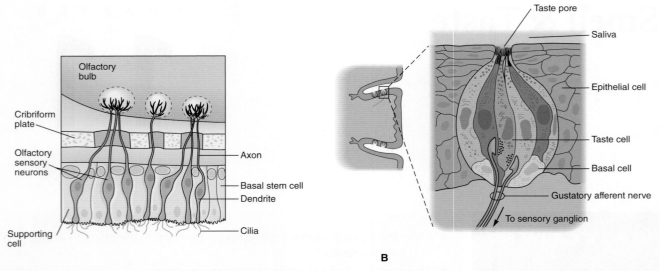

FIGURE 11–1 **Sensory components for smell and taste. (A)** There are three cell types in the olfactory epithelium: olfactory sensory neurons (odorant receptors), supporting (sustentacular) cells, and basal stem cells. Each olfactory sensory neuron has a dendrite that projects to the epithelial surface. Numerous cilia protrude into the mucus layer lining the nasal lumen. Odorants bind to specific odorant receptors on the cilia and initiate a cascade of events leading to generation of action potentials in the sensory axon. **(B)** Taste buds are composed of basal stem cells and three types of taste cells (dark, light, and intermediate). Taste cells extend from the base of the taste bud to the taste pore, where microvilli contact tastants dissolved in saliva and mucus. (Modified with permission from Kandel ER, Schwartz JH, Jessell TM [editors]: *Principles of Neural Science*, 4th ed. New York, NY: McGraw-Hill; 2000.)

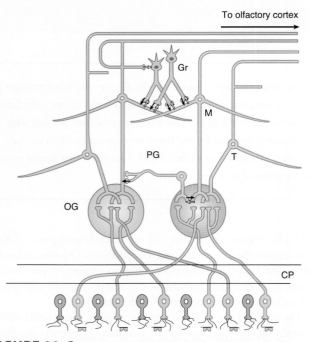

FIGURE 11–2 **Basic neural circuits in the olfactory bulb.**
Note that olfactory receptor cells with one type of odorant receptor project to one olfactory glomerulus (OG) and olfactory receptor cells with another type of receptor project to a different OG. Solid black arrows signify inhibition via GABA release, and white arrows signify excitatory connections via glutamate release. CP, cribriform plate; Gr, granule cell; M, mitral cell; PG, periglomerular cell; T, tufted cell. (Adapted with permission from Mori K, et al: The olfactory bulb: coding and processing of odor molecular information, *Science*. 1999 Oct 22; 286(5440):711–715.)

Free endings of many trigeminal pain fibers are found in the olfactory epithelium. They are stimulated by nasal irritants, which lead to the characteristic "odor" of substances like peppermint, menthol, and chlorine. Activation of these endings also initiates sneezing, lacrimation, and respiratory inhibition.

OLFACTORY CORTEX

The axons of the mitral and tufted cells pass posteriorly through the lateral olfactory stria to terminate on apical dendrites of pyramidal cells in five regions of the olfactory cortex: anterior olfactory nucleus, olfactory tubercle, piriform cortex, amygdala, and entorhinal cortex **(Figure 11–3)**. From these regions, information travels directly to the frontal cortex or via the thalamus to the orbitofrontal cortex. The pathway to the orbitofrontal cortex relays the conscious discrimination of odors; the pathway to the amygdala relays the emotional responses to olfactory stimuli; and the pathway to the entorhinal cortex carries olfactory memories. The sense of smell is more acute in women than in men, and in women it is most acute at the time of ovulation.

ODORANT RECEPTORS & SIGNAL TRANSDUCTION

There are ~500 olfactory genes, accounting for 2% of the human genome. The amino acid sequences of odorant receptors are diverse, but all odorant receptors are G-protein–coupled receptors (GPCRs). When an odorant binds to its receptor, the G-protein subunits (α, β, γ) dissociate. The α-subunit activates adenylyl

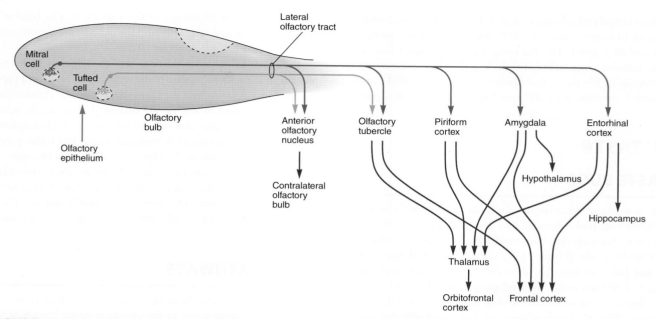

FIGURE 11–3 Diagram of the olfactory pathway. Information is transmitted from the olfactory bulb by axons of mitral and tufted relay neurons in the lateral olfactory tract. Mitral cells project to five regions of the olfactory cortex: anterior olfactory nucleus, olfactory tubercle, piriform cortex, and parts of the amygdala and entorhinal cortex. Tufted cells project to anterior olfactory nucleus and olfactory tubercle; mitral cells in the accessory olfactory bulb project only to the amygdala. Conscious discrimination of odor depends on the neocortex (orbitofrontal and frontal cortices). Emotive aspects of olfaction derive from limbic projections (amygdala and hypothalamus). (Reproduced with permission from Kandel ER, Schwartz JH, Jessell TM [editors]: *Principles of Neural Science*, 4th ed. New York, NY: McGraw-Hill; 2000.)

cyclase to catalyze the production of cAMP which acts as a second messenger to open cation channels, increasing the permeability to Na$^+$, K$^-$, and Ca^{2+}. The net effect is an inward-directed Ca^{2+} current that produces a graded receptor potential that opens Ca^{2+}-activated Cl$^-$ channels, further depolarizing the cell due to the high intracellular Cl$^-$ levels in olfactory sensory neurons. If the stimulus is sufficient for the receptor potential to exceed its threshold, an action potential in the olfactory nerve is triggered.

Although there are millions of olfactory sensory neurons, each expresses only one of the 500 olfactory genes. Each neuron projects to one or two glomeruli (Figure 11–2). This provides a distinct two-dimensional map in the olfactory bulb that is unique to the odorant. The mitral cells with their glomeruli project to different parts of the olfactory cortex. The olfactory glomeruli demonstrate lateral inhibition mediated by periglomerular cells and granule cells to sharpen and focus olfactory signals.

ODOR DETECTION THRESHOLD

Odorants are generally small, containing from 3 to 20 carbon atoms; and molecules with the same number of carbon atoms but different structural configurations have different odors. Relatively high water and lipid solubility is characteristic of substances with strong odors. Some common abnormalities in odor detection are described in **Clinical Box 11–1**.

The odor detection thresholds are the lowest concentration of a chemical that can be detected. The wide range of thresholds illustrates the remarkable sensitivity of the odorant receptors.

CLINICAL BOX 11–1

Abnormalities in Odor Detection

Anosmia (inability to smell) and hyposmia (diminished olfactory sensitivity) can result from simple nasal congestion or nasal polyps. It may also be a sign of a more serious problem such as damage to the olfactory nerves due to fractures of the cribriform plate or head trauma, tumors (eg, neuroblastomas, meningiomas), and respiratory tract infections (such as abscesses). Congenital anosmia is a rare disorder in which an individual is born without the ability to smell. Prolonged use of nasal decongestants can also lead to anosmia and damage to the olfactory nerves is often seen in patients with Alzheimer disease. Aging is associated with abnormalities in smell sensation; 50% of individuals between the ages of 65 and 80 and more than 75% of those over the age of 80 have an impaired ability to identify smells. Because of the close relationship between taste and smell, anosmia is associated with a reduction in taste sensitivity. Anosmia is generally permanent if the olfactory nerve or other neural elements in the olfactory neural pathway are damaged. Individuals with anosmia are not able to detect the odor from gas leaks and spoiled food. Hyperosmia (enhanced olfactory sensitivity) is less common than loss of smell, but pregnant women often become oversensitive to smell. Dysosmia (distorted sense of smell) can be due to sinus infections, partial damage to the olfactory nerves, and poor oral hygiene. Topical corticosteroids have also been shown to be effective in reversing the loss of smell due to nasal and sinus diseases.

Some examples of substances detected at very low concentrations include hydrogen sulfide (0.0005 parts per million, ppm) and gasoline (0.3 ppm). On the other end of the spectrum, some toxic substances are essentially odorless; they have odor detection thresholds higher than lethal concentrations. For example, carbon dioxide is detected at 74,000 ppm but is lethal at 50,000 ppm.

■ TASTE

TASTE BUDS

The specialized sense organ for taste (gustation) consists of ~10,000 taste buds; there are four morphologically distinct types of cells within each taste bud: basal cells, dark cells, light cells, and intermediate cells (Figure 11–1B). Each taste bud has between 50 and 100 taste cells. The three cell types may represent various stages of differentiation of developing taste cells, with the light cells being the most mature or they may represent different cell lineages. The apical ends of taste cells have microvilli that project into the taste pore, a small opening on the dorsal surface of the tongue where tastes cells are exposed to the oral contents. Each taste bud is innervated by ~50 nerve fibers, and each nerve fiber receives input from an average of five taste buds. The basal cells differentiate into new taste cells, and the old cells are continuously replaced with a half-life of about 10 days.

Taste buds are located in the mucosa of the epiglottis, palate, and pharynx in the walls of papillae of the tongue. The fungiform papillae are most numerous near the tip of the tongue; the circumvallate papillae are arranged in a V on the back of the tongue; the foliate papillae are on the posterior edge of the tongue. Each fungiform papilla has up to five taste buds, and each vallate and foliate papilla contains up to 100 taste buds. The von Ebner glands (gustatory or serous glands) secrete saliva into the cleft around the circumvallate and foliate papillae that cleanses the mouth to prepare the taste receptors for a new stimulant. The circumvallate papilla and von Ebner glands form a functional complex that is important in taste detection.

TASTE PATHWAYS

The sensory nerve fibers from the taste buds on the anterior two-thirds of the tongue travel in the chorda tympani branch of the facial nerve, and those from the posterior third of the tongue reach the brainstem via the glossopharyngeal nerve (**Figure 11–4**). The fibers from areas other than the tongue (eg, pharynx) reach the

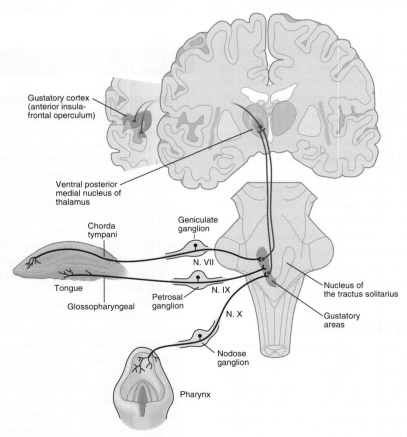

FIGURE 11–4 Diagram of taste pathways. Signals from the taste buds travel via different nerves to gustatory areas of the nucleus of the tractus solitarius, which relays information to the thalamus; the thalamus projects to the gustatory cortex. (Modified with permission from Kandel ER, Schwartz JH, Jessell TM [editors]: *Principles of Neural Science*, 4th ed. New York, NY: McGraw-Hill; 2000.)

brainstem via the vagus nerve. On each side, the myelinated taste fibers in the three nerves unite in the gustatory portion of the nucleus of the tractus solitaries (NTS). From there, axons of second-order neurons ascend in the ipsilateral medial lemniscus and project directly to the ventral posteromedial nucleus of the thalamus. From the thalamus, the axons project to the anterior insula and the frontal operculum in the ipsilateral cerebral cortex. This region is rostral to the face area of the postcentral gyrus, which may mediate conscious perception of taste and taste discrimination.

TASTE MODALITIES, RECEPTORS, & TRANSDUCTION

Humans have five basic tastes: sweet, sour, bitter, salt, and umami. Salt and sour tastes are triggered by activation of ionotropic receptors; sour, bitter, and umami tastes are triggered by activation of GPCR. Many GPCR in the human genome are taste receptors type (T1R1, T1R2, and T1R3 families). Some of these receptors couple to the heterotrimeric G-protein gustducin, which lowers cAMP and increases the formation of inositol phosphates (IP_3) to produce depolarization.

Salt-sensitive taste, triggered by NaCl, is mediated by an epithelial sodium channel (ENaC). Na^+ entry into these receptors depolarizes the membrane, generating a receptor potential. The sour taste is triggered by H^+; ENaCs permit the entry of protons and contribute to the sensation of sour taste. H^+ can also bind to and block a K^+-sensitive channel, which can depolarize the membrane. A hyperpolarization-activated cyclic nucleotide-gated cation channel (HCN) may also contribute to sour transduction.

Substances that taste sweet are detected by at least two types of GPCRs: T1R2 and T1R3. Natural sugars and synthetic sweeteners may act on gustducin via different receptors. Sweet-responsive receptors act via cyclic nucleotides and inositol phosphate metabolism.

Bitter taste is produced by many unrelated compounds, many of which are poisons; the bitter taste serves as a warning to avoid them. Some bitter compounds bind to and block K^+-selective channels. Many GPCRs (T2R family) that interact with gustducin are stimulated by bitter substances (eg, strychnine). Some bitter compounds are membrane permeable and their detection may not involve G-proteins (eg, quinine).

Umami taste is due to the activation of a truncated metabotropic glutamate receptor (mGluR4) in the taste buds. Glutamate in food may also activate ionotropic glutamate receptors to depolarize umami receptors. It is likely that T1R1 and T1R3 receptors also detect umami taste.

TASTE THRESHOLDS & INTENSITY DISCRIMINATION

A 30% change in the concentration of the substance being tasted is needed before an intensity difference can be detected. Taste threshold refers to the minimum concentration at which a substance can be perceived. Some toxic substances such as strychnine

have a bitter taste at very low concentrations, preventing accidental ingestion of the chemical. Some common abnormalities in taste detection are described in **Clinical Box 11–2**.

CHAPTER SUMMARY

- The olfactory epithelium in the upper portion of the nasal cavity contains olfactory sensory neurons, supporting (sustentacular) cells, and basal stem cells.
- The cilia on the dendritic knob of the olfactory sensory neuron contain odorant receptors that are coupled to G-proteins. Axons of olfactory sensory neurons contact the dendrites of mitral and tufted cells in the olfactory bulbs to form olfactory glomeruli.
- Information from the olfactory bulb travels via the lateral olfactory stria to the olfactory cortex, including the anterior olfactory nucleus, olfactory tubercle, piriform cortex, amygdala, and entorhinal cortex.
- Taste buds are composed of basal stem cells and three types of taste cells (dark, light, and intermediate). The three types of taste cells may represent various stages of differentiation of developing taste cells, with the light cells being the most mature. Taste buds are located in the mucosa of the epiglottis, palate, and pharynx and in the walls of papillae of the tongue.
- There are taste receptors for sweet, sour, bitter, salt, and umami. Signal transduction mechanisms include passage

through ion channels and binding to and blocking ion channels and GPCRs.

■ Afferents from taste buds in the tongue travel via the seventh, ninth, and tenth cranial nerves to synapse in the NTS. From there, axons ascend via the ipsilateral medial lemniscus to the ventral posteromedial nucleus of the thalamus, and onto the anterior insula and frontal operculum in the ipsilateral cerebral cortex.

MULTIPLE-CHOICE QUESTIONS

For all questions, select the single best answer unless otherwise directed.

1. A young boy was diagnosed with congenital anosmia, a rare disorder in which an individual is born without the ability to smell. Which parts of the nervous system might be defective in an individual with congenital anosmia to account for the inability to detect odors?
   A. Glossopharyngeal nerve, ventral posterior medial nucleus of the thalamus, and anterior insula-frontal operculum
   B. Nodose ganglion, nucleus of the tractus solitarius, and ventral posterior lateral nucleus of the thalamus
   C. Olfactory nerve, olfactory bulb, and anterior insula-frontal operculum
   D. Olfactory nerve, piriform cortex, and frontal cortex
   E. Trigeminal nerve, olfactory tubercle, and entorhinal cortex

2. A 37-year-old female was diagnosed with multiple sclerosis. One of the potential consequences of this disorder is diminished taste sensitivity. Which three cranial nerves might be defective in an individual with diminished taste sensitivity?
   A. Trigeminal, facial, and vagal nerves
   B. Abducens, trigeminal, and glossopharyngeal nerves
   C. Trigeminal, trochlear, and facial
   D. Trochlear, glossopharyngeal, and vagal nerves
   E. Facial, glossopharyngeal, and vagal nerves

3. A medical student was doing research in a laboratory that studied olfaction. She is intrigued by the fact that a simple sense organ like the human olfactory epithelium can discriminate more than 10,000 odors. What factors contribute to the ability of the human olfactory system to discriminate so many odors?
   A. There are 500 types of odorant receptors and over 1000 types of odorant-binding proteins that sequester odorants to enhance sensory discrimination.
   B. A given odorant binds to a particular subset of odorant receptors and different mitral cells connect to different parts of the olfactory cortex.
   C. Odorants bind to a mixture of GPCR and ion channel receptors on olfactory sensory neurons and the axons of these sensory neurons form anatomically discrete synaptic units called olfactory glomeruli.
   D. Lateral inhibition within olfactory glomeruli sharpen and focus olfactory signals and granule cells within the olfactory glomerulus make specific projections to the postcentral gyrus in the somatosensory cortex
   E. There are about 5000 types of odorant receptors and each odorant binds to only one of these.

4. A 10-year-old boy had removed his seatbelt in order to reach for the toy he had dropped just as a vehicle traveling in the opposite crossed the median causing a head-on collision with the car in which the boy was riding. He was thrown from the car and suffered a head trauma. An MRI showed damage to the periamygdaloid, piriform, and entorhinal cortices. Which of the following sensory deficits is he most likely to experience?
   A. Visual and taste disturbances
   B. Hyperosmia and hypergeusia
   C. Auditory and odorant detection problems
   D. Taste and odor abnormalities
   E. Hyperosmia and ageusia

5. A physician collected data on the ability of his patients to detect various odors. During the course of a week he did an analysis of the following cohort of subjects who came to his office for a routine physical. Amongst his patients he evaluated a 10-year-old boy, a 22-year-old woman during the ovulation phase of her menstrual cycle; a 35-year-old pregnant woman, a 50-year-old woman diagnosed with early-onset Alzheimer disease, a 60-year-old man, and an 85-year-old woman. Which of the following is a likely outcome of his evaluation?
   A. The 10-year-old boy will have a similar sense of smell as the 22-year-old woman during ovulation, and the 85-year-old woman will have the least sense of smell.
   B. The 10-year-old boy will have the greatest sense of smell and the 50-year-old woman diagnosed with early-onset Alzheimer disease will have the least sense of smell.
   C. The 35-year-old pregnant woman will have a greater sense of smell than the 10-year-old boy; a 60-year-old man will have a greater sense of smell than a 50-year-old woman diagnosed with early-onset Alzheimer disease and the 85-year-old woman.
   D. The 22-year-old-woman during ovulation will have a greater sense of smell than the 10-year-old boy, and the 50-year-old woman diagnosed with early-onset Alzheimer disease will have a better sense of smell than the 60-year-old man.
   E. The 10-year-old boy will have a similar sense of smell as the 35-year-old pregnant woman, and the 50-year-old woman diagnosed with early-onset Alzheimer disease will have the least sense of smell.

6. A medical student was doing research on the changes that occur in the olfactory system when a chemical molecule reaches the nasal mucosa. What is the sequence of events that occur after the chemical odorant is dissolved in the mucus and is bound to the odorant receptor through the development of a graded receptor potential?
   A. G-protein subunits dissociate, and the α-subunit inhibits adenylyl cyclase to decrease cAMP which increases the permeability to Ca^{2+}; the inward-directed Ca^{2+} current produces a graded receptor potential.
   B. G-protein subunits dissociate, and the β,γ-subunit activates phospholipase C which leads to the formation of inositol 1,4,5-trisphosphate and diacylglycerol and an inward-directed Na^+ current that produces a graded receptor potential.
   C. G-protein subunits dissociate, and the β,γ-subunit inhibits adenylyl cyclase to increase cGMP which increases the permeability to Ca^{2+}; the inward-directed Ca^{2+} current produces a graded receptor potential.
   D. G-protein subunits dissociate, and the α-subunit activates adenylyl cyclase to produce cAMP which increases the permeability to Na^+, K^-, and Ca^{2+}; the inward-directed Ca^{2+} current produces a graded receptor potential.
   E. G-protein subunits dissociate, and the α-subunit activates phospholipase C which leads to the formation of inositol 1,4,5-trisphosphate and diacylglycerol and an

inward-directed Ca^{+2} current that produces a graded receptor potential.

7. After watching the movie *Christmas Story*, a 10-year-old boy wanted to see if his tongue would really stick to a frozen pole. Much to his surprise, it did stick. No one was around to get warm water, so he pulled hard to remove his tongue from the pole. He was successful in doing so but the anterior one-third of his tongue was injured. What sensory nerve arises from this portion of the tongue, where are the cell bodies of these sensory neurons, and where does the nerve terminate?
    A. Chorda tympani branch of the facial nerve, geniculate ganglion, and nucleus of the tractus solitarius
    B. Chorda tympani branch of the facial nerve, petrosal ganglion, and nucleus of the tractus solitarius
    C. Chorda tympani branch of the facial nerve, taste buds, and gustatory area of the nucleus ambiguus
    D. Glossopharyngeal nerve, petrosal ganglion, and gustatory area of the nucleus ambiguus
    E. Glossopharyngeal nerve, taste buds, and nucleus of the tractus solitaries
    F. Glossopharyngeal nerve, geniculate ganglion, and nucleus of the tractus solitaries

8. A 9-year-old boy had frequent episodes of uncontrollable nose bleeds. At the advice of his pediatrician, he underwent surgery to correct a problem in his nasal septum. A few days after the surgery, he told his mother he could not smell the cinnamon rolls she was baking in the oven. After she gave him one to eat, he said he could barely taste it. What is the relationship between the sensations of smell and taste?
    A. Odorant receptors and taste receptors are innervated by the same sensory nerve fibers.
    B. The afferent fibers from odorant receptors and taste receptors terminate on the same second-order neurons in the brainstem.
    C. Odors from food enter our nasal passages at the same time that the taste receptors in our mouth are stimulated by the food, and the two chemosensory systems interact to establish the flavor of what we ingest.
    D. Olfaction is closely related to gustation because odorant and gustatory receptors send signals to adjacent regions of the postcentral gyrus of the cortex which are connected via axon collaterals.

9. A 31-year-old woman is a smoker who has had poor oral hygiene for most of her life. In the past few years she has noticed a reduced sensitivity to the flavors in various foods which she used to enjoy eating. What types of receptors are likely malfunctioning if she has difficulty sensing sweet and bitter substances?
    A. Epithelial sodium channel (sweet) and hyperpolarization-activated cyclic nucleotide-gated cation channel (bitter)
    B. Hyperpolarization-activated cyclic nucleotide-gated cation channel (sweet) and epithelial sodium channel (sour)
    C. T2R family of GPCRs (sweet) and metabotropic glutamate receptor (mGluR4, bitter)
    D. T1R2 and T1R3 family of GPCRs (sweet) and T2R family of GPCRs (sour)
    E. Metabotropic glutamate receptor (mGluR4, sweet) and epithelial sodium channel (sour)

10. A 25-year-old woman was diagnosed with Bell palsy (damage to facial nerve) after recovering from a flu-like illness. Which of the following symptoms is she most likely to exhibit?

A. Ageusia and anosmia, bilateral facial muscle twitching, and drooping eyelids
B. Hypogeusia, unilateral facial muscle weakness, a drooping eyelid, dryness of one eye, and drooling
C. Anosmia and ageusia, unilateral facial muscle weakness, and contralateral drooping eyelid
D. Hypogeusia, drooping eyelids and excessive tearing bilaterally, drooling, and facial muscle paralysis
E. Hypogeusia, drooping eyelids and dry eyes bilaterally, drooling, and facial muscle weakness

ANSWERS

1. The best answer is **D.** The olfactory nerve innervates mitral and tufted cells in the olfactory bulb; the axons of mitral and tufted cells pass through the lateral olfactory stria to terminate in five regions of the olfactory cortex (anterior olfactory nucleus, olfactory tubercle, piriform cortex, amygdala, and entorhinal cortex). From these regions, information travels directly to the frontal cortex or via the thalamus to the orbitofrontal cortex. The glossopharyngeal nerve, nodose ganglion, nucleus of the tractus solitarius, ventral posterior medial nucleus of the thalamus, and anterior insula-frontal operculum are components of the pathway mediating the sensation of taste (rules out **A, B,** and **C**). The trigeminal nerve terminals in the olfactory epithelium are activated by irritant stimulants (eg, peppermint) that initiates sneezing and other reflexes (rules out **E**).

2. The best answer is **E.** Taste buds on the anterior two-thirds of the tongue relay information via the facial nerve, those on the posterior third of the tongue relay information via the glossopharyngeal nerve, and taste buds located elsewhere (eg, pharynx) relay information via the vagus nerve. Options A–D are ruled out because the trigeminal nerve mediates information about facial pain, and the trochlear nerves contains motor fibers controlling eye movement.

3. The best answer is **B.** Although there are millions of olfactory sensory neurons, each expresses only one of the 500 olfactory receptors. Each sensory neuron projects to one or two glomeruli to provide a distinct two-dimensional map in the olfactory bulb that is unique to the odorant, and the mitral cells with their glomeruli project to different parts of the olfactory cortex. Option **A** is ruled out because there are only one or two types of odorant binding proteins in the olfactory epithelium; one of their functions is to sequester odorants away from the site of odor recognition to allow for odor clearance. All odorant receptors and GPCR, and the olfactory glomeruli are composed of the mitral and tufted cells that are innervated by the terminals of olfactory sensory neurons (rules out option **C**). Granule cells do not have axons that project to the cortex; they make reciprocal synapses with the lateral dendrites of the mitral and tufted cells (rules out option **D**). There are 500 functional odorant receptors in the human olfactory epithelium, and a given odorant binds to a subset of them (rules out option **E**).

4. The best answer is **D.** The periamygdaloid, piriform, and entorhinal cortices are components of the olfactory sensory pathway, so he is likely to have problems detecting odors. Because of the link between taste and odor sensations, he is also likely to have problems discerning flavors from food. There is no reason to expect problems with vision or sound

detection following this injury (rules out **A** and **C**). Hyperosmia and hypergeusia are increases senses of smell and taste, respectively; hyperosmia may be due to genetic or environmental factors, and hyperageusia can result from damage to the posterior fossa (rules out **B** and **E**).

5. The best answer is **C**. The sense of smell peaks sometime between the late teens to early 30s; women have a greater sense of smell than men, and it increases during the ovulation phase of the menstrual cycle and during pregnancy; 50% of individuals between the ages of 65 and 80 and more than 75% of those over the age of 80 have an impaired ability to identify smells; and it is common for loss of smell to be an early sign of Alzheimer disease. The greatest sense of smell would likely be in either the 22-year-old woman during menstruation or the 35-year-old pregnant woman (rules out **A**, **B**, and **E**). Either the 50-year-old woman diagnosed with early-onset Alzheimer disease or the 85-year-old woman will have the least sensitivity to odors (rules out **D**).

6. The best answer is **D**. When an odorant molecule binds to its receptor, the G-protein subunits (α, β, γ) dissociate. The α-subunit activates adenylyl cyclase to catalyze the production of cAMP, which acts as a second messenger to open cation channels, increasing the permeability to Na^+, K^-, and Ca^{2+}. The net effect is an inward-directed Ca^{2+} current which produces the graded receptor potential. The binding of the odorant to the receptor does not inhibit adenylyl cyclase (rules out option **A** and **C**), does not involve the phospholipase C and IP_3/DAG pathway (rules out options **B** and **E**).

7. The best answer is **A**. The sensory nerve fibers from the taste buds on the anterior two-thirds of the tongue travel in the chorda tympani branch of the facial nerve (cell bodies in the geniculate ganglion), and those from the posterior third of the tongue reach the brainstem via the glossopharyngeal nerve (cell bodies in the petrosal ganglion). Both sets of fibers terminate in the rostral portion of the nucleus of the tractus solitarius.

8. The best answer is **C**. Physiologically, the sensations of taste and smell are related to each other. The flavors of various foods are in large part a combination of their taste and smell. This is likely associated with the similar timing of stimuli arriving at the odorant receptors in the olfactory epithelium and the taste receptors in our mouth. Odorant receptors are connected to the CNS via olfactory nerve to the olfactory cortex, and taste receptors are relayed via the facial, glossopharyngeal, and vagal nerves to the nucleus of the tractus solitarius (rules out **A** and **B**). Neither the sense of smell nor the taste is relayed to the postcentral gyrus; conscious discrimination of odors is dependent on the orbitofrontal and frontal cortices; taste is relayed to the anterior insula-frontal operculum (rules out **D**).

9. The best answer is **D**. Substances that taste sweet are detected by at least two types of GPCRs, T1R2 and T1R3. Bitter taste is produced by many unrelated compounds; some bitter compounds bind to and block K^+-selective channels and others bind to GPCRs (T2R family).

10. The best answer is **B**. Symptoms of Bell palsy vary but include facial muscle twitching, weakness, or even paralysis; ageusia or hypogeusia, drooping of the eyelid and corner of the mouth, drooling, dryness of the eye or excessive tearing in one eye. Symptoms are typically on only side of the face (rules out options **A, C, D**, and **E**).

Reflex & Voluntary Control of Posture & Movement

- Describe the elements of the stretch reflex and how the activity of γ-motor neurons alters the response to muscle stretch.
- Describe the role of Golgi tendon organs in control of skeletal muscle.
- Describe the elements of the withdrawal reflex.
- Define spinal shock and describe the initial and long-term changes in spinal reflexes that follow transection of the spinal cord.
- Describe how skilled movements are planned and carried out.
- Compare the organization of the central pathways involved in the control of axial (posture) and distal (skilled movement, fine motor movements) muscles.
- Define decerebrate and decorticate rigidity, and comment on the cause and physiologic significance of each.
- Identify the components of the basal ganglia and the pathways that interconnect them, along with the neurotransmitters in each pathway.
- Explain the pathophysiology and symptoms of Parkinson disease and Huntington disease.
- Discuss the functions of the cerebellum and the neurologic abnormalities produced by diseases of this part of the brain.

INTRODUCTION

All neural influences affecting muscle contraction ultimately funnel through spinal or cranial motor neurons to skeletal muscles. To voluntarily move a limb, the brain must plan a movement, arrange appropriate motion at many different joints at the same time, and adjust the motion by comparing plan with performance. The motor system "learns by doing" and performance improves with repetition. Sensory fibers provide information to the central nervous system (CNS) to promote reflex-induced changes in muscle contraction. The integrated activity of inputs from spinal, medullary, midbrain, and cortical levels as well as peripheral afferents determines the posture of the body and makes coordinated movement possible. This chapter reviews the way the brain, spinal cord, and peripheral afferents work together to regulate the activity of motor neurons for voluntary and reflex-induced movements.

■ MONOSYNAPTIC REFLEX: THE MYOTATIC (STRETCH) REFLEX

When a skeletal muscle is stretched, it initiates a monosynaptic reflex to contract that muscle (stretch reflex or myotatic reflex).

The sense organ is the muscle spindle located within the fleshy part of the muscle. The impulses from the spindle are transmitted to the CNS by sensory fibers that project directly on α-motor neurons that supply the same muscle. Glutamate is the neurotransmitter at the central synapse. The stretch reflex is typified by the knee jerk reflex (**Clinical Box 12–1**).

CLINICAL BOX 12–1

Knee Jerk Reflex

Tapping the patellar tendon stretches the muscle to elicit the knee jerk, a stretch reflex of the quadriceps femoris muscle. Stretch reflexes can be elicited from most of the large muscles of the body. The knee jerk reflex is an example of a deep tendon reflex (DTR) in a neurologic examination and is graded on the following scale: 0 (absent), 1+ (hypoactive), 2+ (brisk, normal), 3+ (hyperactive without clonus), 4+ (hyperactive with mild clonus), and 5+ (hyperactive with sustained clonus). Absence of the knee jerk can signify an abnormality anywhere within the reflex arc, including the muscle spindle, the Ia afferent nerve fibers, or the motor neurons to the quadriceps muscle. The most common cause is a peripheral neuropathy from such things as diabetes, alcoholism, and toxins. A hyperactive reflex can signify an interruption of corticospinal and other descending pathways that suppress the activity in the reflex arc.

STRUCTURE & FUNCTION OF MUSCLE SPINDLES

The muscle spindle functions to maintain muscle length. Each muscle spindle has three elements: (1) intrafusal muscle fibers with contractile polar ends and a noncontractile center, (2) large diameter myelinated afferent nerves (types Ia and II) originating in the central portion of the intrafusal fibers, and (3) small diameter myelinated efferent nerves (γ-motor neurons) supplying the contractile polar ends of the intrafusal fibers (**Figure 12–1A**).

The intrafusal fibers serve a sensory function (proprioception) and are located in parallel to the extrafusal fibers (contractile unit of skeletal muscles); the ends of the spindle capsule are attached to the tendons. There are two types of intrafusal fibers: nuclear bag fibers (dynamic and static subtypes) in a dilated central area and the thinner and shorter nuclear chain fibers (**Figure 12–1B**).

Each spindle has one primary (group Ia) sensory fiber and up to eight secondary (group II) sensory fibers (**Figure 12–2B**). The Ia afferent fiber wraps around the center of the nuclear bag and nuclear

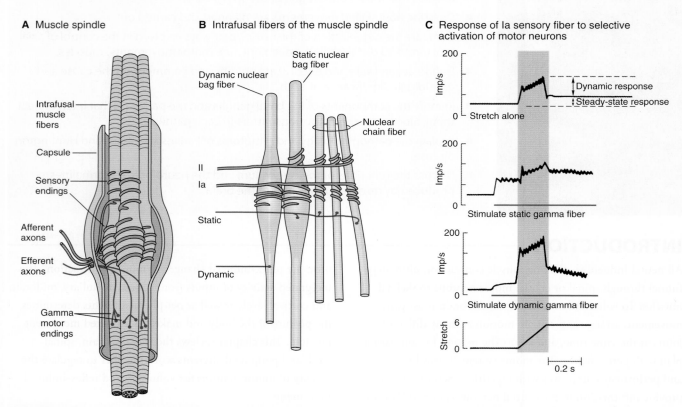

FIGURE 12–1 Mammalian muscle spindle. (A) Diagrammatic representation of the main components of mammalian muscle spindle including intrafusal muscle fibers, afferent sensory fiber endings, and efferent motor fibers (γ-motor neurons). **(B)** Three types of intrafusal muscle fibers: dynamic nuclear bag, static nuclear bag, and nuclear chain fibers. A single Ia afferent fiber innervates all three types of fibers to form a primary sensory ending. A group II sensory fiber innervates nuclear chain and static bag fibers to form a secondary sensory ending. Dynamic γ-motor neurons innervate dynamic bag fibers; static γ-motor neurons innervate combinations of chain and static bag fibers. **(C)** Comparison of discharge pattern of Ia afferent activity during stretch alone and during stimulation of static or dynamic γ-motor neurons. Without γ-stimulation, Ia fibers show a small dynamic response to muscle stretch and a modest increase in steady-state firing. When static γ-motor neurons are activated, the steady-state response increases and the dynamic response decreases. When dynamic γ-motor neurons are activated, the dynamic response is markedly increased but the steady-state response gradually returns to its original level. (Reproduced with permission from Gray H: *Gray's Anatomy: The Anatomical Basis of Clinical Practice*, 40th ed. St. Louis, MO: Churchill Livingstone/Elsevier; 2009.)

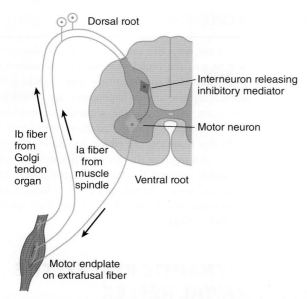

FIGURE 12–2 **Diagram illustrating the pathways responsible for the stretch reflex and the inverse stretch reflex.** Stretch stimulates the muscle spindle, which activates Ia fibers that excite the motor neuron. Stretch also stimulates the Golgi tendon organ, which activates Ib fibers that excite an interneuron that releases the inhibitory mediator glycine. With strong stretch, the resulting hyperpolarization of the motor neuron is so great that it stops discharging.

chain fibers; they synapse directly on motor neurons supplying the extrafusal fibers of the same muscle (**Figure 12–2**). Group II sensory fibers are adjacent to the centers of the static nuclear bag and nuclear chain fibers. Ia afferents are sensitive to the velocity of the change in muscle length during a stretch (dynamic response), so they provide information about the speed of movements. The tonic activity of group Ia and II afferents provides information on steady-state length of the muscle (static response). **Figure 12–1C** shows the dynamic and static components of activity in the Ia afferent during muscle stretch. They discharge most rapidly while the muscle is being stretched and less rapidly during sustained stretch.

There are two types of γ-motor neurons: dynamic (to dynamic nuclear bag fibers) and static (to static nuclear bag fibers and nuclear chain fibers). Activation of dynamic γ-motor neurons increases the dynamic sensitivity of the Ia fibers. Activation of the static γ-motor neurons increases the tonic level of activity in both Ia and II fibers, decreases the dynamic sensitivity of Ia fibers, and can prevent silencing of Ia afferents during muscle stretch (**Figure 12–1C**).

EFFECTS OF γ-MOTOR NEURON DISCHARGE

Because the spindle is parallel to the extrafusal fibers, passive stretch of the muscle pulls on the spindles (loading the spindle) to initiate reflex contraction of the muscle. The spindle afferents normally stop firing when the muscle is made to contract by electrical stimulation of α-motor neurons because the muscle shortens while the spindle is unloaded (**Figure 12–3**). Stimulation of

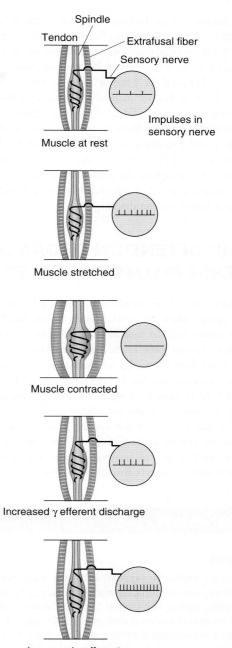

FIGURE 12–3 **Effect of various conditions on muscle spindle discharge.** When the whole muscle is stretched, the muscle spindle is also stretched and its sensory endings are activated at a frequency proportional to the degree of stretching ("loading the spindle"). Spindle afferents stop firing when the muscle contracts ("unloading the spindle"). Stimulation of γ-motor neurons cause the contractile ends of the intrafusal fibers to shorten. This stretches the nuclear bag region, initiating impulses in sensory fibers. If the whole muscle is stretched during stimulation of the γ-motor neurons, the rate of discharge in sensory fibers is further increased.

γ-motor neurons causes the contractile ends of the intrafusal fibers to shorten which stretches the nuclear bag portion of the spindles, deforming the endings, and initiating impulses in the Ia fibers that lead to contraction of the muscle. If the whole muscle is stretched during stimulation of the γ-motor neurons, the rate of discharge in the Ia fibers is further increased. Increased γ-motor neuron activity thus increases spindle sensitivity during stretch.

Descending excitatory input to spinal motor circuits can activate both α- and γ-motor neurons (α-γ coactivation). Thus, intrafusal and extrafusal fibers shorten together, and spindle afferent activity occurs throughout the period of muscle contraction. The spindle remains capable of responding to stretch and reflexively adjusting α-motor neuron discharge.

■ GOLGI TENDON ORGAN & INVERSE MYOTATIC REFLEX

The harder a muscle is stretched, the stronger is the reflex contraction except when the tension is excessive; then contraction suddenly ceases and the muscle relaxes due to the inverse myotatic reflex. The receptor is the Golgi tendon organ. Group Ib sensory fibers from the Golgi tendon organ terminate on spinal inhibitory interneurons that in turn terminate on motor neurons (Figure 12–2). Because the Golgi tendon organs are in series with the muscle fibers, they are stimulated by both passive stretch and active contraction of the muscle. It functions to regulate muscle force. The interaction of spindle discharge, tendon organ discharge, and reciprocal innervation determines the level of α-motor neuron activity (Clinical Box 12–2).

CLINICAL BOX 12–2

Clonus

Clonus is a neurologic sign defined by the occurrence of regular, repetitive, rhythmic contractions of a muscle subjected to sudden, maintained stretch. Sustained clonus with five or more beats is considered abnormal. Ankle clonus is initiated by brisk, maintained dorsiflexion of the foot; the response is rhythmic plantar flexion at the ankle. The spindles of the tested muscle are hyperactive, which simultaneously activates all the motor neurons supplying the muscle. The resultant muscle contraction stops spindle discharge, but the stretch has been maintained, and as soon as the muscle relaxes it is again stretched and the spindles stimulated. The causes of abnormal clonus include amyotrophic lateral sclerosis, traumatic brain injury, brain tumors, stroke, multiple sclerosis, spinal cord injury, epilepsy, liver or kidney failure, and hepatic encephalopathy. Immunosuppressants, anticonvulsants, and tranquilizers can be beneficial in the treatment of clonus. Botulinum toxin is a toxin that acts by binding to receptors on the cholinergic nerve terminals to decrease the release of acetylcholine, causing neuromuscular blockade to prevent clonus.

MUSCLE TONE

Tone or tonus is the resistance of a muscle to stretch. If the motor nerve to a muscle is cut, the muscle has minimal resistance to stretch and becomes flaccid. A spastic muscle is one in which the resistance to stretch is high because of hyperactive stretch reflexes. When the muscles are hypertonic, the sequence of moderate stretch → muscle contraction, strong stretch → muscle relaxation is evident. Passive flexion of the elbow, for example, meets immediate resistance as a result of the stretch reflex in the triceps muscle. Further stretch activates the inverse stretch reflex. The resistance to flexion suddenly collapses, and the arm flexes. Continued passive flexion stretches the muscle again, and the sequence is repeated (clasp-knife effect).

■ POLYSYNAPTIC REFLEX: THE WITHDRAWAL REFLEX

The polysynaptic withdrawal reflex occurs in response to a noxious stimulus to the skin or subcutaneous tissues and muscle. The response is flexor muscle contraction and relaxation of extensor muscles, so the body part stimulated is flexed and withdrawn from the stimulus. When a strong stimulus is applied to a limb, in addition to flexion and withdrawal of that limb the opposite limb is extended (crossed extensor response). Strong stimuli can generate activity in the interneuron pool that spreads to all four extremities. This reflex serves a protective function to move a limb away from the source of irritation, and extension of the other limb supports the body.

■ SPINAL CORD INJURY

The deficits seen after spinal cord injury (SCI) vary, depending on the level of the injury (Clinical Box 12–3). After transection of the spinal cord, there is a period of spinal shock during which spinal reflex responses are profoundly depressed. It usually lasts for a minimum of 2 weeks in humans. The withdrawal reflex is often the first reflex to reappear as spinal shock wears off. Once the spinal reflexes begin to reappear, their threshold steadily drops.

■ MOTOR CORTEX & VOLUNTARY MOVEMENT

MOTOR REGIONS OF THE CORTEX

Within the primary motor cortex (M1) representation of each body part is proportional in size to the skill with which the part is used in fine, voluntary movement. The cells in M1 are arranged in a column, and neurons in several cortical columns project to the same muscle. M1 neurons represent movements of groups of muscles for different tasks.

CLINICAL BOX 12–3

Spinal Cord Injury

The worldwide annual incidence of sustaining spinal cord injury (SCI) is between 10 and 83 per million of the population. Leading causes are vehicular accidents, violence, and sports injuries. The mean age of those who sustain an SCI is 33 years old; men outnumber women with a 4:1 ratio. With quadriplegia, stretch reflexes are hyperactive and the threshold of the withdrawal reflex is very low. Even minor noxious stimuli can cause prolonged withdrawal of one extremity and marked flexion–extension patterns in the other limbs. Minor noxious stimulus applied to the skin may activate autonomic neurons and produce evacuation of the bladder and rectum, sweating, pallor, and blood pressure swings. If the cord section is incomplete, flexor spasms initiated by noxious stimuli can induce bursts of pain. The spasms can be treated with baclofen, a $GABA_B$ receptor agonist that crosses the blood–brain barrier and facilitates inhibition. Because SCI patients are immobile, a negative nitrogen balance develops and large amounts of body protein are catabolized. They experience hypercalcemia, hypercalciuria, and formation of calcium stones in the urinary tract. The combination of stones and bladder paralysis cause urinary stasis, which predisposes to urinary tract infection, the most common complication of SCI. The use of brain–computer interface devices is being explored as a way to bypass the site of SCI.

CLINICAL BOX 12–4

Cerebral Palsy

Cerebral palsy (CP) is a term used to describe any one of several nonprogressive neurologic disorders that occur before or during childbirth or during early childhood. Prenatal factors (eg, exposure of the developing brain to hypoxia, infections, or toxins) account for most cases of CP. Symptoms include spasticity, ataxia, deficits in fine motor control, and abnormal gait. Sensory deficits include loss of vision and hearing; and learning difficulties and seizures often occur in children with CP. In developed countries, the prevalence of CP is 2–2.5 cases per 1000 live births; the incidence in children who are born prematurely is much higher compared with children born at term. CP is classified into different groups. The most prevalent type is spastic CP; it is characterized by spasticity, hyperreflexia, clonus, and a positive Babinski sign due to damage to the corticospinal tract. Dyskinetic CP is characterized by chorea and athetosis that may reflect damage to the basal ganglia. The rarest type is hypotonic CP; it presents with truncal and extremity hypotonia, hyperreflexia, and persistent primitive reflexes.

THERAPEUTIC HIGHLIGHTS

Treatment of CP includes physical and occupational therapy. Botulinum toxin injection into affected muscles reduces muscle spasticity, especially in the gastrocnemius muscle. Other drugs used to treat muscle spasticity include diazepam (a benzodiazepine that binds to $GABA_A$ receptor), baclofen (an agonist at presynaptic $GABA_B$ receptors in the spinal cord), and dantrolene (a direct muscle relaxant). Various surgeries have been used to treat CP, including dorsal root rhizotomy and tenotomy in the gastrocnemius muscles.

The supplementary motor area projects to the primary motor cortex and is involved in organizing or planning motor sequences, while M1 executes the movements. The premotor cortex receives input from sensory regions of the parietal cortex and projects to M1, the spinal cord, and the brainstem reticular formation. This region is concerned with setting posture at the start of a planned movement and with preparing the individual to move. It is most involved in control of proximal limb muscles needed to orient the body for movement.

The somatic sensory area and related portions of the posterior parietal lobe project to the premotor cortex. Lesions of the somatic sensory area cause defects in motor performance that are characterized by inability to execute learned sequences of movements such as eating with a knife and fork. Neurons in this region contribute to the descending pathways involved in motor control.

Damage to the cerebral cortex before or during childbirth or during the first 2–3 years of development can lead to cerebral palsy, a disorder that affects muscle tone, movement, and coordination (**Clinical Box 12–4**).

■ CONTROL OF AXIAL & DISTAL MUSCLES

Within the brainstem and spinal cord, pathways and neurons that control skeletal muscles of the trunk (axial) and proximal portions of the limbs are located medially or ventrally; pathways and neurons that control skeletal muscles in the distal portions of the limbs are located laterally. Axial muscles are concerned with postural adjustments and gross movements; distal limb muscles mediate fine, skilled movements.

CORTICOSPINAL & CORTICOBULBAR TRACTS

The axons of neurons from the motor cortex that project to spinal motor neurons form the corticospinal tract that passes through the corona radiata to the posterior limb of the internal capsule. About 31% of the corticospinal tract neurons are from the primary motor cortex, 29% are from the premotor and supplementary motor cortex, and 40% originate in the parietal lobe and primary somatosensory area.

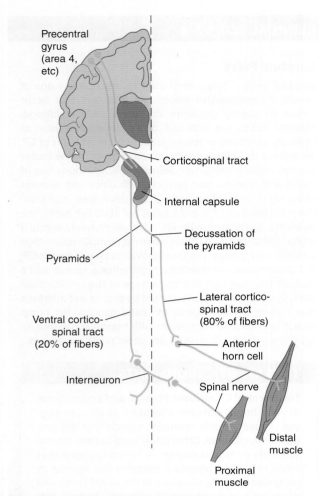

FIGURE 12–4 The corticospinal tracts. This tract originates in the precentral gyrus and passes through the internal capsule. Most fibers decussate in the pyramids and descend in the lateral white matter of the spinal cord to form the lateral division of the tract which can make monosynaptic connections with spinal motor neurons. The ventral division of the tract remains uncrossed until reaching the spinal cord where axons terminate on spinal interneurons antecedent to motor neurons.

The corticospinal tract fibers traverse the cerebral peduncle and basilar pons to reach the medullary pyramids where ~80% of the fibers cross the midline to form the lateral corticospinal tract (Figure 12–4). The other 20% form the ventral corticospinal tract that crosses the midline at the level of the spinal cord at which it terminates. Lateral corticospinal tract neurons make monosynaptic connections to motor neurons, especially those concerned with skilled voluntary movements. Many corticospinal tract neurons synapse on spinal interneurons; this indirect pathway coordinates groups of muscles.

The corticobulbar tract is fibers that pass from the motor cortex to motor neurons in the trigeminal, facial, and hypoglossal nuclei. Corticobulbar neurons end either directly on these nuclei or on brainstem interneurons. Their axons traverse through the genu of the internal capsule, the cerebral peduncle (medial to corticospinal tract neurons), to descend with corticospinal tract fibers in the pons and medulla.

Lower motor neurons refer to the spinal and cranial motor neurons that directly innervate skeletal muscles. Upper motor neurons are those in the cortex and brainstem that activate the lower motor neurons. The pathophysiologic responses to damage to lower and upper motor neurons are very distinctive (**Clinical Box 12–5**).

MEDIAL & LATERAL BRAINSTEM PATHWAYS

The pontine and medullary reticulospinal, vestibulospinal, and tectospinal tracts are the medial brainstem pathways that descend ipsilaterally in the ventral spinal cord and terminate on interneurons and long propriospinal neurons in the ventromedial part of the ventral horn to control axial and proximal muscles (**Figure 12–5**).

The medial and lateral vestibulospinal tracts are involved in vestibular function (see Chapter 10). The medial tract projects bilaterally to cervical spinal motor neurons that control neck muscles; the lateral tract projects ipsilaterally to neurons at all spinal levels to control muscles needed for posture and balance.

The reticulospinal tracts project to all spinal levels and are involved in the maintenance of posture and modulation of muscle tone, especially via an input to γ-motor neurons. Pontine reticulospinal neurons are primarily excitatory and medullary reticulospinal neurons are primarily inhibitory. The tectospinal tract from the superior colliculus of the midbrain projects to the contralateral cervical spinal cord to control head and eye movements.

Neurons in the red nucleus of the midbrain cross the midline and project via the lateral brainstem to interneurons in the dorsolateral part of the spinal ventral horn (Figure 12–5). This rubrospinal tract excites flexor motor neurons and inhibits extensor motor neurons that control distal limb muscles. This pathway is not very prominent in humans, but it may have a role in the posture typical of decorticate rigidity (see below).

■ POSTURE-REGULATING SYSTEMS

When the neural axis is transected, the activities integrated below the section lose the control of higher brain centers. In some cases, activity below the transection can be accentuated due to removal of an inhibitory effect of higher neural centers. Research using animal models has led to information on the role of cortical and brainstem mechanisms involved in control of voluntary movement and posture. The deficits in motor control seen after various lesions mimic those seen in humans with damage in the same structures.

Lower versus Upper Motor Neuron Damage

Lower motor neurons are those whose axons terminate on skeletal muscles. Damage to these neurons is associated with flaccid paralysis, muscle atrophy, fasciculations, hypotonia, and hyporeflexia or areflexia. Amyotrophic lateral sclerosis (ALS) is an example of a lower motor neuron disease. ALS is a selective, progressive degeneration of α-motor neurons. The worldwide annual incidence of ALS is estimated to be 0.5–3 cases per 100,000 people. The disease has no racial, socioeconomic, or ethnic boundaries. The life expectancy of ALS patients is usually 3–5 years after diagnosis. ALS is most commonly diagnosed in middle age and affects men more often than women. Most cases of ALS are sporadic in origin; but 5–10% of the cases have a familial link. Possible causes include viruses, neurotoxins, heavy metals, immune system abnormalities, and enzyme abnormalities. About 40% of the familial cases have a mutation in the gene for Cu/Zn superoxide dismutase (SOD-1) on chromosome 21. SOD is a free radical scavenger that reduces oxidative stress. A defective SOD-1 gene permits free radicals to accumulate and kill neurons. An increase in the excitability of deep cerebellar nuclei due to the inhibition of small-conductance calcium-activated potassium (SK) channels may contribute to the development of cerebellar ataxia.

Upper motor neurons refer to corticospinal tract or brainstem neurons that innervate spinal motor neurons. Damage to these neurons initially causes muscles to become weak and flaccid but eventually leads to spasticity, hypertonia, hyperactive stretch reflexes, and abnormal plantar extensor reflex (positive Babinski sign). The Babinski sign is dorsiflexion of the great toe and fanning of the other toes when the lateral aspect of the sole of the foot is scratched. In adults, the normal response to this stimulation is plantar flexion in all the toes. The Babinski sign is a flexor withdrawal reflex that is normally held in check by the lateral corticospinal system. It is of value in the localization of disease processes, but its physiologic significance is unknown. In infants whose corticospinal tracts are not well developed, dorsiflexion of the great toe and fanning of the other toes is the natural response to stimuli applied to the sole of the foot.

THERAPEUTIC HIGHLIGHTS

Riluzole is one of the few drugs to modestly slow the progression of ALS; it acts by opening the SK channels and may prevent nerve damage caused by excessive release of glutamate. Spasticity can be reduced by the muscle relaxant baclofen; it can be administered via a subarachnoid infusion with an implanted lumbar pump. Botulinum toxin is also approved for the treatment of spasticity.

DECEREBRATION & DECORTICATION

After a complete transection of the brainstem between the superior and inferior colliculi (midcollicular decerebration), the brainstem pathways function independent of their input from higher brain structures (**Figure 12–6**, dashed line A). This lesion interrupts all input from the cortex and red nucleus, primarily to distal limb muscles. The excitatory and inhibitory reticulospinal pathways (primarily to postural extensor muscles) remain intact. The dominance of drive from ascending sensory pathways to the excitatory reticulospinal pathway leads to hyperactivity in extensor muscles in all four extremities (decerebrate rigidity). This resembles what ensues after uncal herniation in patients with large tumors or a hemorrhage in the cerebral hemisphere (**Clinical Box 12–6**). In decerebrate posturing, lower extremities are extended with toes pointed inward, upper limbs are extended with fingers flexed and forearms pronate, and the neck and head are extended.

Removal of the cerebral cortex (decortication; dashed line D in Figure 12–6) causes upper limbs to flex at the elbow (due to rubrospinal excitation of flexor muscles), lower limbs extend with toes pointed slightly inward, and the head is extended. Decorticate rigidity is seen on the hemiplegic side after hemorrhages or thromboses in the internal capsule. The small arteries in the internal capsule are especially prone to rupture or thrombotic obstruction; 60% of intracerebral hemorrhages occur in the internal capsule, the others are equally distributed in the cerebral cortex, pons, thalamus, and cerebellum.

■ BASAL GANGLIA

ORGANIZATION & FUNCTION OF THE BASAL GANGLIA

The basal ganglia include the caudate nucleus and putamen that collectively form the striatum, globus pallidus, subthalamic nucleus, and substantia nigra. The globus pallidus is divided into external and internal segments (GPe and GPi) that contain GABAergic neurons. The substantia nigra is divided into a pars compacta (dopaminergic neurons) and a pars reticulata (GABAergic neurons). About 95% of striatal neurons are medium spiny GABAergic neurons; the other neurons are aspiny interneurons that differ in terms of size and neurotransmitters: large (acetylcholine), medium (somatostatin), and small (GABA).

Figure 12–7 shows the major connections to and from and within the basal ganglia. The excitatory inputs are the corticostriate pathway (from the cerebral cortex) and the thalamostriatal pathway (from intralaminar nuclei). The inhibitory outputs are from GPi and substantia nigra pars reticulata to the thalamus. There is an excitatory projection from the thalamus to the prefrontal and premotor cortex to complete a full cortical-basal ganglia-thalamic-cortical loop.

The connections within the basal ganglia include a dopaminergic nigrostriatal projection and a GABAergic projection

A Medial brainstem pathways

B Lateral brainstem pathways

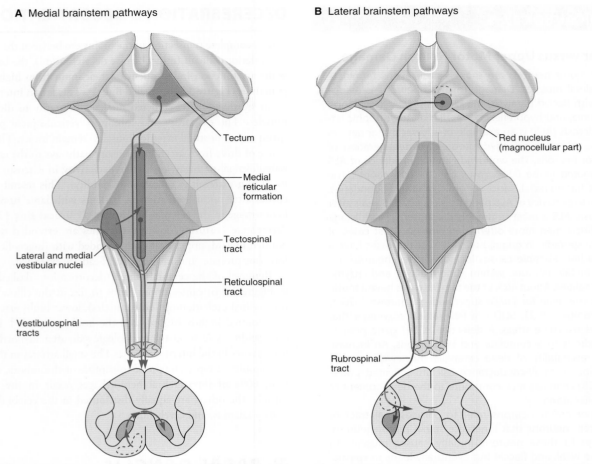

FIGURE 12–5   Medial and lateral descending brainstem pathways involved in motor control. (A) Medial pathways (reticulospinal, vestibulospinal, and tectospinal) terminate in ventromedial area of spinal gray matter and control axial and proximal muscles. **(B)** Lateral pathway (rubrospinal) terminates in dorsolateral area of spinal gray matter and controls distal muscles. (Reproduced with permission from Kandel ER, Schwartz JH, Jessell TM [editors]: *Principles of Neural Science*, 4th ed. New York, NY: McGraw-Hill; 2000.)

from the striatum to substantia nigra pars reticulata. There is an inhibitory projection from the striatum to GPe and GPi. The subthalamic nucleus receives an inhibitory input from GPe, and in turn the subthalamic nucleus has an excitatory projection to GPe and GPi.

The basal ganglia are involved in the planning and programming of movement. The basal ganglia, particularly the caudate nuclei, also play a role in some cognitive processes. Lesions of the caudate nuclei disrupt performance on tests involving object reversal and delayed alternation. Lesions of the head of the left caudate nucleus and nearby white matter are associated with a dysarthric form of aphasia that resembles Wernicke aphasia (see Chapter 15).

DISEASES OF THE BASAL GANGLIA

Three biochemical pathways in the basal ganglia normally operate in a balanced manner: (1) the nigrostriatal dopaminergic system, (2) the intrastriatal cholinergic system, and (3) the

GABAergic system from the striatum to the globus pallidus and substantia nigra. When one or more of these pathways become dysfunctional, characteristic motor abnormalities occur.

Diseases of the basal ganglia lead to two general types of disorders: hyperkinetic (chorea, athetosis, and ballism) and hypokinetic (akinesia and bradykinesia). Chorea is characterized by rapid, involuntary "dancing" movements; athetosis is characterized by continuous, slow writhing movements. In ballism, involuntary flailing, intense, and violent movements occur. Akinesia is difficulty in initiating movement and decreased spontaneous movement; bradykinesia is slowness of movement.

Parkinson disease results from the degeneration of dopaminergic neurons in the substantia nigra pars compacta; fibers to the putamen are most severely affected (**Clinical Box 12–7**). It has both hypokinetic and hyperkinetic features. The hypokinetic features are akinesia and bradykinesia, and the hyperkinetic features are cogwheel rigidity and tremor at rest. The absence of motor activity and the difficulty in initiating voluntary movements are

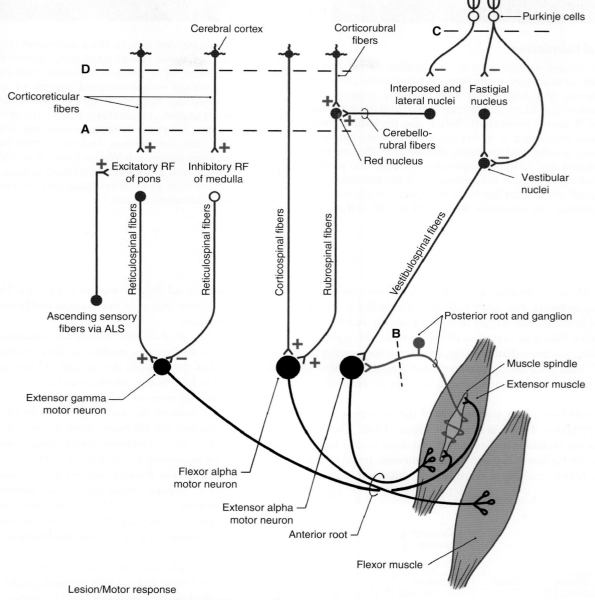

Lesion/Motor response

A = Extensor rigidity in all limbs, decerebrate rigidity/posturing
A+B = Relaxation of extensor rigidity in limb with sectioned root
A+C = Slight enhancement of decerebrate rigidity compared to A
A+C+B = No relaxation of decerebrate rigidity
D = Flexion of upper limbs, extension of lower limbs, decorticate rigidity/posturing

FIGURE 12–6 A circuit drawing representing lesions produced in experimental animals to replicate decerebrate and decorticate deficits seen in humans. Bilateral transections are indicated by dashed lines A, B, C, and D. Decerebration is at a midcollicular level (A), dorsal roots sectioned for one extremity (B), removal of anterior lobe of cerebellum (C), and decortication is rostral to the superior colliculus (D). The objective was to identify anatomic substrates responsible for decerebrate or decorticate rigidity/posturing seen in humans with lesions that either isolate the forebrain from the brainstem or separate rostral from caudal brainstem and spinal cord. (Reproduced with permission from Haines DE (ed): *Fundamental Neuroscience for Basic and Clinical Applications*, 3rd ed. St. Louis, MO: Elsevier; 2006.)

Uncal Herniation

Space-occupying lesions from large tumors, hemorrhages, strokes, or abscesses in the cerebral hemisphere can drive the uncus of the temporal lobe over the edge of the cerebellar tentorium, compressing the ipsilateral cranial nerve III (uncal herniation). Before the herniation these patients experience a decreased level of consciousness, lethargy, poorly reactive pupils, deviation of the eye to a "down and out" position, hyperactive reflexes, and a bilateral Babinski sign (due to compression of the ipsilateral corticospinal tract). After the brain herniates, the patients are decerebrate and comatose, have fixed and dilated pupils, and eye movements are absent. Once damage extends to the midbrain, a Cheyne–Stokes respiratory pattern develops, characterized by a pattern of waxing-and-waning depth of respiration with interposed periods of apnea. Eventually, medullary function is lost, breathing ceases, and recovery is unlikely. Hemispheric masses closer to the midline compress the thalamic reticular formation and can cause coma before eye findings develop (central herniation). As the mass enlarges, midbrain function is affected, the pupils dilate, and a decerebrate posture ensues. With progressive herniation, pontine vestibular and then medullary respiratory functions are lost.

striking. There is a decrease in the normal, unconscious movements (eg, swinging arms while walking). The rigidity is due to increased motor neuron activity to both the agonist and antagonist muscles. Passive motion of an extremity meets with a plastic, dead-feeling resistance (lead pipe rigidity). Sometimes a series of "catches" takes place during passive motion (cogwheel rigidity), but the sudden loss of resistance seen in a spastic extremity is absent.

A current view of the pathogenesis of the movement disorders in Parkinson disease is shown in Figure 12–8. The balance between inhibition and excitation maintains normal motor function. In Parkinson disease, the dopaminergic input to the putamen is lost, resulting in decreased inhibition and increased excitation from the subthalamic nucleus to the GPi. The overall increase in inhibitory output to the thalamus and brainstem disorganizes movement.

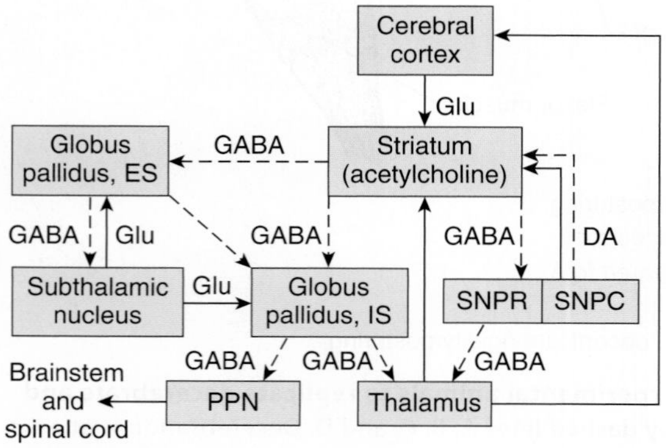

Familial cases of Parkinson disease are uncommon. The genes for at least five proteins involved in ubiquitination can be mutated. Two of the proteins, α-synuclein and barkin, interact and are found in Lewy bodies, which are inclusion bodies in neurons that occur in all forms of Parkinson disease.

The balance between the excitatory discharge of cholinergic interneurons and the inhibitory dopaminergic input in the striatum is important in Parkinson disease. Some improvement is produced by decreasing the cholinergic influence with anticholinergic drugs. More dramatic improvement is produced by administration of L-dopa (levodopa). Unlike dopamine, this dopamine precursor crosses the blood–brain barrier and helps repair the dopamine deficiency. However, the degeneration of these neurons continues and in 5–7 years the beneficial effects of L-dopa disappear.

In addition to Parkinson disease, there are several other disorders that involve a malfunction within the basal ganglia. A few of these are described in Clinical Box 12–8. Huntington disease is one of an increasing number of human genetic diseases affecting the nervous system that are characterized by trinucleotide repeat expansions (Table 12–1).

FIGURE 12–7 Diagrammatic representation of the principal connections of the basal ganglia. Solid lines indicate excitatory pathways, dashed lines inhibitory pathways. The transmitters are indicated in the pathways, where they are known. DA, dopamine; Glu, glutamate. Acetylcholine is the transmitter produced by interneurons in the striatum. ES, external segment; IS, internal segment; PPN, pedunculopontine nuclei; SNPC, substantia nigra, pars compacta; SNPR, substantia nigra, pars reticulata. The subthalamic nucleus also projects to the pars compacta of the substantia nigra; this pathway has been omitted for clarity.

■ CEREBELLUM

The posterolateral fissure separates the medial nodulus and the lateral flocculus on either side from the rest of the cerebellum; the primary fissure divides the remainder into the anterior and posterior lobes. The vermis is subdivided into 10 primary lobules numbered I–X from superior to inferior. The cerebellum is connected to the brainstem by the superior cerebellar peduncle (fibers from deep cerebellar nuclei to the brainstem, red nucleus, and thalamus), middle cerebellar peduncle (afferent fibers from the contralateral pontine nuclei), and inferior cerebellar peduncle

CLINICAL BOX 12–7

Parkinson Disease

Between 7 and 10 million people worldwide have been diagnosed with Parkinson disease; it is 1.5 times more prevalent in men than women. Parkinsonism occurs in sporadic idiopathic form in many middle-aged and elderly individuals and is one of the most common neurodegenerative diseases. It occurs in 1–2% of individuals over age 65. Dopaminergic neurons and dopamine receptors are steadily lost with age in the basal ganglia in healthy individuals, and an acceleration of these losses precipitates parkinsonism. Symptoms appear when 60–80% of the nigrostriatal dopaminergic neurons degenerate. Parkinsonism is also seen as a complication of treatment with the phenothiazine group of antipsychotic drugs and other drugs that block D_2 receptors.

THERAPEUTIC HIGHLIGHTS

Sinemet, a combination of levodopa (L-dopa) and carbidopa, is the most commonly used drug for the treatment of Parkinson disease. The addition of carbidopa to L-dopa increases its effectiveness and prevents the conversion of L-dopa to dopamine in the periphery to reduce some of the adverse side effects (nausea, vomiting, and cardiac rhythm disturbances). Dopamine agonists (eg, apomorphine) are effective in some patients. Taken in combination with levodopa, catechol-O-methyltransferase (COMT) inhibitors (eg, entacapone) exert their therapeutic effects by blocking the breakdown of L-dopa, allowing more of it to reach the brain to increase the level of dopamine. MAO-B inhibitors (eg, selegiline) also prevent the breakdown of dopamine and can be given soon after diagnosis to delay the need for levodopa.

Deep brain stimulation (DBS) is approved by the US Food and Drug Administration for treating Parkinson disease. It reduces the amount of L-dopa needed and thus reduces its adverse side effects (eg, dyskinesias). DBS reduces tremors, slowness of movements, and gait problems. Surgical treatments are reserved for those who have exhausted drug therapies or who have not responded favorably to them. Lesions in GPi or in the subthalamic nucleus have been done to restore the output balance of the basal ganglia toward normal (see Figure 12–8). Transplants of dopamine-secreting tissue (eg, adrenal medullary tissue or carotid body) in or near the basal ganglia works for a while, but long-term results have been disappointing. Results with transplantation of fetal striatal tissue have been better; the transplanted cells survive and make appropriate connections in the host's basal ganglia. Some patients with transplants develop dyskinesias due to excessive levels of dopamine.

(mixture of afferent fibers from the brainstem and spinal cord and efferent fibers to the vestibular nuclei). The middle and inferior cerebellar peduncles carry afferent mossy and climbing fibers that emit collaterals to the deep cerebellar nuclei and pass to the cortex. There are four deep nuclei: dentate, fastigial, globose, and emboliform nuclei.

ANATOMICAL & FUNCTIONAL ORGANIZATION OF THE CEREBELLUM

The cerebellar cortex has three layers: an external molecular layer, a Purkinje cell layer that is only one cell thick, and an internal granular layer. There are five types of neurons in the cortex: Purkinje, granule, basket, stellate, and Golgi cells. The large Purkinje cells have extensive dendritic arbors that extend throughout the molecular layer. Their axons (the only output from the cerebellar cortex) form inhibitory synapses in the deep cerebellar nuclei.

The cerebellar granule cells receive excitatory input from the mossy fibers and innervate the Purkinje cells (Figure 12–9). Each sends an axon to the molecular layer, where the axon bifurcates to form a T, the branches are called parallel fibers. The parallel fibers form excitatory synapses

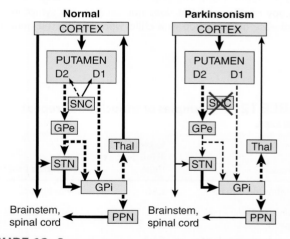

FIGURE 12–8 Probable basal ganglia-thalamocortical circuitry in Parkinson disease. Solid arrows indicate excitatory outputs and dashed arrows inhibitory outputs. The strength of each output is indicated by the width of the arrow. GPe, external segment of the globus pallidus; GPi, internal segment of the globus pallidus; PPN, pedunculopontine nuclei; SNC, pars compacta of the substantia nigra; STN, subthalamic nucleus; Thal, thalamus. See text for details. (Modified with permission from Grafton SC, DeLong M: Tracing the brain circuitry with functional imaging. *Nat Med.* 1997 Jun;3(6):602–603.)

CLINICAL BOX 12–8

Basal Ganglia Diseases

Medium spiny neurons in the striatum are the first to be damaged in Huntington disease. The loss of this GABAergic pathway to the globus pallidus releases inhibition and the hyperkinetic features of the disease develop. An early sign is a jerky trajectory of the hand when reaching to touch something. Later, hyperkinetic choreiform movements appear and gradually increase until they incapacitate the patient. Speech becomes slurred and incomprehensible; a progressive dementia is followed by death, usually within 10–15 years after the onset of symptoms. Huntington disease affects 5 out of 100,000 people worldwide. It is inherited as an autosomal dominant disorder with an onset between the ages of 30 and 50. The abnormal gene responsible for the disease codes for the protein huntingtin. It normally contains 11–34 cytosine-adenine-guanine (CAG) repeats. In patients with Huntington disease, there are 42–86 or more copies; the greater the number of repeats, the earlier the age of onset and the more rapid the progression of the disease. Poorly soluble toxic protein aggregates form in cell nuclei. The loss of the function of huntingtin is proportional to the size of the CAG insert. Tissue caspase-1 activity is increased in the brains of humans with the disease.

Wilson disease is a rare disorder of copper metabolism that has an onset between 6 and 25 years of age, affecting about four times as many females as males and ~30,000 people worldwide. It is a genetic autosomal recessive disorder due to a mutation on the long arm of chromosome 13q. It affects the copper-transporting ATPase gene (*ATP7B*) in the liver; copper accumulates in the liver, causing progressive liver damage. About 1% of the population carries a single abnormal copy of this gene but does not develop any symptoms; the disease may develop in a child who inherits the gene from both parents. In affected individuals, copper accumulates in the periphery of the cornea in the eye accounting for the characteristic yellow Kayser–Fleischer rings. The dominant neuronal pathology is degeneration of the putamen. Motor disturbances include "wing-beating" tremor or asterixis, dysarthria, unsteady gait, and rigidity. Another disease that involves the basal ganglia is tardive dyskinesia; it is an adverse effect of the use of neuroleptic drugs, so it is iatrogenic in origin. These drugs block dopaminergic transmission; their prolonged use leads to hypersensitivity of D_3 receptors and an imbalance in nigrostriatal influences on motor control. Motor disturbances include temporary or permanent uncontrolled involuntary movements of the face and tongue and cogwheel rigidity.

THERAPEUTIC HIGHLIGHTS

Treatment for Huntington disease is directed at treating the symptoms and maintaining quality of life as there is no cure. In general, the drugs used have side effects such as fatigue, nausea, and restlessness. In August 2008, the US Food and Drug Administration approved the use of tetrabenazine to reduce choreiform movements. This drug binds reversibly to vesicular mono-amine transporters (VMAT) to inhibit the uptake of monoamines into synaptic vesicles. It also is a dopamine receptor antagonist. Tetrabenazine is also used to treat other hyperkinetic movement disorders (eg, tardive dyskinesia). Chelating agents are used to reduce the copper in the body in individuals with Wilson disease. Clozapine is an atypical neuroleptic drug that has been an effective substitute for traditional neuroleptic drugs but with less risk for development of tardive dyskinesia.

TABLE 12–1 Examples of trinucleotide repeat diseases.

Disease	Expanded Trinucleotide Repeat	Affected Protein
Huntington disease	CAG	Huntingtin
Spinocerebellar ataxia, types 1, 2, 3, 7	CAG	Ataxin 1, 2, 3, 7
Spinocerebellar ataxia, type 6	CAG	α_{1A} subunit of Ca^{2+} channel
Dentatorubral-pallido-luysian atrophy	CAG	Atrophin
Spinobulbar muscular atrophy	CAG	Androgen receptor
Fragile X syndrome	CGG	FMR-1
Myotonic dystrophy	CTG	DM protein kinase
Friedreich ataxia	GAA	Frataxin

on the dendrites of many Purkinje cells. Basket cells in the molecular layer receive excitatory input from parallel fibers and synapse on the cell body and axon hillock of Purkinje cells. Stellate cells are similar to the basket cells but are in the more superficial molecular layer. Golgi cells in the granular layer have dendrites that project into the molecular layer and they receive excitatory input from the parallel fibers. Their cell bodies receive excitatory input via collaterals from the incoming mossy fibers. Their axons project to the dendrites of the granule cells where they form an inhibitory synapse.

The fundamental circuits of the cerebellar cortex are thus relatively simple (Figure 12–9). Climbing fiber inputs exert a strong excitatory effect on single Purkinje cells, whereas mossy fiber inputs exert a weak excitatory effect on many Purkinje cells via the granule cells. The primary afferent systems that converge to form the mossy fiber or climbing fiber input to the cerebellum are listed in Table 12–2. The basket and stellate cells are also excited

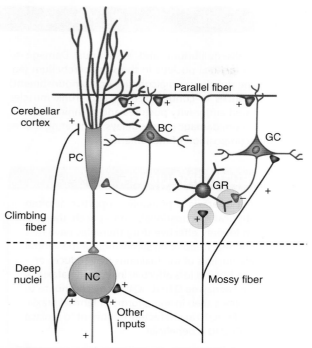

FIGURE 12–9 **Diagram of neural connections in the cerebellum.** Plus (+) and minus (–) signs indicate whether endings are excitatory or inhibitory. BC, basket cell; GC, Golgi cell; GR, granule cell; NC, cell in deep nucleus; PC, Purkinje cell. Note that PCs and BCs are inhibitory. The connections of the stellate cells, which are not shown, are similar to those of the basket cells, except that they end for the most part on Purkinje cell dendrites.

TABLE 12–2 Function of principal afferent systems to the cerebellum.[a]

Afferent Tracts	Transmits
Vestibulocerebellar	Vestibular impulses from labyrinths, direct and via vestibular nuclei
Dorsal spinocerebellar	Proprioceptive and exteroceptive impulses from muscle spindles, Golgi tendon organ, and joint receptors of lower limbs and trunk
Ventral spinocerebellar	Proprioceptive and exteroceptive impulses from muscle spindles, Golgi tendon organ, and joint receptors of upper and lower l imbs
Cuneocerebellar	Proprioceptive impulses from muscle spindles, Golgi tendon organ, and joint receptors of upper limb and upper thorax
Tectocerebellar	Auditory and visual impulses via inferior and superior colliculi, respectively
Pontocerebellar	Impulses from motor and other parts of cerebral cortex via pontine nuclei
Olivocerebellar	Proprioceptive input from whole body via relay in inferior olive

by granule cells via their parallel fibers; and the basket and stellate cells inhibit the Purkinje cells. Golgi cells are excited by the mossy fiber collaterals and parallel fibers, and they inhibit transmission from mossy fibers to granule cells. The neurotransmitter released by the stellate, basket, Golgi, and Purkinje cells is GABA; granule cells release glutamate.

From a functional point of view, the cerebellum is divided into three parts (**Figure 12–10**). The vestibulocerebellum is concerned with equilibrium and eye movements. The spinocerebellum receives proprioceptive input from the body as well as a copy of the "motor plan" from the motor cortex. By comparing plan with performance, it smooths and coordinates movements that are ongoing. The vermis projects to the brainstem area concerned with control of axial and proximal limb muscles (medial brainstem pathways), and the hemispheres of the spinocerebellum project to the brainstem areas concerned with control of distal limb muscles (lateral brainstem pathways). The cerebrocerebellum interacts with the motor cortex in planning and programming movements. The deep nuclei provide the only output for the spinocerebellum and the cerebrocerebellum.

Damage to the cerebellum leads to several characteristic abnormalities, including hypotonia, ataxia, and intention tremor. Motor abnormalities associated with cerebellar damage vary depending on the region involved (**Clinical Box 12–9**).

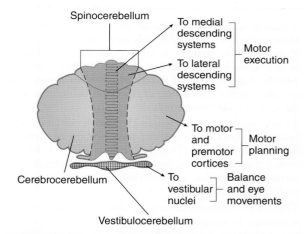

FIGURE 12–10 **Three functional divisions of the cerebellum.** The nodulus in the vermis and the flanking flocculus in the hemisphere on each side form the vestibulocerebellum, which has vestibular connections and is concerned with equilibrium and eye movements. The rest of the vermis and the adjacent medial portions of the hemispheres form the spinocerebellum, the region that receives proprioceptive input from the body as well as a copy of the "motor plan" from the motor cortex. The lateral portions of the cerebellar hemispheres are called the cerebrocerebellum, which interacts with the motor cortex in planning and programming movements. (Modified with permission from Kandel ER, Schwartz JH, Jessell TM (eds): *Principles of Neural Science*, 4th ed. New York, NY: McGraw-Hill; 2000.)

Cerebellar Disease

Most abnormalities linked to cerebellar damage are apparent during movement. The marked ataxia is manifested as a wide-based, unsteady, "drunken" gait and slurred, scanning speech. Many types of ataxia are hereditary (eg, Friedreich ataxia). Voluntary movements are also highly abnormal when the cerebellum is damaged. For example, attempting to touch an object with a finger results in overshooting. This dysmetria promptly initiates a gross corrective action, but the correction overshoots to the other side, and the finger oscillates back and forth (intention tremor). Cerebellar disease prevents the ability to stop movement promptly, contributing to the appearance of dysdiadochokinesia (inability to perform rapidly alternating opposite movements such as repeated pronation and supination of the hands). Patients with cerebellar disease also have difficulty performing actions that involve simultaneous motion at more than one joint. They dissect such movements and carry them out one joint at a time (decomposition of movement). Motor abnormalities associated with cerebellar damage vary depending on the region involved. Damage to the vestibulocerebellum causes ataxia, disequilibrium, and nystagmus. Damage to the vermis and fastigial nucleus in the spinocerebellum (eg, due to thiamine deficiency in alcoholics or malnourishment) causes disturbances in control of axial and trunk muscles during attempted antigravity postures and scanning speech. Cerebrocerebellum damage causes delays in initiating movements and decomposition of movement.

THERAPEUTIC HIGHLIGHTS

Management of ataxia is primarily supportive; it often includes physical, occupational, and speech therapy. Attempts to identify effective drug therapies have met with little success. Deep brain stimulation of the ventral intermediate nucleus of the thalamus may reduce cerebellar tremor, but it is less effective in reducing ataxia. A deficiency in coenzyme Q10 (CoQ10) may contribute to the abnormalities seen in some forms of familial ataxia. If low levels of CoQ10 are detected, treatment to replace the missing CoQ10 is beneficial.

CHAPTER SUMMARY

- A muscle spindle is a group of specialized intrafusal muscle fibers with contractile polar ends and a noncontractile center. It is located in parallel to the extrafusal muscle fibers and is innervated by types Ia and II afferent fibers and efferent γ-motor neurons. Muscle stretch activates the muscle spindle to initiate reflex contraction of the extrafusal muscle fibers in the same muscle (stretch reflex).

- A Golgi tendon organ is within the fascicles of a tendon; it is located in series with extrafusal muscle fibers and innervated by type Ib afferents. They are stimulated by both passive stretch and active contraction of the muscle to relax the muscle (inverse stretch reflex) and function as a transducer to regulate muscle force.

- The flexor withdrawal reflex is a polysynaptic spinal reflex that is initiated by nociceptive stimuli.

- Spinal cord transection is followed by a period of spinal shock during which all spinal reflex responses are profoundly depressed. In humans, recovery begins about 2 weeks after the injury.

- The supplementary cortex, basal ganglia, and cerebellum participate in the planning of skilled movements. Commands from the primary motor cortex and other cortical regions are relayed via the corticospinal and corticobulbar tracts to spinal and brainstem motor neurons.

- The ventral corticospinal tract and medial descending brainstem pathways (tectospinal, reticulospinal, and vestibulospinal tracts) regulate proximal muscles and posture. The lateral corticospinal and rubrospinal tracts control distal limb muscles for fine motor control and skilled voluntary movements.

- Decerebrate rigidity leads to hyperactivity in extensor muscles in all four extremities due to facilitation of the stretch reflex.

It resembles what is seen with uncal herniation due to a supratentorial lesion. Decorticate rigidity is flexion of the upper extremities at the elbow and extensor hyperactivity in the lower extremities. It occurs on the hemiplegic side after hemorrhage or thrombosis in the internal capsule.

- The basal ganglia include the caudate nucleus, putamen, globus pallidus, subthalamic nucleus, and substantia nigra. The connections between the parts of the basal ganglia include a dopaminergic nigrostriatal projection from the substantia nigra to the striatum and a GABAergic projection from the striatum to substantia nigra.

- Parkinson disease is due to degeneration of the nigrostriatal dopaminergic neurons and is characterized by akinesia, bradykinesia, cogwheel rigidity, and tremor at rest. Huntington disease is characterized by choreiform movements due to the loss of the GABAergic inhibitory pathway to the globus pallidus.

- The cerebellar cortex contains five types of neurons: Purkinje, granule, basket, stellate, and Golgi cells. The two main inputs to the cerebellar cortex are climbing fibers and mossy fibers. The only output neurons are the Purkinje cells; they generally project to the deep nuclei. Damage to the cerebellum leads to several characteristic abnormalities, including hypotonia, ataxia, and intention tremor.

MULTIPLE-CHOICE QUESTIONS

For all questions, select the single best answer unless otherwise directed.

1. A medical student was doing research in a neurophysiology laboratory that studied the role of γ-motor neurons in control of group Ia spindle sensitivity. As an initial project he

recorded the group Ia muscle spindle afferent activity during stimulation of only α-motor neurons to the same muscle with that seen during simultaneous stimulation of α- and γ-motor neurons to that muscle. What is he likely to observe?

A. During stimulation of only α-motor neurons, group Ia spindle afferent activity will be markedly increased; during stimulation of both α- and γ-motor neurons, group Ia spindle afferent activity will be suppressed.

B. During stimulation of only α-motor neurons, group Ia spindle afferent activity will be inhibited; during stimulation of both α- and γ-motor neurons, group Ia spindle afferent activity will increase.

C. During stimulation of only α-motor neurons, group Ia spindle afferent activity will be moderately reduced; during stimulation of both α- and γ-motor neurons, group Ia spindle afferent activity will be further reduced.

D. During stimulation of only α-motor neurons, group Ia spindle afferent activity will be moderately increased; during stimulation of both α- and γ-motor neurons, group Ia spindle afferent activity will be markedly increased.

E. During stimulation of only α-motor neurons, group Ia spindle afferent activity will be moderately increased; during stimulation of both α- and γ-motor neurons, group Ia spindle afferent activity will be further increased.

2. An MD/PhD candidate was interested in studying factors that control skeletal muscle force, including the inverse myotatic reflex. In her thesis proposal she outlines the fundamental elements of this reflex. What are these elements?

A. Muscle spindles, group Ia spindle afferents, and α-motor neurons

B. Muscle spindles, group II spindle afferents, spinal excitatory interneurons, and α-motor neurons

C. Golgi tendon organ, group II tendon afferents, spinal excitatory interneurons, and α-motor neurons

D. Golgi tendon organ, group Ib afferents, spinal inhibitory interneurons, and α-motor neurons

E. Golgi tendon organ, group Ia afferents, spinal inhibitory interneurons, and α-motor neurons

3. Following recovery from a stroke, a 47-year-old man was at his neurologist's office for a follow-up examination. The neurologic examination showed that this individual had ankle clonus that is sustained at a frequency of 8 Hz. What is the definition of clonus, and when does it qualify as pathological rather than physiological?

A. Clonus is the occurrence of regular, repetitive, rhythmic contractions of a muscle when subjected to a noxious stimulus; sustained clonus greater than or equal to 10 Hz is considered pathological.

B. Clonus is the resistance of muscle to stretch; sustained clonus greater than or equal to 10 Hz is considered pathological.

C. Clonus is the occurrence of regular, repetitive, rhythmic contractions of a muscle when subjected to sudden, maintained stretch; sustained clonus greater than or equal to 5 Hz is considered pathological.

D. Clonus is a sequence of resistance followed by a sudden decrease in resistance when a limb is moved passively; sustained clonus greater than or equal to 5 Hz is considered pathological.

E. Clonus is an involuntary low amplitude trembling of a body part at a frequency of 10 Hz; sustained clonus greater than or equal to 20 Hz is considered pathological.

4. While exercising, a 42-year-old woman developed sudden onset of tingling from her waist to her toe on the right side and an inability to control movement in that limb. A neurologic exam showed a hyperactive knee jerk reflex and a positive Babinski sign. What is a possible basis for these findings?

A. She had a lower thoracic disk rupture that damaged the right side of her spinal cord.

B. She had a mid-cervical disk rupture that damaged the right side of her spinal cord.

C. She had a lower lumbar disk rupture that compressed the spinal nerve at that segmental level.

D. She had a sacral disk rupture that put pressure on the ventral root at that segmental level.

E. She was experiencing the cauda equina syndrome.

5. A 6-year-old girl had severe physical and cognitive disabilities due to cerebral palsy thought to be related to a prolonged period of hypoxia during a difficult delivery. She had very limited voluntary movements. Increased neural activity before a skilled voluntary movement is *first* seen in the

A. spinal motor neurons.

B. premotor cortex.

C. basal ganglia.

D. cerebellum.

E. cortical association areas.

6. A 58-year-old woman was brought to the emergency department of her local hospital because of a sudden change of consciousness. All four limbs were extended, suggestive of decerebrate rigidity. A brain CT showed a rostral pontine hemorrhage. What are the underlying neurophysiological changes that lead to the appearance of decerebrate rigidity?

A. Destruction of the rubrospinal tract eliminates inhibition of the cerebellar fastigial nucleus and secondarily increases excitation to vestibular nuclei to activate extensor muscles in the limbs.

B. Loss of the corticospinal pathway disrupts excitatory input to motor neurons controlling flexor muscles, leaving extensor muscles to undergo sustained contraction.

C. Sensory input activates the medullary reticulospinal pathway, which then directly activates motor neurons to extensor muscles in all four extremities.

D. Sensory input activates neurons in the rubrospinal tract that inhibit flexor α-motor neurons and excite extensor α-motor neurons in all four limbs.

E. Sensory input activates the pontine reticulospinal pathway, which then activates primarily γ-motor neurons to extensor muscles in all four extremities.

7. A 38-year-old woman with a very large space-occupying metastatic brain tumor was brought to the emergency department of her local hospital because of irregular breathing and progressive loss of consciousness. She also showed signs of decerebrate posturing. Over the next hour, these and other signs progressed to the point that the emergency department physician diagnosed her with an uncal herniation. What changes in the eye likely occurred that contribute to this diagnosis?

A. She had fixed and dilated pupils.

B. Her pupils were constricted and unresponsive to light.

C. She shows nystagmus and deviation of the eye to an up and out position.

D. Her eyes constrict when stimulated by light but are dilated in normal room light.

E. Eyes are deviated toward the left and pupils are hyperreactive to light.

8. Starting about 6 months ago, 30-year-old elementary teacher began noticing various motor abnormalities that were worsening over time. For example, she experienced uncontrolled movement of her arms and legs; she also noticed some memory loss and difficulty when trying to develop lesson plans for her class. After a thorough neurological exam, she also underwent genetic testing that confirmed the presence of the defective gene for huntingtin protein. What group of neurons is among the first to show damage in Huntington disease, and what is the normal function of this group of neurons?
   A. Medium spiny neurons in the striatum are among the first to be damaged; these neurons normally excite the globus pallidus external segment.
   B. The substantia nigra pars reticulata are among the first to be damaged; these neurons normally inhibit the thalamus.
   C. Medium spiny neurons in the striatum are among the first to be damaged; these neurons normally inhibit the globus pallidus external segment.
   D. Subthalamic neurons are among the first to be damaged; these neurons normally excite the globus pallidus.
   E. Globus pallidus external segment neurons are among the first to be damaged; these neurons normally inhibit the motor cortex.

9. At the age of 50, a man was diagnosed with Parkinson disease, the first in his family to develop this neurological disorder. He has been taking carbidopa and L-dopa (Sinemet) since shortly after the diagnosis; until recently, he has been able to continue to work and help with routine jobs around the house. Now, 10 years after initial diagnosis, his tremor and rigidity interfere with these activities. The therapeutic effect of L-dopa in patients with Parkinson disease eventually wears off because
   A. antibodies to dopamine receptors develop.
   B. inhibitory pathways grow into the basal ganglia from the frontal lobe.
   C. there is an increase in circulating α-synuclein.
   D. the number of CAG repeats triggering symptoms of Parkinson disease have increase over time.
   E. the dopaminergic neurons in the substantia nigra continue to degenerate.

10. An 8-year-old girl was brought to her pediatrician because her parents noted frequent episodes of gait unsteadiness and speech difficulties. Her mother was concerned because of a family history of Friedreich ataxia. This is an example of a human genetic disease affecting the nervous system that is characterized by trinucleotide repeat expansion. What type of trinucleotide repeat is expanded in this disorder, and what is the name of the affected protein?
   A. CGG and FMR-1
   B. GAA and frataxin
   C. CTG and DM protein kinase
   D. CAG and the androgen receptor
   E. CAG and ataxin

11. A 75-year-old man presented to his physician with an unsteady gait, repetitive eye movements, tremor when reaching, slurred speech, and dizziness. After a series of tests, he was diagnosed with cerebellar ataxia. Loss of Purkinje cells in the cerebellum is linked to the appearance of cerebellar ataxia. What cerebellar neurons make excitatory and inhibitory connections with the cerebellar Purkinje cells, and where do the axons of Purkinje cells project?
   A. Granule cells excite Purkinje cells, climbing fibers and mossy fibers inhibit Purkinje cells; Purkinje cells excite the vestibular nuclei.
   B. Climbing fiber excite Purkinje cells, mossy fibers inhibit Purkinje cells; Purkinje cells inhibit vestibular nuclei.
   C. Granule cells excite Purkinje cells, basket cells inhibit Purkinje cells; Purkinje cells inhibit deep cerebellar nuclei.
   D. Basket cells excite Purkinje cells, granule cells inhibit Purkinje cells; Purkinje cells inhibit deep cerebellar nuclei.
   E. Granule cells excite Purkinje cells, stellate cells inhibit Purkinje cells; Purkinje cells excite deep cerebellar nuclei.

12. After falling down a flight of stairs, a young woman is found to have partial loss of voluntary movement on the right side of her body and loss of pain and temperature sensation on the left side below the mid-thoracic region. Imaging tests showed evidence for a spinal cord lesion. What is the likely location of this spinal lesion?
   A. On the left half of the spinal cord in the lumbar region.
   B. On the left half of the spinal cord in the upper thoracic region.
   C. On the right half of the spinal cord in the upper thoracic region.
   D. On the dorsal half of the spinal cord in the upper thoracic region.
   E. On the ventral half of the spinal cord in the lumbar region.

13. At the age of 30, a male postal worker reported weakness in his right leg. Within a year the weakness had spread to his entire right side. A neurologic examination revealed flaccid paralysis, muscular atrophy, fasciculations, hypotonia, and hyperreflexia of muscles in the right arm and leg. Sensory and cognitive function tests were normal. Which of the following diagnosis is likely?
   A. A large tumor in the left primary motor cortex
   B. A cerebral infarct in the region of the corona radiate
   C. A vestibulocerebellar tumor
   D. Damage to the basal ganglia
   E. Amyotrophic lateral sclerosis

14. Medical students became concerned when they began to notice changes in the behavior of their 65-year-old dean that have worsened during the past academic year. They noticed that he walked slowly and with very short steps, his posture had become stooped, his speech was slurred, and his writing was so small it was hard to read. Which neurodegenerative disorder could account for these behavioral changes and what is the underlying neuropathology of this disorder?
   A. Huntington disease due to loss of a GABAergic pathway to the globus pallidus
   B. Parkinson disease due to degeneration of nigrostriatal dopaminergic neurons
   C. Cerebellar ataxia due to damage to cerebellar Purkinje fibers
   D. Huntington disease due to loss of cholinergic neurons in the striatum
   E. Parkinson disease due to degeneration of dopaminergic neurons in the globus pallidus

15. An MD/PhD candidate was doing her doctoral work on cerebellar diseases. For her thesis proposal she included a summary of the functional divisions of the cerebellum. What are the three functional divisions of the cerebellum, and what is the major function of each of these divisions?
    A. The nodulus controls eye movements; the vermis controls distal limb muscles; and the cerebellar hemispheres control axial muscles.
    B. The vestibulocerebellum smooths and coordinates ongoing movements; the spinocerebellum controls distal limb muscles; and the cerebrocerebellum is involved in planning and programming movements.
    C. The nodulus controls eye movements; the vermis controls equilibrium; and the cerebellar hemispheres control distal and axial muscles.
    D. The vestibulocerebellum is concerned with equilibrium and eye movements; the spinocerebellum smooths and coordinates ongoing movements; and the cerebrocerebellum is involved in planning and programming movements.
    E. The nodulus controls head movements; the vermis controls equilibrium; and the cerebellar hemispheres are involved in planning and programming movements.

16. An 8-year-old girl was brought to her pediatrician's office by her mother after the child had been complaining of fatigue, lack of appetite, a tendency to bruise easily, difficulty with speech and swallowing, muscle stiffness, and jaundice. An ophthalmology exam revealed the presence of Kayser–Fleischer rings in the periphery of the cornea. She was diagnosed with Wilson disease, a genetic autosomal recessive disorder due to a mutation on the long arm of chromosome 13q. What is the underlying pathology of this disease, and what is the dominant neuronal pathology?
    A. A mutation in the gene for Cu/Zn superoxide dismutase and degeneration within the vestibulocerebellum
    B. A disorder of copper metabolism and degeneration of the putamen
    C. A deficiency in coenzyme Q10 and degeneration of the globus pallidus
    D. A disorder of copper metabolism and degeneration of the substantia nigra
    E. A CAG trinucleotide repeat expansion and degeneration within the spinocerebellum

17. A 43-year-old man was recently diagnosed with Parkinson disease and is being seen by his neurologist today to evaluate how his medication is controlling his motor abnormalities. His physician is assessing (a) his difficulty in initiating movement and decreased spontaneous movement, (b) his slowness of movement, (c) the tension in his muscle that gives way in little jerks when the muscle is passively stretched, and (d) and the muscle contractions in his hands while seated with hands on the arm of a chair. What are the medical (scientific) terms for (a) through (d), respectively?
    A. Bradykinesia, chorea, clasp-knife effect, and intention tremor
    B. Akinesia, athetosis, ballism, and tremor at rest
    C. Athetosis, bradykinesia, dysdiadochokinesia, and ballism
    D. Akinesia, bradykinesia, cogwheel rigidity, and tremor at rest
    E. Akinesia, bradykinesia, lead-pipe rigidity, and fasciculations

ANSWERS

1. The best answer is **B.** The Ia spindle afferents characteristically stop firing when the muscle contracts during electrical stimulation of only the α-motor neurons to the extrafusal fibers because the muscle shortens and the spindle is unloaded (rules out options **A, D**, and **E**). Stimulation of γ-motor neurons cause the contractile ends of the intrafusal fibers to shorten and therefore stretches the nuclear bag portion of the spindles, deforming the endings, and initiating impulses in the Ia fibers (rules out options **A** and **C**).

2. The best answer is **D.** Muscle relaxation in response to a strong stretch is called the inverse myotatic reflex which is the opposite of the stretch reflex. The receptor for the inverse stretch reflex is in the Golgi tendon organ; the sensory fibers from the Golgi tendon organs are the Ib group of myelinated, rapidly conducting sensory nerve fibers that synapse on spinal inhibitory interneurons that in turn terminate directly on the α-motor neurons. Activation of muscle spindles initiates the myotatic (stretch) reflex not the inverse myotatic reflex (rules out options **A** and **B**). Group Ia and II afferents are from the muscle spindle not Golgi tendon organ (rules out options **B, C**, and **E**).

3. The best answer is **C.** Clonus is a repetitive series of contraction and relaxation of a muscle when subjected to sudden, maintained stretch; sustained clonus with five or more beats is considered abnormal. A noxious stimulus induces a withdrawal reflex, not clonus (rules out option **A**). Option **B** includes a definition of tonus; option **D** includes a definition of clasp-knife effect; and option **E** includes a definition of physiological tremor.

4. The best answer is **A.** Hyperactive reflexes and a positive Babinski sign are indicative of "upper motor neuron" (corticospinal tract) damage. This rules out compression of a spinal nerve (rules out options **C** and **D**). Even a lower lumbar disk rupture would not damage the spinal cord as the spinal cord ends at about the L1 or L2 level of the vertebra (also rules out option **C**). The combination of sensory (tingling) and motor abnormalities over an extensive area (waist to toe) indicates that the damage was within the spinal cord. The lumbar spinal cord controls the waist to the toe; but the upper lumbar spinal cord is in the region of the lower thoracic vertebral column. Damage at a mid-cervical level should lead to abnormalities in the arm as well (rules out option **B**). Cauda equina syndrome is a medical emergency due to compression of the lumbosacral nerve bundle at a level below the conus medullaris; symptoms include low back pain, sciatica (typically bilateral), sensory disturbances in the inner thighs, buttocks, back of legs, and sacral region (called saddle sensory disturbances), bladder and bowel dysfunction, and motor abnormalities in the leg (rules out option **E**).

5. The best answer is **E.** Commands for voluntary movement originate in cortical association areas. This region then connects with the basal ganglia and the lateral portions of the cerebellar hemispheres that are also involved in motor planning as indicated by increased activity before the movement begins (rules out option **C** and **D**). The basal ganglia and cerebellum then funnel information to the premotor and motor cortex via the thalamus (rules out option **B**). Motor commands from the motor cortex are relayed via the corticospinal tracts to the spinal motor neurons (rules out option **A**).

6. The best answer is **E.** The dominance of drive from ascending sensory pathways to the excitatory pontine reticulospinal pathway leads to hyperactivity in extensor muscles in all four extremities primarily by activation of γ-motor neurons, which indirectly activate α-motor neurons. Disruption of the anterior lobe of the cerebellum (not the rubrospinal tract) eliminates inhibition of the cerebellar fastigial nucleus and secondarily increases excitation to vestibular nuclei to activate extensor muscles in the limbs (rules out option **A**). Damage to corticospinal tract neurons initially causes muscles to become weak and flaccid but eventually leads to spasticity, hypertonia, hyperactive stretch reflexes, and abnormal plantar extensor reflex (rules out option **B**). Activation of medullary reticulospinal neurons would inhibit not excite primarily γ-motor neurons to extensor muscles (rules out option **C**). The rubrospinal tract is disrupted by a midcollicular lesion that causes decerebrate rigidity; moreover, this pathway excites flexor motor neurons and inhibits extensor motor neurons (rules out **D**).

7. The best answer is **A.** Before the herniation these patients have poorly reactive pupils (rules out option **E**) and the eyes deviate to a "down and out" position (rules out options **C** and **E**). After the brain herniates, the patients have fixed and dilated pupils (rules out option **B** and **D**), and eye movements are absent.

8. The best answer is **C.** The initial detectable damage in Huntington disease is to medium spiny neurons in the striatum. The loss of this GABAergic pathway to the globus pallidus external segment releases inhibition, permitting the hyperkinetic features of the disease to develop (rules out option **A**). The substantia nigra pars reticulata neurons are not damaged in Huntington disease, but normally release GABA to inhibit the thalamus (rules out option **B**). Subthalamic neurons release glutamate to excite both the globus pallidus external segment and internal segment; damage to the subthalamic region causes hemiballismus or the appearance of flailing, ballistic, undesired movements of the limb (rules out option **D**). Globus pallidus external segment neurons is not destroyed by Huntington disease; in fact it is activated due to loss of inhibitory input from the medium spiny neurons of the striatum; these neurons release GABA to inhibit the subthalamic nuclei (rules out option **E**).

9. The best answer is **E.** L-dopa crosses the blood–brain barrier and helps repair the dopamine deficiency; however, the degeneration of the dopaminergic substantia nigra neurons continues and in 5–7 years the beneficial effects of L-dopa disappear. There is no evidence for development of antibodies to dopamine receptors in Parkinson disease, but dopamine receptor-autoantibody interactions may be the basis of neuropsychiatric symptoms in patients diagnosed with Sydenham chorea (rules out option **A**). The pathway from the cortex to the basal ganglia (striatum) is excitatory not inhibitory (rules out option **B**). A major component of Lewy bodies, α-synuclein, is linked to familial forms of Parkinson disease; there is no evidence that α-synucleins interfere with L-dopa (rules out option **C**). Parkinson disease is not an example of a neurological disorder characterized by trinucleotide repeat expansion (rules out option **D**).

10. The best answer is **B.** The gene responsible for Friedreich ataxia codes for the production of a protein called frataxin. In the normal version of this gene, a sequence of GAA is repeated between 7 and 22 times. The defect in the gene causing this disorder, the sequence of GAA repeats hundreds or even a thousand times. A CGG repeat impacting the protein FMR-1 is associated with Fragile X syndrome (rules out **A**). A CTG repeat impacting DM protein kinase is associated with myotonic dystrophy (rules out **C**). A CAG repeat impacting the androgen receptor is associated with spinobulbar muscular atrophy (rules out **D**). A CAG repeat impacting the protein ataxin is associated with spinocerebellar ataxia (rules out **E**).

11. The best answer is **C.** The axons of granule cells (parallel fibers) form excitatory synapses on the dendrites of many Purkinje cells; the axons of the inhibitory basket cells form a basket around the cell body and axon hillock of each Purkinje cell they innervate (rules out option **D**). Stellate cells also inhibit Purkinje cells via a synapse on dendrites. The axons of Purkinje cells (the only output from the cerebellar cortex) project to the deep cerebellar nuclei, especially the dentate nucleus, where they form inhibitory synapses; they also make inhibitory connections with neurons in the vestibular nuclei. Climbing fibers (from inferior olive) and mossy fibers (from pontine nuclei) do not originate in the cerebellum (rules out options **A** and **B**); they both provide excitatory input to the Purkinje cells. Purkinje cells are inhibitory (rules out options **A** and **E**).

12. The best answer is **C.** Damage to the right half of the spinal cord would lead to loss of motor function in limbs innervated by motor neurons below the level of injury; since the ascending pathways mediating pain and temperature cross shortly after entry of afferent fibers in the spinal cord, these sensations are lost from body parts located on the side opposite to the injury. So damage to the right spinal cord at an upper thoracic level could account for the finding in this patient, which is the opposite of what would occur if the injury was on the left half of the spinal cord at an upper thoracic level (rules out option **B**). Damage to left half of the spinal cord in the lumbar region would impact motor function of the left leg and pain and sensation from the right leg (rules out option **A**). Damage to the dorsal half of the upper thoracic spinal cord would interrupt transmission in the dorsal column-medial lemniscal tract (fine touch and proprioception) from body parts located below the level of injury on both sides (rules out option **D**). Damage to the ventral half of the lumbar spinal cord would interrupt transmission in the ventral spinothalamic tract (pain) and corticospinal tract (motor function) from body parts located below the level of injury on both sides (rules out option **E**).

13. The best answer is **E.** Amyotrophic lateral sclerosis is an example of a lower motor neuron disease and is associated with flaccid paralysis, muscular atrophy, fasciculations (visible muscle twitches that appear as flickers under the skin), hypotonia (decreased muscle tone), and hyporeflexia or areflexia. Upper motor neuron diseases (eg, primary motor cortex, corona radiata) does not cause atrophy or fasciculations; it is associated with hypertonia and hyperreflexia (rules out options **A** and **B**). A vestibulocerebellar tumor causes disturbances of posture and a staggering gait (rules out option **C**). Diseases of the basal ganglia lead to two general types of disorders: hyperkinetic and hypokinetic. The hyperkinetic conditions are those in which movement is excessive and abnormal, including chorea, athetosis, and ballism; hypokinetic abnormalities include akinesia and bradykinesia (rules out option **D**).

14. The best answer is **B.** In addition to a tremor at rest, the symptoms experienced by this patient are typical of Parkinson disease which results from the degeneration of dopaminergic neurons in the substantia nigra pars compacta (not globus pallidus neurons, rules out **E**); the fibers to the putamen are most severely affected. See the response to Question 8 for common symptoms and cause of Huntington disease (rules out option **A** and **D**). See Question 11 for an explanation of symptoms and pathology of cerebellar ataxia (rules out option **C**).

15. The best answer is **D.** The three functional divisions of the cerebellum are the vestibulocerebellum, spinocerebellum, and cerebrocerebellum (rules out options **A, C,** and **E**). The vestibulocerebellum is comprised of the nodulus in the vermis and the flanking flocculus in the hemisphere on each side. This lobe has vestibular connections and is concerned with equilibrium and eye movements (rules out option **B**). The spinocerebellum is comprised of the rest of the vermis and the adjacent medial portions of the hemispheres; this region receives proprioceptive input from the body as well as a copy of the "motor plan" from the motor cortex. By comparing plan with performance, it smooths and coordinates ongoing movements. The vermis projects to the medial brainstem pathways to control axial and proximal limb muscles, and the hemispheres of the spinocerebellum project to the lateral brainstem pathways that control distal limb muscles. The cerebrocerebellum is in the lateral portions of the cerebellar hemispheres; it interacts with the motor cortex in planning and programming movements.

16. The best answer is **B.** Wilson disease is a rare disorder of copper metabolism that has an onset between 6 and 25 years of age, affecting about four times as many females as males. It affects the copper-transporting ATPase gene in the liver, leading to an accumulation of copper in the liver and progressive liver damage. Copper accumulates in the periphery of the cornea in the eye (Kayser–Fleischer rings). The dominant neuronal pathology is degeneration of the putamen (not the substantia nigra; rules out option **D**); motor disturbances include "wing-beating" tremor or asterixis, dysarthria, unsteady gait, and rigidity. About 40% of the familial cases of amyotrophic lateral sclerosis have a mutation in the gene for Cu/Zn superoxide dismutase (SOD-1) on chromosome 21 (rules out option **A**). A deficiency in coenzyme Q10 contributes to the abnormalities seen in some forms of familial cerebellar ataxia (rules out option **C**). Spinocerebellar ataxia is associated with a CAG trinucleotide repeat expansion (rules out option **E**).

17. The best answer is **D.** Akinesia, bradykinesia, cogwheel rigidity, and tremor at rest are correctly defined by (a) through (d), respectively. Options **A, B, C,** and **E** can be ruled out as follows. Chorea is involuntary, unpredictable body movements that can range from minor movements such as fidgeting to profound, uncontrolled movements of the arms and legs. Clasp-knife effect is the sequence of resistance followed by a sudden decrease in resistance when a limb is moved passively. Intention tremor (cerebellar tremor) is slow a tremor of the extremities that occurs at the end of a purposeful movement. Athetosis is characterized by continuous, slow writhing movements. Dysdiadochokinesia is the inability to perform rapidly alternating opposite movements such as repeated pronation and supination of the hands. Ballism is involuntary flailing, intense, and violent movements of the limbs. Lead-pipe rigidity is a posture adopted when the rigidity of the limb is maintained equally throughout a passive flexion. Fasciculations are visible muscle twitches that appear as flickers under the skin.

Autonomic Nervous System

O B J E C T I V E S

After studying this chapter, you should be able to:

- Describe the location of the cell bodies and axonal trajectories of preganglionic and postganglionic sympathetic and parasympathetic neurons.
- Name the neurotransmitters that are released by preganglionic autonomic neurons, postganglionic sympathetic neurons, postganglionic parasympathetic neurons, and adrenal medullary cells.
- Name the types of receptors on autonomic ganglia and on their target organs and list the ways that drugs can act to alter autonomic neurotransmission.
- Describe functions of the sympathetic and parasympathetic nervous systems.
- Describe the composition and functions of the enteric nervous system.

INTRODUCTION

The autonomic nervous system (ANS) is responsible for homeostasis via its innervation of smooth muscle (eg, blood vessels, the wall of the gastrointestinal tract, and urinary bladder), cardiac muscle, and glands (eg, sweat glands and salivary glands). It is comprised of the sympathetic, parasympathetic, enteric nervous systems. The sympathetic and parasympathetic divisions include preganglionic and postganglionic neurons. Although survival is possible without an ANS, the ability to adapt to environmental stressors and other challenges is severely compromised. The importance of understanding the functions of the ANS is underscored by the fact that so many commonly prescribed and over-the-counter drugs exert their actions on elements of the ANS or its effector organs. Some neurologic diseases result directly from a loss of preganglionic sympathetic neurons (eg, multiple system atrophy and Shy–Drager syndrome) and others (eg, Parkinson disease) are associated with autonomic dysfunction (**Clinical Box 13–1**).

■ ANATOMIC ORGANIZATION OF AUTONOMIC OUTFLOW

SYMPATHETIC DIVISION

Preganglionic sympathetic neurons are located in the intermediolateral (IML) column of the first thoracic to third or fourth lumbar segments (**Figure 13–1**). They are small-diameter, myelinated, relatively slowly conducting B fibers. After exiting the spinal cord as part of the ventral root, the axons branch off to form the white ramus that can synapse on a postganglionic neuron in a sympathetic paravertebral ganglion. These ganglia are located adjacent to each thoracic and upper lumbar spinal segments and some cervical and sacral spinal segments within the sympathetic chain (**Figure 13–2**). Besides the paravertebral ganglia, the chain includes the axons of preganglionic neurons that travel rostrally or caudally to terminate in the ganglia located at some distance. Some preganglionic axons pass through a paravertebral ganglion to synapse on postganglionic neurons within prevertebral ganglia close to the viscera (eg, celiac, superior mesenteric, and inferior mesenteric ganglia). Other preganglionic axons terminate directly on an effector organ, the adrenal medulla.

Multiple System Atrophy & Shy–Drager Syndrome

Multiple system atrophy (MSA) is a sporadic, progressive, adult-onset disorder characterized by autonomic dysfunction, parkinsonism, and cerebellar ataxia in any combination. Autonomic failure is due to loss of preganglionic autonomic neurons, making it difficult to regulate body temperature, fluid and electrolyte balance, and blood pressure. Shy–Drager syndrome is a subtype of MSA in which autonomic failure dominates. The pathologic hallmark of MSA is cytoplasmic and nuclear inclusions in oligodendrocytes and neurons in central motor and autonomic areas. There is also depletion of monoaminergic, cholinergic, and peptidergic markers in some brain regions and in the cerebrospinal fluid. MSA may result from a neuroinflammatory process that activates microglia and produces toxic cytokines. Basal levels of sympathetic activity and plasma norepinephrine are normal in MSA patients, but they do not increase upon standing, leading to severe orthostatic hypotension. In addition to the fall in blood pressure, orthostatic hypotension leads to dizziness, dimness of vision, and fainting. MSA is also accompanied by parasympathetic dysfunction, including urinary and sexual dysfunction. MSA is most often diagnosed in individuals 50–70 years of age; it affects more men than women. Erectile dysfunction is often the first symptom of the disease. There are also abnormalities in baroreceptor reflex and respiratory control mechanisms. About 75% of patients with MSA experience motor disturbances.

THERAPEUTIC HIGHLIGHTS

There is no cure for MSA but various therapies are used to treat specific signs and symptoms. Corticosteroids help retain salt and water to increase blood pressure. Parkinsonian-like signs can be alleviated by administration of levodopa and carbidopa (Sinemet). Clinical trials are underway to test the effectiveness of using intravenous immunoglobulins to counteract the neuroinflammatory process that occurs in MSA, fluoxetine (a serotonin uptake inhibitor) to prevent orthostatic hypotension, improve mood, and alleviate sleep, pain, and fatigue; and rasagiline (a monoamine oxidase inhibitor) to reduce parkinsonism.

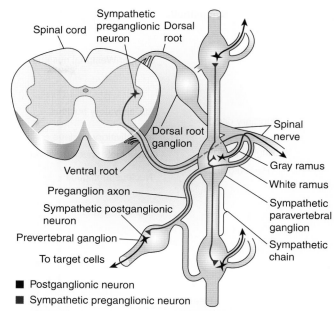

FIGURE 13–1 Projection of sympathetic preganglionic and postganglionic fibers. The axons of the sympathetic preganglionic neurons (red) leave the spinal cord at the level at which their cell bodies are located and exit via the ventral root along with axons of α- and γ-motor neurons. The axons separate from the ventral root via the white ramus to terminate on postganglionic neurons in adjacent or distal paravertebral ganglion or in prevertebral ganglia. The axons of postganglionic neurons (blue) leave the chain ganglia to form the gray ramus or project through the thoracic cavity to innervate visceral organs. Postganglionic fibers from prevertebral ganglia also terminate in visceral targets.

PARASYMPATHETIC DIVISION

Preganglionic neurons located in cranial nerve nuclei (III, VII, IX, and X) and in the second through fourth sacral IML. Figure 13–2 details the location of preganglionic and postganglionic parasympathetic neurons and the effector organs innervated by this division of the ANS. In some cases (eg, heart, lungs) the postganglionic neurons are within the wall of the effector organ.

◼ NEUROTRANSMISSION AT AUTONOMIC JUNCTIONS

ACETYLCHOLINE & NOREPINEPHRINE

Acetylcholine and norepinephrine are the main autonomic neurotransmitters. Cholinergic neurons include all preganglionic neurons, all parasympathetic postganglionic neurons, and a few sympathetic postganglionic neurons (eg, sweat glands). Most sympathetic postganglionic neurons are noradrenergic. Adrenal medullary cells are modified postganglionic neurons that secrete both norepinephrine and epinephrine directly into the bloodstream.

The axons of the postganglionic neurons are mostly unmyelinated C fibers. Some of them reenter the ventral root via the gray ramus to terminate on blood vessels, hair follicles, and sweat glands in the limbs (Figure 13–1). Other postganglionic fibers enter the thoracic cavity to terminate in visceral organs. Postganglionic fibers from prevertebral ganglia also terminate in visceral targets.

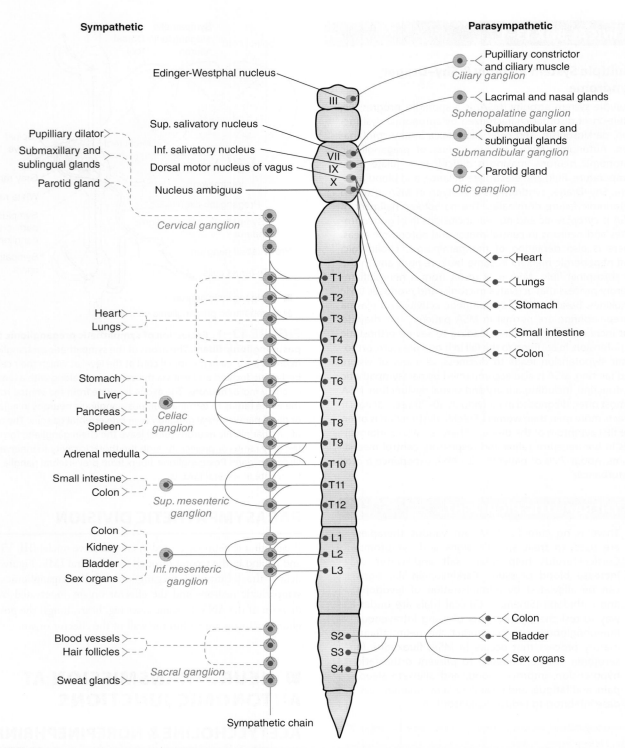

FIGURE 13–2 **Organization of sympathetic (left) and parasympathetic (right) nervous systems.** Cholinergic nerves are shown in red and noradrenergic nerves are shown in blue. Preganglionic nerves are solid lines; postganglionic nerves are dashed lines.

Table 13–1 lists the types of cholinergic and adrenergic receptors at various junctions within the ANS which are common targets for pharmacologic manipulation. The neurotransmitters are synthesized, stored in the nerve endings, and released near their targets where they bind to ion channels or G-protein–coupled receptors (GPCR) to initiate their characteristic actions. The neurotransmitters are then removed from the area by reuptake or metabolism. Each of these steps can be stimulated or inhibited, with predictable consequences. Table 13–2 lists how drugs can affect autonomic neurotransmission.

TABLE 13–1 Responses of some effector organs to autonomic nerve activity.

Effector Organs	Parasympathetic Nervous System	Sympathetic Nervous System	
		Receptor Type	Response
Eyes			
Radial muscle	—	α_1	Mydriasis
Sphincter muscle	Miosis		—
Ciliary muscle	Contraction for near vision		—
Heart			
SA node	↓ Heart rate	β_1	↑ Heart rate
Atria and ventricle	↓ Atrial contractility	β_1, β_2	↑ Contractility
AV node and Purkinje fibers	Decreased conduction velocity	β_1	↑ Conduction velocity
Arterioles			
Skin, splanchnic vessels	—	α_1	Constriction
Skeletal muscle	—	α_1/β_2, M	Constriction/Dilation
Systemic veins	—	$\alpha_1, \alpha_2/\beta_2$	Constriction/Dilation
Respiratory tract			
Bronchial smooth muscle	Contraction	β_2	Relaxation
Bronchial glands	↑ Secretion	α_1	↑ Secretion
Stomach and Intestine			
Motility and tone	Increased	$\alpha_1, \alpha_2, \beta_2$	Decreased
Sphincters	Relaxation	α_1	Contraction
Secretion	Stimulation	—	
Gallbladder	Contraction	β_2	Relaxation
Urinary bladder			
Detrusor	Contraction	β_2	Relaxation
Sphincter	Relaxation	α_1	Contraction
Uterus (pregnant)	—	α_1/β_2	Contraction/Relaxation
Male sex organs	Erection	α_1	Ejaculation
Skin			
Pilomotor muscles	—	α_1	Contraction
Sweat glands	—	M	Secretion
Liver	—	α_1, β_2	Glycogenolysis
Pancreas			
Acini	↑ Secretion	α	↓ Secretion
Islet cells	—	α_2/β_2	↓/↑ Secretion
Salivary glands	Profuse, watery secretion	α_1/β	Thick, viscous secretion/Amylase secretion
Lacrimal glands	Secretion		—
Adipose tissue	—	β_3	Lipolysis

A dash means the target tissue is not innervated by this division of the ANS. Data from Brunton LL, Chabner BA, Knollmann BC (eds): *Goodman and Gilman's The Pharmacological Basis of Therapeutics,* 12th ed. New York, NY: McGraw-Hill; 2011.

CHOLINERGIC NEUROTRANSMISSION

The fast excitatory postsynaptic potential (EPSP) that leads to depolarization of postganglionic neurons is mediated by an action of acetylcholine on nicotinic receptors which are ligand-gated ion channels. The acetylcholine released from postganglionic fibers acts on muscarinic receptors. Muscarinic receptors are GPCR; subtypes M_1–M_3 are found in autonomic target organs. The heart has primarily M_2 receptors; binding of an agonist to these receptors opens K^+ channels and inhibits adenylyl cyclase and cyclic adenosine monophosphate (cAMP). Smooth muscle and glands have primarily M_3 receptors; binding of an agonist to these receptors leads to the formation of inositol 1,4,5-triphosphate (IP_3) and diacylglycerol (DAG) and an increase in intracellular Ca^{2+}. Acetylcholine has a short duration of action because of the high concentration of acetylcholinesterase at cholinergic nerve endings. See Table 13–2 for the effects mediated by drugs acting at these cholinergic synapses. Compounds with

TABLE 13–2 Drugs that affect processes involved in autonomic neurotransmission.

Transmission Process	Drug	Site of Drug Action	Drug Action
Neurotransmitter synthesis	Hemicholinium	Membrane of cholinergic nerve terminals	Blocks choline uptake; slows synthesis
	Metyrosine	Cytoplasm of noradrenergic nerve terminals	Inhibits tyrosine hydroxylase; blocks synthesis
Neurotransmitter storage mechanism	Vesamicol	Vesicles in cholinergic nerve terminals	Prevents storage of acetylcholine
	Reserpine	Vesicles in noradrenergic nerve terminals	Prevents storage of norepinephrine
Neurotransmitter release mechanism	Norepinephrine, dopamine, acetylcholine, prostaglandins	Receptors on cholinergic and adrenergic nerve terminals	Modulates transmitter release
Neurotransmitter reuptake mechanism	Cocaine, tricyclic antidepressants	Noradrenergic nerve terminals	Inhibits uptake; prolongs transmitter's action on postsynaptic receptors
	Amphetamine	NET on noradrenergic nerve terminals	NET substrate and reuptake blocker, causing reverse transport and $\uparrow$ NE release
Inactivation of neurotransmitter	Edrophonium, neostigmine, physostigmine,	Acetylcholinesterase in cholinergic synapses	Inhibits enzyme; prolongs and intensifies actions of acetylcholine
Adrenoceptor agonist	α_1: Phenylephrine	Sympathetic postganglionic nerve–effector organ junctions (eg, blood vessels, hair follicles, and radial muscle)	Binds to and activates α-adrenoceptors; $\uparrow$IP$_3$/DAG cascade (α_1) or $\downarrow$cAMP (α_2)
	α_2: Clonidine		
	β_1: Dobutamine	Sympathetic postganglionic nerve–effector organ junctions (eg, heart, bronchial smooth muscle, and uterine smooth muscle)	Binds to and activates β-adrenoceptors; $\uparrow$cAMP
	β_2: Albuterol, ritodrine, salmeterol, terbutaline		
Adrenoceptor antagonist	Nonselective: Phenoxybenzamine	Sympathetic postganglionic nerve–effector organ junctions (eg, blood vessels)	Binds to and blocks α-adrenoceptors
			Binds to and blocks β-adrenoceptors
	α_1: Prazosin, terazosin	Sympathetic postganglionic nerve–effector organ junctions (eg, heart and bronchial smooth muscle)	
	α_2: Yohimbine		
	β_1, β_2: Propranolol		
	$\beta_1 > \beta_2$: Atenolol, esmolol		
Nicotinic receptor agonist	Nicotine	Receptors on autonomic ganglia	Binds to nicotinic receptors; opens Na$^+$, K$^+$ channels
Nicotinic receptor antagonist	Hexamethonium, trimethaphan	Receptors on autonomic ganglia	Binds to and blocks nicotinic receptors
Muscarinic receptor agonist	Bethanechol	Cholinergic receptors on smooth muscle, cardiac muscle, and glands	Binds to and activates muscarinic receptors; $\uparrow$IP$_3$/DAG cascade or $\downarrow$cAMP
Muscarinic receptor antagonist	Atropine, ipratropium, scopolamine, tropicamide	Cholinergic receptors on smooth muscle, cardiac muscle, and glands	Binds to and blocks muscarinic receptors

cAMP, cyclic adenosine monophosphate; IP$_3$/DAG, inositol 1,4,5-triphosphate, and diacylglycerol.

muscarinic actions include drugs that inhibit acetylcholinesterase. **Clinical Box 13–2** describes some of the signs and strategies for the treatment of acute intoxication from organophosphate cholinesterase inhibitors. **Clinical Box 13–3** describes cholinergic poisoning resulting from digestion of toxic mushrooms.

NORADRENERGIC NEUROTRANSMISSION

Norepinephrine, epinephrine, and dopamine and their metabolites are found in plasma. The norepinephrine released from sympathetic postganglionic fibers binds to GPCRs (adrenoceptors) that include subtypes α_1, α_2, β_1, β_2, and β_3. Table 13–1 shows the locations of

these receptors on smooth muscles, cardiac muscle, and glands. See Table 13–2 for the effects mediated by drugs acting at these noradrenergic synapses. **Clinical Box 13–4** describes Horner syndrome, which is due to interruption of sympathetic nerves to the face. **Clinical Box 13–5** describes a vasospastic condition (Raynaud phenomenon) in which blood flow to the fingers and toes is transiently reduced when a sensitive individual is exposed to stress or cold.

NONADRENERGIC & NONCHOLINERGIC TRANSMITTERS

The small granulated vesicles in postganglionic noradrenergic neurons also contain adenosine triphosphate (ATP), and the large granulated vesicles contain neuropeptide Y (NPY). Many

CLINICAL BOX 13-2

Organophosphates: Pesticides & Nerve Gases

The World Health Organization estimates that 1–3% of agricultural workers worldwide suffer from acute pesticide poisoning; it accounts for significant morbidity and mortality, especially in developing countries. Like organophosphate pesticides (eg, parathion and malathion), nerve gases (eg, soman and sarin) used in chemical warfare and terrorism inhibit acetylcholinesterase at peripheral and central cholinergic synapses, prolonging the actions of acetylcholine at these synapses. The organophosphate cholinesterase inhibitors are readily absorbed by the skin, lung, gut, and conjunctiva, making them very dangerous. They bind to the enzyme and undergo hydrolysis, resulting in a phosphorylated active site on the enzyme. The covalent phosphorous-enzyme bond is very stable and hydrolyzes at a very slow rate. The phosphorylated enzyme complex may undergo a process called aging in which one of the oxygen-phosphorous bonds breaks down, which strengthens the phosphorous-enzyme bond. This process takes only 10 min to occur after exposure to soman. The earliest signs of organophosphate toxicity are usually indicative of excessive activation of autonomic muscarinic receptors; these include miosis, salivation, sweating, bronchial constriction, vomiting, and diarrhea. CNS signs of toxicity include cognitive disturbances, convulsions, seizures, and even coma; these signs are often accompanied by nicotinic effects such as depolarizing neuromuscular blockade.

THERAPEUTIC HIGHLIGHTS

The muscarinic cholinergic receptor antagonist atropine is given parenterally in large doses to control signs of excessive activation of muscarinic cholinergic receptors. When given soon after exposure to the organophosphate and before aging has occurred, nucleophiles such as pralidoxime are able to break the bond between the organophosphate and the acetylcholinesterase. Thus, this drug is called a "cholinesterase regenerator." If pyridostigmine is administered in advance of exposure to a cholinesterase inhibitor, it binds to the enzyme and prevents binding by the toxic organophosphate agent. The protective effects of pyridostigmine dissipate within 3–6 h, but this provides enough time for clearance of the organophosphate from the body. Since the drug cannot cross the blood–brain barrier, protection is limited to peripheral cholinergic synapses. A mixture of pyridostigmine, carbamate, and atropine can be administered prophylactically to soldiers and civilians who are at risk for exposure to nerve gases. Benzodiazepines can be used to abort the seizures caused by exposure to organophosphates.

CLINICAL BOX 13-3

Mushroom Poisoning

Of more than 5000 species of mushrooms found in the United States, about 100 are poisonous and ingestion of 10% of these can result in death. Estimates are an annual incidence of five cases per 100,000 individuals. Mushroom poisoning is divided into rapid-onset (15–30 min after ingestion) and delayed-onset (6–12 h after ingestion) types. In rapid-onset cases caused by mushrooms of the *Inocybe* genus, the symptoms are due to excessive activation of muscarinic synapses. The major signs of muscarinic poisoning include nausea, vomiting, diarrhea, urinary urgency, vasodilation, sweating, and salivation. Ingestion of mushrooms such as the *Amanita muscaria* have signs of the antimuscarinic syndrome because they also contain alkaloids that block muscarinic receptors. The classic symptoms of this syndrome are being "red as a beet" (flushed skin), "hot as a hare" (hyperthermia), "dry as a bone" (xerostomia, anhidrosis), "blind as a bat" (blurred vision, cycloplegia), and "mad as a hatter" (confusion, delirium). The delayed-onset type of mushroom poisoning occurs after ingestion of *Amanita phalloides*, *Amanita virosa*, *Galerina autumnalis*, and *Galerina marginata* which contain amatoxins that inhibit RNA polymerase. These mushrooms cause abdominal cramping, nausea, vomiting, and profuse diarrhea; but the major toxic effects are due to hepatic injury (jaundice and bruising) and associated central effects (confusion, lethargy, and coma). There is a 60% mortality rate associated with ingestion of these mushrooms.

THERAPEUTIC HIGHLIGHTS

The rapid-onset type muscarinic poisoning can be treated effectively with atropine. Individuals who exhibit the antimuscarinic syndrome can be treated with physostigmine, a cholinesterase inhibitor with a 2–4 h duration of action that acts centrally and peripherally. The delayed-onset of toxicity does not respond to cholinergic drugs; treatment of amatoxin ingestion includes intravenous administration of fluids and electrolytes to maintain adequate hydration. Administering a combination of a high dose of penicillin G and silibinin (a flavonolignan found in certain herbs with antioxidant and hepatoprotective properties) has been shown to improve survival. If necessary, vomiting can also be induced by using activated charcoal to reduce the absorption of the toxin.

CLINICAL BOX 13–4

Horner Syndrome

Horner syndrome is a rare disorder resulting from interruption of preganglionic or postganglionic sympathetic innervation to the face. The problem can result from injury to the nerves, injury to the carotid artery, a stroke or lesion in the brainstem, or a tumor in the lung. In most cases the problem is unilateral, with symptoms occurring only on the side of the damage. The hallmark of Horner syndrome is the triad of anhidrosis (reduced sweating), ptosis (drooping eyelid), and miosis (constricted pupil). Symptoms also include enophthalmos (sunken eyeball) and vasodilation.

THERAPEUTIC HIGHLIGHTS

There is no pharmacologic treatment for Horner syndrome, but drugs affecting noradrenergic neurotransmission can be used to determine whether the source of the problem is interruption of the preganglionic or postganglionic innervation to the face. Since the iris of the eye responds to topical sympathomimetic drugs (ie, adrenoceptor agonists or drugs that increase the release or prevent reuptake of norepinephrine from the nerve terminal), a clinician can easily test the viability of the noradrenergic nerves to the eye. If the postganglionic sympathetic fibers are damaged, their terminals would degenerate and there would be a loss of stored catecholamines. If the preganglionic fibers are damaged, the postganglionic noradrenergic nerve would remain intact (but be inactive) and would still have stored catecholamines in its terminal. If administration of a drug that causes release of catecholamine stores (eg, hydroxyamphetamine) and the constricted pupil does not dilate, one would conclude that the noradrenergic nerve is damaged. If the eye dilates in response to this drug, the catecholamine stores are still able to be released, so the damage must be preganglionic. Administration of phenylephrine (α-adrenoceptor agonist) would dilate the pupil regardless of the site of injury as the drug binds to the receptor on the radial muscle of the iris.

sympathetic fibers to the vasculature of viscera, skin, and skeletal muscles release NPY along with norepinephrine. Vasoactive intestinal polypeptide (VIP), calcitonin gene-related peptide (CGRP), or substance P is co-released with acetylcholine from the sympathetic innervation to sweat glands (sudomotor fibers). VIP is co-localized with acetylcholine in parasympathetic postganglionic neurons supplying glands. Vagal postganglionic neurons in the gastrointestinal tract release VIP and nitric oxide synthase.

CLINICAL BOX 13–5

Raynaud Phenomenon

About 5% of men and 8% of women experience an episodic reduction in blood flow primarily to the fingers during exposure to cold or a stressful situation. Vasospasms in the toes, tip of nose, ears, and penis can also occur. Smoking is associated with an increase in the incidence and severity of the symptoms of Raynaud phenomenon. The symptoms begin to occur between the age of 15 and 25; it is most common in cold climates. The symptoms often include a triphasic change in color of the skin of the digits. First, the skin becomes pale or white (pallor), cold, and numb. Second, the skin turns blue or purple (cyanosis) and the reduced blood flow can cause intense pain. Third, with recovery of blood flow, the digits turn deep red (rubor) and there can be swelling and tingling. Raynaud disease refers to the idiopathic appearance of the symptoms in individuals who do not have another underlying disease to account for the symptoms. Raynaud syndrome refers to the presence of these symptoms due to another disorder such as scleroderma, lupus, rheumatoid arthritis, Sjögren syndrome, carpel tunnel syndrome, and anorexia. Although initially thought to reflect an increase in sympathetic activity to the vasculature of the digits, this is no longer regarded as the mechanism underlying the episodic vasospasms.

THERAPEUTIC HIGHLIGHTS

The first treatment strategy for Raynaud phenomenon is to avoid exposure to the cold, reduce stress, quit smoking, and avoid the use of medications that are vasoconstrictors (eg, β-adrenoceptor antagonists, cold medications, caffeine, and opioids). If the symptoms are severe, drugs may be needed to prevent tissue damage. These include calcium channel blockers (eg, nifedipine) and α-adrenoceptor antagonists (eg, prazosin). In individuals who do not respond to pharmacologic treatments, surgical sympathectomy has been done.

■ RESPONSES OF EFFECTOR ORGANS TO AUTONOMIC NERVE ACTIVTY

GENERAL PRINCIPLES

The ANS regulates many physiologic functions including blood flow, blood pressure, heart rate, airflow through the bronchii, gastrointestinal motility, urinary bladder contraction, glandular secretions, pupillary diameter, body temperature, and sexual physiology. Table 13–1 lists the effects of stimulation of sympathetic and parasympathetic nerves. In some cases, the two divisions of the ANS function as physiological antagonists (ie, exert opposite actions on a target organ). In other cases, both divisions of the ANS activate a target organ (eg, parasympathetic nerves release of watery saliva; sympathetic nerves release thick, viscous saliva). The two divisions of the ANS can act in a synergistic manner in the control of some functions (eg, pupil diameter in the eye). Both sympathetic and parasympathetic nerves are excitatory, but the former contracts the radial (dilator) muscle to cause mydriasis and the latter contracts the sphincter (constrictor) muscle to cause miosis. Also, activation of parasympathetic nerves to the penis causes erection and activation of sympathetic nerves causes ejaculation. Some organs are innervated by only one division of the ANS.

AUTONOMIC DYSFUNCTION

Drugs, neurodegenerative diseases, trauma, inflammatory processes, and neoplasia are a few examples of factors that can lead to dysfunction of the ANS (Clinical Boxes 13–1 through 13–4). The types of dysfunction can range from complete autonomic failure to autonomic hyperactivity. Among disorders associated with autonomic failure are orthostatic hypotension, neurogenic syncope (vasovagal response), erectile dysfunction, neurogenic bladder, gastrointestinal dysmotility, sudomotor failure, and Horner syndrome. Autonomic hyperactivity can be the basis for neurogenic hypertension, cardiac arrhythmias, neurogenic pulmonary edema, myocardial injury, hyperhidrosis, hyperthermia, and hypothermia.

■ ENTERIC NERVOUS SYSTEM

The enteric nervous system is located within the wall of the digestive tract from the esophagus to the anus. It is composed of the myenteric plexus (between longitudinal and circular layers of muscle), which controls digestive tract motility and the submucosal plexus (between the circular muscle and the luminal mucosa) that regulates gastrointestinal blood flow and epithelial cell function.

The enteric nervous system contains as many neurons as the entire spinal cord. This "mini brain" contains all the elements of a nervous system including sensory neurons, interneurons, and motor neurons. Sensory neurons innervate receptors in the mucosa that respond to mechanical, thermal, osmotic, and chemical stimuli. Motor neurons control motility, secretion, and absorption by acting on smooth muscle and secretory cells. Interneurons integrate information from sensory neurons and feedback to the enteric motor neurons.

Parasympathetic and sympathetic nerves connect the CNS to the enteric nervous system or directly to the digestive tract. Although the enteric nervous system can function autonomously, normal digestive function often requires communication between the CNS and the enteric nervous system (see Chapter 25).

CHAPTER SUMMARY

- Preganglionic sympathetic neurons are located in the IML of the thoracolumbar spinal cord and project to postganglionic neurons in the paravertebral or prevertebral ganglia or the adrenal medulla. Preganglionic parasympathetic neurons are located in motor nuclei of cranial nerves III, VII, IX, and X and the sacral IML. Postganglionic nerve terminals are located in smooth muscle (eg, blood vessels, gut wall, and urinary bladder), cardiac muscle, and glands (eg, sweat gland and salivary glands).
- Acetylcholine is released at nerve terminals of all preganglionic neurons, postganglionic parasympathetic neurons, and a few postganglionic sympathetic neurons (eg, sweat glands). Most sympathetic postganglionic neurons release norepinephrine.
- Ganglionic transmission is mediated by activation of nicotinic receptors. Activation of muscarinic cholinergic receptors and α_1-, β-, or β_2-adrenoceptors mediates autonomic effects on target organs. Many common drugs exert their therapeutic actions by serving as agonists or antagonists at autonomic synapses.
- The ANS regulates many physiologic functions including blood flow, blood pressure, heart rate, airflow through the bronchii, gastrointestinal motility, urinary bladder contraction, glandular secretions, pupillary diameter, body temperature, and sexual physiology.
- The enteric nervous system is located within the wall of the digestive tract and is composed of the myenteric plexus (control of digestive tract motility) and the submucosal plexus (regulates gastrointestinal blood flow and epithelial cell function).

MULTIPLE-CHOICE QUESTIONS

For all questions, select the single best answer unless otherwise directed.

1. Hypertension and tachycardia developed in a 26-year-old man after he began taking an amphetamine to boost his energy and to suppress his appetite. What is the mechanism(s) of action by which amphetamine would cause an increase in blood pressure and heart rate?
    A. Amphetamine is both a norepinephrine reuptake blocker and it enhances the release of norepinephrine from sympathetic postganglionic nerves.
    B. Amphetamine is both a β_1-adrenoceptor agonist which stimulates the heart and a α_1-adrenoceptor agonist which causes contraction of blood vessels.
    C. Amphetamine is a selective β-adrenoceptor agonist, which increases renin release from the kidney and stimulates the heart.

D. Amphetamine activates preganglionic sympathetic neurons in the thoracolumbar spinal cord.

E. Amphetamine is a direct stimulant of postganglionic sympathetic neurons in the paravertebral ganglia.

2. A 68-year-old man visited his physician's office after experiencing several recent episodes getting very lightheaded as he went from a lying to a standing position. He has become worried especially since he also has been experiencing episodes of loss of balance. When reviewing past medical history, he mentions that he has had erectile dysfunction for the past year or so and that he no longer sweats very much when outside on a hot day. The physical examination does not show any evidence of tremor at rest or cogwheel rigidity. Which of the following is a potential diagnosis?
   A. He is in the late stages of Parkinson disease.
   B. He has Raynaud phenomenon.
   C. He has multiple system atrophy.
   D. There is no known neurologic disorder that can account for all of these signs and symptoms, so he must have more than one underlying problem.

3. A 9-year-old boy is rushed to the hospital after being severely injured when the car in which he was a passenger was struck by a train. His blood pressure is 50/30 mm Hg due to internal bleeding. While attempting intubation for surgery, the doctor notices considerable airway secretions. Which type of drug would be the best choice for reducing the amount of secretions in this patient?
   A. A α_1-adrenoceptor agonist
   B. A α_1-adrenoceptor antagonist
   C. A nonselective α-adrenoceptor antagonist
   D. A muscarinic receptor agonist
   E. A muscarinic receptor antagonist

4. A 45-year-old man had a meal containing wild mushrooms that he picked in a field earlier in the day. Within 30 min after eating, he experienced nausea, vomiting, diarrhea, urinary urgency, vasodilation, sweating, and salivation. What type of chemical in the mushroom is likely responsible for the appearance of these symptoms?
   A. A chemical that stimulated the release of epinephrine from the adrenal medulla
   B. A chemical that blocked nicotinic receptors on autonomic ganglia
   C. A chemical that caused excessive activation of muscarinic receptors
   D. A chemical that blocked muscarinic receptors
   E. A chemical that inhibited RNA polymerase

5. A medical student was doing autonomic research in an animal laboratory. While recording blood pressure in an animal, she first injected a dose of epinephrine (an agonist at α- and β-adrenoceptors) that caused blood pressure to increase from 130/85 to 190/125 mm Hg. After recovery from these effects, she injected a dose of prazosin (a selective α_1-adrenoceptor antagonist) and blood pressure fell from 130/85 to 120/60 mmHg. While blood pressure was still reduced due to prazosin, she injected the same dose of epinephrine but now blood pressure fell further to 100/35 mmHg. Explain the mechanism responsible for the rise in blood pressure with the first dose of epinephrine and why the same dose of epinephrine in the presence of prazosin resulted in a fall in blood pressure.

A. Binding of epinephrine to α_1-adrenoceptors on blood vessels is responsible for the rise in blood pressure. After α_1-adrenoceptor blockade, binding of epinephrine to α_2-adrenoceptors on the blood vessels relaxes vascular smooth muscle to reduce blood pressure.

B. Binding of epinephrine to both α_1- and α_2-adrenoceptors on blood vessels contributes equally to the rise in blood pressure. After α_1-adrenoceptor blockade, binding of epinephrine to β_2-adrenoceptors in the heart reduces cardiac output and thus blood pressure.

C. Binding of epinephrine to α_1-adrenoceptors on blood vessels is responsible for the rise in blood pressure. After α_1-adrenoceptor blockade, binding of epinephrine to β_2-adrenoceptors on the blood vessels relaxes vascular smooth muscle to reduce blood pressure.

D. Binding of epinephrine to both α_1- and α_2-adrenoceptors on blood vessels contributes equally to the rise in blood pressure. After α_1-adrenoceptor blockade, binding of epinephrine to β_1-adrenoceptors on the blood vessels relaxes vascular smooth muscle to reduce blood pressure.

6. When a pheochromocytoma (tumor of the adrenal medulla) suddenly releases a large amount of norepinephrine and epinephrine into the circulation, the patient's heart rate would be expected to
   A. decrease because the increase in blood pressure stimulates the carotid and aortic chemoreceptors.
   B. decrease because of a reflex-induced increase in parasympathetic nerve activity to the heart.
   C. increase because the increase in blood pressure stimulates the carotid and aortic baroreceptors.
   D. increase because epinephrine has a direct positive inotropic effect on the heart.
   E. increase because epinephrine has a direct positive chronotropic effect on the heart.

7. A 20-year-old woman was standing outside for several hours with some friends on a very hot summer day when she suddenly fainted. She gained consciousness within a few minutes, and her friends recalled that a similar incident happened a couple of years ago under similar circumstances. During her next annual physical exam, she mentioned these episodes to her primary care physician who recommended she undergo a stress test. After ruling out any cardiac problems, she was diagnosed with a type of neurally mediated syncope (vasovagal syncope). What is the location of the vagal preganglionic nerves that were activated to induce this response, what type of receptor in the heart was activated, and what second messengers contribute to the action of acetylcholine on this receptor?
   A. Dorsal motor nucleus of the vagus, M_3 muscarinic receptors, formation of IP3 and DAG
   B. Dorsal motor nucleus of the vagus, M_2 muscarinic receptors, inhibits adenylyl cyclase and cAMP
   C. Nucleus ambiguus, M_3 muscarinic receptors, formation of IP3 and DAG
   D. Nucleus ambiguus, M_2 muscarinic receptors, inhibits adenylyl cyclase and cAMP

8. A 68-year-old woman was in an automobile accident that resulted in a blunt trauma injury to her neck. Over the next few days she developed a headache, neck and face pain, vision disturbances. Soon after she had signs of a stroke and was taken to the emergency department, where imaging showed

a carotid artery dissection. Her physician also noted that she had developed Horner syndrome. What signs likely led to the diagnosis of Horner syndrome?
A. Mydriasis, xerostomia, cycloplegia
B. Miosis, ptosis, facial anhidrosis
C. Miosis, blurred vision, facial anhidrosis
D. Mydriasis, cycloplegia, blurred vision
E. Miosis, xerostomia, ptosis

9. Diabetic autonomic neuropathy was diagnosed a few years ago in a 53-year-old woman after many years of poorly controlled diabetes. She recently noted abdominal distension and a feeling of being full after eating only a small portion of food, suggesting that the neuropathy had extended to her enteric nervous system to cause gastroparesis. What are the components of the enteric nervous system?
A. The enteric nervous system is a specialized subdivision of the parasympathetic nervous system for control of gastrointestinal function and includes specialized preganglionic and postganglionic cholinergic neurons.
B. The enteric nervous system is composed of the myenteric plexus that regulates gastrointestinal motility and the submucosal plexus that regulates gastrointestinal blood flow and epithelial cell function. Neuronal types include motor neurons, sensory neurons, and interneurons.
C. The enteric nervous system is composed of a submucosal plexus that contains motor neurons that control gastric secretions and motility and a myenteric plexus that contains sensory neurons that signal information about the environment, and mucosal interneurons that relay sensory information to the central nervous system.
D. The enteric nervous system contains motor neurons within the circular muscle, sensory neurons within the longitudinal muscle, and interneurons within the mucosa that relay sensory information to the central nervous system.
E. The enteric nervous system is composed of the myenteric plexus that contains only motor neurons that regulate gastrointestinal motility and the submucosal plexus that contains only sensory neurons transmit information about the contents of the gastrointestinal tract to the central nervous system.

10. A retiree from the military was telling his son who is a medical student that as a young soldier heading to war, he was given a drug called pyridostigmine as a prophylactic measure in case of an exposure to nerve gas. He also mentioned that he was told he would be given another drug called pralidoxime soon after exposure to the nerve gas. He asked his son to explain how these chemicals worked. What is the mechanism of action of nerve gas, pyridostigmine, and pralidoxime?
A. An irreversible muscarinic receptor antagonist, a reversible muscarinic receptor agonist, and a cholinesterase inhibitor
B. An irreversible cholinesterase inhibitor, a reversible cholinesterase inhibitor, a cholinesterase regenerator
C. An irreversible reversible muscarinic receptor antagonist, cholinesterase regenerator, a reversible cholinesterase inhibitor
D. An irreversible cholinesterase inhibitor, a reversible muscarinic receptor agonist, and a cholinesterase inhibitor
E. An irreversible cholinesterase inhibitor, a reversible muscarinic receptor antagonist, and a cholinesterase regenerator

ANSWERS

1. The best answer is **A.** Amphetamines inhibit the norepinephrine transporter (NET) on sympathetic postganglionic nerve terminals to prevent the reuptake of norepinephrine. This increases the synaptic concentration of norepinephrine. Drugs that block NET also cause "reverse transport" meaning that additional norepinephrine is actually released. The increased levels of norepinephrine lead to greater stimulation of α_1-adrenoceptors on blood vessels to increase in blood pressure and on β_1-adrenoceptors in the heart to increase heart rate. Drugs that act in this way are called indirect sympathomimetics as they do not act directly on adrenoceptors (rules out options **B** and **C**); they also do not directly activate spinal preganglionic neurons or postganglionic sympathetic neurons (rules out options D and E).

2. The best answer is C. Multiple system atrophy (MSA) is a sporadic, progressive, adult-onset disorder characterized by autonomic dysfunction, parkinsonism, and cerebellar ataxia in any combination. A loss of preganglionic autonomic neurons makes it difficult to maintain homeostasis. Although resting levels of sympathetic activity are normal in MSA patients, it does not increase upon standing, leading to orthostatic hypotension. Parasympathetic dysfunction includes urinary and sexual dysfunction. Erectile dysfunction is often the first symptom of the disease. Option A can be ruled out since although Parkinson disease can be associated with autonomic dysfunction, the patent does not have other signs typical of Parkinson disease including cogwheel rigidity and tremor at rest. Option B can be ruled out since Raynaud phenomenon is associated with episodic vasospasms in the fingers, toes, nose, ears, or penis particularly during exposure to cold or a stressful situation. Although it is possible that this individual has more than one pathology to explain the constellation of signs and symptoms; option D can be ruled out because there is a known pathology (MSA) that can account for them.

3. The best answer is **E.** Activation of the parasympathetic nervous system increases bronchial secretions due to an action of acetylcholine on muscarinic receptors. Thus, blocking these receptors would reduce the secretions. A muscarinic agonist would increase the secretions (rules out option **D**). Bronchial secretions are also increased by an action of norepinephrine on α_1-adrenoceptors, so α_1-adrenoceptor antagonist could reduce the secretions, but it would also block sympathetic control of the vasculature which would be contraindicated in this patient (rules out options **A, B,** and **C**).

4. The best answer is **C.** These symptoms are consistent with activation of muscarinic receptors on autonomic effector organs to induce muscarinic poisoning. The rapid onset (within 30 min of consuming the mushrooms) of these symptoms suggests consumption of the mushrooms of the *Inocybe* genus. Other mushrooms (eg, *Amanita muscaria*) contain alkaloids that block muscarinic cholinergic receptors, but ingestion of these causes the antimuscarinic syndrome including hyperthermia, xerostomia, anhidrosis, blurred vision, and confusion (ruling out option **D**). Some mushrooms (eg, *Amanita phalloides*) contain amatoxins that inhibit RNA polymerase, and ingestion of these cause abdominal cramping, nausea, vomiting, and profuse diarrhea but with a delayed onset (at least 6 hours after ingestion). This rules out option **E.** Option **A** can be ruled out because if a chemical in mushrooms stimulated the release of epinephrine from the

adrenal medulla, the major signs would mimic activation of the sympathetic nervous system (eg, tachycardia, mydriasis, urinary retention). If mushrooms contained a chemical that blocked nicotinic receptors on autonomic ganglia, the signs of intoxication might include cycloplegia, tachycardia, hypotension, constipation, urinary retention, and reduced sweating (rules out option **B**).

5. The best answer is **C**. Epinephrine is a nonselective adrenoceptor agonist with similar affinity to α_1- and α_2-adrenoceptors and β_1- and β_2-adrenoceptors. Most blood vessels contain α_1-adrenoceptors, and activation of these receptors caused contraction of the smooth muscle of the vasculature and thus an increase in blood pressure. A contribution of α_2-adrenoceptors on blood vessels to vasoconstriction is minimal (rules out options **B** and **D**); and blood vessels do not contain β_1-adrenoceptors (also rules out option **D**). Some veins contain α_2-adrenoceptors, activation of which causes venoconstriction not relaxation (rules out option **A**). Blood vessels in skeletal muscle have both α_1- and β_2-adrenoceptors; activation of the latter causes vasodilation and a fall in blood pressure. When the α_1-adrenoceptors on blood vessels are blocked by prazosin, the action of epinephrine on these β_2-adrenoceptors is unmasked causing a fall in blood pressure. The experiment by the medical student is a demonstration of the "epinephrine reversal" response. The dominant adrenoceptor in the heart is β_1-adrenoceptors; activation causes an increase not a decrease in cardiac output (also rules out option **B**).

6. The best answer is **E**. Norepinephrine and epinephrine act on β_1-adrenoceptors to increase the rate of depolarization of the sinoatrial node in the heart to increase heart rate (a positive chronotropic effect). They also have a positive inotropic effect on the heart, but this increases contractility not rate (rules out option **D**). Chemoreceptors are activated by reductions in the partial pressure of oxygen in the blood not to increases in blood pressure (rules out option **A**). The catecholamine-induced increase in blood pressure will stimulate the carotid and aortic baroreceptors to increase parasympathetic nerve activity to the heart. Although this can reduce (not increase) heart rate (rules out options **E**), the direct stimulant effect of a potent β_1-adrenoceptor agonist like epinephrine on the heart will not be overcome; thus heart rate will increase but to a lesser extent than if the reflex was not engaged (rules out option **B**).

7. The best answer is **D**. Cardiac vagal preganglionic neurons are located in the nucleus ambiguus, and acetylcholine is released by vagal postganglionic neurons; the heart has primarily M_2 receptors; binding of an agonist to these receptors opens K^+ channels and inhibits adenylyl cyclase and cyclic cAMP (rules out option **C**). Vagal preganglionic neurons within the dorsal motor nucleus of the vagus innervate the smooth muscle and gland of the gastrointestinal tract; the gastrointestinal tract has primarily M3 receptors; binding of an agonist to these receptors leads to the formation of IP3 and DAG (rules out options **A** and **B**).

8. The best answer is **B**. The hallmark of Horner syndrome is the triad of anhidrosis (reduced sweating), ptosis (drooping eyelid), and miosis (constricted pupil) resulting from interruption of preganglionic or postganglionic sympathetic innervation to the face. Causes include injury to the carotid artery, a stroke or lesion in the brainstem, or a tumor in the lung. The combination of signs in options **A** and **D** would result from interruption of the parasympathetic nerve activity. The combination of signs listed in options **C** and **E** would result from a mix of parasympathetic and sympathetic disturbances.

9. The best answer is **B**. The enteric nervous system is composed of a myenteric plexus (between longitudinal and circular layers of muscle), which controls digestive tract motility and a submucosal plexus (between the circular muscle and the luminal mucosa) that regulates gastrointestinal blood flow and epithelial cell function. Within enteric plexuses are three types of neurons: motor neurons that regulate gastrointestinal motility and secretions; sensory neurons that respond to mechanical, thermal, osmotic, and chemical stimuli; and interneurons that link sensory and motor neurons. The enteric nervous system is distinct from the parasympathetic division of the ANS (rules out option **A**). The above description also explains why options **C**, **D**, and **E** are incorrect.

10. The best answer is **B**. Nerve gases (eg, soman and sarin) are irreversible cholinesterase inhibitors that prevent the breakdown of acetylcholine. These and other organophosphates bind to the enzyme and form a stable covalent phosphorous-enzyme bond. By giving a reversible cholinesterase inhibitor (eg, pyridostigmine) prophylactically, less of the nerve gas would be able to bind to cholinesterase. When given soon after exposure to the organophosphate, nucleophiles (eg, pralidoxime) break the bond between the organophosphate and the enzyme, acting as a cholinesterase regenerator. There is no drug that acts as an irreversible muscarinic receptor antagonist (rules out **A** and **C**), neither a reversible muscarinic receptor agonist nor antagonist would be an effective strategy to minimize the binding of an organophosphate to acetylcholinesterase (rules out **A**, **D**, and **E**).

Electrical Activity of the Brain, Sleep–Wake States, & Circadian Rhythms

- Describe the primary types of rhythms that make up the electroencephalogram (EEG).
- List the main clinical uses of the EEG.
- Summarize the behavioral and EEG characteristics of each of the stages of non-rapid eye movement (NREM) and rapid eye movement (REM) sleep and the mechanisms responsible for their production.
- Describe the pattern of normal nighttime sleep in adults and the variations in this pattern from birth to old age.
- Describe the interplay between brainstem neurons that contain norepinephrine, serotonin, and acetylcholine as well as GABA and histamine in mediating transitions between sleep and wakefulness.
- Discuss the circadian rhythm and the role of the suprachiasmatic nuclei (SCN) in its regulation.

INTRODUCTION

The sensory pathways described in Chapters 8–11 relay impulses from sense organs to particular sites in the cerebral cortex. These impulses must be processed in the awake brain to be perceived. Behavioral states range from wakefulness through deep sleep. Discrete patterns of brain electrical activity correlate with each behavioral state. Changes in brain electrical activity also can signify pathologies (eg, seizures). This chapter reviews the neurophysiological basis for the electroencephalogram, changes in the sleep–wake states, and the circadian rhythms.

■ SLEEP–WAKE CYCLE: ALPHA, BETA, & GAMMA RHYTHMS

The electroencephalogram (EEG) recorded from the scalp is a measure of the summation of dendritic postsynaptic potentials rather than action potentials (Figure 14–1). Propagated potentials can be generated in dendrites, and recurrent axon collaterals end on dendrites in the superficial layers. When the sum of the dendritic activity is negative relative to the cell body, the neuron is depolarized and hyperexcitable; when it is positive, the neuron is hyperpolarized and less excitable.

In adult who are awake but at rest with the mind wandering and the eyes closed, the most prominent pattern of the EEG is an alpha rhythm that is a fairly regular sequence of waves at a frequency of 8–13 Hz and amplitude of 50–100 μV (Figure 14–1). It is most marked in the parietal and occipital lobes and is associated with decreased levels of attention. **Clinical Box 14–1** describes some variations in the alpha rhythm. In an awake, alert individual with their eyes open, the alpha rhythm is replaced by an irregular 13–30 Hz low-voltage activity, the beta rhythm (arousal or alerting response) that can be produced by any form of sensory stimulation or mental concentration.

(A)   Alpha rhythm (relaxed with eyes closed)

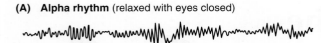

(B)   Beta rhythm (alert)

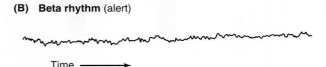

Time ⟶

FIGURE 14–1   EEG records showing the alpha and beta rhythms. When attention is focused on something, the 8–13 Hz alpha rhythm is replaced by an irregular 13–30 Hz low-voltage activity, the beta rhythm. This phenomenon is referred to as alpha block, arousal, or the alerting response. (Reproduced with permission from Widmaier EP, Raff H, Strang KT: *Vander's Human Physiology*, 11th ed. New York, NY: McGraw-Hill; 2008.)

SLEEP STAGES

Rapid eye movement (REM) sleep is named for the characteristic eye movements that occur during this stage of sleep. The non-REM (NREM) or slow-wave sleep is divided into four stages (**Figure 14–2**). As a person begins to fall asleep and enters stage 1, the EEG shows a low-voltage, mixed frequency pattern, the theta rhythm (4–7 Hz). Throughout NREM sleep, there is some activity of skeletal muscle but no eye movements. In stage 2, sleep spindles (12–14 Hz) and occasional high-voltage biphasic K complexes appear. In stage 3, a high-amplitude delta rhythm (0.5–4 Hz) dominates. Maximum slowing with large waves is seen in stage 4. Thus, the characteristic of deep sleep is a pattern of rhythmic slow waves, indicating marked synchronization or slow-wave sleep. While the occurrence of theta and delta rhythms is normal during sleep, their appearance during wakefulness is a sign of brain dysfunction.

REM SLEEP

REM sleep is characterized by the appearance of rapid, low-voltage EEG activity that resembles that seen in the awake, aroused state (Figure 14–2); thus, REM sleep is also called paradoxical sleep. Rapid, roving movements of the eyes occur during paradoxical sleep. The threshold for arousal by sensory stimuli is elevated during REM sleep. Another characteristic of REM sleep is the occurrence of large phasic potentials that originate in the cholinergic neurons in the pons and pass rapidly to the lateral geniculate body and from there to the occipital cortex. They are called pontogeniculo-occipital (PGO) spikes. The tone of the skeletal muscles in the neck is markedly reduced during REM sleep.

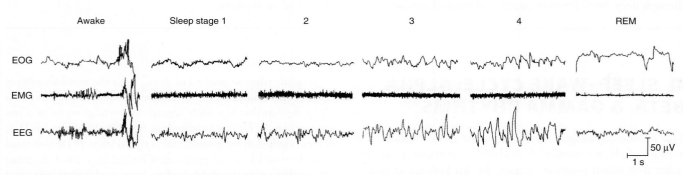

FIGURE 14–2   EEG and muscle activity during various stages of the sleep–wake cycle. NREM sleep has four stages. Stage 1 is characterized by a slight slowing of the EEG. Stage 2 has high-amplitude K complexes and spindles. Stages 3 and 4 have slow, high-amplitude delta waves. REM sleep is characterized by eye movements, loss of muscle tone, and a low-amplitude, high-frequency activity pattern. The higher voltage activity in the EOG tracings during stages 2 and 3 reflect high-amplitude EEG activity in the prefrontal areas rather than eye movements. EOG, electro-oculogram registering eye movements; EMG, electromyogram registering skeletal muscle activity. (Reproduced with permission from Rechtschaffen A, Kales A: *A Manual of Standardized Terminology, Techniques and Scoring System and Sleep Stages of Human Subjects.* Los Angeles: University of California Brain Information Service, 1968.)

Positron emission tomography (PET) scans of humans in REM sleep show increased activity in the pontine area, amygdala, and anterior cingulate gyrus, but decreased activity in the prefrontal and parietal cortex. Activity in visual association areas and primary visual cortex is increased and decreased, respectively. Dreams can occur in both REM and NREM sleep stages; dreams that occur during REM sleep tend to be longer and more visual and emotional than those that occur during NREM sleep.

DISTRIBUTION OF SLEEP STAGES

In a typical night of sleep, a young adult first enters NREM sleep, passes through stages 1 and 2, and spends 70–100 min in stages 3 and 4. Sleep then lightens, and a REM period follows. This cycle is repeated at intervals of about 90 min throughout the night (**Figure 14–3**). The cycles are similar, though there is less

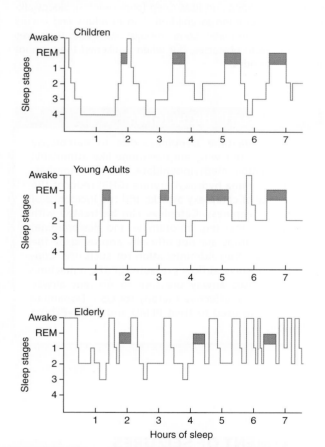

FIGURE 14–3 Normal sleep cycles at various ages. REM sleep is indicated by the darker colored areas. In a typical night of sleep, a young adult first enters NREM sleep, passes through stages 1 and 2, and spends 70–100 min in stages 3 and 4. Sleep then lightens, and a REM period follows. This cycle is repeated at intervals of about 90 min throughout the night. The cycles are similar, though there is less stage 3 and 4 sleep and more REM sleep toward morning. REM sleep occupies 50% of total sleep time in neonates; this proportion declines rapidly and plateaus at ~25% until it falls further in the elderly. (Reproduced with permission from Kales AM, Kales JD: Sleep disorders. *N Engl J Med*. 1974; Feb 28; 290(9):487–499.)

stage 3 and 4 sleep and more REM sleep toward morning. Thus, 4–6 REM periods occur per night. REM sleep occupies 80% of total sleep time in premature infants and 50% in full-term neonates. Thereafter, the proportion of REM sleep falls rapidly and plateaus at about 25% until it falls to about 20% in the elderly. Children have more total sleep time (8–10 h) compared to most adults (about 6 h). Various studies imply that sleep is needed to maintain metabolic–caloric balance, thermal equilibrium, and immune competence. **Clinical Box 14–2** describes several common sleep disorders.

■ CLINICAL USES OF THE EEG

The EEG can be of value in diagnosing pathologies. When fluid collects in a portion of the cortex, activity over this area is dampened; this can aid in diagnosing and localizing conditions such as subdural hematomas. Lesions in the cerebral cortex cause local formation of transient disturbances in brain activity, marked by high-voltage abnormal waves in an EEG recording. Seizure activity can occur because of increased firing of excitatory neurons or decreased firing of inhibitory neurons.

TYPES OF SEIZURES

Epilepsy is a syndrome with multiple causes and is characterized by recurring unprovoked seizures that reflect abnormal, highly synchronous neuronal activity. Seizures are divided into partial (focal) seizures and generalized seizures. Release of glutamate from astrocytes may contribute to the pathophysiology of epilepsy. Also, a combination of reorganization of astrocytes, dendritic sprouting, and new synapse formation may account for recurrent excitation in the epileptic brain. **Clinical Box 14–3** describes the role of genetic mutations in some forms of epilepsy.

Partial seizures originate in a small group of neurons and can result from head injury, brain infection, stroke, or tumor; often the cause is unknown. Symptoms depend on the seizure focus. They are further subdivided into simple partial seizures (without loss of consciousness) and complex partial seizures (with altered consciousness). An example of a simple partial seizure is localized jerking movements in one hand progressing to clonic movements of the entire arm lasting about 60–90 s. Auras typically precede the onset of a partial seizure and include abnormal sensations. The time after the seizure until normal neurologic function returns is called the postictal period.

Generalized seizures are associated with widespread electrical activity and involve both brain hemispheres simultaneously. They are further subdivided into convulsive and nonconvulsive categories depending on whether tonic or clonic movements occur. Absence seizures (formerly called petit mal seizures) are a form of nonconvulsive generalized seizures characterized by a momentary loss of consciousness. They are associated with 3/s doublets, each consisting of a typical spike-and-wave pattern of activity that lasts for about 10 s (**Figure 14–4**). They are not accompanied by auras

CLINICAL BOX 14–2

Sleep Disorders

Narcolepsy is a chronic neurologic disorder caused by the brain's inability to regulate sleep–wake cycles normally. The affected individual experiences a sudden loss of voluntary muscle tone (cataplexy), an eventual irresistible urge to sleep during daytime, and possibly brief episodes of total paralysis at the beginning or end of sleep. Narcolepsy is also characterized by a sudden onset of REM sleep, unlike normal sleep that begins with NREM, slow-wave sleep. The prevalence of narcolepsy is about 1 in 1000 Americans. Narcolepsy has a familial incidence strongly associated with a class II antigen of the major histocompatibility complex on chromosome 6 at the HLA-DR2 or HLA-DQW1 locus, implying a genetic susceptibility to narcolepsy. The HLA complexes are interrelated genes that regulate the immune system. Compared to brains from healthy persons, the brains of persons with narcolepsy often contain fewer hypocretin (orexin)-producing hypothalamic neurons.

Obstructive sleep apnea (OSA) is the most common cause of daytime sleepiness due to fragmented sleep at night; it affects 24% of middle-aged men and 9% of women in the United States. Breathing ceases for more than 10 s during frequent episodes of upper airway obstruction due to reduced muscle tone. The apnea causes brief arousals from sleep that reestablish upper airway tone. An individual with OSA typically begins to snore soon after falling asleep; the snoring gets progressively louder until it is interrupted by an episode of apnea, which is followed by a loud snort and gasp as the individual tries to breathe. OSA is not associated with a reduction in total sleep time, but individuals with OSA experience a much greater time in stage 1 NREM sleep (from an average of 10% of total sleep to 30–50%) and less slow-wave sleep (stages 3 and 4 NREM sleep). The pathophysiology of OSA includes both a reduction in neuromuscular tone at the onset of sleep and a change in the central respiratory drive.

Periodic limb movement disorder (PLMD) is a stereotypical rhythmic extension of the big toe and dorsiflexion of the ankle and knee during sleep lasting for about 0.5–10 s and recurring at intervals of 20–90 s. Movements can range from shallow continual movement of the ankle or toes to wild and strenuous kicking and flailing of the legs and arms. Electromyograph (EMG) recordings show bursts of activity during the first hours of NREM sleep associated with brief EEG signs of arousal. The duration of stage 1 NREM sleep may be increased and that of stages 3 and 4 decreased compared to age-matched controls. PLMD occurs in 5% of individuals between the ages of 30 and 50 years and increases to 44% of those over the age of 65. PLMD is similar to restless leg syndrome or Willis–Ekbom disease in which individuals have an irresistible urge to move their legs while at rest all day long.

Sleepwalking (somnambulism), bed-wetting (nocturnal enuresis), and night terrors are sleep disorders associated with arousal from NREM and REM sleep (parasomnias). Sleepwalking is more common in children than in adults and occurs predominantly in males. Somnambulists walk with their eyes open and avoid obstacles, but when awakened they cannot recall the episodes.

THERAPEUTIC HIGHLIGHTS

Excessive daytime sleepiness due to narcolepsy can be treated with amphetamine-like stimulants (eg, modafinil, methylphenidate, and methamphetamine). Gamma hydroxybutyrate (GHB) reduces the frequency of cataplexy attacks and the incidence of daytime sleepiness. Cataplexy can be treated with antidepressants (eg, imipramine and desipramine) but these drugs are not officially approved by the US Federal Drug Administration for such use. Continuous positive airflow pressure (CPAP), a machine that increases airway pressure to prevent airway collapse, is an effective therapy for OSA. Dopamine agonists are used to treat PLMD and Willis–Ekbom disease.

---

or postictal periods. These spike and waves are generated by low threshold T-type Ca^{2+} channels in thalamic neurons.

The most common convulsive generalized seizure is tonic-clonic seizure (formerly called grand mal seizure). This is associated with sudden onset of contraction of limb muscles (tonic phase) and sudden loss of consciousness lasting about 30 s, followed by symmetric jerking of the limbs as a result of alternating contraction and relaxation (clonic phase) lasting 1–2 min. There is fast EEG activity during the tonic phase. Slow waves, each preceded by a spike, occur at the time of each clonic jerk. For a while after the attack, slow waves are present.

TREATMENT OF SEIZURES

Only about two-thirds of individuals that have seizure activity respond to drug therapies. Some respond to surgical interventions (eg, temporal lobe seizures), and some respond to vagal nerve stimulation (eg, partial seizures). Prior to the 1990s, the most common drugs used to treat seizures (anticonvulsants) included phenytoin, valproate, and barbiturates. Newer drugs have become available but they are palliative rather than curative. Clinical Box 14–3 describes mechanisms of actions of some drugs used to treat seizures.

■ CIRCADIAN RHYTHMS & THE SLEEP–WAKE CYCLE

CIRCADIAN RHYTHMS

Many behaviors have rhythmic fluctuations on a circadian cycle. Normally they become entrained (synchronized) to the day-night light cycle. If they are not entrained, they become progressively

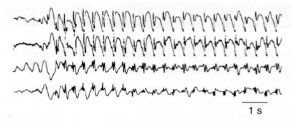

FIGURE 14–4 Absence seizures. This is a recording of four cortical EEG leads from a 6-year-old boy who, during the recording, had one of his "blank spells" in which he was transiently unaware of his surroundings and blinked his eyelids. Absence seizures are associated with 3/s doublets, each consisting of a typical spike-and-wave pattern of activity that lasts for about 10 s. Time is indicated by the horizontal calibration line. (Reproduced with permission from Waxman SG: *Neuroanatomy with Clinical Correlations*, 25th ed. New York, NY: McGraw-Hill; 2003.)

more out of phase with the light–dark cycle because they are longer or shorter than 24 h. The entrainment process usually relies on the suprachiasmatic nuclei (SCN) that receive information about the light–dark cycle via retinohypothalamic fibers. SCN neurons initiate neural and humoral signals that entrain many circadian rhythms including the sleep–wake cycle and the secretion of the pineal hormone melatonin.

Exposure to bright light can advance, delay, or have no effect on the sleep–wake cycle in humans, depending on the time of day when it is experienced. Just after dark, light exposure delays the onset of the sleep period; just before dawn, it accelerates the onset of the next sleep period. Injection of melatonin has similar effects. Exposure to light turns on immediate-early genes in the SCN, but only at times during the circadian cycle when light is capable of influencing entrainment. Stimulation during the day is ineffective. **Clinical Box 14–4** describes circadian rhythm disorders that impact the sleep–wake state.

NEUROCHEMICAL MECHANISMS PROMOTING SLEEP & AROUSAL

Transitions between sleep and wakefulness have a circadian rhythm of 6–8 h of sleep and 16–18 h of wakefulness. Brainstem and hypothalamic neurons are critical for the transitions between these states of consciousness. The brainstem contains several groups of neurons that release norepinephrine, serotonin, or acetylcholine. Hypothalamic neurons involved in control of the sleep–wake cycles include GABAergic preoptic neurons and histaminergic posterior hypothalamic neurons. Also, orexin-containing hypothalamic neurons are involved in sleep–wake transitions.

One theory regarding the basis for transitions from sleep to wakefulness involves alternating reciprocal activity of different groups of brainstem neurons. In this model **(Figure 14–5)**, wakefulness and REM sleep are at opposite extremes. When the activity of norepinephrine- and serotonin-containing neurons (locus coeruleus and raphe nuclei) is dominant, there is a reduced level of activity in acetylcholine-containing neurons in the pontine

CLINICAL BOX 14-4

Insomnia & Circadian Rhythm Disturbances of the Sleep–Wake State

Insomnia is defined as difficulty in initiating and/or maintaining sleep several times a week; ~30% of adults report episodes of insomnia, and more than 50% of those aged 65 or older experience sleep problems. Those with persistent episodes of insomnia are more likely to have accidents, a diminished work experience, and a poorer quality of life. Insomnia is often comorbid with depression; abnormal regulation of corticotropin-releasing factor occurs in both disorders. Two types of sleep disorders are associated with disruption of the circadian rhythm: transient sleep disorders (jet lag, altered sleep cycle because of shift work, and illness) and chronic sleep disorders (delayed or advanced sleep phase syndrome). Those with delayed sleep phase syndrome are unable to fall asleep in the evenings and awaken in the mornings, but they have a normal total sleep time. Those with advanced sleep phase syndrome consistently fall asleep in early evening and awaken in early morning; it is seen primarily in the elderly and the depressed.

THERAPEUTIC HIGHLIGHTS

Light therapy can be an effective treatment in individuals who experience disturbances in their circadian cycle. Melatonin can be used to treat jet lag and insomnia in elderly individuals. Ramelteon is an MT_1 and MT_2 receptor agonist that is more effective than melatonin in treating insomnia. Zolpidem (Ambien) is a sedative-hypnotic that slows brain activity to promote sleep onset. In addition to treating daytime sleepiness in narcolepsy, modafinil has been effective in the treatment of daytime sleepiness due to shift work and delayed sleep disorder syndrome.

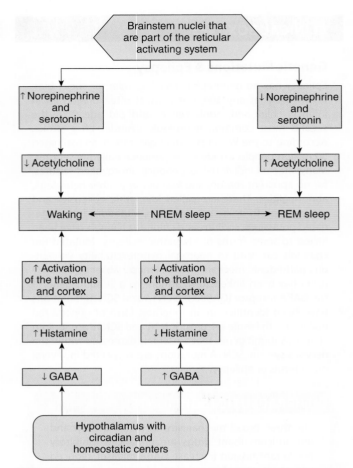

FIGURE 14–5 A model of how alternating activity of brainstem and hypothalamic neurons may influence the different states of consciousness. In this model, wakefulness and REM sleep are at opposite extremes. When the activity of norepinephrine- and serotonin-containing neurons (locus coeruleus and raphe nuclei) is dominant, there is a reduced level of activity in acetylcholine-containing neurons in the pontine reticular formation leading to wakefulness. The reverse of this pattern leads to REM sleep. A more even balance in the activity of these groups of neurons is associated with NREM sleep. Increases in GABA and decreases in histamine promote NREM sleep via deactivation of the thalamus and cortex. Wakefulness occurs when GABA is reduced and histamine is released. (Reproduced with permission from Widmaier EP, Raff H, Strang KT: Vander's Human Physiology, 11th ed. New York, NY: McGraw-Hill; 2008.)

reticular formation. This pattern of activity contributes to the appearance of the awake state. The reverse of this pattern leads to REM sleep. When there is a more even balance in the activity of the aminergic and cholinergic neurons, NREM sleep occurs. The orexin released from hypothalamic neurons may regulate the changes in activity in these brainstem neurons.

In addition, an increased release of GABA and reduced release of histamine increase the likelihood of NREM sleep via deactivation of the thalamus and cortex. Wakefulness occurs when GABA release is reduced and histamine release is increased.

MELATONIN & THE SLEEP–WAKE STATE

The pineal gland contains pinealocytes that synthesize and secrete melatonin into the blood and the cerebrospinal fluid. Neurons in the SCN have two melatonin receptors (MT_1 and MT_2); both are

G-protein–coupled receptors. Activation of MT_1 receptors inhibit adenylyl cyclase and promote sleepiness. MT_2 receptors stimulate phosphoinositide hydrolysis and may help synchronize the light–dark cycle. Melatonin synthesis and secretion are increased during the dark phase and maintained at a low level during daylight hours. This diurnal variation in secretion is brought about by norepinephrine secreted by the postganglionic sympathetic nerves that innervate the pineal gland.

Sympathetic nerve activity to the pineal gland is entrained to the light–dark cycle via the retinohypothalamic fibers to the SCN. GABAergic SCN neurons inhibit hypothalamic paraventricular neurons. These hypothalamic neurons excite preganglionic sympathetic neurons that innervate the superior cervical ganglion, the site of origin of the postganglionic neurons to the pineal gland.

Small concretions of calcium phosphate and carbonate (pineal sand) appear in the pineal gland. Since they are radiopaque, the gland is visible on radiographs of the skull. Displacement of a calcified pineal from its normal position indicates the presence of a space-occupying lesion such as a tumor in the brain.

CHAPTER SUMMARY

- The major rhythms in the EEG are alpha (8–13 Hz), beta (13–30 Hz), theta (4–7 Hz), delta (0.5–4 Hz), and gamma (30–80 Hz) oscillations.
- The EEG is of some value in localizing pathologic processes, and it is useful in characterizing different types of seizures.
- NREM sleep can be divided into 4 stages. A theta rhythm is seen in stage 1. Stage 2 is marked by the appearance of sleep spindles and occasional K complexes. In stage 3, a delta rhythm is dominant. Maximum slowing with large slow waves is seen in stage 4. REM sleep is characterized by low-voltage, high-frequency EEG activity and rapid movements of the eyes.
- A young adult typically passes through stages 1 and 2, and spends 70–100 min in stages 3 and 4. Sleep then lightens, and a REM period follows. This cycle repeats at 90-min intervals throughout the night. REM sleep occupies 50% of total sleep time in full-term neonates; this proportion declines rapidly and plateaus at about 25% until it falls further in old age.
- Transitions from sleep to wakefulness may involve alternating reciprocal activity of different groups of neurons. When the activity of norepinephrine- and serotonin-containing neurons is dominant, the activity in acetylcholine-containing neurons is reduced, leading to the appearance of wakefulness. The reverse of this pattern leads to REM sleep. Also, wakefulness occurs when GABA release is reduced and histamine release is increased.
- The entrainment of biologic processes to the light–dark cycle is regulated by the SCN.
- The diurnal change in melatonin secretion from serotonin in the pineal gland may function as a timing signal to coordinate events with the light–dark cycle, including the sleep–wake cycle.

MULTIPLE-CHOICE QUESTIONS

For all questions, select the single best answer unless otherwise directed.

1. A healthy 23-year-old male medical student volunteered to have his EEG recorded as part of a class demonstration of cortical activity patterns. An electrode was placed over his occipital lobes and the activity was recorded initially while awake, sitting restfully with his eyes closed and then after opening his eyes and he is alert. The dominant EEG patterns observed during these two behaviors is expected to be
   A. beta (18–30 Hz) rhythm and then alpha (8–13 Hz) rhythm, respectively.
   B. delta (0.5–4 Hz) rhythm and then beta (18–30 Hz) rhythm, respectively.
   C. alpha (8–13 Hz) and then beta (18–30 Hz) rhythm, respectively.
   D. delta (0.5–4 Hz) rhythm and then fast, irregular low-voltage activity, respectively.
   E. beta (18–30 Hz) rhythm and then fast, irregular low-voltage activity, respectively.

2. A 35-year-old man reported frequent episodes of daytime sleepiness over the course of the past year or so. His primary care physician recommended that he go to a sleep clinic to determine whether he has obstructive sleep apnea. An EEG recorded during an evening at the sleep clinic showed that NREM sleep accounted for over 30% of his total sleep time. What neurochemical changes in the brain trigger the transition from wakefulness to NREM sleep and does this lead to an increase or a decrease in thalamocortical activity?
   A. A decrease in norepinephrine and serotonin release to increase thalamocortical activity.
   B. A decrease in norepinephrine and serotonin release to decrease thalamocortical activity.
   C. An increase in histamine release and a decrease in GABA release to increase thalamocortical activity.
   D. An increase in GABA and melatonin release to decrease thalamocortical activity.
   E. An increase in GABA release and a decrease in histamine release to decrease thalamocortical activity.

3. A 45-year-old woman spent the evening in a sleep clinic after her husband had repeatedly expressed concern about her restlessness during the night which was keeping him awake. Which of the following pattern of changes in central neurotransmitters or neuromodulators are associated with transitioning from NREM to REM sleep?
   A. Decrease in norepinephrine, increase in serotonin, and increase in acetylcholine.
   B. Decrease in norepinephrine, increase in acetylcholine, and increase in histamine.
   C. Decrease in norepinephrine, decrease in serotonin, and increase in acetylcholine.
   D. Increase in norepinephrine, increase in serotonin, and decrease in GABA.
   E. Increase in norepinephrine, decrease in serotonin, and decrease in GABA.

4. For the past several months, a 67-year-old woman experienced difficulty initiating and/or maintaining sleep several times each week. A friend suggested that she take melatonin to help her fall asleep and stay asleep. Endogenous melatonin secretion would be increased by
   A. reducing the synthesis of serotonin.
   B. inhibition of the paraventricular nucleus.
   C. stimulation of the superior cervical ganglion.
   D. stimulation of the optic nerve.
   E. by blockade of hydroxyindole-O-methyltransferase.

5. Childhood absence epilepsy was diagnosed in a 10-year-old boy. His EEG showed a bilateral synchronous, symmetric 3-Hz spike-and-wave discharge. Absence seizures are a form of
   A. nonconvulsive generalized seizures accompanied by momentary loss of consciousness.
   B. complex partial seizures accompanied by momentary loss of consciousness.

C.   nonconvulsive generalized seizures without a loss of consciousness.

D.   simple partial seizures without a loss of consciousness.

E.   convulsive generalized seizures accompanied by momentary loss of consciousness.

6. Childhood absence epilepsy was diagnosed in a 10-year-old boy. His EEG showed a bilateral synchronous, symmetric 3-Hz spike-and-wave discharge. He began treatment with ethosuximide. What is the mechanism of action by which ethosuximide is an effective antiseizure drug?

A.   It is a GABA analog that decreases Ca^{2+} entry into cells.

B.   It blocks voltage-gated Na^+ channels associated with glutamate receptors.

C.   It potentiates GABA transmission.

D.   It is a dopamine receptor agonist.

E.   It inhibits T-type Ca^{2+} channels.

7. A 57-year-old professor at a medical school experienced numerous episodes of a sudden loss of muscle tone and an irresistible urge to sleep in the middle of the afternoon. The diagnosis was narcolepsy, which

A.   is characterized by a sudden onset of NREM sleep.

B.   has a familial incidence associated with a class II antigen of the major histocompatibility complex.

C.   may be due to the presence of an excessive number of orexin-producing neurons in the hypothalamus.

D.   is often effectively treated with dopamine receptor agonists.

E.   is the most common cause of daytime sleepiness.

8. A 69-year-old man went to a sleep clinic after his wife expressed concerns about his behavioral pattern during his sleep despite having normal behavioral patterns during the daytime. Both electromyograph (EMG) and EEG recordings were made. EMG recordings showed bursts of activity during the first hours of NREM sleep associated with brief signs of arousal. Compared to healthy age-matched controls, he spent more time in stage 1 NREM sleep and less time in stages 3 and 4. The likely diagnosis is

A.   somnambulism.

B.   nocturnal enuresis.

C.   night terrors.

D.   periodic limb movement disorder.

E.   restless leg syndrome.

9. A 21-year-old woman was talking with her friends when she suddenly experienced the onset of strong contraction of her left and right limb muscles that lasted about 30 s which was accompanied by a grunting sound and momentary loss of consciousness causing her to collapse; this was immediately followed by jerking of her limbs that lasted for about 2 min. This description is consistent with

A.   a complex partial seizure.

B.   a simple partial seizure.

C.   tonic-clonic seizure.

D.   periodic limb movement disorder.

E.   restless leg syndrome.

10. A 57-year-old woman was being seen by a neurologist after reporting several episodes of abnormal hand and arm movements that lasted for less than 2 min. She reports that she first experiences an unusual feeling that has served as a warning that something is about to happen. This is followed by

jerking movements in the fingers of her right hand and then her entire arm begins to shake. She indicates that she does not lose consciousness during these episodes, but they frighten her. This description is consistent with

A.   a complex partial seizure.

B.   a simple partial seizure.

C.   tonic-clonic seizure.

D.   absence epilepsy.

E.   temporal lobe epilepsy.

11. An 11-month-old boy was brought to an urgent care facility by his mother because he had a fever (103.5°F) for the past 24 hours or so that was not reduced by ibuprofen. While being examined by a physician, the infant suddenly began to jerk his arms and legs and briefly lost consciousness. When the seizure ended, he fell asleep. The physician explained to the mother that her child likely experienced a febrile seizure. The mother then indicated that she has a family history of children that develop febrile seizures, including one of her siblings. All family members that experienced these febrile seizures eventually outgrew them, but not until the age of 10–12 but experienced no developmental disorders. What genetic mutation(s) have been linked to an inherited form of generalized epilepsy with febrile seizures plus?

A.   TNK2 and ST3GAL5

B.   PCDH19

C.   GRIN2A

D.   CNA1 and SCNB1

E.   GABRB3

12. A 35-year-old man with a history of epilepsy was brought to the emergency department by a family member who found him on the ground shaking. Typically his seizures would last no more than a few minutes, but this episode of rhythmic shaking has persisted for the past 30 min. It was determined that he was experiencing a tonic-clonic seizure. Blood was dripping from his mouth because he bit his tongue during the convulsion. After making certain his airway was patent, the physician requested that an intravenous dose of phenytoin be administered to the patient. What is the mechanism of action of phenytoin?

A.   Blocks Na^+ channels and decreases synaptic release of glutamate

B.   Blocks N-type voltage-gated Ca^{2+} channels and decreases glutamate release

C.   Blocks Na^+ channels, inhibits T-type Ca^{2+} channels, and enhances GABA transmission

D.   A GABA analog, blocks N-type voltage-gated Ca^{2+} channels, and reduces synaptic release of glutamate

E.   Potentiates GABA transmission, decreases glutamate receptor activity, and blocks Na^+ channels

ANSWERS

1. The best answer is **C**. In healthy adults who are awake but at rest with their eyes closed, the most prominent component of the EEG is a fairly regular pattern of waves at a frequency of 8–13 Hz (alpha rhythm). When the eyes are opened and attention is focused on something, the alpha rhythm is replaced by fast irregular 13–30 Hz low-voltage activity (beta rhythm). This phenomenon is called alpha block and can be produced by any form of sensory stimulation or mental concentration, such as solving arithmetic problems. Another term for this phenomenon is the arousal or alerting response

because it is correlated with the aroused, alert state. It has also been called desynchronization because it represents breaking up of the obviously synchronized neural activity necessary to produce regular waves. Option **A** can be ruled out as the description is the opposite of the behavioral-induced changes in the EEG pattern. A high-amplitude delta rhythm (0.5–4 Hz) dominates in stage 3 of NREM sleep (rules out options **B** and **D**). The appearance of these large amplitude rhythmic slow waves is indicative of marked synchronization of cortical activity during deep sleep; their appearance is also the reason that sometimes deep sleep is referred to as slow-wave sleep. Option **E** suggests that there was no behavioral-induced change in the EEG because beta rhythm is also described as fast, irregular low-voltage activity.

2. The best answer is **E**. An increased release of GABA and reduced release of histamine increase the likelihood of NREM sleep via deactivation of the thalamus and cortex. A decrease in norepinephrine and serotonin leads to REM sleep not NREM sleep (rules out options **A** and **B**). An increase in histamine release and a decrease in GABA release would lead to increased thalamocortical activity and wakefulness (rules out option **C**). Changes in melatonin occur on the timescale of a circadian rhythm not on the timescale of transitions between sleep stages (rules out option **D**).

3. The best answer is **C**. REM sleep occurs with a decrease in the activity of norepinephrine- and serotonin-containing neurons and an increase in the activity of acetylcholine-containing neurons. The directional change in norepinephrine and serotonin release is the same and opposite to that of acetylcholine release across different sleep–wake states (rules out options **A** and **E**). Changes in GABA and histamine are related to transitioning between wakefulness and NREM rather than REM sleep (rules out options **B**, **D**, and **E**).

4. The best answer is **C**. The superior cervical ganglion is the site of origin of the postganglionic neurons to the pineal gland, where melatonin is synthesized and released. All other options would decrease the levels of melatonin in the circulation. Specifically, serotonin is a precursor for melatonin, stimulation of the paraventricular nucleus activates preganglionic neurons that synapse in the superior cervical ganglia, activation of the optic nerve by light is a trigger to reduce the synthesis and release of melatonin in the pinealocytes, and hydroxyindole-O-methyltransferase is the enzyme that converts N-acetylserotonin to melatonin in the pinealocytes (rules out options **A**, **B**, **D**, and **E**).

5. The best answer is **A**. Absence seizures (formerly called petit mal seizures) are a form of nonconvulsive generalized seizures characterized by a momentary loss of consciousness. The momentary loss of consciousness rules out option **C**. A complex partial seizure originates in a small group of neurons and causes impaired consciousness; it often represents temporal lobe epilepsy (rules out option **B**). An example of a simple partial seizure without a loss of consciousness is jerking movements in one hand progressing to clonic movements of the entire arm lasting about 60–90 s (rules out option **D**). The most common convulsive generalized seizure is tonic-clonic seizure, formerly called grand mal seizure (rules out option **E**).

6. The best answer is **E**. Ethosuximide reduces the low threshold T-type Ca^{2+} currents in thalamic neurons, and thus is particularly effective in treatment of absence seizures. Gabapentin is

an example of an anticonvulsant (antiepileptic drug) that is a GABA analog and blocks N-type voltage-gated Ca^{2+} channels and reduces glutamate release (rules out option **A**). Topiramate is an example of an anticonvulsant that blocks voltage-gated Na^+ channels associated with glutamate receptors and potentiates GABA transmission (rules out options **B** and **C**). Dopamine receptor agonists are not used to treat seizures (rules out option **D**).

7. The best answer is **B**. Narcolepsy has a familial incidence strongly associated with a class II antigen of the major histocompatibility complex on chromosome 6 at the HLA-DR2 or HLA-DQW1 locus, implying a genetic susceptibility to narcolepsy. Narcolepsy is also characterized by a sudden onset of REM sleep, unlike normal sleep that begins with NREM, slow-wave sleep (rules out option **A**). Compared to brains from healthy persons, the brains of those with narcolepsy often contain fewer hypocretin (orexin)-producing hypothalamic neurons; the HLA complex may increase susceptibility to an immune attack on these neurons, leading to their degeneration (rules out option **C**). Dopamine agonists are used to treat PLMD and Willis–Ekbom disease not narcolepsy; excessive daytime sleepiness due to narcolepsy can be treated with amphetamine-like stimulants such as modafinil (rules out option **D**). OSA is the most common cause of daytime sleepiness (rules out option **E**).

8. The best answer is **D**. The description is consistent with periodic limb movement disorder, a stereotypical rhythmic extension of the big toe and dorsiflexion of the ankle and knee during sleep lasting for about 0.5–10 s and recurring at intervals of 20–90 s. This occurs in 44% of those over the age of 65. It is similar to restless leg syndrome; but in the latter case, the individual has an irresistible urge to move their legs while at rest all day long (rules out option **E**). Sleepwalking (somnambulism), bed-wetting (nocturnal enuresis), and night terrors are parasomnias, which are sleep disorders associated with arousal from NREM and REM sleep (rules out options **A**, **B**, and **C**).

9. The best answer is **C**. The most common generalized convulsive seizure is tonic-clonic seizure (formerly called grand mal seizure). This is associated with sudden onset of contraction of limb muscles (tonic phase) lasting about 30 s and accompanied by a grunt (the tonic contraction of the diaphragm causes a forced expiration) and loss of consciousness, followed by symmetric jerking of the limbs as a result of alternating contraction and relaxation (clonic phase) lasting 1–2 min. A complex partial seizure begins in a localized region of the brain and causes impaired consciousness (rules out option **A**). A simple partial seizure occurs without a loss of consciousness is jerking movements in one hand progressing to clonic movements of the entire arm lasting about 60–90 s (rules out option **B**). Periodic limb movement disorder is a stereotypical rhythmic extension of the big toe and dorsiflexion of the ankle and knee during sleep (rules out option **D**). With restless leg syndrome, an individual has an irresistible urge to move their legs at rest (rules out option **E**).

10. The best answer is **B**. A simple partial seizure occurs without a loss of consciousness and can present as jerking movements in one hand progressing to clonic movements of the entire arm lasting about 60–90 s. Auras can precede the onset of a partial seizure; these include abnormal sensations. A complex partial seizure is accompanied by a loss

of consciousness; an example is temporal lobe epilepsy (rules out options **A** and **E**). Both tonic-clonic seizures and absence epilepsy are generalized (not partial) seizures and are associated with widespread electrical activity of both brain hemispheres simultaneously; they also include a loss of consciousness (rules out options **C** and **D**).

11. The best answer is **D**. The syndrome of generalized epilepsy with febrile seizures plus (GEFS+) can be caused by mutations affecting the voltage-gated sodium channel subunits SCN1A (sodium channel, voltage gated, type I alpha subunit) and SCN1B (sodium channel, voltage gated, type I beta subunit) or GABRG2 (gamma 2-subunit of the GABA$_A$ receptor). A mutation of TNK2 (tyrosine kinase, nonreceptor, 2) gene or the ST3GAL5 (ST3 beta-galactoside alpha-2,3-sialyltransferase 5) gene is linked with the development of an autosomal recessive infantile-onset symptomatic epilepsy syndrome associated with developmental stagnation and blindness (rules out option **A**). PCDH19 Epilepsy includes a wide spectrum of severity in seizures (eg, generalized tonic-clonic, complex partial seizures, myoclonic), cognitive delays, autism spectrum disorder (60% of the cases), and other problems (eg, sleep disturbances, hypotonia, dysautonomia) that are due to a mutation of the PCDH19 gene on the x chromosome (rules out option **B**). A mutation in the GRIN2A (glutamate receptor, ionotropic, N-methyl D-aspartate 2A) gene is linked with the development of several types of acquired epileptic aphasia and related childhood focal epilepsies including acquired epileptic aphasia (Landau–Kleffner syndrome, LKS) whose onset is typically between the ages of 3 and 7 (rules out option **C**). A mutation in the GABR3A (beta 3-subunit of the GABA$_A$ receptor) gene is linked to the development of childhood absence epilepsy (CAE) in which the seizure is often expressed by staring spells during which the child is not responsive (rules out option **E**).

12. The best answer is **A**. Phenytoin can be used to treat both partial and generalized seizures and it acts via blockade of Na$^+$ channels and reduced the amount of glutamate released from neurons. Carbamazepine is an example of an anticonvulsant that blocks N-type voltage-gated Ca^{2+} channels and decreases glutamate release; it is used for the treatment of partial seizures (rules out option **B**). Lamotrigine is an example of an anticonvulsant that blocks Na$^+$ channels, inhibits T-type Ca^{2+} channels, and enhances GABA transmission; it is used to treat both partial and generalized seizures (rules out option **C**). Gabapentin and pregabalin are examples of a GABA analog anticonvulsant that block N-type voltage-gated Ca^{2+} channels and reduce synaptic release of glutamate (rules out option **D**). Topiramate is an example of an anticonvulsant that potentiates GABA transmission, decreases glutamate receptor activity, and blocks Na$^+$ channels (rules out option **E**).

Learning, Memory, Language, & Speech

15

After studying this chapter,
you should be able to:

- Describe the various forms of memory.
- Identify the parts of the brain involved in memory processing and storage.
- Define synaptic plasticity, long-term potentiation (LTP), long-term depression (LTD), habituation, and sensitization, and their roles in learning and memory.
- Describe the abnormalities of brain structure and function found in Alzheimer disease.
- Define the terms categorical hemisphere and representational hemisphere and summarize the difference between these hemispheres.
- Summarize the differences between fluent and nonfluent aphasia, and explain each type on the basis of its pathophysiology.

INTRODUCTION

The understanding of brain function in humans has been revolutionized by the use of positron emission tomographic (PET), functional magnetic resonance imaging (fMRI), computed tomography (CT) scanning, and other imaging and diagnostic techniques. These techniques provide an index of the level of the activity in various parts of the brain in healthy humans and in those with different diseases or brain injuries (Clinical Box 15–1). They have been used to study learning, memory, and sensory perception. Learning is acquisition of the information that makes it possible for humans to alter

their behavior on the basis of experience. Memory is the retention and storage of that information. The two are closely related and are considered together in this chapter. Experience-dependent growth of new granule cells in the dentate gyrus of the hippocampus may contribute to learning and memory. Memory and learning are functions of large parts of the brain, but the centers controlling some of the other "higher functions of the nervous system" such as the mechanisms related to language are localized to the neocortex. Speech and other intellectual functions are especially well developed in humans.

■ FORMS OF MEMORY

Explicit (declarative) memory is associated with awareness and is dependent on the hippocampus and other parts of the medial temporal lobes. It allows one to retain knowledge about people, places, and things and is subdivided into semantic memory for facts and episodic memory for events. Implicit (nondeclarative) memory is important for training reflexive motor or perceptual skills and is subdivided into four types. Priming (facilitation of

the recognition of words or objects by prior exposure to them) requires the neocortex. Procedural memory (skills and habits, which, once acquired, become unconscious and automatic) is processed in the striatum. Associative learning (classical and operant conditioning) uses the amygdala for its emotional responses and the cerebellum for the motor responses. Nonassociative learning (habituation and sensitization) is dependent on reflex pathways.

Explicit memories that are initially required for activities such as riding a bicycle can become implicit once the task is thoroughly

CLINICAL BOX 15–1

Traumatic Brain Injury

Traumatic brain injury (TBI) is an insult to the brain due to an excessive mechanical force or penetrating injury to the head. It can lead to permanent or temporary impairment of cognitive, physical, emotional, and behavioral functions; and it can be associated with a diminished or altered state of consciousness. TBI is one of the leading causes of death or disability worldwide. According to the Centers for Disease Control and Prevention, each year at least 1.5 million persons in the United States sustain a TBI. It is most common in children under age 4, in adolescents aged 15–19 years of age, and in adults over the age of 65. In all age groups, TBI occurs more often in males than in females (2:1). In 75% of the cases, the TBI is mild and manifests as a concussion. Adults with severe TBI who are treated have a mortality rate of about 30%, but 50% regain most of their functions with therapy. The leading causes of TBI include falls, motor vehicle accidents, being struck by an object, and assaults. TBI can be divided into primary and secondary stages. Primary injury is that caused by the mechanical force (eg, skull fracture and surface contusions) or acceleration-deceleration due to unrestricted movement of the head leading to shear, tensile, and compressive strains. These injuries can cause intracranial hematoma (epidural, subdural, or subarachnoid) and diffuse axonal injury. Secondary injury is often a delayed response and may be due to impaired cerebral blood flow that can eventually lead to cell death. A Glasgow Coma Scale is often used to define the severity of TBI and evaluates motor responses, verbal responses, and eye opening to assess the levels of consciousness and neurologic functioning after an injury. Symptoms of mild TBI include headache, confusion, dizziness, blurred vision, tinnitus, a bad taste in the mouth, fatigue, sleep disturbances, mood changes, and problems with memory, concentration, or thinking. Individuals with moderate or severe TBI also experience vomiting or nausea, convulsions or seizures, an inability to be roused, fixed and dilated pupils, slurred speech, limb weakness, loss of coordination, and increased confusion, restlessness, or agitation. In the most severe cases of TBI, the affected individual may go into a permanent vegetative state.

THERAPEUTIC HIGHLIGHTS

The advancements in brain imaging technology have improved the ability of medical personnel to diagnose and evaluate the extent of brain damage. Therapy is initially directed at stabilizing the patient and trying to prevent further injury. Diuretics (to reduce pressure in the brain), anticonvulsant drugs during the first week post injury (to avoid additional brain damage resulting from a seizure), and coma-inducing drugs (to reduce oxygen demands) can be administered. This is followed by rehabilitation that includes physical, occupational, and speech/language therapies. Recovery of brain function can be due to several factors: brain regions that were suppressed but not damaged can regain their function, axonal sprouting and redundancy allows other areas of the brain to take over the functions lost due to the injury, and behavioral substitution, by learning new strategies to compensate for the deficits.

learned. Explicit memory and many forms of implicit memory involve (1) short-term memory, lasting seconds to hours, during which processing in the hippocampus and elsewhere creates long-term changes in synaptic strength; and (2) long-term memory, which stores memories for years and sometimes for life. Short-term memory can be disrupted by trauma and drugs; long-term memory traces are remarkably resistant to disruption. Working memory is a form of short-term memory that keeps information available for very short periods while the individual plans action based on it.

NEURAL BASIS OF MEMORY, SYNAPTIC PLASTICITY & LEARNING

Learning and memory are linked to alterations in cellular membrane channels, the synthesis of proteins, and the activation of genes that occur during the change from short-term working memory to long-term memory. Interrupting the ability to make these alterations can contribute to retrograde amnesia, the loss of memory for the events immediately preceding a concussion.

Short- and long-term changes in presynaptic or postsynaptic function can be influenced by the history of activity at a synapse; that is, synaptic conduction can be strengthened or weakened due to past experiences. These changes are forms of learning and memory. Post-tetanic potentiation is the enhancement (up to 60 s) of postsynaptic potentials after a brief period of tetanizing stimulation of the presynaptic neuron that causes Ca^{2+} to accumulate in the presynaptic neuron to a level that overwhelms the intracellular binding sites that keep cytoplasmic Ca^{2+} low.

Habituation is an example of nonassociative learning. A novel stimulus evokes a reaction, but after frequent repetition, one becomes habituated to the stimulus and ignores it. This is linked to decreased release of neurotransmitter from the presynaptic terminal because of reduced intracellular Ca^{2+} due to a gradual inactivation of Ca^{2+} channels.

Sensitization is the prolonged occurrence of augmented post-synaptic responses after a stimulus to which one has become habituated is paired with a noxious stimulus; sensitization is due to presynaptic facilitation and can have features of short-term or long-term memory. The short-term prolongation of sensitization is due to a Ca^{2+}-mediated change in adenylyl cyclase that increases production of cAMP.

Long-term potentiation (LTP) involves protein synthesis and growth of the presynaptic and postsynaptic neurons and their connections. LTP is a rapidly developing persistent enhancement of the postsynaptic response after a brief period of rapidly repeated stimulation of the presynaptic neuron. The basis for LTP at the connection of a pyramidal cell in the CA3 region and a pyramidal cell in the CA1 region via the Schaffer collateral is shown in Figure 15–1.

Long-term depression (LTD) is characterized by a decrease in synaptic strength produced by slower stimulation of presynaptic neurons. It is linked to a smaller rise in intracellular Ca^{2+} than occurs in LTP. In the cerebellum, its occurrence requires the phosphorylation of the GluR2 subunit of the AMPA receptors.

ASSOCIATIVE LEARNING: CONDITIONED REFLEXES

A conditioned reflex is an example of associative learning; it is a reflex response to a stimulus (conditioned stimulus) that previously elicited little or no response, acquired by repeatedly pairing the stimulus with one that normally produces a response (unconditioned stimulus). After the two stimuli are paired a sufficient number of times, the conditioned stimulus produces the response originally evoked only by the unconditioned stimulus.

HIPPOCAMPUS & MEDIAL TEMPORAL LOBE

Removal of the hippocampus in the medial temporal lobes leads to marked memory deficits. Long-term memory for events that occurred prior to surgery is maintained, but anterograde amnesia can ensue. Short-term memory is intact, but one cannot commit new events to long-term memory or learn new motor tasks. The temporal lobe, in particular the hippocampus, is critical in the formation of long-term declarative memories and for the conversion of short-term to long-term memories.

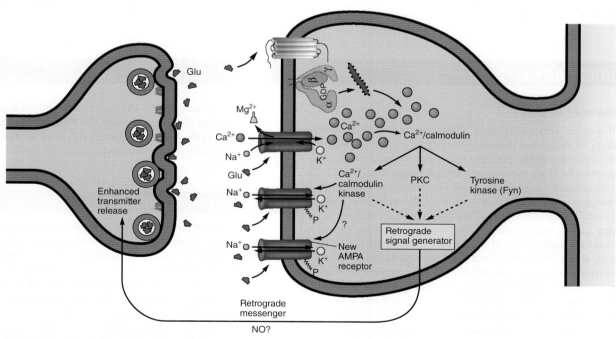

FIGURE 15–1 Production of LTP in Schaffer collaterals in the hippocampus. Glutamate (Glu) released from the presynaptic neuron binds to AMPA and NMDA receptors in the membrane of the postsynaptic neuron. Na$^+$ and K$^-$ can flow only through the AMPA receptor because the presence of Mg^{2+} on the NMDA receptor blocks it. However, the membrane depolarization that occurs in response to high-frequency tetanic stimulation of the presynaptic neuron is sufficient to expel the Mg^{2+} from the NMDA receptor, allowing the influx of Ca^{2+} into the postsynaptic neuron. This leads to activation of Ca^{2+}/calmodulin kinase, protein kinase C, and tyrosine kinase which together induce LTP. The Ca^{2+}/calmodulin kinase phosphorylates the AMPA receptors, increasing their conductance, and moves more of these receptors into the synaptic cell membrane from cytoplasmic storage sites. In addition, once LTP is induced, a chemical signal (possibly nitric oxide, NO) is released by the postsynaptic neuron and passes retrogradely to the presynaptic neuron, producing a long-term increase in the quantal release of glutamate.

LONG-TERM MEMORY

Long-term memories are stored in various parts of the neocortex. The various parts of the memories (visual, olfactory, auditory, etc) are located in the cortical regions concerned with these functions. These pieces are tied together by long-term changes in the strength of transmission at relevant synaptic junctions so that all the components are brought to consciousness when the memory is recalled. Once long-term memories have been established, they can be recalled by many associations. For example, the memory of a vivid scene can be evoked not only by a similar scene but also by a sound or smell associated with the scene. Many memories have an emotional component (pleasant or unpleasant).

STRANGENESS & FAMILIARITY

The occurrence of a sense of familiarity or a sense of strangeness in appropriate situations may help an individual adjust to the environment. In strange surroundings, one is alert and on guard, whereas in familiar surroundings, vigilance is relaxed. An inappropriate feeling of familiarity with new events or in new surroundings is known clinically as the déjà vu phenomenon, from the French words meaning "already seen." The phenomenon occurs from time to time in healthy individuals, but it also may occur as an aura (a sensation immediately preceding a seizure) in patients with temporal lobe epilepsy.

ALZHEIMER DISEASE & SENILE DEMENTIA

Alzheimer disease is the most common age-related neurodegenerative disorder. Memory decline initially manifests as a loss of episodic memory for recent events and is followed by general loss of cognitive and other brain functions, agitation, depression, the need for constant care, and, eventually, death. **Clinical Box 15–2** describes the etiology and therapeutic strategies for the treatment of Alzheimer disease. The cytopathologic hallmarks of Alzheimer disease are intracellular neurofibrillary tangles, made up in part of hyperphosphorylated forms of the tau protein that normally binds to microtubules, and extracellular amyloid plaques, which have a core of β-amyloid peptides surrounded by altered nerve fibers and reactive glial cells (**Figure 15–2**).

The β-amyloid peptides are products of APP, a normal transmembrane protein that projects into the extracellular fluid from neurons. This protein is hydrolyzed at three sites by α-secretase, β-secretase, and γ-secretase, respectively. When APP is hydrolyzed by α-secretase, it produces nontoxic peptide products. However, when it is hydrolyzed by β-secretase and γ-secretase, polypeptides with 40–42 amino acids are produced; the actual length varies depending on the site at which γ-secretase cuts the protein chain. These polypeptides are toxic; the most toxic is $A\beta\sigma^{1-42}$. The polypeptides form extracellular aggregates, which can stick to AMPA receptors and Ca^{2+} ion channels, increasing

---

CLINICAL BOX 15–2

Alzheimer Disease

Both genetic and environmental factors contribute to the etiology of Alzheimer disease. Risk factors for the development of Alzheimer disease include genetic mutations in apolipoprotein E4 allele (ApoE4), amyloid precursor protein (APP, chromosome 21), presenilin (PS-1, chromosome 14), PS-2 (chromosome 1), and Down syndrome (trisomy 21). Environmental factors include low education level, head trauma, prions, toxins, and viruses. Most cases are sporadic, but a familial form accounts for about 5% of the cases and is seen in an early-onset form of the disease. It is transmitted in an autosomal dominant mode, so offspring in the same generation have a 50/50 chance of developing familial Alzheimer disease if one of their parents is affected. Genetic mutations lead to an overproduction of the β-amyloid protein found in neuritic plaques. Senile dementia can be caused by vascular disease and other disorders, but Alzheimer disease is the most common cause, accounting for 50–60% of the cases. The most common risk factor for developing Alzheimer disease is age. This neurodegenerative disease is present in 8–17% of the population over the age of 65, with the incidence increasing steadily with age (nearly doubling every 5 years after reaching the age of 60). In those who are 95 years of age and older, the incidence is 40–50%. It is estimated that by the year 2050,

up to 16 million people age 65 and older in the United States will have Alzheimer disease. Although the prevalence of the disease appears to be higher in women, this may be due to their longer life span as the incidence rates are similar for men and women.

THERAPEUTIC HIGHLIGHTS

Research is aimed at identifying strategies to prevent the occurrence, delay the onset, slow the progression, or alleviate the symptoms of Alzheimer disease. The use of acetylcholinesterase inhibitors (eg, donepezil) in early stages of the disease increases the availability of acetylcholine in the synaptic cleft. This class of drugs has shown some promise in ameliorating global cognitive dysfunction, but not learning and memory impairments in these patients. These drugs also delay the worsening of symptoms for up to 12 months in about half of the cases studied. Memantine (an NMDA receptor antagonist) prevents glutamate-induced excitotoxicity in the brain and is used to treat moderate to severe Alzheimer disease. It delays but does not prevent worsening of symptoms (eg, loss of memory and confusion).

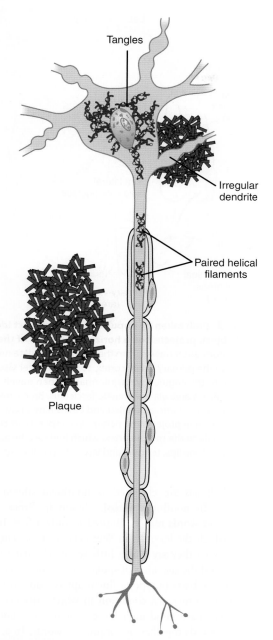

FIGURE 15–2 Abnormalities in a neuron that are associated with Alzheimer disease. The cytopathologic hallmarks are intracellular neurofibrillary tangles, extracellular amyloid plaques that have a core of β-amyloid peptides surrounded by altered nerve fibers and reactive glial cells, and brain atrophy. (Modified with permission from Kandel ER, Schwartz JH, Jessell TM (eds): *Principles of Neural Science*, 5th ed. McGraw-Hill, 2013.)

Ca^{2+} influx. The polypeptides also initiate an inflammatory response with production of intracellular tangles. The damaged cells eventually die, leading to a third characteristic of this brain pathology—atrophy associated with narrowing of the gyri, widening of the sulci, enlargement of the ventricles, and reduction in brain weight.

■ LANGUAGE & SPEECH

There is complementary specialization of the hemispheres, one for sequential-analytic processes and language functions (categorical hemisphere) and one for visuospatial relations (representational hemisphere). Clinical Box 15–3 describes deficits that occur in those with representational or categorical hemisphere lesions.

CLINICAL BOX 15–3

Lesions of Representational & Categorical Hemispheres

Lesions in the categorical hemisphere produce language disorders, and lesions in the representational hemisphere produce astereognosis (inability to identify objects by feeling them) and other agnosias. Agnosia is the inability to recognize objects by a particular sensory modality even though the sensory modality itself is intact. Lesions producing these defects are generally in the parietal lobe. Especially when they are in the representational hemisphere, lesions of the inferior parietal lobule close to the occipital lobe cause unilateral inattention and neglect. Individuals with such lesions ignore stimuli from the contralateral portion of their bodies, leading to failure to care for half their bodies. This inability to put together a picture of visual space on one side is due to a shift in visual attention to the side of the brain lesion and can be improved by wearing eyeglasses that contain prisms. Patients with lesions in the categorical hemisphere are disturbed about their disability and often depressed, whereas patients with lesions in the representational hemisphere are sometimes unconcerned and even euphoric. Lesions of different parts of the categorical hemisphere produce fluent, nonfluent, and anomic aphasias. Although aphasias are produced by lesions of the categorical hemisphere, lesions in the representational hemisphere also have effects. For example, they may impair the ability to tell a story or make a joke. They may also impair a subject's ability to comprehend the meaning of differences in inflection and the "color" of speech.

THERAPEUTIC HIGHLIGHTS

Treatments for agnosia and aphasia are symptomatic and supportive. Individuals with agnosia can be taught exercises to help them identify objects that are a necessity for independence. Therapy for individuals with aphasia helps them use remaining language abilities, compensate for language problems, and learn other methods of communicating. Factors that influence the degree of improvement include the cause and extent of the brain damage, the area of the brain that was damaged, and the age and health of the individual. Computer-assisted therapies improve retrieval of certain parts of speech as well as allowing an alternative way to communicate.

Hemispheric specialization is related to handedness which is genetically determined. In 96% of right-handed individuals (91% of the human population), the left hemisphere is the dominant or categorical hemisphere; in the other 4%, the right hemisphere is dominant. In ~15% of left-handed individuals, the right hemisphere is the categorical hemisphere and in 15%, there is no clear lateralization. However, in 70% of left-handers, the left hemisphere is the categorical hemisphere. Learning disabilities such as **dyslexia** (Clinical Box 15–4), an impaired ability to learn to read, are 12 times more common in left-handers than in right-handers. However, the spatial talents of left-handers may be well above average; a disproportionately large number of artists, musicians, and mathematicians are left-handed.

The primary brain areas concerned with language are near the sylvian fissure (lateral cerebral sulcus) of the categorical hemisphere. A region at the posterior end of the superior temporal gyrus (Wernicke area) is concerned with comprehension of auditory and visual information. It projects via the arcuate fasciculus to the Broca area in front of the inferior end of the motor cortex. Broca area processes the information received from Wernicke area into a detailed and coordinated pattern for vocalization and then projects the pattern via a speech articulation area in the insula to the motor cortex. This then initiates the appropriate movements of the lips, tongue, and larynx to produce speech. Figure 15–3 shows the probable sequence of events that occurs when a subject names a visual object. The angular gyrus behind Wernicke area processes information from words that are read in such a way that they can be converted into the auditory forms of the words.

Aphasias are abnormalities of language functions that are caused by lesions in the categorical hemisphere (Clinical Box 15–3). The most common cause is embolism or thrombosis of a cerebral

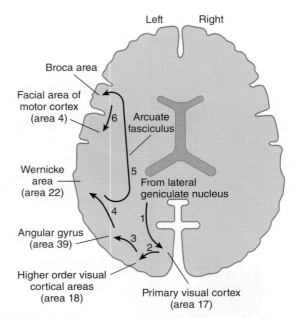

FIGURE 15–3 Path taken by impulses when a subject identifies a visual object, projected on a horizontal section of the human brain. Information travels from the lateral geniculate nucleus in the thalamus to the primary visual cortex, to higher order visual critical areas, and to the angular gyrus. Information then travels from Wernicke area to Broca area via the arcuate fasciculus. Broca area processes the information into a detailed and coordinated pattern for vocalization and then projects the pattern via a speech articulation area in the insula to the motor cortex, which initiates the appropriate movements of the lips, tongue, and larynx to produce speech.

blood vessel. Aphasias are classified as nonfluent, fluent, and anomic aphasias. In nonfluent aphasia (lesion in Broca area), speech is slow, and words may be limited to only a few. In fluent aphasia in which the lesion is in Wernicke area, patients talk excessively, but what they say makes little sense. The patient also fails to comprehend the meaning of spoken or written words.

In conduction aphasia (a type of fluent aphasia due to lesions near the auditory cortex) is a condition in which patients speak relatively well and have good auditory comprehension but cannot put parts of words together or conjure up words. In anomic aphasia (lesion of the angular gyrus in the categorical hemisphere without affecting Wernicke or Broca areas), there is trouble understanding written language or pictures, because visual information is not processed and transmitted to Wernicke area.

CHAPTER SUMMARY

- Memory is either explicit (declarative) or implicit (nondeclarative). Explicit is divided into semantic and episodic. Implicit is divided into priming, procedural, associative learning, and nonassociative learning.
- Declarative memory involves the hippocampus and the medial temporal lobe for retention. Priming is dependent on the neocortex. Procedural memory is processed in the striatum.

CLINICAL BOX 15–4

Dyslexia

Dyslexia, which is a broad term applied to impaired ability to read, is characterized by difficulties with learning how to decode at the word level, to spell, and to read accurately and fluently despite having a normal or even higher than normal level of intelligence. It is often due to an inherited abnormality that affects 5% of the population with a similar incidence in boys and girls. Dyslexia is the most common and prevalent learning disability. It often coexists with attention deficit disorder. Many individuals with dyslexic symptoms also have problems with short-term memory skills and problems processing spoken language. Acquired dyslexia is often due to brain damage in the language area of the left hemisphere and a decreased blood flow in the angular gyrus in the categorical hemisphere. Treatments for children with dyslexia frequently rely on modified teaching strategies that include the involvement of various senses (hearing, vision, and touch) to improve reading skills. The sooner the diagnosis is made and interventions are applied, the better the prognosis.

Associative learning requires the amygdala for emotional responses and the cerebellum for motor responses. Nonassociative learning uses various reflex pathways.

- Synaptic plasticity is the ability of neural tissue to change as reflected by LTP (an increased effectiveness of synaptic activity) or LTD (a reduced effectiveness of synaptic activity) after continued use. Habituation is a simple form of learning in which a neutral stimulus is repeated many times. Sensitization is the prolonged occurrence of augmented postsynaptic responses after a stimulus to which one has become habituated is paired once or several times with a noxious stimulus.

- Alzheimer disease is characterized by progressive loss of short-term memory followed by general loss of cognitive function. The cytopathologic hallmarks of Alzheimer disease are intracellular neurofibrillary tangles and extracellular amyloid plaques.

- Categorical and representational hemispheres are for sequential-analytic processes and visuospatial relations, respectively. Lesions in the categorical hemisphere produce language disorders; lesions in the representational hemisphere produce astereognosis.

- Aphasias are abnormalities of language functions caused by lesions in the categorical hemisphere. They are classified as fluent (Wernicke area), nonfluent (Broca area), and anomic (angular gyrus) based on the location of brain lesions.

MULTIPLE-CHOICE QUESTIONS

For all questions, select the single best answer unless otherwise directed.

1. A 27-year-old man suffered a traumatic brain injury as a result of a motorcycle accident. He was unconscious and was rushed to the emergency department of the local hospital. A CT scan was performed and appropriate interventions were taken. About 6 months later he still had memory deficits. Specifically, he could no longer facilitate the recognition of words by prior exposure to them. What type of memory is this and what part of the brain is likely to have been damaged by the traumatic brain injury?
   A. Episodic memory and hippocampus
   B. Priming memory and neocortex
   C. Associative learning and amygdala
   D. Semantic memory and medial temporal lobe
   E. Procedural memory and striatum

2. A 25-year-old man who was not wearing a helmet was in a motorcycle accident. He was rushed to the emergency department of the local hospital where it was determined that he had a traumatic brain injury. Based on the Glasgow Coma Scale, the trauma was defined as being moderate to severe. Which of the following symptoms are consistent with this level of traumatic brain injury?
   A. Problems with memory, concentration, or thinking
   B. Fatigue, sleep disturbances, and mood changes
   C. Convulsions or seizures, an inability to be roused, and fixed and dilated pupils
   D. A permanent vegetative state
   E. Slurred speech, limb weakness, loss of coordination, and increased confusion

3. A 32-year-old man had medial temporal lobe epilepsy for over 10 years. This caused bilateral loss of hippocampal function. As a result, this individual might be expected to experience a

   A. disappearance of remote memories.
   B. loss of working memory.
   C. loss of the ability to encode events of the recent past into long-term memory.
   D. loss of the ability to recall faces and forms but not the ability to recall printed or spoken words.
   E. production of inappropriate emotional responses when recalling events of the recent past.

4. A 70-year-old woman fell down a flight of stairs, hitting her head on the concrete sidewalk. The trauma caused a severe intracranial hemorrhage resulting in brain damage. Following this injury, she seemed to ignore her left side; for example, she would only wash the right side of her body or only put a shoe on her right foot. What area of the brain was most likely damaged as a result of this fall down the stairs?
   A. Inferior parietal lobe of the representational hemisphere
   B. Nucleus basalis of Meynert and related areas of the forebrain
   C. Mammillary bodies
   D. Angular gyrus in the categorical hemisphere
   E. Parietal lobe of the categorical hemisphere

5. A 65-year-old woman with long-standing, uncontrolled hypertension developed a cerebral aneurysm that caused damage to the angular gyrus in her categorical hemisphere without affecting Wernicke or Broca areas. Which of the following symptoms is she likely to develop as a result of damage to this region of the brain?
   A. The inability to identify objects by feeling them
   B. Impaired ability to tell a story or make a joke
   C. Speech that is full of jargon and neologisms that make little sense
   D. Slowed speech, use of very few words
   E. Trouble understanding written language or pictures

6. A medical student wanted to join a laboratory that studied differences between the functions of the categorical and representational hemispheres. In an effort to prepare for this experience, she did some reading and learned that the representational hemisphere is better than the categorical hemisphere at
   A. expressing ideas in speech and writing and recognizing faces.
   B. identifying objects by their form and recognizing faces.
   C. understanding printed words and expressing ideas in speech.
   D. understanding spoken words and recognizing objects by their form.
   E. making mathematical calculations and recognizing musical themes.

7. A medical student wanted to join a laboratory that studied differences between the functions of the categorical and representational hemispheres. In an effort to prepare for this experience, she did some reading to find out how hemispheric specialization is related to handedness. She would have learned the following from these readings.
   A. In 96% of right-handed individuals, the left hemisphere is the categorical hemisphere; and in 70% of left-handed individuals, the left hemisphere is the categorical hemisphere.
   B. In 96% of right-handed individuals, the right hemisphere is the categorical hemisphere; and in 70% of

left-handed individuals, the right hemisphere is the categorical hemisphere.

C.   In 96% of right-handed individuals, the left hemisphere is the representational hemisphere; and in 70% of left-handed individuals, the left hemisphere is the representational hemisphere.

D.   In 96% of right-handed individuals, the left hemisphere is the categorical hemisphere; and in 15% of left-handed individuals, the left hemisphere is the categorical hemisphere.

E.   In 96% of right-handed individuals, the left hemisphere is the representational hemisphere; and in 15% of left-handed individuals, the right hemisphere is the categorical hemisphere.

8.   A 67-year-old woman suffered a stroke that damaged the posterior end of the superior temporal gyrus on the left side of her brain. A lesion of Wernicke area in this region of her categorical hemisphere will likely cause her to
A.   lose her short-term memory.
B.   experience nonfluent aphasia in which she speaks in a slow, halting voice.
C.   experience déjà vu.
D.   talk rapidly but make little sense, which is characteristic of fluent aphasia.
E.   lose the ability to recognize faces, which is called prosopagnosia.

9.   An MD/PhD candidate was doing her doctoral research on the role of long-term potentiation (LTP) in the connection between a pyramidal cell in the CA3 region and a pyramidal cell in the CA1 region via the Schaffer collateral. Which of the following factors likely contribute to the production of LTP in this synapse?
A.   Binding of glutamate to NMDA and AMPA receptors, membrane hyperpolarization, and activation of Ca^{2+}/calmodulin kinase, protein kinase C, and tyrosine kinase
B.   Activation of non-NMDA receptors, membrane depolarization, and efflux of Ca^{2+} from the postsynaptic neuron
C.   Activation of NMDA but not non-NMDA receptors, membrane depolarization, and an efflux of Ca^{2+} from the postsynaptic neuron
D.   Activation of AMPA receptors, membrane depolarization, and activation of Ca^{2+}/calmodulin kinase, protein kinase C, and tyrosine kinase
E.   Activation of NMDA receptors, membrane hyperpolarization, and deactivation of Ca^{2+}/calmodulin kinase

10.   A 79-year-old woman has been experiencing difficulty finding her way back home after her morning walks. Her husband has also noted that she takes much longer to do routine chores around the home and often appears to be confused. He is hoping that this is just due to "old age" but fears it may be a sign of Alzheimer disease. Which of the following are the definitive signs of this disease?
A.   Loss of short-term memory, inability to form new long-term memories, and depression
B.   The presence of intracellular neurofibrillary tangles and extracellular neuritic plaques with a core of β-amyloid peptides and brain atrophy
C.   A mutation in genes for amyloid precursor protein (APP) on chromosome 21 and the presence of intracellular neurofibrillary tangles and extracellular amyloid plaques

D.   The inability to form new long-term memories, rapid reversal of all symptoms with the use of acetylcholinesterase inhibitors, and brain atrophy
E.   A loss of cholinergic neurons in the nucleus basalis of Meynert, rapid reversal of symptoms with the use of acetylcholinesterase inhibitors, and brain atrophy

11.   A 63-year-old man was hospitalized after having an ischemic stroke. In the days following the stroke it was evident that he had difficulty expressing himself in both oral and written forms of communication; and he had difficulty reading. What type of aphasia does he likely have, and what part of his brain was likely damaged by the stroke?
A.   Global aphasia, Broca's area
B.   Conduction aphasia, posterior perisylvian gyrus
C.   Conduction aphasia, arcuate fasciculus
D.   Global aphasia, perisylvian cortex
E.   Anomic aphasia, CA1 neurons in the hippocampus

12.   A 6-year-old boy with above average intelligence had difficulty reading because he was unable to decode at the word level, to spell, and to read accurately. What is the likely diagnosis and what other disorder often coexists in these individuals?
A.   Global aphasia, temporal lobe epilepsy
B.   Conduction aphasia, temporal lobe epilepsy
C.   Dyslexia, attention deficit disorder
D.   Anomic aphasia, stuttering
E.   Dyslexia, stuttering

ANSWERS

1.   The best answer is **B.** Priming is a subtype of implicit or nondeclarative memory; it refers to the facilitation of the recognition of words or objects by prior exposure to them and is dependent on the neocortex. Episodic (for events) and semantic (for words) memory are subtypes of explicit (declarative) memory for factual knowledge about people, places, and things and is dependent on the hippocampus and other parts of the medial temporal lobes for retention (rules out options **A** and **D**). Associative learning relates to classical and operant conditioning in which one learns about the relationship between one stimulus and another; it is dependent on the amygdala for its emotional responses and the cerebellum for the motor responses (rules out option **C**). Procedural memory includes skills and habits, which, once acquired, become unconscious and automatic; it is processed in the striatum (rules out option **E**).

2.   The best answer is **C.** Individuals with moderate to severe traumatic brain injury show the following symptoms vomiting or nausea, convulsions or seizures, an inability to be roused, fixed and dilated pupils, slurred speech, limb weakness, loss of coordination, and increased confusion, restlessness, or agitation. Symptoms of mild traumatic brain injury include headache, confusion, dizziness, blurred vision, ringing in the ears, a bad taste in the mouth, fatigue, disturbances in sleep, mood changes, and problems with memory, concentration, or thinking (rules out options **A, B,** and **E**). In the most severe cases of traumatic brain injury, the affected individual may go into a permanent vegetative state (rules out option **D**).

3.   The best answer is **C.** The hippocampus is important for conversion of short-term memory to long-term memory. Remote memory, the ability to recall events from the distant

past, is retained after damage to the hippocampus, but the anatomical region involved in remote memory is uncertain (rules out option **A**). The prefrontal cortex is important for working memory which is a type of short-term memory that keeps information available for very short periods of time while the individual plans action based on it (rules out option **B**). An important part of the visual input goes to the inferior temporal lobe, where representations of objects, particularly faces, are stored (rules out option **D**). Emotional responses are mediated via the amygdala (rules out option **E**).

4. The best answer is **A**. A lesion of the inferior parietal lobe of the representational hemisphere causes unilateral inattention and neglect on the side contralateral to the lesion. A lesion of the nucleus basalis of Meynert and related areas of the forebrain occurs in Alzheimer disease (rules out option **B**). Damage to the mammillary bodies is associated with impairment of recent memory (rules out option **C**). A lesion that damages the angular gyrus in the categorical hemisphere leads to anomic aphasia (rules out option **D**). A lesion of the inferior parietal lobe of the categorical hemisphere causes dysphasia, apraxia, agnosia, and dyslexia (rules out option **E**).

5. The best answer is **E**. When a lesion damages the angular gyrus in the categorical hemisphere without affecting Wernicke or Broca areas, the individual may develop anomic aphasia characterized by trouble understanding written language or pictures, because visual information is not processed and transmitted to Wernicke area. Damage to the representational hemisphere can lead to the inability to identify objects by feeling them or the inability to tell a story or make a joke (rules out options **A** and **B**). A lesion in Wernicke area of the categorical hemisphere can result in fluent aphasia in which speech is full of jargon and neologisms that make little sense (rules out option **C**). A lesion in Broca area of the categorical hemisphere can result in nonfluent aphasia in which speech is slow and words are hard to come by (rules out option **D**).

6. The best answer is **B**. The representational hemisphere specializes in the identification of objects by their form, the recognition of musical themes, and the recognition of faces. The categorical hemisphere specializes in the understanding of the spoken and printed word, expressing ideas in speech and writing, and making mathematical calculations (rules out options **A, C, D,** and **E**).

7. The best answer is **A**. In 96% of right-handed individuals, which constitutes 91% of the population, the left hemisphere is the dominant or categorical hemisphere; and in the remaining 4%, the right hemisphere is dominant. In about 15% of left-handed individuals, the right hemisphere is the categorical hemisphere and in 15%, there is no clear lateralization. However, in the remaining 70% of left-handers, the left hemisphere is the categorical hemisphere. This explanation rules out options **B, C, D,** and **E**.

8. The best answer is **D**. Damage to Wernicke area in the categorical hemisphere can cause one to talk rapidly but make little sense, which is characteristic of fluent aphasia. Damage to CA1 neurons in the hippocampus cause loss of short-term memory (rules out option **A**). A lesion in Broca area of the categorical hemisphere can result in the development of a nonfluent aphasia in which she might speak in a slow, halting voice (rules out option **B**). An inappropriate feeling of familiarity with new events or in new surroundings is known clinically as the déjà vu phenomenon; it can occur in healthy individuals, but it also may occur as an aura (a sensation immediately preceding a seizure) in patients with temporal lobe epilepsy (rules out option **C**). Damage to the right inferior temporal lobe can cause prosopagnosia, the inability to recognize faces (rules out option **E**).

9. The best answer is **D**. At the resting membrane potential, glutamate release from a presynaptic neuron binds to both NMDA and non-NMDA receptors on the postsynaptic neuron. In the case of the Schaffer collateral the non-NMDA receptor is the α-amino-3-hydroxy-5-methylisoxazole-4 propionic acid (AMPA) receptor. Na^+ and K^- can flow only through the AMPA receptor because the presence of Mg^{2+} on the NMDA receptor blocks it. However, the membrane depolarization that occurs in response to high frequency tetanic stimulation of the presynaptic neuron is sufficient to expel the Mg^{2+} from the NMDA receptor, allowing the influx of Ca^{2+} into the postsynaptic neuron. This leads to activation of Ca^{2+}/calmodulin kinase, protein kinase C, and tyrosine kinase which together induce LTP. LTP does not involve membrane hyperpolarization, an efflux of Ca^{2+} from the postsynaptic neuron, or deactivation of Ca^{2+}/calmodulin kinase (rules out options **A, B, C,** and **E**).

10. The best answer is **B**. The cytopathologic hallmarks of Alzheimer disease are intracellular neurofibrillary tangles, comprised of tau proteins that normally bind to microtubules, and extracellular amyloid plaques with a core of β-amyloid peptides that are products of a normal protein, amyloid precursor protein (APP). When APP is hydrolyzed by β-secretase and γ-secretase, toxic polypeptides are produced, the most toxic being $A\beta\sigma^{1-42}$. The polypeptides form extracellular aggregates, which can stick to AMPA receptors and Ca^{2+} ion channels, increasing Ca^{2+} influx. The polypeptides also initiate an inflammatory response, with production of intracellular tangles. The damaged cells eventually die, leading to a third characterization of the brain pathology in individuals with this neurodegenerative disease, atrophy associated with narrowing of the gyri, widening of the sulci, enlargement of the ventricles, and reduction in brain weight. Although other symptoms (eg, loss of short-term memory, inability to form new long-term memories, and depression occur in Alzheimer disease, these symptoms are not specifically diagnostic for it (rules out options **A** and **D**). A mutation in genes for amyloid precursor protein (APP) on chromosome 21 can lead to the development of Alzheimer disease, but is not involved in all cases (rules out option **C**). Treatment with acetylcholinesterase inhibitors has shown some promise in ameliorating global cognitive dysfunction, but not learning and memory impairments in these patients (rules out **D**). A loss of cholinergic neurons in the nucleus basalis of Meynert is contributory but not a hallmark of this disease (rules out **E**).

11. The best answer is **D**. Global aphasia involves loss of both receptive and expressive functions and is due to damage of a large area of the brain in the perisylvian cortex, including frontal, temporal, and parietal lobes. These individuals have an impairment of both comprehension and expression of language; they are unable to say or understand more than a few words and are unable to read or write. Damage restricted to Broca's area would lead to the development of a nonfluent aphasia (rules out option **A**). Conduction aphasia results from damage near the auditory cortex in the posterior perisylvian gyrus; it was formerly thought to be due to lesion of the arcuate fasciculus connecting the Wernicke and Broca areas. With

conduction aphasia, patients can speak relatively well and have good auditory comprehension but cannot put parts of words together or conjure up words (rules out options **B** and **C**). Damage to CA1 neurons in the hippocampus cause loss of short-term memory not speech and language impairments (rules out option **E**).

12. The best answer is **C**. Dyslexia, which is a broad term applied to impaired ability to read, is characterized by difficulties with learning how to decode at the word level, to spell, and to

read accurately and fluently despite having a normal or even higher than normal level of intelligence. It is frequently due to an inherited abnormality that affects 5% of the population with a similar incidence in boys and girls. Dyslexia is the most common and prevalent of all known learning disabilities. It often coexists with attention deficit disorder but not stuttering (rules out option **E**). See the response to Question 11 for explanations of the impairments experienced by individuals with various aphasias (rules out options **A, B,** and **D**).

SECTION III ENDOCRINE & REPRODUCTIVE PHYSIOLOGY

The role of the endocrine system is to maintain whole body homeostasis. This is accomplished via the coordination of hormonal signaling pathways that regulate cellular activity in target organs. Classic **endocrine glands** are scattered throughout the body and secrete **hormones** into the circulatory system. **Target organs** express receptors that bind the specific hormone to initiate a cellular response. The endocrine system can be contrasted with the neural regulation of physiologic function that was the focus of the previous section. Endocrine effectors typically provide "broadcast" regulation of multiple tissues and organs simultaneously, with specificity provided for by the expression of relevant receptors. Neural regulation, on the other hand, is often exquisitely spatially delimited. Nevertheless, both systems must work collaboratively to allow for minute-to-minute as well as longer term stability of the body's interior milieu.

Hormones are the soluble messengers of the endocrine system and are classified into steroids, peptides, and amines (see Chapters 1 and 2). Steroid hormones can cross the lipid-containing plasma membrane of cells and usually bind to intracellular receptors. Peptide and amine hormones bind to cell surface receptors. The majority of hormones are peptides and usually synthesized as preprohormones before being cleaved first to prohormones in the endoplasmic reticulum and then to the active hormone in secretory vesicles.

Endocrine and metabolic disorders are among the most common afflictions in developed countries. At least 11 endocrine and metabolic disorders are present in 5% or more of the adult US population, including diabetes mellitus, osteopenia, dyslipidemia, metabolic syndrome, and thyroiditis. In large part, the high and increasing prevalence of diabetes and other metabolic disorders may be related to the substantial prevalence of obesity in developed countries. Overall, the burden of endocrine and metabolic disorders, with their protean manifestations and complications, is a serious public health crisis.

Basic Concepts of Endocrine Regulation

- Describe hormones and their contribution to whole body homeostasis.
- Understand the chemical nature of different classes of hormones and how this determines their mechanism of action.
- Define how hormones are synthesized and secreted.
- Explain the relevance of protein carriers in the blood for hydrophobic hormones, and the mechanisms that determine the level of free circulating hormones.
- Understand the principles of feedback control for hormone release and its relevance for homeostasis.
- Understand disease states that result from over- or underproduction of key hormones.

INTRODUCTION

This section of the text deals with the various endocrine glands that control the function of multiple organ systems of the body. In general, endocrine physiology is concerned with the maintenance of **homeostasis**. The mediators of such control mechanisms are soluble factors known as **hormones**. In preparation for specific discussions of the various endocrine systems and their hormones, this chapter addresses common concepts of endocrine regulation.

■ EVOLUTION OF HORMONES & THEIR ACTIONS ON TARGET CELLS

Many hormones can be grouped into families reflecting their structural similarities as well as the similarities of the receptors they activate. The number of hormones and their diversity increases as one moves from simple to higher life forms. This molecular evolution implies that hormone receptors also needed to evolve to allow for spreading of hormone actions/specificity. This was accomplished by coevolution of the G-protein–coupled receptors (GPCR) and receptor tyrosine kinases that mediate the effects of peptide and amine hormones that act at the cell surface (see Chapter 2).

Steroids and thyroid hormones are distinguished by their predominantly intracellular sites of action, since they can diffuse freely through the cell membrane. They bind to a family of largely cytoplasmic proteins known as nuclear receptors. Upon ligand binding, the receptor–ligand complex translocates to the nucleus. The complex binds to DNA to either increase or decrease gene transcription in the target tissue. Individual members of the nuclear receptor family have a considerable degree of homology and share many functional domains, such as the zinc fingers that permit DNA binding. However, sequence variations allow for ligand specificity as well as binding to specific DNA motifs. In this way, the transcription of distinct genes is regulated by individual hormones.

■ HORMONE SECRETION

SYNTHESIS & PROCESSING

For peptide hormones as well as hormone receptors, synthesis is controlled predominantly at the level of transcription. For amine and steroid hormones, synthesis is controlled indirectly by regulating the production of key synthetic enzymes as well as by substrate availability.

The majority of peptide hormones are synthesized initially as much larger polypeptide chains, and then processed intracellularly by specific proteases to yield the final hormone molecule. The hormone precursors themselves are typically inactive. This may provide for an additional measure of regulatory control, or dictate the site of highest hormone availability.

The synthesis of all of the proteins/peptides discussed above is subject to the normal mechanisms of transcriptional control (see Chapter 2). In addition, there is provision for specific regulation by other hormones, since the regulatory regions of many peptide hormone genes contain binding motifs for nuclear receptors. These mechanisms are essential to the function of feedback loops. In some cases, the abundance of selected hormones may also be regulated via effects on translation, allowing for more precise and timely regulation of hormone levels than could be accomplished with transcriptional regulation alone.

Peptide hormone precursors are processed through the cellular machinery for exported proteins, including trafficking through specific vesicles where the propeptide form can be cleaved to the final active hormones. Mature hormones are also subjected to posttranslational processing, which can influence their biologic activity and/or stability.

SECRETION

Many hormones are secreted by exocytosis, as discussed in Chapter 2. Exocytosis is activated when the cell type that synthesizes the hormone is activated by a specific signal, such as a neurotransmitter or peptide releasing factor. Other hormones are continually released by diffusion (eg, steroids). Their secretion is influenced by regulation of their synthetic enzymes or carrier proteins.

Some hormones are secreted in a pulsatile manner, with secretion rates that peak and ebb relative to circadian rhythms, in response to the timing of meals, or other pattern generators whose periodicity may range from milliseconds to years. Pulsatile secretion is often related to the activity of oscillators in the hypothalamus that trigger bursts of hormone releasing factors in the hypophysial blood flow that then cause the release of pituitary and other downstream hormones in a similar pulsatile manner (see Chapters 17 and 18). Hormone pulses convey different information compared to steady exposure to a single concentration of the hormone.

■ HORMONE TRANSPORT IN THE BLOOD

In addition to the rate of secretion and its nature (steady vs pulsatile), a number of factors influence the circulating levels of hormones. These include the rates of hormone degradation and/or uptake, receptor binding and availability of receptors, and the affinity of a given hormone for plasma carriers (Figure 16–1).

Plasma carriers for specific hormones have a number of important physiologic functions. First, they serve as a reservoir of

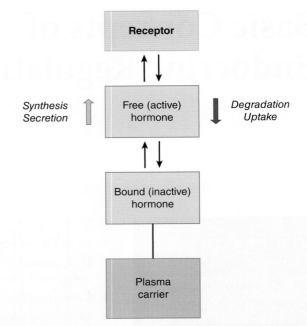

FIGURE 16–1 Summary of factors that determine the level of free hormones circulating in the bloodstream. Factors that increase (green upward arrow) or decrease (red downward arrow) hormone levels are shown. Free hormones also equilibrate with the forms bound to either receptors or plasma carrier proteins.

inactive hormone since bound hormones are typically prevented from degradation or uptake. This bound hormone reservoir smooths fluctuations in hormonal levels over time. Plasma carriers also restrict the access of the hormone to some sites. Typically, it is only the free hormone that is biologically active in target tissues or can mediate feedback regulation (see below).

Catecholamine and most peptide hormones are soluble in plasma and are transported as such. In contrast, steroid hormones are hydrophobic and are mostly bound to large proteins called **steroid binding proteins**, which are synthesized in the liver. As a result, only small amounts of the free hormone are dissolved in the plasma. The SBP-hormone complex and the free hormone are in equilibrium in the plasma, and only the free hormone is able to diffuse across cell membranes.

In a pathophysiologic setting, some medications can alter levels of binding proteins or displace hormones that are bound to them. In addition, some binding proteins are promiscuous and bind multiple hormones.

Finally, the relationship of the sites of release and action of hormones may play a key role in their regulation. For example, hormones may be destroyed by passage through the pulmonary circulation or the liver.

■ HORMONE ACTION

Hormones exert a wide range of actions such as changes in metabolism, release of other hormones and regulatory substances, changes in ion channel activity, and cell growth, among others

Breast Cancer

Breast cancer is the most common malignancy of women. The majority of breast tumors proliferate in response to estrogen because they express high levels of posttranslationally modified estrogen receptors (ER). The clinical significance of these molecular findings has been known for more than 100 years, since Sir Thomas Beatson reported delayed breast cancer progression following removal of the ovaries. In modern times, determination of whether a given breast cancer is, or is not, **ER-positive** is a critical diagnostic test. ER-positive tumors are typically of lower grade, and patients with such tumors have improved survival (although the latter is likely due, at least in part, to the availability of excellent treatment options for ER-positive tumors).

THERAPEUTIC HIGHLIGHTS

Estrogen-responsive breast tumors are dependent on the hormone for growth. Cells can be deprived of the effects of estrogen pharmacologically using **tamoxifen** and related agents that inhibit the ER and may also hasten its degradation. In postmenopausal women, where estrogen is derived from the metabolism of testosterone in extragonadal tissues rather than from the ovaries, **aromatase inhibitors** inhibit the conversion of androgens to estrogen, and thereby deprive tumor cells of their signal for proliferation.

(Clinical Box 16–1). Ultimately, the concerted action of the hormones of the body ensures the maintenance of homeostasis. A subset of the hormones, including thyroid hormone, cortisol, parathyroid hormone, vasopressin, the mineralocorticoids, and insulin, are the key contributors to homeostasis (Table 16–1).

■ PRINCIPLES OF FEEDBACK CONTROL

A final general principle that is critical for endocrine physiology is that of **feedback regulation**. This holds that the responsiveness of target cells to hormonal action subsequently "feeds back" to control the inciting endocrine organ. Feedback can regulate the further release of the hormone in either a negative feedback or (much more rarely) a positive feedback loop. Negative feedback involves the inhibition or dampening of the initial hormone release mechanism/stimulus, and serves to maintain a steady state. A general scheme for feedback inhibition of endocrine axes is depicted in **Figure 16–2**.

TABLE 16–1 Major hormonal contributors to homeostasis.

Hormone	Source	Action
Thyroid hormone	Thyroid	Controls basal metabolism in most tissues
Cortisol	Adrenal cortex	Energy metabolism; permissive action for other hormones
Mineralocorticoids	Adrenal cortex	Regulate plasma volume via effects on serum electrolytes
Vasopressin	Posterior pituitary	Regulates plasma osmolality via effects on water excretion
Parathyroid hormone	Parathyroids	Regulates calcium and phosphorus levels
Insulin	Pancreas	Regulates plasma glucose concentration

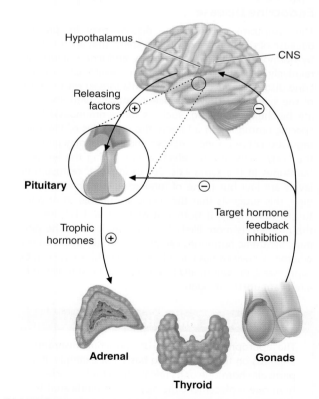

FIGURE 16–2 Summary of feedback loops regulating endocrine axes. CNS, central nervous system. (Reproduced with permission from Jameson JL (ed): *Harrison's Endocrinology*, 2nd ed. New York, NY: McGraw Hill; 2010.)

■ TYPES OF ENDOCRINE DISORDERS

It is pertinent also to discuss briefly the types of disease states where endocrine physiology can become deranged. A general approach to the patient with a suspected endocrine disorder is discussed in Clinical Box 16-2.

HORMONE DEFICIENCY

Deficiencies of particular hormones are most commonly seen in the setting where there is destruction of the glandular structure responsible for their production. Similarly, hormonal deficiencies arise when there are inherited mutations in the factors responsible for their release or in the receptors for these releasing factors. Defects in the enzymatic machinery needed for hormone production, or a lack of appropriate precursors, will also reduce the amount of the relevant hormone available.

CLINICAL BOX 16–2

Approach to the Patient with Suspected Endocrine Disease

The symptoms of endocrine disease may be protean because of the number of body systems that are impacted by hormonal action. Further, many endocrine glands are relatively inaccessible to direct physical examination. Endocrine disorders must therefore be diagnosed on the basis of the symptoms they produce in concert with appropriate biochemical testing, such as radioimmunoassays for specific hormones. In addition, the principles of feedback regulation of hormone synthesis and release may pinpoint the likely locus of any defect by comparing the levels of hormones in the same axis. For example, if testosterone levels are low but those of luteinizing hormone (LH) are high, this suggests that the testes are unable to respond to LH. Conversely, if both testosterone and LH are low, the problem is more likely to be at the level of the pituitary. Synthetic hormones can also be administered to test whether increased basal levels of a given hormone can be suppressed, or abnormally low levels can be stimulated by a relevant upstream agent.

THERAPEUTIC HIGHLIGHTS

The appropriate treatment of endocrine disorders depends on their underlying basis. For example, if a particular hormone or its releasing factor is deficient, hormone replacement therapy is often indicated to ameliorate symptoms as well as long-term negative outcomes.

HORMONE RESISTANCE

Many of the consequences of hormone deficiency can be reproduced in disease states where adequate levels of a given hormone are present, but the target tissues become resistant to the hormone's effects. Indeed, there is often overproduction of the implicated hormone in these conditions because the feedback loops that normally shut off hormone synthesis are similarly desensitized. Mutations in hormone receptors (especially nuclear receptors) may result in heritable syndromes of hormone resistance. Functional hormone resistance that develops over time is also seen. Resistance arises from a relative failure of receptor signaling to couple efficiently to downstream effector pathways. The most common example is type 2 diabetes mellitus.

HORMONE EXCESS

The converse of disorders of hormone deficiency or resistance is seen in diseases associated with hormone excess or overstimulation of hormone receptors (or both). Endocrine tumors may produce hormones in an excessive and uncontrolled manner. In addition, other endocrine tumors may secrete hormones other than those characteristic of the cell type or tissue from which they are originally derived. When hormone production is increased, there usually will also be downregulation of upstream releasing factors due to the triggering of negative feedback loops.

Disorders of hormone excess can also be mimicked by antibodies that bind to, and activate, the receptor for the hormone. Diseases associated with hormone excess can also occur in a heritable manner secondary to activating mutations of hormone releasing factor receptors or their downstream targets. These pathophysiologic triggers of excessive hormone release are not subject to dampening by negative feedback loops.

CHAPTER SUMMARY

- The endocrine system consists of a distributed set of glands and the chemical messengers that they produce, referred to as hormones. Hormones play a critical role in ensuring homeostasis.
- Hormones can be grouped into peptide/protein, amine, and steroid categories. Water-soluble hormones (peptides and catecholamines) bind to cell surface receptors; hydrophobic hormones diffuse into the cell and activate nuclear receptors to regulate gene transcription.
- Hormone availability is dictated by synthesis, releasing factors, and rates of degradation or uptake. Free hydrophobic hormones are also in equilibrium with a form bound to plasma protein carriers, the latter representing a hormone reservoir.
- The synthesis and release of many hormones is subject to regulation by negative feedback loops.
- Disease states can arise in the setting of both hormone deficiency and excess.

MULTIPLE-CHOICE QUESTIONS

For all questions, select the single best answer unless otherwise directed.

1. A 40-year-old woman is referred to an endocrinologist for evaluation of persistent lethargy, diminished mentation, and poor tolerance of cold. She reports that the symptoms began after she was prescribed lithium for bipolar disorder. A physical examination reveals that her thyroid gland is enlarged and a diagnosis of hypothyroidism is made. A blood test substantiates that her T_4 thyroid hormone levels are low, while levels of circulating thyroid stimulating hormone (TSH) are markedly increased. The most likely reason for the increase in TSH is
   A. the presence of a tumor that secretes TSH in an uncontrolled fashion.
   B. the presence of a tumor that secretes thyrotropin releasing hormone (TRH, the hormone that stimulates TSH release from the pituitary).
   C. ingestion of excessive amounts of iodide.
   D. lack of the normal suppressive effect of thyroid hormone on TSH and TRH synthesis and secretion.
   E. a decrease in the levels of plasma proteins that bind thyroid hormone.

2. In the patient described in Question 1, assuming her lithium treatment cannot be discontinued, what is likely to be the most effective treatment to reverse her symptoms of hypothyroidism?
   A. T_4
   B. TRH
   C. TSH
   D. Increased dietary iodide
   E. Surgical removal of her enlarged thyroid gland

3. In a laboratory research project, a mouse is treated with a drug that inhibits the activity of the major enzyme responsible for the catabolism of circulating thyroid hormones. Identify the pattern of changes in TSH, free T_4 and protein-bound T_4 that are most likely to be detected in this animal immediately following the drug treatment:
   A. Increased, increased, increased
   B. Increased, decreased, decreased
   C. Increased, decreased, increased
   D. Decreased, increased, increased
   E. Decreased, increased, decreased

4. A scientist in a drug company is trying to develop a replacement therapy for patients who congenitally lack a specific hormone that is normally secreted by the pituitary gland. She develops a peptide analogue that exerts the expected effect on target cells studied in vitro, and can be shown to be stable in the bloodstream. However, in clinical trials, intravenous infusion of the analogue proves ineffective in treating the consequences of loss of the natural hormone. The most likely reason for this therapeutic failure is as follows:
   A. The analogue fails to bind to cell-surface receptors for the natural hormone.
   B. The analogue is metabolized too rapidly to attain sufficient concentrations in the bloodstream for biologic activity.
   C. Secretion of the analogue is not induced by the appropriate releasing factor from the hypothalamus.
   D. The mode of administration fails to reproduce the normal pulsatile secretion of the natural hormone.
   E. The analogue is not appropriately processed in pituitary gland secretory vesicles.

5. A medical student participating in an ultramarathon decides to avoid drinking during the event, believing that it will enhance his performance. When he collapses and is unable to complete the race, he is noted to be dehydrated with an associated increase in his plasma osmolality and a reduction in urine output. The latter homeostatic response is most directly attributable to which of the following hormones:
   A. Insulin
   B. Vasopressin
   C. Aldosterone
   D. Cortisol
   E. Parathyroid hormone

ANSWERS

1. The best answer is **D.** Thyroid hormone is secreted from the thyroid gland in response to TSH coming from the pituitary, which in turn is released in response to TRH from the hypothalamus. In this patient, symptoms of hypothyroidism are likely due to adverse effects of lithium on thyroid hormone synthesis. The lack of circulating thyroid hormone means that the normal negative feedback that suppresses TSH and TRH release as thyroid hormone levels rise is absent (option **D**). Tumors producing TSH or TRH are unlikely because thyroid hormone levels are low (thus eliminating options **A** and **B**). Ingestion of excessive iodide can inhibit organic iodide binding in the thyroid, but the effects are mild and transient and unlikely to be associated with persistent symptoms or a substantial rise in TSH (eliminating option **C**). Finally, if plasma binding proteins are decreased, levels of free thyroid hormone would be expected to increase, in turn suppressing TSH. Thus, option **E** is not consistent with the clinical picture or the blood test findings.

2. The best answer is **A.** The patient's symptoms stem from a deficiency in circulating thyroid hormone, and can best be treated by replacing this (option **A**). TSH is already elevated, so providing more of this hormone or the factor that stimulates its release from the pituitary (TRH) will not be effective, eliminating options **B** and **C.** Because lithium is thought to directly impair thyroid hormone synthesis, increasing the availability of iodide is unlikely to overcome this (ruling out option **D**). Finally, enlargement of the thyroid gland in this patient likely reflects an effort to adapt to the lack of thyroid hormone synthesis, and perhaps the effects of TSH. However, excision of the gland would remove any residual thyroid hormone production, and thus worsen rather than ameliorate the symptoms (ruling out option **E**).

3. The best answer is **D.** A reduction in thyroid hormone catabolism will acutely increase the quantity of free T_4 in the circulation (ruling out options **B** and **C**), which will also equilibrate with plasma binding proteins to increase the levels of bound T_4 (ruling out options **B** and **E**). An increase in circulating free T_4 will feedback on the pituitary to reduce the synthesis and secretion of TSH (ruling out options **A, B,** and **C**). Thus, by a process of elimination, the only possible option is **D.** Of course, if treatment is continued over a longer time period, a new steady state will likely be reached whereby thyroid secretion is suppressed, secondary to the reduction in TSH levels, to reestablish homeostasis.

4. The best answer is **D.** Because the analogue is designed to be administered exogenously, its response to hypothalamic

releasing factors as well as its processing in pituitary cells are irrelevant, ruling out options **C** and **E**. In addition, it is active in vitro, suggesting that receptor binding is unlikely to be a problem (ruling out option **A**) and the question indicates that it is stable in the circulation, ruling out option **B**. On the other hand, many pituitary hormones are secreted in a pulsatile fashion in response to bursts of releasing factors from the hypothalamus, and the oscillating plasma levels of the hormone that are thereby produced encode different signaling outcomes than steady levels of the hormone such as would be produced by infusion at a constant rate.

5. The best answer is **B**. Insulin and cortisol have no direct effects on urine output, ruling out options **A** and **D**. Parathyroid hormone regulates levels of calcium and phosphorus, but these minerals are not major determinants of urine flow, ruling out option **E**. Aldosterone and vasopressin act on the kidney, but aldosterone synthesis is triggered by a decrease in plasma sodium, and acts to increase sodium reabsorption in the kidney. While the latter action would decrease urine flow, plasma sodium would be increased rather than decreased in this dehydrated student, ruling out option **C**. On the other hand, vasopressin is released following stimulation of receptors in the hypothalamus by a rise in plasma osmolality, and increases the reabsorption of water in the kidney tubule, decreasing urine production.

Hypothalamic Regulation of Hormonal Functions

OBJECTIVES

After reading this chapter, you should be able to:

- Describe anatomic connections between the hypothalamus and the pituitary gland and their functional significance.
- List the factors that control water intake, and outline the way in which they exert their effects.
- Describe the synthesis, processing, storage, and secretion of the hormones of the posterior pituitary.
- Discuss the effects of vasopressin, the receptors on which it acts, and how its secretion is regulated.
- Discuss the effects of oxytocin, the receptors on which it acts, and how its secretion is regulated.
- Name the hypophysiotropic hormones, and outline the effects that each has on anterior pituitary function.
- List body temperature-regulating mechanisms, and describe the way in which they are integrated under hypothalamic control to maintain normal body temperature.
- Discuss the pathophysiology of fever.

INTRODUCTION

Many of the complex autonomic mechanisms that maintain the chemical constancy and temperature of the internal environment are integrated in the hypothalamus.

The hypothalamus also functions with the limbic system as a unit that regulates emotional and instinctual behavior.

■ HYPOTHALAMUS: ANATOMIC CONSIDERATIONS

The hypothalamus is the portion of the anterior end of the diencephalon that lies below the hypothalamic sulcus and in front of the interpeduncular nuclei. It is divided into a variety of nuclei and nuclear areas.

AFFERENT & EFFERENT CONNECTIONS OF THE HYPOTHALAMUS

The principal afferent and efferent neural pathways to and from the hypothalamus are mostly unmyelinated. Many connect the hypothalamus to the limbic system. Important connections also exist between the hypothalamus and nuclei in the midbrain tegmentum, pons, and hindbrain.

Norepinephrine-secreting neurons with their cell bodies in the hindbrain end in many different parts of the hypothalamus. Paraventricular neurons that secrete oxytocin and vasopressin project in turn to the hindbrain and the spinal cord. Neurons that secrete epinephrine have their cell bodies in the hindbrain and end in the ventral hypothalamus.

RELATION TO THE PITUITARY GLAND

There are neural connections between the hypothalamus and the posterior lobe of the pituitary gland and vascular connections between the hypothalamus and the anterior lobe. The posterior pituitary is made up in large part of the endings of axons that arise from cell bodies in the supraoptic and paraventricular nuclei and pass to the posterior pituitary (**Figure 17–1**) via the **hypothalamohypophysial tract**. The anterior and intermediate lobes of the pituitary arise from an evagination from the roof of the pharynx (see Chapter 18). Few, if any, nerve fibers pass to the anterior pituitary from the hypothalamus. Rather, the **portal hypophysial vessels** form a direct vascular link. A network of fenestrated capillaries called the **primary plexus** lies on the ventral surface of the hypothalamus (Figure 17–1). Capillary loops also penetrate the median eminence. The capillaries drain into the portal hypophysial vessels that carry blood down the pituitary stalk to the capillaries of the anterior pituitary.

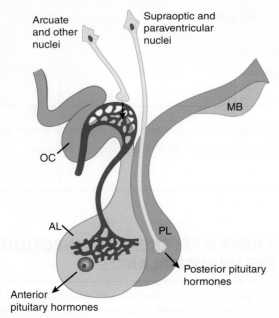

FIGURE 17–1 Secretion of hypothalamic hormones. The hormones of the posterior lobe (PL) are released into the general circulation from the endings of supraoptic and paraventricular neurons, whereas hypophysiotropic hormones are secreted into the portal hypophysial circulation from the endings of arcuate and other hypothalamic neurons. AL, anterior lobe; MB, mamillary bodies; OC, optic chiasm.

HYPOTHALAMIC FUNCTION

The major functions of the hypothalamus are summarized in **Table 17–1**. Some are fairly clear-cut visceral reflexes, and others include complex behavioral and emotional reactions; however, all involve a particular response to a particular stimulus.

RELATION TO AUTONOMIC FUNCTION

Stimulation of the hypothalamus produces autonomic responses, but the hypothalamus does not seem to be concerned with the regulation of visceral function per se. Rather, the autonomic responses triggered in the hypothalamus are part of more complex phenomena such as eating, and emotions such as rage. For example, stimulation of various parts of the hypothalamus, especially the lateral areas, produces diffuse sympathetic discharge and increased adrenal medullary secretion—the mass sympathetic discharge seen in animals exposed to stress (the flight or fight reaction).

The hypothalamus and related parts of the brain play a key role in the regulation of food intake. Obesity is considered in Chapter 26, and the relation of obesity to diabetes mellitus is discussed in Chapter 24. Hypothalamic regulation of sleep and circadian rhythms is discussed in Chapter 14.

THIRST

Another appetitive mechanism under hypothalamic control is thirst. Water intake is increased by increased effective osmotic pressure of the plasma, by decreases in extracellular fluid (ECF) volume, and by psychological and other factors. Osmolality acts via **osmoreceptors** in the anterior hypothalamus.

Decreases in ECF volume can stimulate thirst by a pathway independent of that mediated by increased plasma osmolality (**Figure 17–2**). Thus, hemorrhage causes increased drinking even if there is no change in osmolality. The effect of volume depletion is mediated in part via the renin–angiotensin system (see Chapter 38). Baroreceptors in the heart and blood vessels are also involved. Renin secretion is increased by hypovolemia and results in an increase in circulating angiotensin II. The angiotensin II acts on the **subfornical organ**, a specialized receptor area in the diencephalon, to stimulate the neural areas concerned with thirst. Some evidence suggests that it acts on the **organum vasculosum of the lamina terminalis (OVLT)** as well. These areas are highly permeable and are two of the circumventricular organs located outside the blood–brain barrier (see Chapter 33).

When the sensation of thirst is obtunded, patients stop drinking adequate amounts of fluid. Dehydration results if measures are not instituted to maintain water balance. Most cases of **hypernatremia** are actually due to simple dehydration in patients with psychoses or hypothalamic disease who do not or cannot increase their water intake when thirst is stimulated. Lesions of the anterior communicating artery can also obtund thirst because branches of this artery supply the hypothalamic areas concerned with thirst.

TABLE 17–1 Summary of principal hypothalamic regulatory mechanisms.

Function	Afferents From	Integrating Areas
Temperature regulation	Temperature receptors in the skin, deep tissues, spinal cord, hypothalamus, and other parts of the brain	Anterior hypothalamus, response to heat; posterior hypothalamus, response to cold
Neuroendocrine control of:		
Catecholamines	Limbic areas concerned with emotion	Dorsal and posterior hypothalamus
Vasopressin	Osmoreceptors, "volume receptors," others	Supraoptic and paraventricular nuclei
Oxytocin	Touch receptors in breast, uterus, genitalia	Supraoptic and paraventricular nuclei
Thyroid-stimulating hormone (thyrotropin, TSH) via TRH	Temperature receptors in infants, perhaps others	Paraventricular nuclei and neighboring areas
Adrenocorticotropic hormone (ACTH) and β-lipotropin (β-LPH) via CRH	Limbic system (emotional stimuli); reticular formation ("systemic" stimuli); hypothalamic and anterior pituitary cells sensitive to circulating blood cortisol level; suprachiasmatic nuclei (diurnal rhythm)	Paraventricular nuclei
Follicle-stimulating hormone (FSH) and luteinizing hormone (LH) via GnRH	Hypothalamic cells sensitive to estrogens, eyes, touch receptors in skin and genitalia of reflex ovulating species	Preoptic area; other areas
Prolactin via PIH and PRH	Touch receptors in breasts, other unknown receptors	Arcuate nucleus; other areas (hypothalamus inhibits secretion)
Growth hormone via somatostatin and GHRH	Unknown receptors	Periventricular nucleus, arcuate nucleus
"Appetitive" behavior		
Thirst	Osmoreceptors, probably located in the organum vasculosum of the lamina terminalis; angiotensin II uptake in the subfornical organ	Lateral superior hypothalamus
Hunger	Glucostat cells sensitive to rate of glucose utilization; leptin receptors; receptors for other polypeptides	Ventromedial, arcuate, and paraventricular nuclei; lateral hypothalamus
Sexual behavior	Cells sensitive to circulating estrogen, androgen, and others	Anterior ventral hypothalamus plus, in the male, piriform cortex
Defensive reactions (fear, rage)	Sense organs and neocortex, paths unknown	Diffuse, in limbic system and hypothalamus
Control of body rhythms	Retina via retinohypothalamic fibers	Suprachiasmatic nuclei

OTHER FACTORS REGULATING WATER INTAKE

A number of other well-established factors contribute to the regulation of water intake. Psychological and social factors are important. Dryness of the pharyngeal mucous membrane also causes a sensation of thirst.

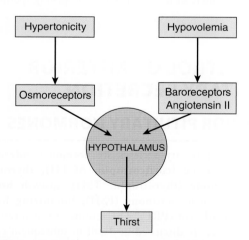

FIGURE 17–2 Diagrammatic representation of the way in which changes in plasma osmolality and changes in ECF volume affect thirst by separate pathways.

■ CONTROL OF POSTERIOR PITUITARY SECRETION

VASOPRESSIN & OXYTOCIN

In most mammals, the hormones secreted by the posterior pituitary are **arginine vasopressin (AVP)** and **oxytocin.**

BIOSYNTHESIS, INTRANEURONAL TRANSPORT, & SECRETION

The hormones of the posterior pituitary are synthesized in the cell bodies of the magnocellular neurons and transported down the axons of these neurons to their endings in the posterior lobe, where they are secreted in response to electrical activity. Some of the neurons make oxytocin and others make vasopressin. Oxytocin and vasopressin are typical **neural hormones,** that is, hormones secreted into the circulation by nerves.

Like other peptide hormones, the posterior lobe hormones are synthesized as part of larger precursor molecules. The leader sequences of the precursor molecules are removed in the endoplasmic reticulum, then the products are packaged into secretory granules in the Golgi apparatus and transported down the axons by axoplasmic flow to the endings in the posterior pituitary. The secretory granules are called **Herring bodies**. Cleavage of the precursor molecules occurs as they are being transported, and the storage granules in the endings contain free vasopressin or oxytocin.

ELECTRICAL ACTIVITY OF MAGNOCELLULAR NEURONS

The oxytocin-secreting and vasopressin-secreting neurons also generate and conduct action potentials, and action potentials reaching their endings trigger the release of hormones by Ca^{2+}-dependent exocytosis. At least in anesthetized rats, these neurons are silent at rest or discharge at low, irregular rates (0.1–3 spikes/s). However, their response to stimulation varies. Stimulation of the nipples causes a synchronous, high-frequency discharge of the oxytocin neurons after an appreciable latency. This discharge causes release of a pulse of oxytocin and consequent milk ejection in postpartum females. On the other hand, stimulation of vasopressin-secreting neurons by a stimulus such as an increase in blood osmolality causes an initial steady increase in firing rate followed by a prolonged pattern of phasic discharge in which periods of high-frequency discharge alternate with periods of electrical quiescence (**phasic bursting**). These phasic bursts are generally not synchronous in different vasopressin-secreting neurons. They are well suited to maintain a prolonged increase in the output of vasopressin.

Vasopressin Receptors

There are at least three kinds of vasopressin receptors: V_{1A}, V_{1B}, and V_2. All are G-protein coupled. The V_{1A} and V_{1B} receptors act through phosphatidylinositol hydrolysis to increase intracellular Ca^{2+} concentrations. The V_2 receptors act through G_s to increase cyclic adenosine monophosphate levels.

Effects of Vasopressin

Because one of its principal physiologic effects is the retention of water by the kidney, vasopressin is often called the **antidiuretic hormone (ADH)**. It increases the permeability of the collecting ducts of the kidney so that water enters the hypertonic interstitium of the renal pyramids (see Chapter 37). The urine becomes concentrated and its volume decreases. The overall effect is therefore retention of water in excess of solute. In the absence of vasopressin, the urine is hypotonic to plasma, urine volume is increased, and there is a net water loss.

Effects of Oxytocin

In humans, oxytocin acts primarily on the breasts and uterus. A G-protein–coupled oxytocin receptor has been identified in human myometrium, and a similar or identical receptor is found in mammary tissue and the ovary. It triggers increases in intracellular Ca^{2+} levels.

The Milk Ejection Reflex

Oxytocin causes contraction of the **myoepithelial cells** that line the ducts of the breast. This squeezes the milk out of the alveoli of the lactating breast into the large ducts (sinuses) and thence out of the nipple (**milk ejection**). Many hormones acting in concert are responsible for breast growth and the secretion of milk, but milk ejection in most species requires oxytocin.

Milk ejection is normally initiated by a neuroendocrine reflex initiated by the suckling infant. The receptors involved are touch receptors, which are plentiful around the nipple. Impulses generated in these receptors are relayed from the somatic touch pathways to the supraoptic and paraventricular nuclei. Discharge of the oxytocin-containing neurons causes secretion of oxytocin. In lactating women, genital stimulation and emotional stimuli also produce oxytocin secretion, sometimes causing milk to spurt from the breasts.

Other Actions of Oxytocin

Oxytocin causes contraction of the smooth muscle of the uterus. The sensitivity of the uterine musculature to oxytocin is enhanced by estrogen and inhibited by progesterone. The inhibitory effect of progesterone is due to a direct action of the steroid on uterine oxytocin receptors. In late pregnancy, the uterus becomes very sensitive to oxytocin coincident with a marked increase in the number of oxytocin receptors. Oxytocin secretion is then increased during labor. After dilation of the cervix, descent of the fetus down the birth canal initiates impulses in the afferent nerves that are relayed to the supraoptic and paraventricular nuclei, causing secretion of sufficient oxytocin to enhance labor.

Circulating oxytocin increases at the time of ejaculation in males, and it is possible that this causes increased contraction of the smooth muscle of the vas deferens, propelling sperm toward the urethra.

■ CONTROL OF ANTERIOR PITUITARY SECRETION

ANTERIOR PITUITARY HORMONES

The anterior pituitary secretes six hormones: **adrenocorticotropic hormone (corticotropin, ACTH), thyroid-stimulating hormone (thyrotropin, TSH), growth hormone, follicle-stimulating hormone (FSH), luteinizing hormone (LH)**, and **prolactin (PRL)**. The actions of the anterior pituitary hormones are discussed in detail in subsequent chapters. The hypothalamus plays an important stimulatory role in secretion of ACTH, TSH, growth hormone, FSH, and LH.

It also regulates prolactin secretion, but its effect is predominantly inhibitory.

NATURE OF HYPOTHALAMIC CONTROL

Anterior pituitary secretion is controlled by chemical agents carried in the portal hypophysial vessels from the hypothalamus to the pituitary. These substances are called **hypophysiotropic hormones**. Small amounts escape into the general circulation, but they are at their highest concentration in portal hypophysial blood.

HYPOPHYSIOTROPIC HORMONES

There are six established hypothalamic releasing and inhibiting hormones: **corticotropin-releasing hormone (CRH); thyrotropin-releasing hormone (TRH); growth hormone-releasing hormone (GHRH); growth hormone–inhibiting hormone (GIH**, now generally called **somatostatin); luteinizing hormone-releasing hormone (LHRH**, now generally known as **gonadotropin-releasing hormone [GnRH]); and prolactin-inhibiting hormone** (PIH, widely considered to be represented by dopamine). In addition, hypothalamic extracts contain prolactin-releasing activity, and a **prolactin-releasing hormone (PRH)** has been postulated to exist. GnRH stimulates the secretion of FSH as well as that of LH, and it seems unlikely that a separate FSH-releasing hormone exists.

The hypothalamic releasing and inhibiting hormones are secreted from the median eminence. This region contains few nerve cell bodies, but many nerve endings are in close proximity to the capillary loops from which the portal vessels originate. The GnRH-secreting neurons are primarily in the medial preoptic area, the somatostatin-secreting neurons are in the periventricular nuclei, the TRH-secreting and CRH-secreting neurons are in the medial parts of the paraventricular nuclei, and the GHRH-secreting (and dopamine-secreting) neurons are in the arcuate nuclei.

Most, if not all, of the hypophysiotropic hormones affect the secretion of more than one anterior pituitary hormone. The FSH-stimulating activity of GnRH has been mentioned previously. TRH stimulates the secretion of prolactin as well as TSH. Somatostatin inhibits the secretion of TSH as well as growth hormone.

SIGNIFICANCE & CLINICAL IMPLICATIONS

The hypothalamus helps to match endocrine secretion to the demands of a changing environment. The nervous system receives information about changes in the internal and external environment from the sense organs. It brings about adjustments to these changes, in part, by changes in the rate at which hormones are secreted.

The manifestations of hypothalamic disease are neurologic defects, endocrine changes, and metabolic abnormalities such as hyperphagia and hyperthermia. The possibility of hypothalamic pathology should be kept in mind in evaluating all patients with pituitary dysfunction, especially those with isolated deficiencies of single pituitary tropic hormones.

◼ TEMPERATURE REGULATION

In the body, heat is produced by muscular exercise, assimilation of food, and all the vital processes that contribute to the basal metabolic rate. It is lost from the body by radiation, conduction, and vaporization of water in the respiratory passages and on the skin. Small amounts of heat are also removed in the urine and feces. The balance between heat production and heat loss determines the body temperature. Normal body function depends on a relatively constant body temperature.

Vertebrates have evolved mechanisms for maintaining body temperature by adjusting heat production and heat loss. In reptiles, amphibians, and fish, the adjusting mechanisms are relatively rudimentary, and these species are called "cold-blooded" (**poikilothermic**) because their body temperature fluctuates over a considerable range. In "warm-blooded" (**homeothermic**) birds and mammals, a group of reflex responses that are primarily integrated in the hypothalamus maintain body temperature within a narrow range. The hibernating mammals are a partial exception. While awake they are homeothermic, but during hibernation their body temperature falls.

NORMAL BODY TEMPERATURE

In humans, the traditional normal value for the oral temperature is 37°C (98.6°F) but likely ranges from 36.3 to 37.1°C in healthy young adults. Various parts of the body are at different temperatures, and the magnitude of the temperature difference between the parts varies with the environmental temperature. The extremities are generally cooler than the rest of the body. The temperature of the scrotum is carefully regulated at 32°C. The rectal temperature is representative of the temperature at the core of the body and varies least with changes in environmental temperature. The oral temperature is normally 0.5°C lower than the rectal temperature, but it is affected by many factors, including ingestion of hot or cold fluids, gum chewing, smoking, and mouth breathing.

The core temperature undergoes a circadian fluctuation of 0.5–0.7°C, being lowest at about 6:00 AM and highest in the evenings. In women, an additional monthly cycle of temperature variation is characterized by a rise in basal temperature at the time of ovulation. Temperature regulation is less precise in young children and they may normally have a temperature that is 0.5°C higher than adults.

During exercise, the heat produced by muscular contraction accumulates and the rectal temperature rises as high as

TABLE 17–2 Body heat production and heat loss.

Body heat is produced by	
Basic metabolic processes	
Food intake (specific dynamic action)	
Muscular activity	
body heat is lost by	**Percentage of heat lost at 21°c**
Radiation and conduction	70
Vaporization of sweat	27
Respiration	2
Urination and defecation	1

40°C (104°F). This rise is due in part to the inability of the heat-dissipating mechanisms to keep pace with the amount of heat produced, but exercise likely also elevates the temperature at which heat-dissipating mechanisms are activated. Body temperature also rises slightly during emotional excitement, probably owing to unconscious tensing of the muscles. It is chronically elevated by as much as 0.5°C when the metabolic rate is high, as in hyperthyroidism, and lowered when the metabolic rate is low, as in hypothyroidism.

HEAT PRODUCTION

The major source of heat is the contraction of skeletal muscle (Table 17–2). Heat production can be varied by endocrine mechanisms in the absence of food intake or muscular exertion. Epinephrine and norepinephrine produce a rapid but short-lived increase in heat production; thyroid hormones produce a slowly developing but prolonged increase.

Another source of considerable heat, particularly in infants, is **brown fat**. This fat has a high rate of metabolism and its thermogenic function has been likened to that of an electric blanket.

HEAT LOSS

The processes by which heat is lost from the body when the environmental temperature is below body temperature are listed in Table 17–2. **Conduction** is heat exchange between objects or substances at different temperatures that are in contact with one another. The amount of heat transferred is proportional to the temperature difference between the objects (**thermal gradient**). Conduction is aided by **convection**, the movement of molecules away from the area of contact. **Radiation** is the transfer of heat by infrared electromagnetic radiation from one object to another. When an individual is in a cold environment, heat is lost by conduction to the surrounding air and by radiation to cool objects in the vicinity.

The temperature of the skin determines to a large extent the degree to which body heat is lost or gained. The amount of heat reaching the skin from the deep tissues can be varied by changing blood flow. When the cutaneous vessels are dilated, warm blood wells into the skin, whereas in the maximally vasoconstricted state, heat is held centrally in the body. Heat loss may also be impeded by the layers of air trapped in hair or clothing. "Goose pimples" are the result of **horripilation**; they are the visible manifestation of cold-induced contraction of the piloerector muscles attached to the rather meager hair supply in an effort to increase the air layer.

The other major process transferring heat from the body is vaporization of water on the skin and mucous membranes of the mouth and respiratory passages. Vaporization of 1 g of water removes about 0.6 kcal of heat. A certain amount of water is vaporized at all times. This **insensible water loss** amounts to 50 mL/h in humans. During muscular exertion in a hot environment, sweat secretion reaches values as high as 1600 mL/h, and in a dry atmosphere, most of this sweat is vaporized. Heat loss by vaporization of water therefore varies from 30 to over 900 kcal/h.

The relative contribution of each of the processes that transfer heat away from the body varies with the environmental temperature. At 21°C, vaporization is a minor component in humans at rest. As the environmental temperature approaches body temperature, radiation losses decline and vaporization losses increase.

TEMPERATURE-REGULATING MECHANISMS

The reflex and semireflex thermoregulatory responses in humans are listed in Table 17–3. They include autonomic, somatic, endocrine, and behavioral changes.

Curling up decreases the body surface exposed to the environment. Shivering is an involuntary response of the skeletal muscles,

TABLE 17–3 Temperature-regulating mechanisms.

Mechanisms activated by cold
Shivering
Hunger
Increased voluntary activity
Increased secretion of norepinephrine and epinephrine
Decreased heat loss
Cutaneous vasoconstriction
Curling up
Horripilation
Mechanisms activated by heat
Increased heat loss
Cutaneous vasodilation
Sweating
Increased respiration
Decreased heat production
Anorexia
Apathy and inertia

but cold also causes a semiconscious general increase in motor activity. Increased catecholamine secretion is an important endocrine response to cold.

Thermoregulatory adjustments involve local responses as well as more general reflex responses. When cutaneous blood vessels are cooled they become more sensitive to catecholamines and the arterioles and venules constrict. This local effect of cold directs blood away from the skin. Another heat-conserving mechanism that is important in animals living in cold water is heat transfer from arterial to venous blood in the limbs. This limits the ability to maintain heat in the tips of the extremities but conserves body heat.

The reflex responses activated by cold are controlled from the posterior hypothalamus. Those activated by warmth are controlled primarily from the anterior hypothalamus. Stimulation of the anterior hypothalamus causes cutaneous vasodilation and sweating, and lesions in this region cause hyperthermia. Posterior hypothalamic stimulation causes shivering, and the body temperature of animals with posterior hypothalamic lesions falls toward that of the environment.

AFFERENTS

The hypothalamus integrates body temperature information from sensory receptors (primarily cold receptors) in the skin, deep tissues, spinal cord, extrahypothalamic portions of the brain, and the hypothalamus itself. There are threshold core temperatures for each of the main temperature-regulating responses and when the threshold is reached the response begins. The threshold is 37°C for sweating and vasodilation, 36.8°C for vasoconstriction, 36°C for nonshivering thermogenesis, and 35.5°C for shivering.

FEVER

Fever is perhaps the oldest and most universally known hallmark of disease. When it occurs in homeothermic animals, the thermoregulatory mechanisms behave as if they were adjusted to maintain body temperature at a higher than normal level. The temperature receptors then signal that the actual temperature is below the new set point, and temperature-raising mechanisms are activated. This usually produces chilly sensations due to cutaneous vasoconstriction and occasionally enough shivering to produce a shaking chill. However, the nature of the response depends on the ambient temperature. The temperature rise in experimental animals injected with a pyrogen is due mostly to increased heat production if they are in a cold environment and decreased heat loss if they are in a warm environment.

The pathogenesis of fever is summarized in Figure 17–3. There is good evidence that IL-1β, IL-6, IFN-β, IFN-γ, and TNF-α (see Chapter 3) can produce fever. These circulating cytokines are polypeptides and it is unlikely that they penetrate the brain. Instead, evidence suggests that they act on the OVLT. This in turn activates the preoptic area of the hypothalamus.

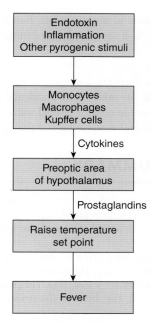

FIGURE 17–3 **Pathogenesis of fever.**

The fever produced by cytokines is probably due to local release of prostaglandins in the hypothalamus. The antipyretic effect of aspirin is exerted directly on the hypothalamus, and aspirin inhibits prostaglandin synthesis. PGE_2 is one of the prostaglandins that causes fever. Knockout of the EP_3 receptor impairs the febrile response to PGE_2, IL-1β, and bacterial lipopolysaccharide (LPS).

The benefit of fever to the organism is uncertain, but a rise in temperature may inhibit the growth of microbes. In addition, antibody production is increased when body temperature is elevated. Hyperthermia also slows the growth of some tumors. However, very high temperatures are harmful. A rectal temperature over 41°C (106°F) for prolonged periods results in some permanent brain damage. When the temperature is over 43°C, heat stroke develops and death is common.

In **malignant hyperthermia**, various mutations of the gene coding for the ryanodine receptor (see Chapter 5) lead to excess Ca^{2+} release during muscle contraction triggered by stress. This in turn leads to contractures of the muscles, increased muscle metabolism, and a great increase in heat production in muscle. The increased heat production causes a marked rise in body temperature that is fatal if not treated.

HYPOTHERMIA

In hibernating mammals, body temperature drops to low levels without causing any demonstrable ill effects. This observation led to experiments on induced hypothermia. When the skin or the blood is cooled enough to lower the body temperature, metabolic and physiologic processes slow down. Respiration and heart rate are very slow, blood pressure is low, and consciousness is lost. At rectal temperatures of about 28°C, the ability to spontaneously return the temperature to normal is lost, but the individual continues to survive and, if rewarmed with external heat, returns to a normal state.

Humans tolerate body temperatures of 21–24°C (70–75°F) without permanent ill effects, and induced hypothermia has been used in surgery. On the other hand, accidental hypothermia due to prolonged exposure to cold air or cold water is a serious condition and requires careful monitoring and prompt rewarming.

CHAPTER SUMMARY

- Neural connections link the hypothalamus and the posterior lobe of the pituitary gland, while vascular connections run between the hypothalamus and the anterior lobe of the pituitary.
- The posterior pituitary gland secretes vasopressin and oxytocin. Vasopressin increases the permeability of the collecting ducts of the kidney to water, thus concentrating the urine. Oxytocin acts on the breasts (lactation) and the uterus (contraction).
- The anterior pituitary secretes six hormones: adrenocorticotropic hormone (corticotropin, ACTH), thyroid-stimulating hormone (thyrotropin, TSH), growth hormone, follicle-stimulating hormone (FSH), luteinizing hormone (LH), and prolactin (PRL).
- Other complex autonomic mechanisms that maintain the chemical constancy and temperature of the internal environment are integrated in the hypothalamus.

MULTIPLE-CHOICE QUESTIONS

For all questions, select the single best answer unless otherwise directed.

1. An athlete competing in an obstacle course event on a hot day sustains a serious cut as he clears the last hurdle on the course. He reports an intense feeling of thirst to responding paramedics. His thirst is most likely is stimulated by
   A. increases in plasma osmolality and volume.
   B. an increase in plasma osmolality and a decrease in plasma volume.
   C. a decrease in plasma osmolality and an increase in plasma volume.
   D. decreases in plasma osmolality and volume.
   E. a decrease in plasma osmolality with no change in plasma volume.

2. In an experiment, a student is asked to sit quietly, unclothed, in a room in which the air temperature is 21°C (69.8°F) and the humidity 80%. The greatest amount of heat lost from their body will be by
   A. elevated metabolism.
   B. respiration.
   C. urination.
   D. vaporization of sweat.
   E. radiation and conduction.

3. In the scenario described above, the rate of heat loss from the subject's body would be increased by which of the following interventions?

   A. Asking the subject to don a white bathrobe
   B. Switching on a fan in the room
   C. Heating the walls of the room to body temperature while keeping the air temperature constant
   D. Asking the subject to curl up in a ball
   E. Asking the subject to don a black bathrobe

4. A 30-year-old woman is referred to a reproductive specialist because of difficulties in conceiving a child. She reports that she has frequently been bothered by a milky discharge from her breasts, and also has experienced irregular periods. A pregnancy test is negative. An MRI scan reveals a mass in her pituitary. A blood test is likely to reveal elevated levels of
   A. vasopressin.
   B. growth hormone.
   C. prolactin-inhibiting hormone.
   D. gonadtropin-releasing hormone (GnRH).
   E. prolactin.

5. In an experiment designed to study mechanisms whereby vasopressin influences renal function, a scientist transfects a renal collecting duct cell line with a vector designed to express V_2 receptors. Stimulation of these cells with vasopressin would be expected to increase which of the following:
   A. Inositol trisphosphate
   B. Free cytosolic calcium
   C. Storage of aquaporins in intracellular vesicles
   D. Cyclic AMP
   E. Nitric oxide

6. A woman whose nursing infant is being cared for in a daycare center following her return to work happens to hear another baby crying as she entertains a business client over lunch. She notices that this triggers leakage of milk from her breasts. The emotional trigger likely stimulated which of the following events in her hypothalamus:
   A. Release of prolactin
   B. Release of vasopressin
   C. Phasic discharge of magnocellular neurons
   D. Synchronous high-frequency discharge of magnocellular neurons
   E. Release of GnRH

7. A scientist studying neuroendocrine regulation in the rat creates a lesion of the portal hypophysial vessels. Compared to the period prior to the surgery, circulating levels of which of the following hormones would be increased?
   A. GnRH
   B. Vasopressin
   C. Luteinizing hormone
   D. Growth hormone
   E. Oxytocin

8. A 22-year-old medical student visits the student health center complaining of an acute febrile illness accompanied by shivering and chills. He is diagnosed with influenza and sent home to rest and recuperate. His chills are ascribable to which of the following:
   A. Cutaneous vasodilation
   B. Horripilation
   C. Decreased heat production
   D. Cutaneous vasoconstriction
   E. Anorexia

9. The patient described in Question 8 is advised to take aspirin until his shaking chills resolve. This drug will be effective because it blocks the action of which class of mediators in which site?
   A. Prostaglandins/hypothalamus
   B. Prostaglandins/skin
   C. Cytokines/hypothalamus
   D. Cytokines/skin
   E. Endotoxin/hypothalamus

10. Various physiological parameters were assessed in a volunteer subjected to a period of hypothermia by being placed in a cold room such that rectal temperature was reduced to 30°C. Compared to an individual with a normal core temperature in a warm room, which of the following would be increased:
    A. Blood pressure
    B. Mentation
    C. Heart rate
    D. Respiration
    E. Difference in temperature of the feet versus core temperature

ANSWERS

1. The correct answer is **B**. Because he has been engaged in vigorous exercise, the athlete likely has lost water in excess of solute by sweating, with an associated increase in plasma osmolality. In addition, plasma volume will be reduced by hemorrhage. As shown in Figure 17–2, hypertonicity activates chemoreceptors in the hypothalamus and hypovolemia activates peripheral baroreceptors that in turn induce renin secretion and an increase in circulating angiotensin II. Angiotensin II then acts on circumventricular organs to signal to the hypothalamus. The hypothalamus integrates these various inputs and triggers brain areas concerned with thirst. Plasma tonicity and volume are independent regulators of the thirst response but the explanation above rules out options **A, C, D**, and **E**. In particular, option **C** would never trigger thirst mechanisms, nor would plasma volume ever be increased in the circumstances described.

2. The correct answer is **E. A** is ruled out because, while metabolism contributes to heat production, it is not responsible for heat loss from the body. All of the remaining mechanisms contribute to heat loss, but the magnitude of heat loss by each route differs considerably. For example, respiration and urination (assuming the latter occurred during the study) would each be responsible for no more than 2% of heat loss (rules out **B** and **C**). Because the subject is at rest and unlikely to be sweating at an increased rate, and the temperature of the room is below body temperature, the significant majority of heat loss (around 70%) will be by conduction to the surrounding air and the chair on which the subject is sitting, as well as radiation to surrounding objects, rather than vaporization of sweat (rules out option **D**). Sweat vaporization will also be impeded by the relatively humid conditions.

3. The correct answer is **B**. A fan will circulate the air around the subject that has been heated by conduction, replacing the heated air with that which is cooler and increasing the rate of conduction. Providing clothing will decrease the rate of heat loss by trapping heat in an air layer next to the skin; the effect will be greatest with the black robe because it will also reduce radiation (rules out **A** and **E**). If the walls of the room are heated, less heat will be lost to them by radiation because of the reduced temperature gradient (rules out option **C**). Curling into a ball will reduce the surface area available for heat loss (rules out option **D**).

4. The correct answer is **E**. The symptoms are consistent with a diagnosis of a secreting prolactinoma. Uncontrolled prolactin production causes milk production and secretion from the breasts in the absence of breast feeding. Excessive prolactin levels feedback to reduce GnRH secretion, affecting the female reproductive cycle (rules out **D**). Prolactin-inhibiting hormone derives from the hypothalamus and would not be increased; indeed, patients suffering from a prolactinoma can often obtain some relief of their symptoms by treatment with a dopamine agonist such as bromocriptine (rules out **C**). Finally, neither vasopressin (primarily involved in the regulation of water balance) nor growth hormone (involved in growth and metabolism) has effects that are consistent with the patient's presentation (rules out **A** and **B**).

5. The correct answer is **D**. V_2 receptors, which are the major mediators of the effects of vasopressin on renal water handling, are linked via G_s proteins to the stimulation of adenylyl cyclase activity and production of cAMP. In vivo, a major response to stimulation of these receptors is the exocytosis of aquaporin from intracellular vesicles and its insertion into the plasma membrane (rules out option **C**). V_{1A} and V_{1B} vasopressin receptors predominantly mediate the effects of the hormone on the vascular smooth muscle and pituitary, respectively, and are linked to G_q proteins, resulting in the turnover of membrane phosphatidylinositol and release of calcium from intracellular stores (rules out **A** and **B**). Vasopressin does increase nitric oxide in the kidney, but this effect is mediated by V_{1A} receptors on smooth muscle cells (rules out option **E**).

6. The correct answer is **D**. The emotional trigger would stimulate milk ejection in this mother in a fashion similar to suckling. Oxytocin is released as a pulse from the endings of magnocellular nerves following a burst of synchronous activation. This can be contrasted with the phasic firing of magnocellular neurons that results in the prolonged output of vasopressin (rules out options **B** and **C**). Prolactin, which is produced by the anterior pituitary rather than the hypothalamus, is involved in milk production in lactating women but not its ejection (rules out option **A**). GnRH is a hypothalamic hormone, but is not directly involved in lactation (rules out option **E**).

7. The correct answer is **A**. Interruption of the blood supply that links the hypothalamus to the anterior pituitary would reduce the release of hormones from this gland, including luteinizing hormone and growth hormone (rules out **C** and **D**). However, the hormones of the posterior pituitary (namely vasopressin and oxytocin), which are produced by hypothalamic magnocellular neurons that project to this site, should be unaffected (rules out **B** and **E**). On the other hand, because secretion of all anterior pituitary hormones should be impaired, they will not be available to trigger feedback inhibitory mechanisms that limit the synthesis and release of hypophysiotropic hormones, such as GnRH. Thus, levels of these hormones that spill over into the systemic circulation should be increased.

8. The correct answer is **D**. An infectious trigger can cause the release of pyrogenic cytokines that act on the hypothalamus

to alter the thermoregulatory set point upwards, such that a stimulation of heat production activities occurs at normal temperatures. Thus, blood vessels in the skin constrict to return blood to the core and limit heat loss, even if the subject is in a warm room, which is perceived as a cooling of the skin and also is accompanied by shivering (rules out option **A**). Horripilation may also occur, but will not lead to chills specifically (rules out option **B**). A decrease in heat production and anorexia are mechanisms normally activated by heat to lower temperature, but these may not be activated in fever due to the altered set point (rules out options **C** and **E**).

9. **The correct answer is A.** The antipyretic action of aspirin is ascribable to its activity as an inhibitor of cyclooxygenase, the enzyme that synthesizes prostaglandins. Prostaglandins of the E-class bind to EP_3 receptors in the hypothalamus to alter the temperature set point. The action of prostaglandins is not in the periphery, because fever can be produced with direct injection of prostaglandins into the hypothalamus (rules out option **B**). Likewise, cytokine production in response to a viral infection is upstream of cyclooxygenase activation (rules out options **C** and **D**). Endotoxin is associated with bacterial infections, and in any event it acts on immune cells in the periphery to trigger cytokine production (rules out option **E**).

10. **The correct answer is E.** Because a drop in core temperature slows all metabolic processes, blood pressure, mentation, heart rate, and respiration will all be reduced (rules out options **A–D**). However, the core temperature will continue to be defended at the expense of the extremities, increasing the gradient between temperatures measured in the rectum and at the feet.

The Pituitary Gland

OBJECTIVES

After studying this chapter, you should be able to:

- Describe the structure of the pituitary gland and how it relates to function.
- Define the cell types present in the anterior pituitary and understand how their numbers are controlled.
- Understand the function of hormones derived from proopiomelanocortin, and how they are involved in regulating pigmentation.
- Define the effects of the growth hormone on growth and metabolic function, and how insulin-like growth factor I (IGF-I) may mediate some of its actions in the periphery.
- List the stimuli that regulate growth hormone secretion and define their underlying mechanisms.
- Understand the relevance of pituitary secretion of gonadotropins and prolactin, and how this is regulated.
- Understand the basis of conditions where pituitary function and growth hormone secretion and function are abnormal, and how they can be treated.

INTRODUCTION

The pituitary gland lies in a pocket of the sphenoid bone at the base of the brain. It is a coordinating center for control of many downstream endocrine glands. In many ways, it can be considered to consist of at least two separate endocrine organs that contain a plethora of hormonally active substances. The anterior pituitary secretes **thyroid-stimulating hormone (TSH, thyrotropin), adrenocorticotropic hormone (ACTH), luteinizing hormone (LH), follicle-stimulating hormone (FSH), prolactin**, and **growth hormone**, and receives almost all of its blood supply from the portal hypophysial vessels. This vascular arrangement positions the anterior pituitary to respond efficiently to regulatory factors released from the hypothalamus. Of the listed hormones, prolactin acts on the breast. The remaining five are **tropic hormones;** that is, they stimulate secretion of hormonally active substances. The tropic

hormones for some endocrine glands are discussed in the chapter on that gland: TSH in Chapter 19; and ACTH in Chapter 20. However, the gonadotropins FSH and LH, along with prolactin, are covered here. To avoid redundancy, this chapter focuses predominantly on growth hormone and its role in growth and facilitating the activity of other hormones, along with general considerations about the pituitary.

The posterior pituitary in mammals consists predominantly of nerves that have their cell bodies in the hypothalamus, and stores **oxytocin** and **vasopressin** in their termini (see Chapter 17). In some species, there is also a well-developed intermediate lobe of the pituitary, whereas in humans it is rudimentary. Nevertheless, the intermediate lobe, as well as the anterior pituitary, contains hormonally active derivatives of the proopiomelanocortin (POMC) molecule that regulate skin pigmentation.

■ MORPHOLOGY

GROSS ANATOMY

The anatomy of the pituitary gland was discussed in detail in Chapter 17. The posterior pituitary is made up largely of the endings of axons from the hypothalamus and arises initially as an extension of this structure. The anterior pituitary contains endocrine cells that store its characteristic hormones and arises embryologically as an invagination of the pharynx (**Rathke pouch**). In species where it is well developed, the intermediate lobe is formed in the embryo from the dorsal half of Rathke pouch, but is closely adherent to the posterior lobe in the adult. It is separated from the anterior lobe by the remains of the cavity in Rathke pouch, the **residual cleft**.

HISTOLOGY

In the posterior lobe, the endings of the axons can be observed in close relation to blood vessels. **Pituicytes**, stellate cells that are modified astrocytes, are also present.

In humans, most of the cells of the intermediate lobe are incorporated in the anterior lobe. Along the residual cleft are small thyroid-like follicles, some containing a little colloid (see Chapter 19). The anterior pituitary is made up of interlacing cell cords and an extensive network of sinusoidal capillaries. The endothelium of the capillaries is fenestrated. The cells contain granules that are extruded from the cells by exocytosis.

CELL TYPES IN THE ANTERIOR PITUITARY

Five types of secretory cells have been identified in the anterior pituitary—somatotropes, which secrete growth hormone; lactotropes (also called mammotropes), which secrete prolactin; corticotropes, which secrete ACTH; thyrotropes, which secrete TSH; and gonadotropes, which secrete FSH and LH. Some cells may contain two or more hormones.

The anterior pituitary also contains folliculostellate cells that send processes between the granulated secretory cells and produce paracrine factors that regulate their growth and function. The relative proportion of secretory cell types can be adjusted to meet varying requirements for different hormones at different life stages. This plasticity is ascribed to the presence of a small number of pluripotent stem cells that persist in the adult gland.

■ PROOPIOMELANOCORTIN & DERIVATIVES

BIOSYNTHESIS

Intermediate-lobe cells, if present, and corticotropes of the anterior lobe synthesize a large precursor protein that is cleaved to form a family of hormones. Removal of the signal peptide results in the formation of the prohormone proopiomelanocortin (POMC). This molecule is also synthesized in the hypothalamus, the lungs, the gastrointestinal tract, and the placenta. In corticotropes, POMC is hydrolyzed to ACTH and β-lipotropin (β-LPH), plus a small amount of β-endorphin, and these substances are secreted. In the intermediate lobe cells, POMC is hydrolyzed to corticotropin-like intermediate-lobe peptide (CLIP), γ-LPH, and appreciable quantities of β-endorphin. β-Endorphin is an opioid peptide (see Chapter 7) that has the five amino acid residues of met-enkephalin at its amino terminal end. The **melanotropins** α- and β-MSH are also formed. It appears that neither α-MSH nor β-MSH is secreted in adult humans. In some species, however, the melanotropins have important physiologic functions.

CONTROL OF SKIN COLORATION & PIGMENT ABNORMALITIES

Fish, reptiles, and amphibia change the color of their skin for thermoregulation, camouflage, and behavioral displays. They do this by moving black or brown granules into or out of the periphery of pigment cells called **melanophores**. The granules are made up of **melanins**. The movement of these granules is controlled by α- and β-MSH, melanin-concentrating hormone, melatonin, and catecholamines.

Mammals have no melanophores, but they do have **melanocytes**, which have multiple processes containing melanin granules and express **melanotropin-1** receptors. Treatment with MSHs accelerates melanin synthesis, causing darkening of the skin. While α- and β-MSH do not circulate in adult humans, ACTH binds to the melanotropin-1 receptor and pigmentary changes in several endocrine diseases are due to changes in circulating ACTH. Abnormal pallor is a hallmark of hypopituitarism whereas hyperpigmentation occurs in adrenal insufficiency due to primary adrenal disease. Other disorders of pigmentation result from peripheral mechanisms. Thus, **albinos** have a congenital inability to synthesize melanin. **Piebaldism** is characterized by patches of skin that lack melanin as a result of congenital defects in the migration of pigment cell precursors from the neural crest during development. **Vitiligo** involves a similar patchy loss of melanin, but the loss develops progressively after birth secondary to autoimmune destruction of melanocytes.

■ GROWTH HORMONE

BIOSYNTHESIS & CHEMISTRY

Growth hormone that is secreted into the circulation by the pituitary gland consists of a complex mixture of the most abundant ("normal") form of growth hormone, hGH-N, peptides derived from this molecule with varying degrees of posttranslational modifications, and a splice variant of hGH-N that lacks amino acids 32–46. The physiologic significance of this complex array of hormones has yet to be fully understood.

PLASMA LEVELS, BINDING, & METABOLISM

A portion of circulating growth hormone is bound to a plasma protein that is a fragment of the extracellular domain of the growth hormone receptor (see below). Its concentration is an index of the number of growth hormone receptors in the tissues. Approximately 50% of the circulating pool of growth hormone activity is in the bound form, providing a reservoir of the hormone.

The basal plasma growth hormone level measured by radioimmunoassay in adult humans is normally less than 3 ng/mL. This represents both the protein-bound and free forms. Growth hormone is metabolized rapidly, at least in part in the liver. The half-life of circulating growth hormone in humans is 6–20 min, and the daily growth hormone output has been calculated to be 0.2–1.0 mg/day in adults.

GROWTH HORMONE RECEPTORS

The growth hormone receptor has a large extracellular portion, a transmembrane domain, and a large cytoplasmic portion. It is a member of the cytokine receptor superfamily discussed in Chapter 3. Growth hormone has two domains that can bind to its receptor, and when it binds to one receptor, the second binding site attracts another, producing a homodimer. Dimerization is essential for receptor activation.

Growth hormone activates many different intracellular signaling cascades. Of particular note is its activation of the JAK2–STAT pathway. JAK2 is a member of the Janus family of cytoplasmic tyrosine kinases. STATs (for signal transducers and activators of transcription) are a family of cytoplasmic transcription factors that, upon phosphorylation by JAK kinases, migrate to the nucleus where they activate various genes. JAK–STAT pathways are known also to mediate the effects of prolactin and various other growth factors.

EFFECTS ON GROWTH

In young animals in which the epiphyses have not yet fused to the long bones (see Chapter 21), growth is inhibited by hypophysectomy and stimulated by growth hormone. Chondrogenesis is accelerated, and as the cartilaginous epiphysial plates widen, they lay down more bone matrix at the ends of long bones. In this way, stature is increased. Prolonged treatment of animals with growth hormone leads to gigantism.

When the epiphyses are closed, linear growth is no longer possible. In this case, an overabundance of growth hormone produces the pattern of bone and soft tissue deformities known as **acromegaly**. The sizes of most of the viscera are increased (Clinical Box 18–1).

CLINICAL BOX 18-1

Gigantism & Acromegaly

Tumors of the somatotropes secrete large amounts of growth hormone, leading to **gigantism** in children and **acromegaly** in adults. If the tumor arises before puberty, the individual may grow to an extraordinary height. After linear growth is no longer possible, on the other hand, the characteristic features of acromegaly arise, including greatly enlarged hands and feet, vertebral changes attributable to osteoarthritis, soft tissue swelling, hirsutism, and protrusion of the brow and jaw. Abnormal growth of internal organs may eventually impair their function such that the condition, which has an insidious onset, can prove fatal if left untreated. Hypersecretion of growth hormone is accompanied by hypersecretion of prolactin in 20–40% of patients with acromegaly. About 25% of patients have abnormal glucose tolerance tests, and 4% develop lactation in the absence of pregnancy. Acromegaly can be caused by extra-pituitary as well as intrapituitary growth hormone–secreting tumors and by hypothalamic tumors that secrete GRH, but the latter are rare.

THERAPEUTIC HIGHLIGHTS

The mainstay of therapy for acromegaly remains the use of somatostatin analogues that inhibit the secretion of growth hormone. A growth hormone receptor antagonist has also become available. Surgical removal of the pituitary tumor is also helpful in both acromegaly and gigantism, but sometimes challenging to perform. In any case, adjuvant pharmacologic therapy must often be continued after surgery to control ongoing symptoms.

EFFECTS ON PROTEIN & ELECTROLYTE HOMEOSTASIS

Growth hormone is a protein anabolic hormone and produces a positive nitrogen and phosphorus balance, a rise in plasma phosphorus, and a fall in blood urea nitrogen and amino acid levels. In adults with growth hormone deficiency, recombinant human growth hormone produces an increase in lean body mass and a decrease in body fat, along with an increase in metabolic rate and a fall in plasma cholesterol. Gastrointestinal absorption of Ca^{2+} is increased. Na^+ and K^+ excretion is reduced by an action independent of the adrenal glands, probably because these electrolytes are diverted from the kidneys to the growing tissues. On the other hand, excretion of the amino acid 4-hydroxyproline is increased during this growth, reflective of the ability of growth hormone to stimulate the synthesis of collagen.

TABLE 18–1 Comparison of insulin and the insulin-like growth factors (IGFs).

	Insulin	IGF-I	IGF-II
Other names	—	Somatomedin C	Multiplication-stimulating activity (MSA)
Number of amino acids	51	70	67
Source	Pancreatic β cells	Liver and other tissues	Diverse tissues
Level regulated by	Glucose	Growth hormone after birth, nutritional status	Unknown
Plasma levels	0.3–2 ng/mL	10–700 ng/mL; peaks at puberty	300–800 ng/mL
Plasma-binding proteins	No	Yes	Yes
Major physiologic role	Control of metabolism	Skeletal and cartilage growth	Growth during fetal development

EFFECTS ON CARBOHYDRATE & FAT METABOLISM

The actions of growth hormone on carbohydrate metabolism are discussed in Chapter 24. Some forms of growth hormone are diabetogenic because they increase hepatic glucose output and exert an anti-insulin effect in muscle. Growth hormone is also ketogenic and increases circulating free fatty acid (FFA) levels. The increase in plasma FFA provides a source of energy for the tissues during hypoglycemia, fasting, and stressful stimuli. Growth hormone does not stimulate β cells of the pancreas directly, but increases the ability of the pancreas to respond to insulinogenic stimuli such as arginine and glucose. This is an additional way growth hormone promotes growth, since insulin has a protein anabolic effect (see Chapter 24).

SOMATOMEDINS

The effects of growth hormone on growth, cartilage, and protein metabolism depend on an interaction between growth hormone and **somatomedins**, which are polypeptide growth factors secreted by the liver and other tissues.

The principal somatomedins are **IGF-I** (also known as somatomedin C) and **IGF-II**. These factors are closely related to insulin. The hormone relaxin (see Chapter 22) is also a member of this family.

The properties of insulin, IGF-I, and IGF-II are compared in Table 18–1. Both IGF-I and IGF-II are tightly bound to proteins in the plasma, which prolongs their half-life in the circulation. The IGF-I receptor is very similar to the insulin receptor and probably uses similar or identical intracellular signaling pathways. The IGF-II receptor has a distinct structure and is involved in the intracellular targeting of acid hydrolases and other proteins to intracellular organelles. Secretion of IGF-I is independent of growth hormone before birth but is stimulated by growth hormone after birth, and it has pronounced growth-stimulating activity. Its concentration in plasma rises during childhood and peaks at the time of puberty, then declines to low levels in old age. IGF-II is largely independent of growth hormone and plays a role in the growth of the fetus before birth. In human fetuses in which it is overexpressed, several organs, especially the tongue, other muscles, kidneys, heart, and liver, develop out of proportion to the rest of the body.

DIRECT & INDIRECT ACTIONS OF GROWTH HORMONE

Growth hormone and IGF-I can act both in cooperation and independently to stimulate pathways that lead to growth. Figure 18–1 is a summary of actions of growth hormone and IGF-I. However, growth hormone probably combines with circulating and locally produced IGF-I in various proportions to produce at least some of the latter effects.

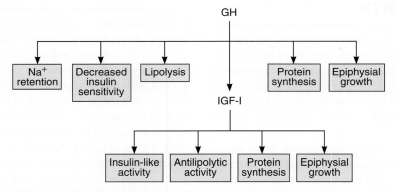

FIGURE 18–1 Direct and indirect actions of growth hormone (GH). The latter are mediated by the ability of GH to induce production of IGF-I. (Used with permission from R Clark and N Gesundheit.)

HYPOTHALAMIC & PERIPHERAL CONTROL OF GROWTH HORMONE SECRETION

Adolescents have the highest circulating levels of growth hormone, followed by children and finally adults. Levels decline in old age. There are also diurnal variations in growth hormone secretion superimposed on these developmental stages. Growth hormone is found at relatively low levels during the day, unless specific triggers for its release are present. During sleep, on the other hand, large pulsatile bursts of growth hormone secretion occur. The hypothalamus controls growth hormone production by secreting growth hormone–releasing hormone (GHRH) as well as somatostatin, which inhibits growth hormone release (see Chapter 17). Thus, the balance between the effects of these hypothalamic factors will determine the level of growth hormone release. Stimuli of growth hormone secretion can therefore act by increasing hypothalamic secretion of GHRH, decreasing secretion of somatostatin, or both. A third regulator of growth hormone secretion is **ghrelin**. The main site of ghrelin synthesis and secretion is the stomach, but it is also produced in the hypothalamus and has marked growth hormone–stimulating activity.

Growth hormone secretion is under feedback control (see Chapter 16), like the secretion of other anterior pituitary hormones. Growth hormone acts on the hypothalamus to antagonize GHRH release. Growth hormone also increases circulating IGF-I, and IGF-I exerts a direct inhibitory action on growth hormone secretion from the pituitary and stimulates somatostatin secretion (Figure 18–2).

Stimuli Affecting Growth Hormone Secretion

The stimuli that increase and decrease growth hormone secretion are summarized in Table 18–2. The stimuli that increase secretion fall

TABLE 18–2 Stimuli that affect growth hormone secretion in humans.

Stimuli that increase secretion
Hypoglycemia
2-Deoxyglucose
Exercise
Fasting
Increase in circulating levels of certain amino acids
Protein meal
Infusion of arginine and some other amino acids
Glucagon
Lysine vasopressin
Going to sleep
L-dopa and α-adrenergic agonists that penetrate the brain
Apomorphine and other dopamine receptor agonists
Estrogens and androgens
Stressful stimuli (including various psychological stresses)
Pyrogen
Stimuli that decrease secretion
REM sleep
Glucose
Cortisol
FFA
Medroxyprogesterone
Growth hormone and IGF-I

FFA, free fatty acid; IGF, insulin-like growth factor; REM, rapid eye movement.

into three general categories: (1) conditions such as hypoglycemia and/or fasting in which there is an actual or threatened decrease in the substrate for energy production, (2) conditions in which certain amino acids are increased in the plasma, and (3) stressful stimuli.

Glucose infusions lower plasma growth hormone levels and inhibit the response to exercise. The increase produced by 2-deoxyglucose is presumably due to intracellular glucose deficiency, since this compound blocks the catabolism of glucose-6-phosphate. Sex hormones induce growth hormone secretion, increase growth hormone responses to provocative stimuli such as arginine and insulin, and also serve as permissive factors for the action of growth hormone in the periphery. This likely contributes to the relatively high levels of circulating growth hormone and associated growth spurt in puberty.

■ PHYSIOLOGY OF GROWTH

Growth hormone, while being essentially unimportant for fetal development, is the most important hormone for postnatal growth. However, growth overall is a complex phenomenon that is affected not only by growth hormone and IGF-I, but also thyroid hormones,

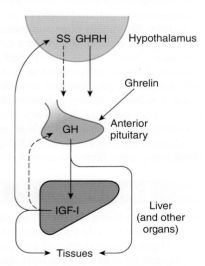

FIGURE 18–2 Feedback control of growth hormone secretion. Solid arrows represent positive effects and dashed arrows represent inhibition. GH, growth hormone; GHRH, growth hormone–releasing hormone; IGF-I, insulin-like growth factor-I; SS, somatostatin.

androgens, estrogens, glucocorticoids, and insulin. It is also affected by genetic factors and depends on adequate nutrition. It is normally accompanied by an orderly sequence of maturational changes, and it involves accretion of protein and an increase in length and size, not just an increase in weight.

ROLE OF NUTRITION

The food supply is the most important extrinsic factor affecting growth. The diet must be adequate not only in protein content but also in essential vitamins and minerals (see Chapter 26) and in calories, so that ingested protein is not burned for energy. However, the age at which a dietary deficiency occurs appears to be an important consideration. For example, once the pubertal growth spurt has commenced, considerable linear growth continues even if caloric intake is reduced. Injury and disease, on the other hand, stunt growth because they increase protein catabolism.

GROWTH PERIODS

Patterns of growth vary somewhat from species to species. Rats continue to grow, although at a declining rate, throughout life. In humans, two periods of rapid growth occur: the first in infancy and the second in late puberty just before growth stops. The second growth spurt is due to growth hormone, androgens, and estrogens, and subsequent cessation of growth is due in large part to closure of the epiphyses in the long bones by estrogens (see Chapter 21). After this time, further increases in height are not possible.

HORMONAL EFFECTS

Plasma growth hormone is elevated in newborns. Subsequently, average resting levels fall but the spikes of growth hormone secretion are larger, especially during puberty, so the mean plasma level over 24 h is increased. Plasma IGF-I levels rise during childhood, reaching a peak at 13–17 years of age. In contrast, IGF-II levels are constant.

The growth spurt that occurs at the time of puberty is due in part to the protein anabolic effect of androgens, and the secretion of adrenal androgens increases at this time in both sexes; however, it is also due to an interaction among sex steroids, growth hormone, and IGF-I. Treatment with estrogens and androgens increases the secretion of growth hormone in response to various stimuli and increases plasma IGF-I secondary to this increase in circulating growth hormone. This, in turn, causes growth.

Patients with sexual precocity are apt to be dwarfed due to premature closure of the epiphyses. On the other hand, men who were castrated before puberty tend to be tall because their estrogen production is decreased and their epiphyses remain open, allowing some growth to continue past the normal age of puberty.

In hypophysectomized animals, growth hormone increases growth but this effect is potentiated by thyroid hormones, which by themselves have no effect on growth. Thyroid hormones also often appear to be necessary for the normal rate of growth hormone secretion; basal growth hormone levels are normal in hypothyroidism, but the response to hypoglycemia may be blunted. Thyroid hormones have widespread effects on the ossification of cartilage, the growth of teeth, the contours of the face, and the proportions of the body. Hypothyroid dwarfs (also known as **cretins**) therefore have infantile features. Patients who are dwarfed because of panhypopituitarism have features consistent with their chronologic age until puberty, but since they do not mature sexually, they have juvenile features in adulthood (Clinical Box 18–2).

CLINICAL BOX 18–2

Dwarfism

Short stature can be due to GHRH deficiency, growth hormone deficiency, or deficient secretion of IGF-I. Isolated growth hormone deficiency is often due to GHRH deficiency, and in these instances, the growth hormone response to GHRH is normal. However, some patients with isolated growth hormone deficiency have abnormalities of their somatotropes. In another group of dwarfed children, plasma growth hormone is normal or elevated but their growth hormone receptors are unresponsive. The resulting condition is known as **growth hormone insensitivity** or **Laron dwarfism**. Plasma IGF-I is markedly reduced, along with IGFBP-3. African pygmies have normal plasma growth hormone levels and a modest reduction in the plasma level of growth hormone–binding protein. However, their plasma IGF-I concentration fails to increase at the time of puberty.

Short stature may also be caused by mechanisms independent of specific defects in the growth hormone axis. It is characteristic of childhood hypothyroidism (cretinism) and occurs in patients with precocious puberty. It is also part of the syndrome of **gonadal dysgenesis** seen in patients who have an XO chromosomal pattern instead of an XX or XY pattern (see Chapter 22). Various bone and metabolic diseases also cause stunted growth, and in many cases there is no known cause. Chronic abuse and neglect can also cause dwarfism in children, independent of malnutrition. This condition is known as **psychosocial dwarfism** or the **Kaspar Hauser syndrome**. Finally, **achondroplasia**, the most common form of dwarfism in humans, is characterized by short limbs with a normal trunk. It is an autosomal dominant condition caused by a mutation in the gene that codes for **fibroblast growth factor receptor 3 (FGFR3)**.

THERAPEUTIC HIGHLIGHTS

The treatment of dwarfism is dictated by its underlying cause. If treatment to replace a relevant hormone is commenced promptly in childhood cases, almost normal stature can often be attained. Thus, the availability of recombinant forms of growth hormone and IGF-I has greatly improved treatment in cases where these hormones are deficient.

Adrenocortical hormones other than androgens exert a permissive action on growth. On the other hand, glucocorticoids are potent inhibitors of growth because of their direct action on cells, and treatment of children with pharmacologic doses of corticosteroids slows or stops growth for as long as the treatment is continued.

■ PITUITARY GONADOTROPINS & PROLACTIN

CHEMISTRY

FSH and LH are each glycoproteins made up of an α and a β subunit. The carbohydrate in the gonadotropin molecules increases their potency by markedly slowing their metabolism. The half-life of human FSH is about 170 min; the half-life of LH is about 60 min. Loss-of-function mutations in the FSH receptor cause hypogonadism.

Human pituitary prolactin has considerable structural similarity to human growth hormone and human chorionic somatomammotropin (hCS). The half-life of prolactin, like that of growth hormone, is about 20 min.

RECEPTORS

The receptors for FSH and LH are G-protein–coupled receptors coupled to adenylyl cyclase through a stimulatory G-protein (G_s; see Chapter 2). The human prolactin receptor resembles the growth hormone receptor. It dimerizes and activates the JAK–STAT pathway and other intracellular enzyme cascades.

ACTIONS

The testes and ovaries become atrophic when the pituitary is removed or destroyed. The actions of prolactin and the gonadotropins FSH and LH, as well as those of the gonadotropin secreted by the placenta, are described in detail in Chapters 22 and 23. In brief, FSH helps maintain the spermatogenic epithelium by stimulating Sertoli cells in the male and is responsible for the early growth of ovarian follicles in the female. LH is tropic for the Leydig cells and, in females, is responsible for the final maturation of the ovarian follicles and estrogen secretion from them. It is also responsible for ovulation, the initial formation of the corpus luteum, and secretion of progesterone.

Prolactin causes milk synthesis and secretion from the breast after estrogen and progesterone priming. Prolactin also inhibits the effects of gonadotropins, possibly by an action at the level of the ovary and prevents ovulation in lactating women. Excess prolactin secreted by tumors in males causes erectile dysfunction.

REGULATION OF PROLACTIN SECRETION

The regulatory factors for prolactin secretion by the pituitary overlap, in part, with those causing secretion of growth hormone, but there are important differences (Table 18–3). The normal

TABLE 18–3 Comparison of factors affecting the secretion of human prolactin and growth hormone.

Factor	Prolactin	Growth Hormone
Sleep	I+	I+
Nursing	I++	N
Breast stimulation in nonlactating women	I	N
Stress	I+	I+
Hypoglycemia	I	I+
Strenuous exercise	I	I
Sexual intercourse in women	I	N
Pregnancy	I++	N
Estrogens	I	I
Hypothyroidism	I	N
TRH	I+	N
Phenothiazines, butyrophenones	I+	N
Opioids	I	I
Glucose	N	D
Somatostatin	N	D+
L-dopa	D+	I+
Apomorphine	D+	I+
Bromocriptine and related ergot derivatives	D+	I

I, moderate increase; I+, marked increase; I++, very marked increase; N, no change; D, moderate decrease; D+, marked decrease; TRH, thyrotropin-releasing hormone.

plasma prolactin concentration is approximately 5 ng/mL in men and 8 ng/mL in women. Secretion is tonically inhibited by the hypothalamus, and section of the pituitary stalk leads to an increase in circulating prolactin. Thus, the effect of the hypothalamic prolactin-inhibiting hormone, dopamine, must normally be dominant. Prolactin secretion is increased by exercise, surgical and psychological stresses, and stimulation of the nipple (Table 18–3). Plasma prolactin rises during sleep, the rise starting after the onset of sleep and persisting throughout the sleep period. Secretion is increased during pregnancy, reaching a peak at the time of parturition. After delivery, the plasma concentration falls to nonpregnant levels in about 8 days. Suckling produces a prompt increase in secretion, but the magnitude of this rise gradually declines after a woman has been nursing for more than 3 months. With prolonged lactation, milk secretion occurs with prolactin levels that are in the normal range.

Chlorpromazine and related drugs that block dopamine receptors increase prolactin secretion. Thyrotropin-releasing hormone (TRH) stimulates the secretion of prolactin in addition to TSH, and additional polypeptides with prolactin-releasing activity are present in hypothalamic tissue. Estrogens produce a slowly developing increase in prolactin secretion as a result of a direct action on lactotropes.

It has now been established that prolactin facilitates the secretion of dopamine in the median eminence. Thus, prolactin acts in the hypothalamus in a negative feedback manner to inhibit its own secretion.

■ EFFECTS OF PITUITARY INSUFFICIENCY

CHANGES IN OTHER ENDOCRINE GLANDS

The widespread changes that develop when the pituitary is removed surgically or destroyed by disease are predictable in terms of the known hormonal functions of the gland. In hypopituitarism, the adrenal cortex atrophies, and the secretion of adrenal glucocorticoids and sex hormones falls to low levels. Stress-induced increases in aldosterone secretion are absent, but basal aldosterone secretion and increases induced by salt depletion are normal, at least for some time. Since no mineralocorticoid deficiency is present, salt loss and hypovolemic shock do not develop, but the inability to increase glucocorticoid secretion makes patients with pituitary insufficiency sensitive to stress. The development of salt loss in long-standing hypopituitarism is discussed in Chapter 20. Growth is inhibited (see above). Thyroid function is depressed to low levels, and cold is tolerated poorly. The gonads atrophy, sexual cycles stop, and some of the secondary sex characteristics disappear.

INSULIN SENSITIVITY

Hypophysectomized animals have a tendency to become hypoglycemic, especially when fasted. Hypophysectomy ameliorates diabetes mellitus and markedly increases the hypoglycemic effect of insulin. This is due in part to the deficiency of adrenocortical hormones, but hypophysectomized animals are more sensitive to insulin than adrenalectomized animals because they also lack the anti-insulin effect of growth hormone.

WATER METABOLISM

Although selective destruction of the supraoptic–posterior pituitary causes diabetes insipidus, removal of both the anterior and posterior pituitary usually causes no more than a transient polyuria. The amelioration of the diabetes insipidus is actually explained by a decrease in the osmotic load presented for excretion. Osmotically active particles hold water in the renal tubules (see Chapter 38). Because of the ACTH deficiency, the rate of protein catabolism is decreased in hypophysectomized animals. Because of the TSH deficiency, the metabolic rate is low. Consequently, fewer osmotically active products of catabolism are filtered and urine volume declines, even in the absence of vasopressin. Growth hormone deficiency contributes to the depression of the glomerular filtration rate in hypophysectomized animals. Finally, because of the glucocorticoid deficiency, there is the same defective excretion of a water load that is seen in adrenalectomized animals.

CAUSES OF PITUITARY INSUFFICIENCY IN HUMANS

Tumors of the anterior pituitary cause pituitary insufficiency. Suprasellar cysts, remnants of Rathke pouch that enlarge and compress the pituitary, are another cause of hypopituitarism. In women

who have an episode of shock due to postpartum hemorrhage, the pituitary may become infarcted, with the subsequent development of postpartum necrosis (**Sheehan syndrome**). The blood supply to the anterior lobe is vulnerable because it descends on the pituitary stalk through the rigid diaphragma sellae, and during pregnancy the pituitary is enlarged. Pituitary infarction is rare in men.

CHAPTER SUMMARY

■ The pituitary gland plays a critical role in regulating the function of downstream glands, and exerts independent endocrine actions on a wide variety of peripheral organs. It consists of two functional sections in humans: the anterior pituitary, which secretes mainly tropic hormones; and the posterior pituitary, which contains nerve endings that release oxytocin and vasopressin.

■ Corticotropes of the anterior lobe synthesize proopiomelanocortin, which is the precursor of ACTH, endorphins, and melanotropins. ACTH is a primary regulator of skin pigmentation in mammals.

■ Growth hormone is synthesized by somatotropes. It is secreted in an episodic manner in response to hypothalamic factors, and subject to feedback inhibition.

■ Growth hormone activates growth and influences protein, carbohydrate, and fat metabolism to react to stressful conditions. Many actions of growth hormone can be attributed to its ability to stimulate production of IGF-I.

■ Growth reflects a complex interplay of growth hormone, IGF-I, and many other hormones as well as extrinsic influences and genetic factors. Deficiencies in components of the growth hormone pathway in childhood lead to dwarfism; overproduction results in gigantism, acromegaly, or both.

■ The pituitary also supplies hormones that regulate reproductive tissues and lactation—follicle-stimulating hormone, luteinizing hormone, and prolactin.

MULTIPLE-CHOICE QUESTIONS

For all questions, select the single best answer unless otherwise directed.

1. An endocrine physiologist is studying communication between the hypothalamus and pituitary in a rat model. She interrupts blood flow emanating from the median eminence and then measures circulating levels of pituitary hormones following appropriate physiologic stimulation. Secretion of which of the following hormones will be unaffected by the experimental manipulation?
   A. Growth hormone
   B. Prolactin
   C. Thyroid-stimulating hormone (TSH)
   D. Follicle-stimulating hormone (FSH)
   E. Vasopressin

2. A 20-year-old African American woman is seen by her primary care physician for evaluation of patches of skin on her face and hands that have lost pigmentation. She denies any injuries to the affected areas and is otherwise healthy. The symptoms have developed over the last few weeks. Blood tests reveal the presence of autoantibodies to tyrosinase. The most likely diagnosis is
   A. albinism.
   B. piebaldism.

C.   primary adrenal insufficiency.
D.   vitiligo.
E.   hypopituitarism.

3. A scientist studying pain processing in a mouse model administers a drug that inhibits proteolytic processing of proopiomelanocortin (POMC) in the pituitary. An increased response to painful stimuli is noted in the treated animals compared to controls. The effect of the drug is due to a lack of effective levels of
A.   α-melanocyte-stimulating hormone (α-MSH).
B.   β-MSH.
C.   ACTH.
D.   growth hormone.
E.   β-endorphin.

4. During childbirth, a woman suffers a serious hemorrhage and goes into shock. After she recovers, she displays symptoms of hypopituitarism. Which of the following will not be expected in this patient?
A.   Cachexia
B.   Infertility
C.   Pallor
D.   Low basal metabolic rate
E.   Intolerance to stress

5. A scientist finds that infusion of growth hormone into the median eminence of the hypothalamus in experimental animals inhibits the secretion of growth hormone and concludes that this proves that growth hormone feeds back physiologically to inhibit GHRH secretion. Do you accept this conclusion?
A.   No, because growth hormone does not cross the blood–brain barrier.
B.   No, because the infused growth hormone could be stimulating dopamine secretion.
C.   No, because substances placed in the median eminence could be transported to the anterior pituitary.
D.   Yes, because systemically administered growth hormone inhibits growth hormone secretion.
E.   Yes, because growth hormone binds GHRH, inactivating it.

6. In a cell culture model of hepatocytes expressing the growth hormone receptor, a scientist administers a mutated form of growth hormone that contains only one binding site for the receptor. The failure of this analogue to stimulate IGF-I secretion from the cell line, compared to native growth hormone, is explained by the fact that the growth factor receptor
A.   activates G_s.
B.   requires dimerization to exert its effects.
C.   must be internalized to exert its effects.
D.   resembles the IGF-I receptor.
E.   resembles the ACTH receptor.

7. A mother brings her 7-year-old son to the pediatrician for an evaluation of his short stature. Blood tests reveal that his average plasma concentration of growth hormone is within the normal range for his age or even slightly elevated, but levels of IGF-I are markedly reduced. The growth failure in this child is most likely due to a defect in
A.   GHRH release from the hypothalamus.
B.   GHRH receptors.
C.   androgen synthesis.
D.   estrogen synthesis.
E.   growth hormone receptors.

8. In patient described in Question 7, treatment with which recombinant peptide, and by which route, would be most likely to increase his growth?
A.   Intravenous GHRH
B.   Intravenous growth hormone
C.   Oral growth hormone
D.   Intravenous IGF-I
E.   Oral IGF-I

9. A 30-year-old man is referred to an endocrinologist for evaluation of a constellation of symptoms that have arisen with an insidious course over a 5-year period. The patient notes that his feet have grown to an extent that he has had to replace all of his shoes; he has persistent headaches and protrusion of his brow and jaw, and frequent joint pain. A physical examination reveals hepatomegaly. The physician suspects a diagnosis of acromegaly caused by a pituitary adenoma but a blood test reveals that the plasma concentration of growth hormone is within the normal range. Assuming the diagnosis is correct, measurement of increased levels of what other substance in the blood might confirm the diagnosis?
A.   GHRH
B.   Prolactin
C.   IGF-I
D.   IGF-II
E.   Insulin

10. Following a diagnosis of acromegaly secondary to a growth hormone-secreting pituitary adenoma in the patient described in Question 9, the endocrinologist reviews possible treatments that might be anticipated to improve his symptoms. The list of options may contain all of the following *except*
A.   surgical removal of the adenoma.
B.   long-acting somatostatin analogue.
C.   growth hormone receptor antagonist.
D.   targeted radiotherapy of the adenoma.
E.   GHRH receptor antagonist.

ANSWERS

1. The correct answer is **E**. Secretion of hormones from the anterior pituitary (including growth hormone, prolactin, TSH, and FSH) is regulated either positively or negatively by factors delivered from the hypothalamus in the portal hypophysial circulation. Thus, the secretion of all anterior pituitary hormones will be influenced by the manipulation described, although it is important to note that secretion of prolactin will be increased rather than decreased since the dominant influence of the hypothalamus on its secretion is inhibitory (mediated by dopamine) (rules out options **A, B, C,** and **D**). Conversely, vasopressin is released from the endings of hypothalamic nerves that make up the posterior pituitary and should be unaffected.

2. The correct answer is **D**. Vitiligo is an autoimmune condition that develops at varying times after birth and results from patchy destruction of melanocytes by antibodies directed against their cellular components (such as tyrosinase, the enzyme responsible for the synthesis of melanin from tyrosine). It can be distinguished from piebaldism, which it otherwise may resemble, because piebaldism is present from birth and results from developmental defects in migration of neural crest cells that become melanocytes (rules out option **B**). Albinism results in a generalized, rather than patchy, loss of pigmentation from birth, ascribable to a genetic defect in tyrosinase activity (rules out option **A**). Pallor does occur in hypopituitarism

due to a loss of circulating ACTH (the circulating trigger for melanin synthesis in adults), but again it is generalized (rules out option **E**). In primary adrenal disease, hyper- rather than hypopigmentation occurs because ACTH levels are increased in the absence of negative feedback on the secretion of ACTH normally exerted by glucocorticoids (rules out option **C**).

3. The correct answer is **E**. In the anterior pituitary, POMC is produced in corticotropes and processed into a number of biologically active peptides in response to stressful situations, such as pain. α-MSH, β-MSH, and ACTH are all cleavage products of POMC, but are not involved in analgesia (rules out options **A, B,** and **C**) whereas β-endorphin is an endogenous opioid peptide. Growth hormone is also produced by the anterior pituitary, but is not derived from POMC (rules out option **D**).

4. The correct answer is **A**. The blood supply to the anterior pituitary is vulnerable in postpartum women because the gland enlarges during pregnancy and the portal hypophysial vessels pass through a rigid orifice. In shock, infarction of the pituitary may lead to postpartum necrosis and a deficit in the hormones of the anterior pituitary. Inadequate levels of GnRH (infertility), ACTH (pallor as well as intolerance to stress), and thyroid stimulating hormone (low basal metabolic rate) can lead to the symptoms noted (rules out options **B, C, D,** and **E**). Cachexia, on the other hand, is defined as weight loss, muscle atrophy, and fatigue that accompanies a chronic illness such as cancer. If anything, weight gain might be expected in this patient due to secondary effects on thyroid function.

5. The correct answer is **C**. Conclusions about whether growth hormone can cross the blood–brain barrier cannot be drawn from these experiments where growth hormone is directly infused into the hypothalamus (rules out option **A**). Further, while dopamine is known to be an important hypothalamic negative regulator of prolactin secretion from the anterior pituitary, it positively regulates growth hormone secretion (rules out option **B**). Systemic growth hormone could impact growth hormone secretion via numerous mechanisms, including the production of somatostatin (rules out option **D**) and there is no known physical interaction, positive or negative, between growth hormone and GHRH (rules out option **E**). On the other hand, it is clear that substances placed in or released from the median eminence can enter the portal hypophysial vessels and be carried to the anterior pituitary, and growth hormone has been shown to inhibit its own release from somatotropes. Overall, the experiment is not definitive and the stated conclusion cannot be drawn, which illustrates the complexity of feedback mechanisms controlling the release of many hormones.

6. The correct answer is **B**. The growth factor receptor is a receptor tyrosine kinase (rather than a G-protein–coupled receptor, ruling out option **A**) that shares at least some downstream signaling components with the IGF-I receptor (as well as receptor for insulin). However, this relationship would not account for the experimental findings (rules out option **D**). The growth hormone receptor does not resemble that for ACTH, which is a G-protein–coupled receptor linked to G_S (rules out option **E**). Further, internalization of the growth hormone receptor is triggered by ligand binding, but is responsible for receptor inactivation rather than mediating its effects (rules out option **C**). On the other hand, the growth hormone receptor must dimerize to exert its effects, and a mutated ligand capable of binding only a single receptor would not be able to induce such dimers by crosslinking.

7. The correct answer is **E**. Because plasma growth hormone levels are normal, it is unlikely that there is a deficit in GHRH, the factor that causes its release from the anterior pituitary, or the response of somatotropes to GHRH (rules out options **A** and **B**). Androgens and estrogens do not play a significant role in growth until the time of puberty, and thus are unlikely to be implicated in this child (rules out options **C** and **D**). However, the markedly reduced levels of IGF-I, a hormone that is normally released by the liver and other tissue in response to growth hormone, suggests a generalized defect in the response to growth hormone most likely attributable to a malfunctioning receptor. In fact, patients with this disease (Laron syndrome) have homozygous deletions or mutations in their gene for the growth hormone receptor.

8. The correct answer is **D**. Because growth hormone levels are normal or even slightly elevated, no therapeutic benefit is likely to be obtained from supplying this hormone intravenously, nor the factor that causes its release (rules out options **A** and **B**). Further, even if their administration is indicated, growth hormone and IGF-I are both peptides, and unlikely to persist in intact form during gastrointestinal passage to be bioavailable via the oral route (rules out **C** and **E**). Growth restoration has been accomplished in Laron syndrome patients, on the other hand, with intravenous treatment with recombinant human IGF-I, because many of the normal effects of growth hormone on growth are mediated indirectly by its ability to cause secretion of IGF-I. Indeed, infusion of IGF-I into hypophysectomized rats restored bone and body growth.

9. The correct answer is **C**. While individual measurements of circulating growth hormone may be uninformative because it is secreted in a pulsatile manner, it also triggers the synthesis and secretion of IGF-I and this hormone is relatively stable in the plasma over time. Evidence for increased levels of GHRH might reveal a rare cause of acromegaly caused by a hypothalamic tumor secreting this substance, but would not confirm a pituitary adenoma (rules out option **A**). Some pituitary adenomas secrete more than one hormone, but measurement of prolactin levels would not be definitive (rules out option **B**). IGF-II is involved in regulating growth during fetal life, and is not regulated by growth hormone (rules out option **D**). Finally, growth hormone can antagonize the effects of insulin and result in glucose intolerance and even diabetes mellitus in acromegaly, but there are many other possible causes of changes in circulating insulin so its measurement also would not be definitive in this case (rules out option **E**).

10. The correct answer is **E**. All of the other modalities listed would be expected to offer benefits at least in a subset of patients (rules out options A, B, C and D), with the use of somatostatin analogues representing the mainstay of medical treatment and often resulting in the regression of symptoms as well as normalization of circulating IGF-I levels. Full surgical resection of these tumors may be challenging, and even highly targeted radiotherapy may result in significant side effects, but each have their place in well-selected patients. A relatively recently approved growth hormone receptor antagonist has also been shown to be beneficial, particularly in those patients found to be refractory to other agents. On the other hand, because secretion of growth hormone from a pituitary adenoma of this type is largely independent of GHRH (and indeed may even arise from a tumor in an extra-pituitary site, not accessible to releasing factors carried in the portal hypophysial circulation), antagonism of GHRH is unlikely to be effective.

The Thyroid Gland

OBJECTIVES

OBJECTIVES

After studying this chapter, you should be able to:

- Describe the structure of the thyroid gland and how it relates to function.
- Define the chemical nature of the thyroid hormones and how they are synthesized.
- Understand the role of iodine in the thyroid gland and how its transport is controlled.
- Describe the role of protein binding in the transport of thyroid hormones and peripheral metabolism.
- Identify the role of the hypothalamus and pituitary in regulating thyroid function.
- Define the effects of the thyroid hormones in homeostasis and development.
- Understand the basis of conditions where thyroid function is abnormal and how they can be treated.

INTRODUCTION

The thyroid gland has two primary functions. The first is to secrete the thyroid hormones, which maintain optimal levels of tissue metabolism. Thyroid hormones stimulate O_2 consumption by most cells, help regulate lipid and carbohydrate metabolism, and influence body mass and mentation. Consequences of thyroid gland dysfunction depend on life stage. The thyroid is not essential for life, but hypofunction during fetal and neonatal life results in severe mental retardation and dwarfism. In adults, hypothyroidism is accompanied by mental and physical slowing and poor resistance to cold. Conversely, excess thyroid secretion leads to body wasting, nervousness, tachycardia, tremor, and excess heat production. Thyroid function is controlled by the thyroid-stimulating hormone (TSH, thyrotropin) of the anterior pituitary. The secretion of this hormone is in turn increased by thyrotropin-releasing hormone (TRH) from the hypothalamus and is also subject to negative feedback control.

The second function of the thyroid gland is to secrete calcitonin, a hormone that regulates circulating levels of calcium. This function of the thyroid gland is discussed in Chapter 21.

■ ANATOMIC CONSIDERATIONS

The thyroid is a butterfly-shaped gland that straddles the trachea in the front of the neck. It develops from an evagination of the floor of the pharynx. The gland is well vascularized, with one of the highest rates of blood flow per gram of tissue of any organ.

The portion of the thyroid concerned with the production of thyroid hormone consists of multiple **acini (follicles)** surrounded by a single layer of polarized epithelial cells and filled with material called **colloid**. Colloid consists predominantly of the glycoprotein, thyroglobulin. Microvilli project into the colloid from the apexes of the thyroid cells and canaliculi extend into them. The endoplasmic reticulum is prominent, a feature common to most glandular cells, and secretory granules containing thyroglobulin are seen. The individual thyroid cells rest on a basal lamina that separates them from the adjacent fenestrated capillaries.

■ FORMATION & SECRETION OF THYROID HORMONES

CHEMISTRY

The primary hormone secreted by the thyroid is **thyroxine (T_4)**, along with much lesser amounts of **triiodothyronine (T_3)**. T_3 has much greater biologic activity than T_4 but is generated at its site of action in peripheral tissues by deiodination of T_4 (see below). Both hormones are iodine-containing amino acids. Small amounts of reverse triiodothyronine (3,3′,5′-triiodothyronine, RT_3) are also found. Whether RT_3 is biologically active remains unclear.

IODINE HOMEOSTASIS

Iodine is an essential raw material for thyroid hormone synthesis. Dietary iodide is absorbed by the intestine and enters the circulation; its subsequent fate is summarized in **Figure 19–1**. The minimum daily iodine intake that will maintain normal thyroid function is 150 μg in adults, but average intake is 500 μg. The principal organs that take up circulating I^- are the thyroid, which uses it to make thyroid hormones, and the kidneys, which excrete it in the urine. Circulating T_3 and T_4 are metabolized in the liver and other tissues. Some thyroid hormone derivatives are excreted in the bile, and some of the iodine in them is reabsorbed (enterohepatic circulation), but there is a net loss of I^- in the stool of approximately 20 μg/day.

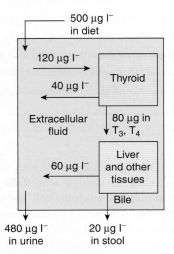

FIGURE 19–1 Iodine metabolism. The figure shows the movement of iodide among various body compartments on a daily basis.

IODIDE TRANSPORT ACROSS THYROCYTES

The basolateral membranes of thyrocytes facing the capillaries contain a **symporter** that transports two Na^+ ions and one I^- ion into the cell with each cycle. This Na^+/I^- symporter (**NIS**) is capable of producing intracellular I^- concentrations that are 20–40 times as great as the concentration in plasma by secondary active transport. NIS is regulated both by transcriptional means and by active trafficking into and out of the basolateral membrane in response to thyroid-stimulating hormone (TSH). Iodide must also exit the thyrocyte across the apical membrane to access the colloid, where the initial steps of thyroid hormone synthesis occur. This transport step is believed to be mediated, at least in part, by a Cl^-/I^- exchanger known as **pendrin**. Iodide is essential for normal thyroid function, but iodide deficiency and iodide excess both inhibit thyroid function.

THYROID HORMONE SYNTHESIS & SECRETION

At the interface between the thyrocyte and the colloid, iodide undergoes a process referred to as organification. First, it is oxidized to iodine, and then incorporated into the carbon 3 position of tyrosine residues that are part of the thyroglobulin molecule in the colloid. **Thyroglobulin** contains 123 tyrosine residues, but only 4–8 of these are normally incorporated into thyroid hormones. Thyroglobulin is synthesized in the thyroid cells and secreted into the colloid by exocytosis. The oxidation and reaction of iodide with the secreted thyroglobulin is mediated by **thyroid peroxidase**, found in the thyrocyte apical membrane. The thyroid hormones produced remain part of the thyroglobulin molecule until needed. As such, colloid represents a reservoir of thyroid hormones, and humans can ingest a diet completely devoid of iodide for up to 2 months before a decline in circulating thyroid hormone levels is seen. When there is a need for thyroid hormone secretion, colloid is internalized by the thyrocytes by endocytosis, and directed toward lysosomal degradation. The peptide bonds of thyroglobulin are hydrolyzed, and free T_4 and T_3 are discharged into cytosol and thence to the capillaries.

Thyroid hormone synthesis is a multistep process. Thyroid peroxidase generates reactive iodine species that can attack thyroglobulin. The first product is monoiodotyrosine (MIT). MIT is next iodinated on the carbon 5 position to form diiodotyrosine (DIT). Two DIT molecules then undergo an oxidative condensation to form T_4 with the elimination of the alanine side chain from the molecule that forms the outer ring. T_3 is formed by condensation of MIT with DIT. In the normal human thyroid, the average distribution of iodinated compounds is 3% MIT, 33% DIT, 35% T_4, and 7% T_3.

The human thyroid secretes about 80 μg (103 nmol) of T_4, 4 μg (7 nmol) of T_3, and 2 μg (3.5 nmol) of RT_3 per day. MIT

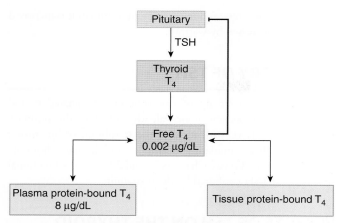

FIGURE 19–2 Regulation of thyroid hormone synthesis. T_4 is secreted by the thyroid in response to TSH. Free T_4 secreted by the thyroid into the circulation is in equilibrium with T_4 bound to both plasma and tissue proteins. Free T_4 also feeds back to inhibit TSH secretion by the pituitary.

and DIT are not secreted. These iodinated tyrosines are deiodinated by a microsomal **iodotyrosine deiodinase**, representing a mechanism to recover iodine and bound tyrosines and recycle them for additional rounds of hormone synthesis.

■ TRANSPORT & METABOLISM OF THYROID HORMONES

PROTEIN BINDING

The normal total **plasma T_4** level in adults is approximately 8 μg/dL (103 nmol/L), and the **plasma T_3** level is approximately 0.15 μg/dL (2.3 nmol/L). T_4 and T_3 are relatively lipophilic; thus, their free forms in plasma are in equilibrium with a much larger pool of protein-bound thyroid hormones in plasma and in tissues. Free thyroid hormones are added to the circulating pool by the thyroid. It is the free thyroid hormones in plasma that are physiologically active and that feed back to inhibit TSH secretion **(Figure 19–2)**. Protein-binding maintains a large pool of hormone that can be mobilized as needed.

In addition, at least for T_3, hormone binding prevents excess uptake by the first cells encountered and promotes uniform tissue distribution. Total T_4 and T_3 can both be measured by radioimmunoassay. There are also direct assays that measure only the free forms of the hormones. The latter are the more clinically relevant.

The plasma proteins that bind thyroid hormones are **albumin**, a prealbumin called **transthyretin**, and a globulin known as **thyroxine-binding globulin (TBG)**. Of the three proteins, albumin has the largest **capacity** to bind T_4 (ie, it can bind the most T_4 before becoming saturated) and TBG has the smallest capacity. However, the **affinities** of the proteins for T_4 are such that most of the circulating T_4 is bound to TBG. Normally, 99.98% of the T_4 in plasma is bound.

T_3 is not bound to quite as great an extent; of the 0.15 μg/dL normally found in plasma, 0.2% (0.3 ng/dL) is free. The remaining 99.8% is protein-bound, 46% to TBG and most of the remainder to albumin, with very little binding to transthyretin. The lesser binding of T_3 correlates with the facts that T_3 has a shorter half-life than T_4 and that its action on the tissues is much more rapid.

FLUCTUATIONS IN BINDING

When a sudden, sustained increase in the concentration of thyroid-binding proteins in the plasma takes place, the concentration of free thyroid hormones falls. This change is temporary, however, because the decrease in free hormones stimulates TSH secretion, which in turn causes an increase in the production of free thyroid hormones. A new equilibrium is eventually reached at which the total quantity of thyroid hormones in the blood is elevated but the concentration of free hormones, the rate of their metabolism, and the rate of TSH secretion are normal. Corresponding changes in the opposite direction occur when the concentration of thyroid-binding protein is reduced.

TBG levels are modulated during pregnancy, as well as after treatment with various drugs **(Table 19–1)**. A number of other drugs inhibit binding of T_4 and T_3 to TBG and consequently produce changes similar to those produced by a decrease in TBG concentration. Changes can also be produced by changes in plasma concentrations of albumin and prealbumin.

TABLE 19–1 Effect of variations in the concentrations of thyroid hormone–binding proteins in the plasma on various parameters of thyroid function after equilibrium has been reached.

Condition	Concentrations of Binding Proteins	Total Plasma T_4, T_3, RT_3	Free Plasma T_4, T_3, RT_3	Plasma TSH	Clinical State
Hyperthyroidism	Normal	High	High	Low	Hyperthyroid
Hypothyroidism	Normal	Low	Low	High	Hypothyroid
Estrogens, methadone, heroin, antipsychotic drugs, clofibrate	High	High	Normal	Normal	Euthyroid
Glucocorticoids, androgens, danazol, asparaginase	Low	Low	Normal	Normal	Euthyroid

METABOLISM OF THYROID HORMONES

T_4 and T_3 are deiodinated in the liver, the kidneys, and many other tissues. These deiodination reactions catabolize the hormones but also provide a local supply of T_3, which is believed to be the primary mediator of the physiologic effects of thyroid secretion.

Three different deiodinases act on thyroid hormones: D_1, D_2, and D_3. All are unique in that they contain the rare amino acid selenocysteine, with selenium in place of sulfur, which is essential for enzymatic activity. D_1 is present in high concentrations in the liver, kidneys, thyroid, and pituitary. It appears primarily to be responsible for maintaining the formation of T_3 from T_4 in the periphery. D_2 is present in the brain, pituitary, and brown fat. It also contributes to the formation of T_3. In the brain, it is located in astroglia and produces a supply of T_3 to neurons. D_3 is also present in the brain and in reproductive tissues. It acts only on the carbon 5 position of T_4 and T_3 and is probably the main source of RT_3 in the blood and tissues. Overall, the deiodinases appear to be responsible for maintaining differences in T_3/T_4 ratios in various tissues.

Some of the T_4 and T_3 is further converted to diiodotyrosines. T_4 and T_3 are also conjugated in the liver to form sulfates and glucuronides. These conjugates enter the bile and pass into the intestine, where some recirculate but others are excreted in the stool.

FLUCTUATIONS IN DEIODINATION

Much more RT_3 and much less T_3 are formed during fetal life. Various drugs inhibit deiodinases, producing a fall in plasma T_3 levels and a reciprocal rise in RT_3. Selenium deficiency has the same effect. A wide variety of nonthyroidal illnesses also suppress deiodinases. These include burns, trauma, advanced cancer, cirrhosis, chronic kidney disease, myocardial infarction, and febrile states. The low-T_3 state produced by these conditions disappears with recovery.

Diet also has a clear-cut effect on conversion of T_4 to T_3. Fasting reduces plasma T_3 with a corresponding rise in RT_3 while free and bound T_4 levels remain essentially normal. The basal metabolic rate (BMR) falls and urinary nitrogen excretion, an index of protein breakdown, is decreased. Thus, the decline in T_3 conserves calories and protein. Conversely, overfeeding increases T_3 and reduces RT_3.

■ REGULATION OF THYROID SECRETION

Thyroid function is regulated primarily by TSH (Figure 19–2). TSH secretion is increased by the hypothalamic TRH (see Chapter 17) and inhibited in a negative feedback manner by circulating free T_4 and T_3. The effect of T_4 is enhanced by production of T_3 in the cytoplasm of the pituitary cells. TSH secretion is also inhibited by stress, and in experimental animals it is increased by cold and decreased by warmth.

CHEMISTRY OF TSH

Human TSH is made up of two subunits, designated α and β. The subunits become noncovalently linked in the pituitary thyrotropes. TSH-α is identical to the α subunit of luteinizing hormone, follicle-stimulating hormone, and human chorionic gonadotropin (hCG) (see Chapters 18 and 22) with the functional specificity of TSH conferred by the β subunit.

EFFECTS OF TSH ON THE THYROID

When the pituitary is removed, thyroid function is depressed and the gland atrophies; when TSH is administered, thyroid function is stimulated. With long-term TSH treatment, the cell hypertrophy and the weight of the gland increase. Whenever TSH stimulation is prolonged, the thyroid becomes detectably enlarged. Enlargement of the thyroid is called a **goiter**.

TSH RECEPTORS

The TSH receptor is a typical G-protein–coupled, seven-transmembrane receptor that activates adenylyl cyclase through G_s. It also activates phospholipase C (PLC). Like other glycoprotein hormone receptors, it has an extended, glycosylated extracellular domain.

OTHER FACTORS AFFECTING THYROID GROWTH

In addition to TSH receptors, thyrocytes express receptors for insulin-like growth factor I (IGF-I), epidermal growth factor (EGF), and other growth factors. IGF-I and EGF promote growth, whereas interferon-γ and tumor necrosis factor-α inhibit growth. Thyroid function might be inhibited in the setting of chronic inflammation, which could contribute to cachexia, or weight loss.

CONTROL MECHANISMS

The mechanisms regulating thyroid secretion are summarized in Figure 19–2. The negative feedback effect of thyroid hormones on TSH secretion is exerted in part at the hypothalamic level, but also on the pituitary, since T_4 and T_3 block the increase in TSH secretion produced by TRH. Infusion of either T_4 or T_3 reduces the circulating level of TSH. The day-to-day maintenance of thyroid secretion depends on the feedback interplay of thyroid hormones with TSH and TRH (Figure 19–2). The adjustments that appear to be mediated via TRH include the increased secretion of thyroid hormones produced by cold and,

CLINICAL BOX 19–1

Reduced Thyroid Function

The syndrome of adult **hypothyroidism** is generally called **myxedema**, although this term is also used to refer specifically to the skin changes in the syndrome. Hypothyroidism may be the end result of a number of diseases of the thyroid gland, or it may be secondary to pituitary or hypothalamic failure. In the latter two conditions, the thyroid remains able to respond to TSH. Thyroid function may be reduced by a number of conditions (Table 19–2). For example, when the dietary iodine intake falls below 50 μg/day, thyroid hormone synthesis is inadequate and secretion declines. As a result of increased TSH secretion, the thyroid hypertrophies, producing an **iodine deficiency goiter** that may become very large. Such "endemic goiters" have been substantially reduced by the practice of adding iodide to table salt. Drugs may also inhibit thyroid function. Most do so either by interfering with the iodide-trapping mechanism or by blocking the organic binding of iodine. In either case, TSH secretion is stimulated by the decline in circulating thyroid hormones, and a goiter is produced. Paradoxically, another substance that inhibits thyroid function under certain conditions is iodide itself. In normal individuals, large doses of iodide act directly on the thyroid to produce a mild and transient inhibition of organic binding of iodide and hence of hormone synthesis. This inhibition is known as the **Wolff–Chaikoff effect**.

In completely athyreotic adults, the BMR falls to about 40%. The hair is coarse and sparse, the skin is dry and yellowish (carotenemia), and cold is poorly tolerated. Mentation is slow, memory is poor, and in some patients there are severe mental symptoms ("myxedema madness"). Plasma cholesterol is elevated. Children who are hypothyroid from birth or before are called **cretins**. They are dwarfed and mentally retarded. Worldwide, congenital hypothyroidism is one of the most common causes of preventable mental retardation. The main causes are included in Table 19–2. They include not only maternal iodine deficiency and various congenital abnormalities of the fetal hypothalamo–pituitary–thyroid axis, but also maternal antithyroid antibodies that cross the placenta and damage the fetal thyroid. T_4 crosses the placenta, and unless the mother is hypothyroid, growth and development are normal until birth. If treatment is started at birth, the prognosis for normal growth and development is good, and mental retardation can generally be avoided; for this reason, screening tests for congenital hypothyroidism are becoming routine. When the mother is hypothyroid as well, as in the case of iodine deficiency, the mental deficiency is more severe and less responsive to treatment after birth. It has been estimated that 20 million people in the world now have various degrees of brain damage caused by iodine deficiency in utero.

Uptake of tracer doses of radioactive iodine can be used to assess thyroid function (contrast this with the use of large doses to ablate thyroid tissue in cases of hyperthyroidism (Clinical Box 19–2).

THERAPEUTIC HIGHLIGHTS

The treatment of hypothyroidism depends on the underlying mechanisms. Iodide deficiency can be addressed by adding it to the diet, as is done routinely in developed countries with the use of iodized salt. In congenital hypothyroidism, levothyroxine—a synthetic form of the thyroid hormone T_4—can be given. It is important that this take place as soon as possible after birth, with levels regularly monitored, to minimize long-term adverse effects.

---

presumably, the decrease produced by heat. However, while cold produces clear-cut increases in circulating TSH in infants, the rise in adults is negligible. Consequently, in adults, increased heat production due to increased thyroid hormone secretion **(thyroid hormone thermogenesis)** plays little if any role in the response to cold. Stress has an inhibitory effect on TRH secretion. Dopamine and somatostatin act at the pituitary to inhibit TSH secretion, but it is not known whether they play a physiologic role in the regulation of TSH secretion. Glucocorticoids also inhibit TSH secretion.

TABLE 19–2 Causes of congenital hypothyroidism.

Maternal iodine deficiency
Fetal thyroid dysgenesis
Inborn errors of thyroid hormone synthesis
Maternal antithyroid antibodies that cross the placenta
Fetal hypopituitary hypothyroidism

Measurement of TSH is now widely regarded as one of the best tests of thyroid function. The amount of T_4 that normalizes plasma TSH in athyreotic individuals averages 112 μg of T_4 by mouth per day in adults. In humans, circulating T_3 rather than T_4 is the principal feedback regulator of TSH secretion (Clinical Boxes 19–1 and 19–2).

■ EFFECTS OF THYROID HORMONES

Some of the widespread effects of thyroid hormones in the body are secondary to stimulation of O_2 consumption (**calorigenic action**), although the hormones also affect growth and development, regulate lipid metabolism, and increase the absorption of carbohydrates from the intestine (Table 19–4). They also increase the dissociation of oxygen from hemoglobin by increasing red cell 2,3-diphosphoglycerate (DPG) (see Chapter 35).

CLINICAL BOX 19-2

Hyperthyroidism

The symptoms of an overactive thyroid gland follow logically from the actions of thyroid hormone discussed in this chapter. Thus, hyperthyroidism is characterized by nervousness; weight loss; hyperphagia; heat intolerance; increased pulse pressure; a fine tremor of the outstretched fingers; warm, soft skin; sweating; and a BMR from +10 to as high as +100. It has various causes (Table 19–3); however, the most common cause is **Graves disease (Graves hyperthyroidism)**, which accounts for 60–80% of the cases. This is an autoimmune disease, more common in women, in which antibodies to the TSH receptor stimulate the receptor. This produces marked T_4 and T_3 secretion and enlargement of the thyroid gland (goiter). However, due to the feedback effects of T_4 and T_3, plasma TSH is low, not high. Another hallmark of Graves disease is the occurrence of swelling of tissues in the orbits, producing protrusion of the eyeballs (**exophthalmos**). This occurs in 50% of patients and often precedes the development of obvious hyperthyroidism. Other antithyroid antibodies are present in Graves disease, including antibodies to thyroglobulin and thyroid peroxidase. In Hashimoto thyroiditis, autoimmune antibodies and infiltrating cytotoxic T cells ultimately destroy the thyroid, but during the early stage the inflammation of the gland causes excess thyroid hormone secretion and thyrotoxicosis similar to that seen in Graves disease.

THERAPEUTIC HIGHLIGHTS

Some of the symptoms of hyperthyroidism can be controlled by the **thioureylenes**. These are a group of compounds related to thiourea, which inhibit the iodination of monoiodotyrosine and block the coupling reaction. The two used clinically are propylthiouracil and methimazole. Iodination of tyrosine is inhibited because propylthiouracil and methimazole compete with tyrosine residues for iodine and become iodinated. In addition, propylthiouracil but not methimazole inhibits D_2 deiodinase, reducing the conversion of T_4 to T_3 in many extrathyroidal tissues. In severe cases, hyperthyroidism can also be treated by the infusion of radioactive iodine, which accumulates in the gland and then partially destroys it. Surgery is also considered if the thyroid becomes so large that it affects swallowing and/or breathing.

MECHANISM OF ACTION

Thyroid hormones enter cells and T_3 binds to TR in the nuclei. T_4 can also bind, but not as avidly. The hormone-receptor complex then binds to DNA via zinc fingers and increases (or in some cases, decreases) the expression of a variety of genes coding for proteins that regulate cell function.

There are two human TR genes: α and β. By alternative splicing, each forms at least two different mRNAs and therefore two different receptor proteins. TRβ2 is found only in the brain, but TRα1, TRα2, and TRβ1 are widely distributed. TRα2 does not bind T_3 and its function is not established. TRs bind to DNA as monomers, homodimers, and heterodimers with other nuclear receptors, particularly the retinoid X receptor (**RXR**). The TR/RXR heterodimer does not bind to the ligand for RXR, 9-*cis* retinoic acid, but binding to of this heterodimer to DNA is greatly enhanced in response to thyroid hormones. There are also coactivator and corepressor proteins that affect the actions of TRs. Presumably, this complexity underlies the ability of thyroid hormones to produce many different effects in the body (Clinical Box 19–3).

In most of its actions, T_3 acts more rapidly and is three to five times more potent than T_4. This is because T_3 is less tightly bound to plasma proteins than is T_4, but binds more avidly to thyroid hormone receptors.

TABLE 19–3 Causes of hyperthyroidism.

Thyroid overactivity
Graves disease
Solitary toxic adenoma
Toxic multinodular goiter
Early stages of Hashimoto thyroiditis[a]
TSH-secreting pituitary tumor
Mutations causing constitutive activation of TSH receptor
Other rare causes
Extrathyroidal
Administration of T_3 or T_4 (factitious or iatrogenic hyperthyroidism)
Ectopic thyroid tissue

[a]Note that ultimately the thyroid will be destroyed in Hashimoto disease, resulting in hypothyroidism. Many patients only present after they become hypothyroid, and do not recall a transient phase of hyperthyroidism.

CALORIGENIC ACTION

T_4 and T_3 increase O_2 consumption by almost all metabolically active tissues. The exceptions are the adult brain, testes, uterus, lymph nodes, spleen, and anterior pituitary. T_4 actually depresses the O_2 consumption by the anterior pituitary, presumably because it inhibits TSH secretion. The increase in metabolic rate produced by a single dose of T_4 becomes measurable after a latent period of several hours and lasts 6 days or more.

Some of the calorigenic effect of thyroid hormones is due to metabolism of the fatty acids they mobilize. In addition, thyroid hormones increase the activity of the membrane-bound Na, K ATPase in many tissues.

CLINICAL BOX 19–3

Thyroid Hormone Resistance

Some mutations in the gene that codes for TRβ are associated with resistance to the effects of T_3 and T_4. Most commonly, there is resistance to thyroid hormones in the peripheral tissues and the anterior pituitary gland. Patients with this abnormality are usually not clinically hypothyroid, because they maintain plasma levels of T_3 and T_4 that are high enough to overcome the resistance, and hTRα is unaffected. However, plasma TSH is inappropriately high relative to the high circulating T_3 and T_4 levels and is difficult to suppress with exogenous thyroid hormone. Some patients have thyroid hormone resistance only in the pituitary. They have hypermetabolism and elevated plasma T_3 and T_4 levels with normal, nonsuppressible levels of TSH. A few patients apparently have peripheral resistance with normal pituitary sensitivity. They have hypometabolism despite normal plasma levels of T_3, T_4, and TSH. An interesting finding is that **attention deficit hyperactivity disorder**, a condition frequently diagnosed in children who are overactive and impulsive, is much more common in individuals with thyroid hormone resistance than in the general population. This suggests that hTRβ may play a special role in brain development.

THERAPEUTIC HIGHLIGHTS

Most patients remain euthyroid in this condition, even in the face of a goiter. It is important to consider thyroid hormone resistance in the differential diagnosis of Graves disease to avoid the inappropriate use of antithyroid medications or even thyroid ablation. Isolated peripheral resistance to thyroid hormones can be treated by supplying large doses of synthetic T_4 exogenously. These are sufficient to overcome the resistance and increase the metabolic rate.

Effects Secondary to Calorigenesis

When the metabolic rate is increased in adults, nitrogen excretion is increased; if food intake is not increased, endogenous protein and fat stores are catabolized and weight is lost. In hypothyroid children, small doses of thyroid hormones cause a positive nitrogen balance because they stimulate growth, but large doses cause protein catabolism similar to that produced in the adult.

When the metabolic rate is increased, the need for vitamins is increased and vitamin deficiency syndromes may be precipitated. Thyroid hormones are necessary for hepatic conversion of carotene to vitamin A, and the accumulation of carotene in the bloodstream (**carotenemia**) in hypothyroidism is responsible for the yellowish tint of the skin.

The skin normally contains a variety of proteins combined with polysaccharides, hyaluronic acid, and chondroitin sulfate. In hypothyroidism, these complexes accumulate, promoting water retention and the characteristic puffiness of the skin (myxedema). When thyroid hormones are administered, the proteins are metabolized, and diuresis continues until the myxedema is cleared.

Milk secretion is decreased in hypothyroidism and stimulated by thyroid hormones. Thyroid hormones do not stimulate the metabolism of the uterus but are essential for normal menstrual cycles and fertility.

TABLE 19–4 Physiologic effects of thyroid hormones.

Target Tissue	Effect	Mechanism
Heart	Chronotropic and inotropic	Increased number of β-adrenergic receptors
		Enhanced responses to circulating catecholamines
		Increased proportion of α-myosin heavy chain (with higher ATPase activity)
Adipose tissue	Catabolic	Stimulated lipolysis
Muscle	Catabolic	Increased protein breakdown
Bone	Developmental	Promote normal growth and skeletal development
Nervous system	Developmental	Promote normal brain development
Gut	Metabolic	Increased rate of carbohydrate absorption
Lipoprotein	Metabolic	Formation of LDL receptors
Other	Calorigenic	Stimulated oxygen consumption by metabolically active tissues (exceptions: testes, uterus, lymph nodes, spleen, anterior pituitary)
		Increased metabolic rate

Modified with permission from McPhee SJ, Lingarra VR, Ganong WF (eds): *Pathophysiology of Disease*, 6th ed. New York, NY: McGraw-Hill; 2010.

EFFECTS ON THE CARDIOVASCULAR SYSTEM

Large doses of thyroid hormones cause enough extra heat production to lead to a slight rise in body temperatures (Chapter 17), which in turn activates heat-dissipating mechanisms. Peripheral resistance decreases because of cutaneous vasodilation, and this increases levels of renal Na^+ and water absorption, expanding blood volume. Cardiac output is increased by the direct action of thyroid hormones, as well as that of catecholamines, on the heart, so that pulse pressure and cardiac rate are increased and circulation time is shortened.

T_3 is not formed from T_4 in cardiac myocytes to any degree, but circulatory T_3 enhances expression of α-myosin heavy chain, sarcoplasmic reticulum Ca^{2+} ATPase, β-adrenergic receptors, G-proteins, Na, K ATPase, and certain K^+ channels. Expression of β-myosin heavy chain, phospholamban, two types of adenylyl cyclase, T_3 nuclear receptors, and NCX, the Na^+–Ca^{2+} exchange is inhibited. The net result is increased heart rate and force of contraction.

EFFECTS ON THE NERVOUS SYSTEM

In hypothyroidism, mentation is slow and cerebrospinal fluid (CSF) protein is elevated. Thyroid hormones reverse these changes, while large doses cause rapid mentation, irritability, and restlessness. Overall, cerebral blood flow and glucose and O_2 consumption by the brain are normal in adult hypothyroidism and hyperthyroidism. Astrocytes in the brain convert T_4 to T_3, and there is a sharp increase in brain D_2 activity after thyroidectomy that is reversed within 4 h by a single intravenous dose of T_3. Some of the effects of thyroid hormones on the brain are probably secondary to increased responsiveness to catecholamines. In addition, thyroid hormones have marked effects on brain development. The parts of the central nervous system (CNS) most affected are the cerebral cortex and the basal ganglia. The cochlea is also affected. Consequently, thyroid hormone deficiency during development causes mental retardation, motor rigidity, and deaf–mutism. Thyroid hormones also exert effects on reflexes. The reaction time of stretch reflexes (see Chapter 12) is shortened in hyperthyroidism and prolonged in hypothyroidism.

RELATION TO CATECHOLAMINES

The actions of thyroid hormones and the catecholamines are intimately interrelated. Catecholamines increase the metabolic rate, stimulate the nervous system, and produce cardiovascular effects similar to those of thyroid hormones, although the duration of these actions is brief. The toxicity of the catecholamines is markedly increased in rats treated with T_4. Although plasma catecholamine levels are normal in hyperthyroidism, the cardiovascular effects, tremulousness, and sweating that are seen can be reduced by sympathectomy or by β-adrenergic blockade. However, even

though β-blockers are weak inhibitors of extrathyroidal conversion of T_4 to T_3, and consequently may produce a small fall in plasma T_3, they have little effect on the other actions of thyroid hormones. Presumably, the functional synergism observed between catecholamines and thyroid hormones arises from their overlapping biologic functions as well as the ability of thyroid hormones to increase expression of catecholamine receptors.

EFFECTS ON SKELETAL MUSCLE

Muscle weakness occurs in most patients with hyperthyroidism **(thyrotoxic myopathy)**, due in part to increased protein catabolism. Hypothyroidism is associated with muscle weakness, cramps, and stiffness.

EFFECTS ON CARBOHYDRATE ABSORPTION

Thyroid hormones increase the rate of absorption of carbohydrates from the gastrointestinal tract. In hyperthyroidism, therefore, the plasma glucose level rises rapidly after a carbohydrate meal.

EFFECTS ON CHOLESTEROL METABOLISM

Thyroid hormones lower circulating cholesterol levels. The plasma cholesterol level drops before the metabolic rate rises, which indicates that this action is independent of the stimulation of O_2 consumption. The decrease in plasma cholesterol concentration is due to increased formation of low-density lipoprotein (LDL) receptors in the liver, resulting in increased hepatic removal of cholesterol from the circulation. However, it has not been possible to produce a thyroid hormone analog that lowers plasma cholesterol without increasing metabolism.

EFFECTS ON GROWTH

Thyroid hormones are essential for normal growth and skeletal maturation (see Chapter 21). In hypothyroid children, bone growth is slowed and epiphysial closure delayed. In the absence of thyroid hormones, growth hormone secretion is also depressed. This further impairs growth and development, since thyroid hormones normally potentiate the effect of growth hormone on tissues.

CHAPTER SUMMARY

- The thyroid gland transports and fixes iodide to amino acids present in thyroglobulin to generate the thyroid hormones thyroxine (T_4) and triiodothyronine (T_3).
- Synthesis and secretion of thyroid hormones is stimulated by pituitary thyroid-stimulating hormone (TSH), which in turn is released in response to thyrotropin-releasing hormone (TRH) from the hypothalamus. These releasing factors are controlled by changes in whole body status (eg, cold or stress).

- Thyroid hormones circulate in the plasma predominantly in protein-bound forms. Only the free hormones are biologically active, and feed back to reduce secretion of TSH.

- The liganded forms of thyroid receptors are nuclear transcription factors that alter gene expression.

- Thyroid hormones stimulate metabolic rate, calorigenesis, cardiac function, and normal mentation, and interact synergistically with catecholamines. Thyroid hormones also play critical roles in development and growth.

- Disease results with both underactivity and overactivity of the thyroid gland. Hypothyroidism is accompanied by mental and physical slowing in adults, and by mental retardation and dwarfism if it occurs in neonatal life. Hyperthyroidism results in body wasting, nervousness, and tachycardia.

MULTIPLE-CHOICE QUESTIONS

For all questions, select the single best answer unless otherwise directed.

1. A 40-year-old woman comes to her primary care clinician complaining of nervousness and an unexplained weight loss of 20 pounds over the past 3 months despite her impression that she is eating all the time. On physical examination, her eyes are found to be protruding, her skin is moist and warm, and her fingers have a slight tremor. Compared to a healthy individual, a biopsy of her thyroid gland would most likely reveal which of the following:
   A. Decreased numbers of reabsorption lacunae
   B. Decreased evidence of endocytosis
   C. A decrease in the cross-sectional area occupied by colloid
   D. Increased levels of NIS in the basolateral membrane of thyrocytes
   E. Decreased evidence of lysosomal activity

2. A scientist studying the normal biosynthesis of thyroid hormones creates a series of mouse models that are deficient in various putative contributors to hormone production. Of the animals tested, those lacking which of the following factors should exhibit normal levels of thyroid hormone synthesis?
   A. Iodine
   B. Ferritin
   C. Thyroglobulin
   D. Protein synthesis
   E. TSH

3. In a cell culture model, a scientist transfects mRNA specific for NIS and shows that the transfected cells take up radioactive iodide at a rate that is faster than that seen in control cells. This increase in intracellular I⁻ due to the action of NIS is an example of
   A. endocytosis.
   B. passive diffusion.
   C. Na^+ and K^+ cotransport.
   D. primary active transport.
   E. secondary active transport.

4. A 50-year-old woman is prescribed hormone-replacement therapy to ameliorate perimenopausal symptoms. She subsequently develops sustained metabolic symptoms consistent with hypothyroidism. Her metabolic rate likely has been *least* affected by a change in the plasma level of
   A. TSH.
   B. TRH.

   C. TBG.
   D. Free T_4.
   E. Free T_3.

5. In a 30-year-old female patient being evaluated for a constellation of symptoms suspected to relate to thyroid dysfunction, TRH is infused and the release of TSH is measured. The TSH response to TRH is found to be reduced compared to a normal individual. Which is the most likely underlying condition?
   A. Hypothyroidism due to tissue resistance to thyroid hormone
   B. Hypothyroidism due to disease destroying the thyroid gland
   C. Hyperthyroidism due to circulating antithyroid antibodies with TSH activity
   D. Hyperthyroidism due to diffuse hyperplasia of thyrotropes of the anterior pituitary
   E. Iodine deficiency

6. A 50-year-old woman comes to her physician complaining of unexplained weight gain and memory problems. Physical examination reveals a yellowing of her skin without a discoloration of her sclera. Circulating levels of TSH are increased. A blood test is likely to reveal increased plasma levels of
   A. cholesterol.
   B. albumin.
   C. RT_3.
   D. Iodide.
   E. TBG.

7. A young woman has puffy skin and a hoarse voice. Her plasma TSH concentration is low but increases markedly when she is given TRH. She probably has
   A. hyperthyroidism due to a thyroid tumor.
   B. hypothyroidism due to a primary abnormality in the thyroid gland.
   C. hypothyroidism due to a primary abnormality in the pituitary gland.
   D. hypothyroidism due to a primary abnormality in the hypothalamus.
   E. hyperthyroidism due to a primary abnormality in the hypothalamus.

8. A scientist studying thyroid physiology creates a series of knock-out mice lacking various enzymes involved in thyroid hormone biochemistry. In one mouse line, she finds that T_4 levels are normal but T_3 is markedly reduced, and signs of hypothyroidism emerge. The enzyme most likely to have been knocked out in this line of mice is
   A. D_1 thyroid deiodinase.
   B. D_2 thyroid deiodinase.
   C. D_3 thyroid deiodinase.
   D. thyroid peroxidase.
   E. None of the above.

9. A group of medical students volunteers for a study in which they are administered injections of TSH over a period of several weeks. They develop weight loss and nervousness. Which of the following would be *least* affected?
   A. Thyroidal uptake of iodine
   B. Synthesis of thyroglobulin
   C. Cyclic adenosine monophosphate (cAMP) in thyroid cells
   D. Cyclic guanosine monophosphate (cGMP) in thyroid cells
   E. Size of the thyroid

10. A scientist treats a hepatocyte cell line with T_3 and measures transcription factors bound to the promoter of thyroid-hormone sensitive genes. In addition to monomers and homodimers of various thyroid hormone receptors (TR), which other form of TR is likely to be found bound to DNA?
    A. A heterodimer with the prolactin receptor
    B. A heterodimer with the growth hormone receptor
    C. A heterodimer with the retinoid X receptor
    D. A heterodimer with the insulin receptor
    E. A heterodimer with the progesterone receptor

ANSWERS

1. The correct answer is **C.** The patient's symptoms are consistent with a diagnosis of hyperthyroidism. Because thyroid hormones are secreted in excess in this patient, the thyroid will show evidence of activation of thyrocytes, including an increase in the numbers of resorption lacunae at their apical membranes as colloid is absorbed, as well as increased endocytosis, and lysosomal activity (rules out options **A, B,** and **E**). However, NIS expression and translocation to the basolateral membrane is regulated by TSH, and TSH levels will likely be decreased secondary to feedback inhibition (rules out option **D**). On the other hand, increased thyroid hormone secretion is accompanied by active resorption of colloid and a decrease in its proportion of the gland as a whole.

2. The correct answer is **B.** Thyroid hormones are synthesized when tyrosine residues in the thyroglobulin molecule are iodinated in the thyroid gland (rules out options **A** and **C**). Further, even though thyroid hormones are not themselves proteinaceous, production of thyroglobulin, as well as thyroid peroxidase that mediates the iodination reaction, requires protein synthesis (rules out option **D**). Thyroid hormone production is also under the control of TSH from the anterior pituitary, and reduced in hypopituitarism (rules out option **E**). On the other hand, ferritin is involved in cellular storage of iron, which is not directly involved in thyroid hormone biosynthesis.

3. The correct answer is **E.** In the experimental model, as well as in native thyrocytes, iodide can be taken up by the sodium/iodide symporter (NIS). Exogenous expression of this molecule alone should not alter rates of nonspecific solute uptake, such as endocytosis or passive diffusion (rules out options **A** and **B**). NIS also is not responsible for the cotransport of potassium ions (rules out option **C**). On the other hand, while the ability of NIS to accumulate iodide above its electrochemical equilibrium relies on the low intracellular sodium concentration established in all cells by the primary active transporter, Na, K ATPase, but NIS does not itself directly consume cellular energy (rules out option **D**). Rather, its mode of action can best be described as secondary active transport.

4. The correct answer is **C.** The change in metabolic rate in this patient implies an alteration in circulating levels of both thyroid hormones, since the less active T_4 can be converted to T_3 in the periphery (rules out options **D** and **E**). Thyroid hormone synthesis and release is under the sequential control of TSH and TRH, and both of these hormones should be increased in the setting of hypothyroidism due to the loss in negative feedback control (rules out options **A** and **B**). Estrogen, contained in hormone-replacement therapy, causes an increase in the levels of TBG. Transiently, this will reduce levels of free T_3 and T_4 due to an increase in the capacity for protein binding of the hormones in the circulation. However, rapidly, a new steady state will be reached, because the loss of negative feedback will increase TSH and TRH. Thus, an increase in TBG secondary to estrogen administration is unlikely to be the cause of her hypothyroid symptoms.

5. The correct answer is **C.** Free T_4 feeds back on the pituitary to reduce the release of TSH in response to TRH coming from the hypothalamus. Because the response of TSH to TRH is reduced, circulating levels of T_4 must be increased and the patient must be hyperthyroid (rules out options **A** and **B**). Similarly, iodine deficiency eventually reduces, rather than increases, T_4 synthesis (rules out option E). In hyperthyroidism due to hyperplasia of pituitary thyrotropes, there is increased capacity for TSH secretion and so the response to TRH should be increased rather than decreased (rules out option **D**). On the other hand, autoantibodies that bind to the TSH receptor and mimic the action of TSH will elevate the secretion of thyroid hormones as well as thyroid enlargement in an autonomous fashion (Graves disease). Nevertheless, the response of TSH itself to TRH will be markedly suppressed by the feedback effects of the oversecretion of thyroid hormones.

6. The correct answer is **A.** The patient has symptoms consistent with hypothyroidism due to dysfunction of the thyroid gland. Levels of albumin and TBG, which each bind a portion of any circulating thyroid hormones that persist, should be unaffected (rules out options **B** and **E**). Iodide is unlikely to be increased—indeed, an important cause of thyroid dysfunction, at least in developing countries, is iodide insufficiency (rules out option **D**). Further, because RT_3 is produced predominantly by conversion of T_4 in the periphery, its levels will be decreased rather than increased (rules out option **C**). On the other hand, because thyroid hormones stimulate the expression of hepatocyte LDL receptors, increasing the removal of cholesterol from the circulation, cholesterol levels will be increased in the setting of hypothyroidism.

7. The correct answer is **D.** Again, the clinical presentation is consistent with hypothyroidism (rules out options **A** and **E**). In hypothyroidism due to a primary thyroid abnormality, TSH levels are high due to the lack of feedback inhibition produced by T_4 on TSH secretion that would otherwise be stimulated by TRH (rules out option **B**). Similarly, because TSH secretion can be stimulated when TRH is given, the anterior pituitary is apparently functioning normally (rules out option **C**). Instead, hypothyroidism in this patient is most likely due to a lack of TRH secretion secondary to an abnormality in the hypothalamus.

8. The correct answer is **A.** Thyroid peroxidase is responsible for generating reactive iodine species that can attack thyroglobulin. Because production of T_4 is apparently normal, option **D** is ruled out. On the other hand, a significant fraction of T_4 is converted to T_3 in the periphery by deiodinase enzymes (rules out option **E**). The D_2 deiodinase is present in the brain, pituitary and brown fat, and is mostly responsible for supplying T_3 to the central nervous system (rules out option **B**) and the D_3 deiodinase, also in the brain, acts to convert thyroid hormones to RT_3 (rules out option **C**). The D_1 deiodinase, on the other hand, is more widely expressed, including in the liver and kidneys, and is the primary means by which T_4 is converted to the more active T_3 in the periphery, close to its sites of action.

9. The correct answer is **D**. TSH, normally released from the anterior pituitary, stimulates both the synthesis and secretion of thyroid hormones, requiring increased uptake of iodine, as well as the synthesis of thyroglobulin (rules out options **A** and **B**). Because the exogenous TSH will not be subject to feedback inhibition, moreover, it will continue to drive thyroid hormone synthesis as if responding to a hypothyroid condition, and the thyroid gland will grow (rules out option **E**). TSH binds to receptors on thyrocytes that are linked to G_s. Thus cAMP, but not cGMP, will be markedly elevated in these cells (rules out option **C**).

10. The correct answer is **C**. TR is activated when it binds T_3 in the cell cytosol and translocates to the nucleus, where it binds specific DNA regions. In addition to the ability of TR to regulate gene transcription in monomeric and dimeric forms, it is particularly active in regulating a subset of genes when in the form of a heterodimer with the retinoid X receptor (RXR, rules out options **A, B, D,** and **E**). This heterodimer no longer binds typical RXR ligands such as retinoic acid derivatives, but rather its DNA binding activity is triggered by T_3 and, to a lesser extent, T_4.

The Adrenal Medulla & Adrenal Cortex

OBJECTIVES

After reading this chapter, you should be able to:

- Name the three catecholamines secreted by the adrenal medulla and summarize their biosynthesis, metabolism, and function.
- List the stimuli that increase adrenal medullary secretion.
- Differentiate between C_{18}, C_{19}, and C_{21} steroids and give examples of each.
- Outline the steps involved in steroid biosynthesis in the adrenal cortex.
- Name the plasma proteins that bind adrenocortical steroids and discuss their physiologic role.
- Name the major site of adrenocortical hormone metabolism and the principal metabolites produced from glucocorticoids, adrenal androgens, and aldosterone.
- Describe the mechanisms by which glucocorticoids and aldosterone produce changes in cellular function.
- List and briefly describe the physiologic and pharmacologic effects of glucocorticoids.
- Contrast the physiologic and pathologic effects of adrenal androgens.
- Describe the mechanisms that regulate secretion of glucocorticoids and adrenal sex hormones.
- List the actions of aldosterone and describe the mechanisms that regulate aldosterone secretion.
- Describe the main features of the diseases caused by excess or deficiency of each of the hormones of the adrenal gland.

■ ADRENAL MORPHOLOGY

There are two endocrine organs in the adrenal gland, one surrounding the other. The main secretions of the inner **adrenal medulla** are the catecholamines **epinephrine, norepinephrine,** and **dopamine;** the outer **adrenal cortex** secretes steroid hormones.

The adrenal cortex secretes **glucocorticoids,** steroids with widespread effects on the metabolism of carbohydrate and protein; and a **mineralocorticoid** essential to the maintenance of Na^+ balance and extracellular fluid (ECF) volume. It is also a secondary site of **androgen** synthesis, secreting sex hormones such as testosterone.

The adrenal medulla, which constitutes 28% of the mass of the adrenal gland, is made up of interlacing cords of densely innervated granule-containing cells that abut on venous sinuses. Two cell types can be distinguished morphologically: an epinephrine-secreting type that has larger, less dense granules; and a norepinephrine-secreting type in which smaller, very dense granules fail to fill the vesicles in which they are contained. In humans, 90% of the cells are the epinephrine-secreting type and 10% are the norepinephrine-secreting type. The type of cell that secretes dopamine is unknown.

The adrenal cortex is divided into three zones: the outer **zona glomerulosa** is made up of whorls of cells that are continuous with the columns of cells that form the **zona fasciculate,** separated by venous sinuses. The inner portion of the zona fasciculata merges into the **zona reticularis,** where the cell columns become interlaced into a network. The zona glomerulosa makes up 15%

of the mass of the adrenal gland; the zona fasciculata, 50%; and the zona reticularis, 7%. The adrenocortical cells contain abundant lipid, especially in the outer portion of the zona fasciculata. All three cortical zones secrete **corticosterone,** but the active enzymatic mechanism for aldosterone biosynthesis is limited to the zona glomerulosa, whereas the enzymatic mechanisms for forming cortisol and sex hormones are found in the two inner zones. Furthermore, subspecialization occurs within the inner two zones, with the zona fasciculata secreting mostly glucocorticoids and the zona reticularis secreting mainly sex hormones.

Arterial blood reaches the adrenal from many small branches of the phrenic and renal arteries and the aorta. From a plexus in the capsule, blood flows through the cortex to the sinusoids of the medulla. The medulla is also supplied by a few arterioles that pass directly to it from the capsule. In most species, including humans, blood from the medulla flows into a central adrenal vein. The blood flow through the adrenal is large, as it is in most endocrine glands.

The cells of the adrenal cortex contain large amounts of smooth endoplasmic reticulum, which is involved in the steroid-forming process.

In the medulla, norepinephrine and epinephrine are stored in granules with ATP. The granules also contain chromogranin A (see Chapter 7). Secretion is initiated by acetylcholine released from the preganglionic neurons that innervate the secretory cells. Acetylcholine activates cation channels allowing Ca^{2+} to enter the cells from the ECF and trigger the exocytosis of the granules. In this manner, catecholamines, ATP, and proteins from the granules are all released into the blood together.

Epinephrine-containing cells of the medulla also contain and secrete opioid peptides (see Chapter 7). The precursor molecule is preproenkephalin. Most of the circulating metenkephalin comes from the adrenal medulla. The circulating opioid peptides do not cross the blood–brain barrier.

Adrenomedullin, a vasodepressor polypeptide found in the adrenal medulla, is discussed in Chapter 32.

EFFECTS OF EPINEPHRINE & NOREPINEPHRINE

In addition to mimicking the effects of noradrenergic nervous discharge, norepinephrine and epinephrine exert metabolic effects that include glycogenolysis in liver and skeletal muscle, mobilization of free fatty acids (FFA), increased plasma lactate, and stimulation of the metabolic rate. The effects of norepinephrine and epinephrine are brought about by actions on two classes of receptors: α- **and** β-**adrenergic receptors.** α-Receptors are subdivided into two groups, α_1- and α_2-receptors, and β-receptors into three groups, β_1-, β_2-, and β_3-receptors. There are three subtypes of α_1-receptors and three subtypes of α_2-receptors.

Norepinephrine and epinephrine both increase the force and rate of contraction of the isolated heart. These responses are mediated by β_1-receptors. The catecholamines also increase myocardial excitability, causing extrasystoles and, occasionally, more serious cardiac arrhythmias. Norepinephrine produces vasoconstriction in

most if not all organs via α_1-receptors, but epinephrine dilates the blood vessels in skeletal muscle and the liver via β_2-receptors. This usually overbalances the vasoconstriction produced by epinephrine elsewhere, and the total peripheral resistance drops.

When norepinephrine is infused slowly in normal animals or humans, the systolic and diastolic blood pressures rise. The **hypertension** stimulates the carotid and aortic baroreceptors, producing reflex bradycardia that overrides the direct cardioacceleratory effect of norepinephrine. Consequently, cardiac output per minute falls. Epinephrine causes a widening of the pulse pressure but because baroreceptor stimulation is insufficient to obscure the direct effect of the hormone on the heart, cardiac rate and output increase.

Catecholamines have several different actions that affect blood glucose. Epinephrine and norepinephrine both cause glycogenolysis, and produce this effect via β-adrenergic receptors that increase cyclic adenosine monophosphate (cAMP), with activation of phosphorylase, and via α-adrenergic receptors that increase intracellular Ca^{2+}. In addition, catecholamines increase secretion of insulin and glucagon via β-adrenergic mechanisms and inhibit the secretion of these hormones via α-adrenergic mechanisms.

EFFECTS OF DOPAMINE

The physiologic function of the dopamine in the circulation is unknown. Dopamine is made in the renal cortex, and causes natriuresis perhaps by inhibiting renal Na, K, ATPase. Injected dopamine produces renal and mesenteric vasodilation, probably by acting on a specific dopaminergic receptor. Elsewhere, it produces vasoconstriction, probably by releasing norepinephrine, and it has a positive inotropic effect on the heart by an action on β_1-adrenergic receptors. The net effect of moderate doses of dopamine is an increase in systolic pressure and no change in diastolic pressure. Because of these actions, dopamine is useful in the treatment of traumatic and cardiogenic shock.

■ ADRENAL CORTEX: STRUCTURE & BIOSYNTHESIS OF ADRENOCORTICAL HORMONES

CLASSIFICATION & STRUCTURE

The hormones of the adrenal cortex are derivatives of cholesterol and contain the **cyclopentanoperhydrophenanthrene nucleus.** Gonadal and adrenocortical steroids are of three types: C_{21} **steroids,** which have a two-carbon side chain at position 17; C_{19} **steroids,** which have a keto or hydroxyl group at position 17; and C_{18} **steroids,** which, in addition to a 17-keto or hydroxyl group, have no angular methyl group attached to position 10. The adrenal cortex secretes primarily C_{21} and C_{19} steroids. Most of the C_{19} steroids have a keto group at position 17 and are therefore called **17-ketosteroids.** The C_{21} steroids that have a hydroxyl group at the 17 position in addition to the side chain are often called 17-hydroxycorticoids or 17-hydroxycorticosteroids.

The C_{19} steroids have **androgenic activity.** The C_{21} steroids are classified as mineralocorticoids or glucocorticoids. All secreted C_{21} steroids have both mineralocorticoid and glucocorticoid activity; **mineralocorticoids** are those in which effects on Na^+ and K^+ excretion predominate and **glucocorticoids** are those in which effects on glucose and protein metabolism predominate.

STEROID BIOSYNTHESIS

The major paths by which the naturally occurring adrenocortical hormones are synthesized in the body are summarized in **Figures 20–1** and **20–2.** The precursor of all steroids is cholesterol. Some of the cholesterol is synthesized from acetate, but most of it is taken up from LDL in the circulation. LDL receptors are especially abundant in adrenocortical cells. The cholesterol is esterified and stored in lipid droplets. **Cholesterol ester hydrolase** catalyzes the formation of free cholesterol in the lipid droplets. Cholesterol is transported to the mitochondria by a sterol carrier protein. In the mitochondria, it is converted to pregnenolone in a reaction catalyzed by an enzyme known as **cholesterol desmolase** or **side-chain cleavage enzyme.** This enzyme, like most of the enzymes involved in steroid biosynthesis, is a member of the cytochrome P450 superfamily and is also known as **P450scc** or **CYP11A1.**

Pregnenolone moves to the smooth endoplasmic reticulum, where some of it is dehydrogenated to form progesterone in a reaction catalyzed by **3β-hydroxysteroid dehydrogenase.** This enzyme also catalyzes the conversion of 17α-hydroxypregnenolone to

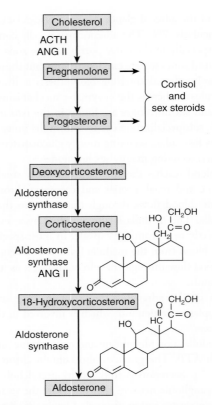

FIGURE 20–2 Hormone synthesis in the zona glomerulosa. The zona glomerulosa lacks 17α-hydroxylase activity, and only the zona glomerulosa can convert corticosterone to aldosterone because it is the only zone that normally contains aldosterone synthase. ANG II, angiotensin II.

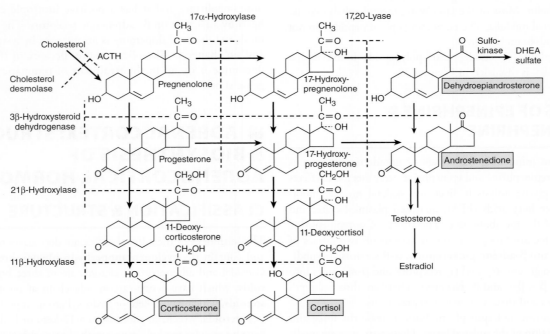

FIGURE 20–1 Outline of hormone biosynthesis in the zona fasciculata and zona reticularis of the adrenal cortex. The major secretory products are underlined. The enzymes for the reactions are shown on the left and at the top of the chart. When a particular enzyme is deficient, hormone production is blocked at the points indicated by the shaded bars. (Data from Sagnella GA, et al: Plasma atrial natriuretic peptide: Its relationship to changes in sodium in-take, plasma renin activity, and aldosterone in man. Clin Sci 1987; 72:25)

17α-hydroxyprogesterone, and dehydroepiandrosterone to androstenedione in the smooth endoplasmic reticulum. The 17α-hydroxypregnenolone and the 17α-hydroxyprogesterone are formed from pregnenolone and progesterone, respectively by the action of **17α-hydroxylase.** This is another mitochondrial P450, and it is also known as **P450c17** or **CYP17.** Located in another part of the same enzyme is **17,20-lyase** activity that breaks the 17,20 bond, converting 17α-pregnenolone and 17α-progesterone to the C_{19} steroids dehydroepiandrosterone and androstenedione.

Hydroxylation of progesterone to 11-deoxycorticosterone and of 17α-hydroxyprogesterone to 11-deoxycortisol occurs in the smooth endoplasmic reticulum. These reactions are catalyzed by 21β-hydroxylase, a cytochrome P450 that is also known as **P450c21** or **CYP21A2.**

11-Deoxycorticosterone and the 11-deoxycortisol move back to the mitochondria, where they are 11-hydroxylated to form corticosterone and cortisol. These reactions occur in the zona fasciculata and zona reticularis and are catalyzed by 11β-hydroxylase, a cytochrome P450 also known as **P450c11** or **CYP11B1.**

In the zona glomerulosa there is no 11β-hydroxylase, but a closely related enzyme called **aldosterone synthase** is present. This cytochrome P450 is 95% identical to 11β-hydroxylase and is also known as **P450c11AS** or **CYP11B2.** However, aldosterone synthase is normally found only in the zona glomerulosa. The zona glomerulosa also lacks 17α-hydroxylase. This is why the zona glomerulosa makes aldosterone but fails to make cortisol or sex hormones.

Furthermore, subspecialization occurs within the inner two zones. The zona fasciculata has more 3β-hydroxysteroid dehydrogenase activity than the zona reticularis, and the zona reticularis has more of the cofactors required for the 17,20-lyase activity of 17α-hydroxylase. Therefore, the zona fasciculata makes more cortisol and corticosterone, and the zona reticularis makes more androgens. Most of the dehydroepiandrosterone that is formed is converted to dehydroepiandrosterone sulfate (DHEAS) by **adrenal sulfokinase,** and this enzyme is localized in the zona reticularis as well.

■ SECRETED STEROIDS

Innumerable steroids have been isolated from adrenal tissue, but the only steroids normally secreted in physiologically significant amounts are the mineralocorticoid **aldosterone,** the glucocorticoids **cortisol** and **corticosterone,** and the androgens **dehydroepiandrosterone (DHEA)** and **androstenedione. Deoxycorticosterone** is a mineralocorticoid that is normally secreted in about the same amount as aldosterone, but has only 3% of the mineralocorticoid activity of aldosterone.

ACTION OF ACTH

ACTH binds to high-affinity receptors on the plasma membrane of adrenocortical cells. This activates adenylyl cyclase via G_s resulting in the increase in pregnenolone and its derivatives, with secretion of the latter. Over longer periods, ACTH also increases the synthesis of the P450s involved in the synthesis of glucocorticoids.

ENZYME DEFICIENCIES

Congenital defects in enzymes that produce adrenal hormones lead to deficient cortisol secretion and the syndrome of **congenital adrenal hyperplasia** due to increased ACTH secretion. Cholesterol desmolase deficiency is fatal in utero because it prevents the placenta from making the progesterone necessary for pregnancy to continue. A cause of severe congenital adrenal hyperplasia in newborns is a loss of function mutation of the gene for the **steroidogenic acute regulatory (StAR) protein.** This protein is essential in the adrenals and gonads but not in the placenta for the normal movement of cholesterol into the mitochondria to reach cholesterol desmolase, which is located on the matrix space side of the internal mitochondrial membrane. In its absence, only small amounts of steroids are formed. The degree of ACTH stimulation is marked, resulting eventually in accumulation of large numbers of lipoid droplets in the adrenal. For this reason, the condition is called **congenital lipoid adrenal hyperplasia.**

21β-hydroxylase deficiency is common, accounting for 90% or more of the enzyme deficiency cases. Mutations occur at many different sites in the gene, and the abnormalities that are produced therefore range from mild to severe. Production of cortisol and aldosterone are generally reduced, so ACTH secretion and consequently production of precursor steroids are increased. These steroids are converted to androgens, producing **virilization.** The characteristic pattern that develops in females in the absence of treatment is the **adrenogenital syndrome.** Masculinization may not be marked until later in life and mild cases can be detected only by laboratory tests. In 75% of the cases, aldosterone deficiency causes appreciable loss of Na^+ (**salt-losing form** of adrenal hyperplasia). The resulting hypovolemia can be severe.

In 11β-hydroxylase deficiency, virilization plus excess secretion of 11-deoxycortisol and 11-deoxycorticosterone take place. Because the former is an active mineralocorticoid, patients with this condition also have salt and water retention and, in two-thirds of the cases, hypertension (**hypertensive form** of congenital adrenal hyperplasia).

Glucocorticoid treatment is indicated in all of the virilizing forms of congenital adrenal hyperplasia because it repairs the glucocorticoid deficit and inhibits ACTH secretion, reducing the abnormal secretion of androgens and other steroids.

■ TRANSPORT, METABOLISM, & EXCRETION OF ADRENOCORTICAL HORMONES

GLUCOCORTICOID BINDING

Cortisol is bound in the circulation to an α globulin called **transcortin** or **corticosteroid-binding globulin (CBG).** Corticosterone is similarly bound but to a lesser degree. The half-life of cortisol in the circulation is longer (about 60–90 min) than that of corticosterone (50 min). Bound steroids are physiologically inactive. In addition, relatively little free cortisol and corticosterone are found in the urine because of protein binding.

Bound cortisol functions as a circulating reservoir of hormone that keeps a supply of free cortisol available to the tissues. At normal levels of total plasma cortisol (13.5 μg/dL or 375 nmol/L), very little free cortisol is present in the plasma, but the binding sites on CBG become saturated when the total plasma cortisol exceeds 20 μg/dL. At higher plasma levels, binding to albumin increases, but the main increase is in the unbound fraction.

CBG is synthesized in the liver and its production is increased by estrogen. CBG levels are elevated during pregnancy and depressed in cirrhosis, nephrosis, and multiple myeloma. When the CBG level rises, more cortisol is bound, and initially the free cortisol level drops. This stimulates ACTH secretion, and more cortisol is secreted until a new equilibrium is reached at which the bound cortisol is elevated but the free cortisol is normal. Changes in the opposite direction occur when the CBG level falls. This explains why pregnant women have high total plasma cortisol levels without symptoms of glucocorticoid excess and, conversely, why some patients with nephrosis have low total plasma cortisol without symptoms of glucocorticoid deficiency.

METABOLISM & EXCRETION OF GLUCOCORTICOIDS

Cortisol is metabolized in the liver, which is the principal site of glucocorticoid catabolism. Most of the cortisol is reduced to dihydrocortisol and then to tetrahydrocortisol, which is conjugated to glucuronic acid. The glucuronyl transferase system responsible for this conversion also catalyzes the formation of the glucuronides of bilirubin.

The liver and other tissues contain the enzyme **11β hydroxysteroid dehydrogenase.** There are at least two forms of this enzyme. **Type 1** catalyzes the conversion of cortisol to cortisone and the reverse reaction, though it functions primarily as a reductase, forming cortisol from corticosterone. **Type 2** catalyzes almost exclusively the one-way conversion of cortisol to cortisone. Cortisone is an active glucocorticoid because it is converted to cortisol. It is not secreted in appreciable quantities by the adrenal glands. Little, if any, of the cortisone formed in the liver enters the circulation, because it is promptly reduced and conjugated to form tetrahydrocortisone glucuronide. The tetrahydroglucuronide derivatives ("conjugates") of cortisol and corticosterone are freely soluble. They enter the circulation, where they do not become bound to protein and are rapidly excreted in the urine.

About 10% of the secreted cortisol is converted in the liver to the 17-ketosteroid derivatives of cortisol and cortisone. The ketosteroids are conjugated for the most part to sulfate and then excreted in the urine. Other metabolites, including 20-hydroxy derivatives, are formed. There is an enterohepatic circulation of glucocorticoids and about 15% of the secreted cortisol is excreted in the stool. The metabolism of corticosterone is similar to that of cortisol, except that it does not form a 17-ketosteroid derivative.

ALDOSTERONE

Aldosterone is bound to protein to only a slight extent, and its half-life is short (about 20 min). The amount secreted is small, and the total plasma aldosterone level in humans is normally about 0.006 μg/dL (0.17 nmol/L), compared with a cortisol level (bound and free) of about 13.5 μg/dL (375 nmol/L). Much of the aldosterone is converted in the liver to the tetrahydroglucuronide derivative, but some is changed in the liver and in the kidneys to an 18-glucuronide. This glucuronide, which is unlike the breakdown products of other steroids, is converted to free aldosterone by hydrolysis at pH 1.0, and it is therefore often referred to as the "acid-labile conjugate." Less than 1% of the secreted aldosterone appears in the urine in the free form. Another 5% is in the form of the acid-labile conjugate, and up to 40% is in the form of the tetrahydroglucuronide.

17-KETOSTEROIDS

The major adrenal androgen is the 17-ketosteroid dehydroepiandrosterone, although androstenedione is also secreted. The 11-hydroxy derivative of androstenedione and the 17-ketosteroids formed from cortisol and cortisone by side chain cleavage in the liver are the only 17-ketosteroids that have an =O or an —OH group in the 11 position ("11-oxy-17-ketosteroids"). Testosterone is also converted to a 17-ketosteroid.

■ PHYSIOLOGIC EFFECTS OF GLUCOCORTICOIDS

ADRENAL INSUFFICIENCY

In untreated adrenal insufficiency, Na^+ loss and shock occur due to lack of mineralocorticoid activity, as well as abnormalities of water, carbohydrate, protein, and fat metabolism due to the lack of glucocorticoids. These metabolic abnormalities are eventually fatal despite mineralocorticoid treatment. Small amounts of glucocorticoids correct the metabolic abnormalities, in part directly and in part by permitting other reactions to occur. It is important to separate these physiologic actions of glucocorticoids from the quite different effects produced by large amounts of the hormones.

EFFECTS ON INTERMEDIARY METABOLISM

Glucocorticoids increase protein catabolism and increase hepatic glycogenesis and gluconeogenesis. Glucose-6-phosphatase activity is increased, and the plasma glucose level rises. Glucocorticoids exert an anti-insulin action in peripheral tissues and make diabetes worse. However, the brain and the heart are spared, so the increase in plasma glucose provides extra glucose to these vital organs. In diabetics, glucocorticoids raise plasma lipid levels and increase ketone body formation, but in normal individuals, the increase in insulin secretion provoked by the rise in plasma glucose obscures these actions. In adrenal insufficiency, the plasma glucose level is normal as long as an adequate caloric intake is maintained, but fasting causes hypoglycemia that can be fatal. The adrenal cortex is not essential for the ketogenic response to fasting.

PERMISSIVE ACTION

Small amounts of glucocorticoids must be present for a number of metabolic reactions to occur, although the glucocorticoids do not produce the reactions by themselves, their **permissive action.** Permissive effects include the requirement for glucocorticoids to be present for glucagon and catecholamines to exert their calorigenic effects, for catecholamines to exert their lipolytic effects, and for catecholamines to produce pressor responses and bronchodilation.

VASCULAR REACTIVITY

In adrenally insufficient animals, vascular smooth muscle becomes unresponsive to norepinephrine and epinephrine. The capillaries dilate and become permeable. Failure to respond to the norepinephrine liberated at noradrenergic nerve endings probably impairs vascular compensation for the hypovolemia of adrenal insufficiency and promotes vascular collapse. Glucocorticoids restore vascular reactivity.

EFFECTS ON WATER METABOLISM

Adrenal insufficiency is characterized by an inability to excrete a water load, causing the possibility of water intoxication. Only glucocorticoids repair this deficit. In patients with adrenal insufficiency who have not received glucocorticoids, glucose infusion may cause high fever ("glucose fever") followed by collapse and death. Presumably, the glucose is metabolized, the water dilutes the plasma, and the resultant osmotic gradient between the plasma and the cells causes the cells of the thermoregulatory centers in the hypothalamus to swell to such an extent that their function is disrupted.

The cause of defective water excretion in adrenal insufficiency is unsettled. Plasma vasopressin levels are elevated in adrenal insufficiency and reduced by glucocorticoid treatment. The glomerular filtration rate is low, and this probably contributes to the reduction in water excretion. The selective effect of glucocorticoids on the abnormal water excretion is consistent with this possibility, because even though the mineralocorticoids improve filtration by restoring plasma volume, the glucocorticoids raise the glomerular filtration rate to a much greater degree.

EFFECTS ON THE BLOOD CELLS & LYMPHATIC ORGANS

Glucocorticoids decrease the number of circulating eosinophils by increasing their sequestration in the spleen and lungs. Glucocorticoids also lower the number of basophils in the circulation and increase the number of neutrophils, platelets, and red blood cells.

Glucocorticoids decrease the circulating lymphocyte count and the size of the lymph nodes and thymus by inhibiting lymphocyte mitotic activity. They reduce secretion of cytokines by inhibiting the effect of NF-κB on the nucleus. The reduced secretion of the cytokine IL-2 leads to reduced proliferation of lymphocytes, and these cells undergo apoptosis.

RESISTANCE TO STRESS

The term **stress** as used in biology has been defined as any change in the environment that changes or threatens to change an existing optimal steady state. Most, if not all, of these stresses activate processes at the molecular, cellular, or systemic level that tend to restore the previous state, that is, they are homeostatic reactions. Some, but not all, of the stresses stimulate ACTH secretion. The increase in ACTH secretion is essential for survival when the stress is severe. If animals are then hypophysectomized, or adrenalectomized but treated with maintenance doses of glucocorticoids, they die when exposed to the same stress.

The reason an elevated circulating ACTH, and hence glucocorticoid level, is essential for resisting stress remains for the most part unknown. Most of the stressful stimuli that increase ACTH secretion also activate the sympathetic nervous system, and part of the function of circulating glucocorticoids may be maintenance of vascular reactivity to catecholamines. Glucocorticoids are also necessary for the catecholamines to exert their full FFA-mobilizing action, and the FFAs are an important emergency energy supply. However, sympathectomized animals tolerate a variety of stresses with relative impunity. Another theory holds that glucocorticoids prevent other stress-induced changes from becoming excessive. At present, all that can be said is that stress causes increases in plasma glucocorticoids to high "pharmacologic" levels that in the short run are lifesaving.

It should also be noted that the increase in ACTH, which is beneficial in the short term, becomes harmful and disruptive in the long term, causing among other things, the abnormalities of Cushing syndrome.

■ PHARMACOLOGIC & PATHOLOGIC EFFECTS OF GLUCOCORTICOIDS

CUSHING SYNDROME

The clinical picture produced by prolonged increases in plasma glucocorticoids was described by Harvey Cushing and is called **Cushing syndrome.** It may be **ACTH-independent** or **ACTH-dependent.** The causes of ACTH-independent Cushing syndrome include glucocorticoid-secreting adrenal tumors, adrenal hyperplasia, and prolonged administration of exogenous glucocorticoids for diseases such as rheumatoid arthritis. Rare but interesting ACTH-independent cases have been reported in which adrenocortical cells abnormally express receptors for gastric inhibitory polypeptide (GIP), vasopressin, β-adrenergic agonists, IL-1, or gonadotropin-releasing hormone, causing these peptides to increase glucocorticoid secretion. The causes of ACTH-dependent Cushing syndrome include ACTH-secreting tumors of the anterior pituitary gland and tumors of other organs, usually the lungs that secrete ACTH (ectopic ACTH syndrome) or corticotropin releasing hormone (CRH).

Patients with Cushing syndrome are protein depleted as a result of excess protein catabolism with thin skin and subcutaneous tissues and poorly developed muscles. Wounds heal poorly, and minor injuries cause bruises and ecchymoses. Hair is thin and scraggly. Body fat is redistributed in a characteristic way. Extremities are thin, but fat collects in the abdominal wall, face, and upper back, where it produces a "buffalo hump." As the thin skin of the abdomen is stretched by the increased subcutaneous fat depots, the subdermal tissues rupture to form prominent reddish purple **striae.** These scars are seen normally whenever a rapid stretching of skin occurs, but in normal individuals the striae are usually inconspicuous and lack the intense purplish color.

Many of the amino acids liberated from catabolized proteins are converted into glucose in the liver and the resultant hyperglycemia and decreased peripheral utilization of glucose may be sufficient to precipitate insulin-resistant diabetes mellitus, especially in patients genetically predisposed to diabetes. Hyperlipidemia and ketosis are associated with the diabetes, but acidosis is usually not severe.

The glucocorticoids are present in such large amounts in Cushing syndrome that they may exert a significant mineralocorticoid action. Deoxycorticosterone secretion is also elevated in cases due to ACTH hypersecretion. Salt and water retention plus facial obesity cause the characteristic plethoric, rounded "moon-faced" appearance, and there may be significant K+ depletion and weakness. About 85% of patients with Cushing syndrome are hypertensive. The hypertension may be due to increased deoxy-corticosterone secretion, increased angiotensinogen secretion, or a direct glucocorticoid effect on blood vessels.

Glucocorticoid excess leads to bone dissolution by decreasing bone formation and increasing bone resorption. This leads to **osteoporosis,** a loss of bone mass that leads eventually to collapse of vertebral bodies and other fractures. Glucocorticoids in excess accelerate the basic electroencephalographic rhythms and produce mental aberrations ranging from increased appetite, insomnia, and euphoria to frank toxic psychoses.

ANTI-INFLAMMATORY & ANTI-ALLERGIC EFFECTS OF GLUCOCORTICOIDS

Glucocorticoids inhibit the inflammatory response to tissue injury. Glucocorticoids also suppress manifestations of allergic reactions that are due to the release of histamine from mast cells and basophils. Both of these effects require high levels of circulating glucocorticoids and cannot be produced by administering steroids without producing the other manifestations of glucocorticoid excess. Furthermore, large doses of exogenous glucocorticoids inhibit ACTH secretion to the point that severe adrenal insufficiency can be a dangerous problem when therapy is stopped. However, local administration of glucocorticoids, for example, by injection into an inflamed joint or near an irritated nerve, produces a high local concentration of the steroid, often without enough systemic absorption to cause serious side effects.

The actions of glucocorticoids in patients with bacterial infections are dramatic but dangerous. For example, in pneumococcal pneumonia or active tuberculosis, the febrile reaction, the toxicity, and the lung symptoms disappear, but unless antibiotics are given at the same time, the bacteria spread throughout the body.

■ REGULATION OF GLUCOCORTICOID SECRETION

ROLE OF ACTH

Both basal and increased secretion (provoked by stress) of glucocorticoids depend on ACTH from the anterior pituitary. Angiotensin II also stimulates the adrenal cortex, but its effect is mainly on aldosterone secretion.

ACTH is a single-chain polypeptide containing 39 amino acids. It originates from proopiomelanocortin (POMC) in the pituitary. The first 23 amino acids in the chain generally constitute the active "core" of the molecule. Amino acids 24–39 constitute a "tail" that stabilizes the molecule.

The half-life of ACTH in the circulation is about 10 min. A large part of an injected dose of ACTH is found in the kidneys, but neither nephrectomy nor evisceration appreciably enhances its in vivo activity, and the site of its inactivation is not known.

After hypophysectomy, glucocorticoid synthesis and output decline within 1 h to very low levels, although some hormone is still secreted. Within a short time after an injection of ACTH, glucocorticoid output is increased. With low doses of ACTH, the relationship between the log of the dose and the increase in glucocorticoid secretion is linear. However, the maximal rate at which glucocorticoids can be secreted is rapidly reached.

ACTH not only produces prompt increases in glucocorticoid secretion but also increases the sensitivity of the adrenal to subsequent doses of ACTH. Conversely, a single dose of ACTH does not increase glucocorticoid secretion in chronically hypophysectomized patients with hypopituitarism, and repeated injections or prolonged infusions of ACTH are necessary to restore normal adrenal responses to ACTH. Decreased responsiveness is also produced by doses of glucocorticoids that inhibit ACTH secretion. The decreased adrenal responsiveness to ACTH is detectable within 24 h after hypophysectomy and increases progressively with time.

ACTH is secreted in irregular bursts throughout the day in a **diurnal (circadian) rhythm** with plasma cortisol levels rising and falling in response to these bursts. Bursts are most frequent in the early morning, and about 75% of the daily production of cortisol occurs between 4:00 AM and 10:00 AM. The bursts are least frequent in the evening. This diurnal rhythm in ACTH secretion is present in patients with adrenal insufficiency receiving constant doses of glucocorticoids. The biologic clock responsible for the diurnal ACTH rhythm is located in the suprachiasmatic nuclei of the hypothalamus.

The morning plasma ACTH concentration in a healthy individual is about 25 pg/mL (5.5 pmol/L). During severe stress, the amount of ACTH secreted exceeds the amount necessary to produce maximal glucocorticoid output. However, prolonged exposure to ACTH in conditions such as the ectopic ACTH syndrome increases the adrenal maximum.

Increases in ACTH secretion to meet emergency situations are mediated almost exclusively through the hypothalamus via release of CRH. This polypeptide is produced by neurons in the paraventricular nuclei. It is secreted in the median eminence and transported in the portal-hypophysial vessels to the anterior pituitary, where it stimulates ACTH secretion. Fibers from the amygdaloid nuclei mediate responses to emotional stresses, fear, anxiety, and apprehension cause marked increases in ACTH secretion. Input from the suprachiasmatic nuclei provides the drive for the diurnal rhythm. Impulses ascending to the hypothalamus via the nociceptive pathways and the reticular formation trigger increased ACTH secretion in response to injury. Baroreceptors exert an inhibitory input via the nucleus of the tractus solitarius.

Free glucocorticoids inhibit ACTH secretion, and the degree of pituitary inhibition is proportional to the circulating glucocorticoid level setting a negative feedback. The inhibitory effect is exerted at both the pituitary and the hypothalamic levels. A drop in resting corticoid levels stimulates ACTH secretion, and in chronic adrenal insufficiency the rate of ACTH synthesis and secretion is markedly increased.

Thus, the rate of ACTH secretion is determined by two opposing forces: the sum of the neural and possibly other stimuli converging through the hypothalamus to increase ACTH secretion, and the magnitude of the braking action of glucocorticoids on ACTH secretion, which is proportional to their level in the circulating blood.

The dangers involved when prolonged treatment with anti-inflammatory doses of glucocorticoids is stopped deserve emphasis. Not only is the adrenal atrophic and unresponsive after such treatment, but even if its responsiveness is restored by injecting ACTH, the pituitary may be unable to secrete normal amounts of ACTH for as long as a month. The cause of the deficiency is presumably diminished ACTH synthesis. Thereafter, ACTH secretion slowly increases to supranormal levels. These in turn stimulate the adrenal, and glucocorticoid output rises, with feedback inhibition gradually reducing the elevated ACTH levels to normal. Thus cessation of steroid therapy should be avoided by slowly decreasing the steroid dose over a long period of time.

■ EFFECTS OF MINERALOCORTICOIDS

Aldosterone and other steroids with mineralocorticoid activity increase the reabsorption of Na^+ from the urine, sweat, saliva, and the contents of the colon. Thus, mineralocorticoids cause retention of Na^+ in the ECF expanding ECF volume. In the kidneys, they act primarily on the **principal cells (P cells)** of the collecting ducts. Under the influence of aldosterone, increased amounts of Na^+ are in effect exchanged for K^+ and H^+ in the renal tubules, producing a K^+ diuresis and an increase in urine acidity.

Aldosterone binds to a cytoplasmic receptor, and the receptor–hormone complex moves to the nucleus where it alters transcription of mRNAs. Aldosterone-stimulated proteins have two effects—a rapid effect, to increase the activity of **epithelial sodium channels** (ENaCs) by increasing the insertion of these channels into the cell membrane from a cytoplasmic pool; and a slower effect to increase the synthesis of ENaCs. Among the genes activated by aldosterone is the gene for **serum and glucocorticoid-regulated kinase (sgk)**, a serine/threonine protein kinase. The gene for sgk is an early response gene, and sgk increases ENaC activity. Aldosterone also increases the mRNAs for the three subunits that make up ENaCs. The fact that sgk is activated by glucocorticoids as well as aldosterone is not a problem because glucocorticoids are inactivated at mineralocorticoid receptor sites. However, aldosterone activates the genes for other proteins in addition to sgk and ENaCs and inhibits others. Therefore, the exact mechanism by which aldosterone-induced proteins increase Na^+ reabsorption is still unsettled.

Evidence is accumulating that aldosterone also binds to the cell membrane and by a rapid, nongenomic action increases the activity of membrane Na^+–K^+ exchangers. This produces an increase in intracellular Na^+, and the second messenger involved is probably IP_3. In any case, the principal effect of aldosterone on Na^+ transport takes 10–30 min to develop and peaks even later, indicating that it depends on the synthesis of new proteins by a genomic mechanism.

RELATION OF MINERALOCORTICOID TO GLUCOCORTICOID RECEPTORS

It is intriguing that in vitro, the mineralocorticoid receptor (MR) has an appreciably higher affinity for glucocorticoids than the glucocorticoid receptor does, and glucocorticoids are present in large amounts in vivo. This raises the question of why glucocorticoids do not bind to the mineralocorticoid receptors in the kidneys and other locations and produce mineralocorticoid effects. At least in part, the answer is that the kidneys and other mineralocorticoid-sensitive tissues also contain the enzyme **11β-hydroxysteroid dehydrogenase type 2,** which converts cortisol to cortisone and corticosterone to its 11-oxy derivative but leaves aldosterone untouched. These 11-oxy derivatives do not bind to the receptor.

EFFECT OF ADRENALECTOMY

In adrenal insufficiency, Na^+ is lost in the urine; K^+ is retained, and the plasma K^+ rises. When adrenal insufficiency develops rapidly, the amount of Na^+ lost from the ECF exceeds the amount excreted in the urine, indicating that Na^+ also must be entering cells.

When the posterior pituitary is intact, salt loss exceeds water loss, and the plasma Na⁺ falls. However, the plasma volume is also reduced, resulting in hypotension, circulatory insufficiency and, eventually, fatal shock. These changes can be prevented to a degree by increasing dietary NaCl intake but the amount of supplementary salt needed is so large that it is almost impossible to prevent eventual collapse and death unless mineralocorticoid treatment is also instituted.

■ REGULATION OF ALDOSTERONE SECRETION

STIMULI

The primary regulatory factors involved in aldosterone secretion are ACTH from the pituitary, renin from the kidney via angiotensin II, and a direct stimulatory effect on the adrenal cortex of a rise in plasma K⁺ concentration.

When first administered, ACTH stimulates the output of aldosterone as well as that of glucocorticoids and sex hormones. Although the amount of ACTH required to increase aldosterone is somewhat greater than the amount that stimulates maximal glucocorticoid secretion, it is well within the range of endogenous ACTH secretion. The effect is transient, and even if ACTH secretion remains elevated, aldosterone output declines in 1 or 2 days. On the other hand, the output of the mineralocorticoid deoxycorticosterone remains elevated. The decline in aldosterone output is partly due to decreased renin secretion secondary to hypervolemia, but it is possible that some other factor also decreases the conversion of corticosterone to aldosterone. After hypophysectomy, the basal rate of aldosterone secretion is normal. The increase normally produced by surgical and other stresses is absent, but the increase produced by dietary salt restriction is unaffected for some time. Later on, atrophy of the zona glomerulosa complicates the picture in long-standing hypopituitarism, and this may lead to salt loss and hypoaldosteronism.

Normally, glucocorticoid treatment does not suppress aldosterone secretion. However, an interesting recently described syndrome is **glucocorticoid-remediable aldosteronism (GRA).** This is an autosomal dominant disorder in which the increase in aldosterone secretion produced by ACTH is no longer transient. The hypersecretion of aldosterone and the accompanying hypertension are remedied when ACTH secretion is suppressed by administering glucocorticoids. The genes encoding aldosterone synthase and 11β-hydroxylase are 95% identical and are close together on chromosome 8. In individuals with GRA, there is unequal crossing over so that the 5′regulatory region of the 11β-hydroxylase gene is fused to the coding region of the aldosterone synthase gene. The product of this hybrid gene is an ACTH-sensitive aldosterone synthase.

Angiotensin II produced by renin and ACE stimulates adrenocortical secretion and, in small doses, affect primarily the secretion of aldosterone. The sites of action of angiotensin II are both early and late in the steroid biosynthetic pathway. The early action is on the conversion of cholesterol to pregnenolone, and the late action is on the conversion of corticosterone to aldosterone. A drop in ECF volume or intra-arterial vascular volume leads to a reflex increase in renal nerve discharge and decreases renal arterial pressure. Both changes increase renin secretion, and the angiotensin II formed by the action of renin increases the rate of secretion of aldosterone. Aldosterone causes Na⁺ and, secondarily, water retention, expanding ECF volume, and shutting off the stimulus that initiated increased renin secretion.

Hemorrhage stimulates ACTH and renin secretion. Like hemorrhage, standing and constriction of the thoracic inferior vena cava decrease intrarenal arterial pressure. Dietary sodium restriction also increases aldosterone secretion via the renin–angiotensin system. Such restriction reduces ECF volume, but aldosterone and renin secretion are increased before any consistent decrease in blood pressure takes place. Consequently, the initial increase in renin secretion produced by dietary sodium restriction is probably due to a reflex increase in the activity of the renal nerves. The increase in circulating angiotensin II produced by salt depletion upregulates the angiotensin II receptors in the adrenal cortex and hence increases the response to angiotensin II, whereas it downregulates the angiotensin II receptors in blood vessels.

An acute decline in plasma Na⁺ of about 20 mEq/L stimulates aldosterone secretion (**Figure 20–3**), but changes of this magnitude are rare. However, the plasma K⁺ level need increase only 1 mEq/L to stimulate aldosterone secretion, and transient increases of this magnitude may occur after a meal, particularly if it is rich in K⁺. Like angiotensin II, K⁺ stimulates the conversion of cholesterol to pregnenolone and the conversion of deoxycorticosterone to aldosterone. It appears to act by depolarizing the cell, which opens voltage-gated Ca²⁺ channels, increasing intracellular Ca²⁺. The sensitivity of the zona glomerulosa to angiotensin II and consequently to a low-sodium diet is decreased by a low-potassium diet.

In normal individuals, plasma aldosterone concentrations increase during the portion of the day that the individual is carrying on activities in the upright position. This increase is due to a decrease in the rate of removal of aldosterone from the circulation by the liver and an increase in aldosterone secretion due to a postural increase in renin secretion. Individuals who are confined to bed show a circadian rhythm of aldosterone and renin secretion, with the highest values in the early morning before awakening. Atrial natriuretic peptide (ANP) inhibits renin secretion and decreases the responsiveness of the zona glomerulosa to angiotensin II.

■ SUMMARY OF THE EFFECTS OF ADRENOCORTICAL HYPER- & HYPOFUNCTION IN HUMANS

Recapitulating the manifestations of excess and deficiency of the adrenocortical hormones in humans is a convenient way to summarize the multiple and complex actions of these steroids. A characteristic clinical syndrome is associated with excess secretion of each of the types of hormones.

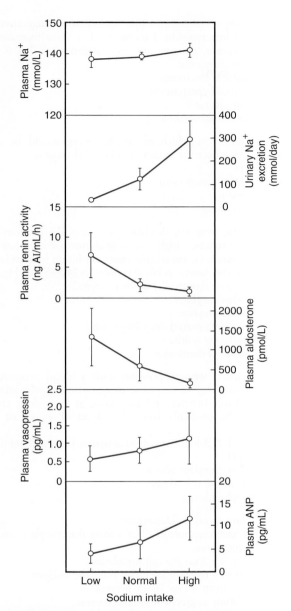

FIGURE 20–3 Effect of low-, normal-, and high-sodium diets on sodium metabolism and plasma renin activity, aldosterone, vasopressin, and ANP in normal humans. (Data from Sagnella GA, et al: Plasma atrial natriuretic peptide: Its relationship to changes in sodium in-take, plasma renin activity, and aldosterone in man. *Clin Sci.* 1987; 72:25.)

Excess androgen secretion causes masculinization (**adrenogenital syndrome**) and precocious pseudopuberty or female pseudohermaphroditism.

Excess glucocorticoid secretion produces a moon-faced, plethoric appearance, with trunk obesity, purple abdominal striae, hypertension, osteoporosis, protein depletion, mental abnormalities and, frequently, diabetes mellitus (**Cushing syndrome**). Excess mineralocorticoid secretion leads to K^+ depletion and Na^+ retention, usually without edema but with weakness, hypertension,

tetany, polyuria, and hypokalemic alkalosis (**hyperaldosteronism**). This condition may be due to primary adrenal disease (**primary hyperaldosteronism; Conn syndrome**) such as an adenoma of the zona glomerulosa, unilateral or bilateral adrenal hyperplasia, adrenal carcinoma, or by GRA. In patients with primary hyperaldosteronism, renin secretion is depressed. **Secondary hyperaldosteronism** with high plasma renin activity is caused by cirrhosis, heart failure, and nephrosis. Increased renin secretion is also found in individuals with the salt-losing form of the adrenogenital syndrome (see earlier), because their ECF volume is low. In patients with elevated renin secretion due to renal artery constriction, aldosterone secretion is increased; in those in whom renin secretion is not elevated, aldosterone secretion is normal. The relationship of aldosterone to hypertension is discussed in Chapter 32.

Primary adrenal insufficiency due to disease processes that destroy the adrenal cortex is called **Addison disease.** The condition used to be a relatively common complication of tuberculosis, but now it is usually due to autoimmune inflammation of the adrenal. Patients lose weight, are tired, and become chronically hypotensive. They have small hearts, probably because the hypotension decreases the work of the heart. Eventually, severe hypotension and shock (**addisonian crisis**) develop. This is due not only to mineralocorticoid deficiency but to glucocorticoid deficiency as well. Fasting causes fatal hypoglycemia, and any stress causes collapse. Water is retained, and there is always the danger of water intoxication. Circulating ACTH levels are elevated. The diffuse tanning of the skin and the spotty pigmentation characteristic of chronic glucocorticoid deficiency are due, at least in part, to the melanocyte-stimulating hormone (MSH) activity of the ACTH in the blood. Pigmentation of skin creases on the hands and the gums are common. Minor menstrual abnormalities occur in women, but the deficiency of adrenal sex hormones usually has little effect in the presence of normal testes or ovaries.

Secondary adrenal insufficiency is caused by pituitary diseases that decrease ACTH secretion, and **tertiary adrenal insufficiency** is caused by hypothalamic disorders disrupting CRH secretion. Both are usually milder than primary adrenal insufficiency because electrolyte metabolism is affected to a lesser degree. In addition, there is no pigmentation because in both of these conditions, plasma ACTH is low, not high.

Cases of isolated aldosterone deficiency have also been reported in patients with renal disease and a low circulating renin level (**hyporeninemic hypoaldosteronism**). In addition, **pseudohypoaldosteronism** is produced when there is resistance to the action of aldosterone. Patients with these syndromes have marked hyperkalemia, salt wasting, and hypotension, and they may develop metabolic acidosis.

CHAPTER SUMMARY

- The adrenal gland consists of the adrenal medulla that secretes dopamine and the catecholamines epinephrine and norepinephrine, and the adrenal cortex that secretes steroid hormones.

■ Norepinephrine and epinephrine act on two classes of receptors, α- and β-adrenergic receptors, and exert metabolic effects that include glycogenolysis in liver and skeletal muscle, mobilization of FFA, increased plasma lactate, and stimulation of the metabolic rate.

■ The hormones of the adrenal cortex are derivatives of cholesterol and include the mineralocorticoid aldosterone, the glucocorticoids cortisol and corticosterone, and the androgens dehydroepiandrosterone (DHEA) and androstenedione.

■ Androgens are the hormones that exert masculinizing effects, and they promote protein anabolism and growth. The adrenal androgen androstenedione is converted to testosterone and to estrogens (aromatized) in fat and other peripheral tissues. This is an important source of estrogens in men and postmenopausal women.

■ The mineralocorticoid aldosterone has effects on Na$^+$ and K$^+$ excretion and glucocorticoids affect glucose and protein metabolism.

■ Glucocorticoid secretion is dependent on ACTH from the anterior pituitary and is increased by stress. Angiotensin II increases the secretion of aldosterone.

MULTIPLE-CHOICE QUESTIONS

For all questions, select the single best answer unless otherwise directed.

1. Which of the following is produced only by *large amounts* of glucocorticoids?
   A. Normal responsiveness of fat depots to norepinephrine
   B. Maintenance of normal vascular reactivity
   C. Increased excretion of a water load
   D. Inhibition of the inflammatory response
   E. Inhibition of ACTH secretion

2. Which of the following are *incorrectly* paired?
   A. Gluconeogenesis : Cortisol
   B. Free fatty acid mobilization : Dehydroepiandrosterone
   C. Muscle glycogenolysis : Epinephrine
   D. Kaliuresis : Aldosterone
   E. Hepatic glycogenesis : Insulin

3. Which of the following hormones has the shortest plasma half-life?
   A. Corticosterone
   B. Renin
   C. Dehydroepiandrosterone
   D. Aldosterone
   E. Norepinephrine

4. A 60-year-old man is brought to the ED with pulmonary symptoms. He is found to have pneumonia and is treated with glucocorticoids. The physician says this treatment will not work immediately due to its actions at what receptor?
   A. G-protein receptors
   B. Intracellular receptors
   C. Cell surface receptors
   D. Tyrosine kinase receptors

5. A 29-year-old woman comes to see her physician with complaints of episodic palpitations and sweating for the past 5 months. She also complains of headaches not relieved by over-the-counter medications. She has a history of kidney stones, but no significant family history. Upon examination, her blood pressure is 210/114 mm Hg, and she has

renal changes ophthalmoscopic examination suggestive of prolonged hypertension. Laboratory data show increases in plasma calcium, glucose, and metanephrines. What is the most likely diagnosis?
   A. Renal cell carcinoma
   B. Essential hypertension
   C. Conn disease
   D. Pheochromocytoma

6. The secretion of which of the following would be *least* affected by a decrease in extracellular fluid volume?
   A. CRH
   B. Arginine vasopressin
   C. Estrogens
   D. Aldosterone

7. A young man presents with a blood pressure of 175/110 mm Hg. He is found to have a high circulating aldosterone but a low circulating cortisol. Glucocorticoid treatment lowers his circulating aldosterone and lowers his blood pressure to 140/85 mm Hg. He probably has an abnormality in what enzyme?
   A. 17α-hydroxylase
   B. 21β-hydroxylase
   C. 3β-hydroxysteroid dehydrogenase
   D. aldosterone synthase
   E. cholesterol desmolase

8. A 32-year-old woman presents with a blood pressure of 155/96 mm Hg. In response to questioning, she admits that she loves licorice and eats some at least three times a week. She probably has a low level of which of the following:
   A. Type 2 11β-hydroxysteroid dehydrogenase activity
   B. ACTH
   C. 11β-hydroxylase activity
   D. Glucuronyl transferase
   E. Norepinephrine

9. In its action in cells, aldosterone
   A. increases transport of ENaCs from the cytoplasm to the cell membrane.
   B. does not act on the cell membrane.
   C. binds to a receptor excluded from the nucleus.
   D. may activate a heat shock protein.
   E. also binds to glucocorticoid receptors.

10. A group of medical students were hiking in Yellowstone National Park and came across a mother bear with two cubs. They managed to escape without being hurt, but what hormone would be expected to be increased in response to the stress of interacting with the bear.
   A. Oxytocin
   B. ACTH
   C. Insulin
   D. Testosterone

11. A medical student is performing a study in which he is infusing norepinephrine acutely into a rat. The norepinephrine causes an increase in both systolic and diastolic blood pressure, but causes a concomitant reduction in heart rate. What is the mechanism responsible for the reduction in heart rate?
   A. Stimulation of α$_2$-receptors
   B. Blockade of β$_1$-receptors
   C. Stimulation of baroreceptors
   D. Inhibition of baroreceptors.

ANSWERS

1. Answer is **D.** High levels of glucocorticoids are necessary to inhibit the immune response and that is why slow weaning off of the glucocorticoids is necessary when they are stopped. Chronic elevated levels of glucocorticoids increase body fat deposition. Vascular reactivity and water reabsorption are increased as well. Glucocorticoids stimulate ACTH secretion.

2. Answer is **B.** Free fatty acids are mobilized by epinephrine and norepinephrine.

3. Answers is **E.** NE half life is approximately 2 min. Corticosterone half life is 60–90 min renin is 10–15 min; DHEA is 15–38 min; aldosterone is 20 min.

4. Answer is **B.** Glucocorticoids bind to receptors in the cytoplasm and move to the nucleus to affect DNA transcription by bind to glucocorticoid response elements (GRE). The time is at least 2–6 h for new protein synthesis to occur.

5. Answer is **D.** Pheochromocytoma is characterized by palpitations, hypertension, headache, and glucosuria.

6. Answer is **C.** Estrogens are little affected by changes in ECF. All the others would change in response to a decrease in ECF.

CRH would cause ACTH release; arginine vasopressin would increase; aldosterone would increase in response to a decrease in ECF because Ang II would increase in response to a drop in ECF thereby increase sodium reabsorption.

7. Answer is **C.** 3-beta-hydroxysteroid hydrogenase is the enzyme responsible for aldosterone synthesis, but not cortisol.

8. Answer is **A.** Licorice is a potent inhibitor of the 11β-hydroxysteroid dehydrogenase.

9. Answer is **A.** Aldosterone increases transport of ENaCs from the cytoplasm to the cell membrane to increase activity and also increases expression of ENaCs.

10. Answer is **B.** Stress first caused short-term activation of the sympathetic nervous system and excretion of adrenal medullary catecholamines. This is supported and continued by secretion of ACTH causes release of cortisol, the "fight or flight" hormone.

11. Answer is **C.** The increase in mean arterial pressure causes stimulation and increased firing rate of the carotid and aortic baroreceptors, which causes a reflex slowing of the heart. This occurs due to the direct stimulation of cardiac β_1-receptors by norepinephrine.

Hormonal Control of Calcium & Phosphate Metabolism & the Physiology of Bone

- Understand the importance of maintaining homeostasis of body calcium and phosphate.
- Describe the body pools of calcium, their rates of turnover, and the organs that regulate movement of calcium between stores.
- Delineate mechanisms of calcium and phosphate absorption and excretion.
- Identify the major hormones that regulate calcium and phosphate homeostasis and their sites of synthesis as well as targets of their action.
- Define the basic anatomy of bone.
- Delineate cells and their functions in bone formation and resorption.

INTRODUCTION

Calcium is an essential intracellular signaling molecule and also plays a variety of extracellular functions, thus the control of body calcium concentrations is vitally important. The system that maintains calcium homeostasis includes cells that sense changes in extracellular calcium and release calcium-regulating hormones, and the targets of these hormones that respond with changes in calcium mobilization, excretion, or uptake. Three hormones primarily regulate calcium homeostasis. Parathyroid hormone (PTH) is secreted by the parathyroid glands. Its main action is to mobilize calcium from bone and increase urinary phosphate excretion. 1,25-Dihydroxycholecalciferol is a steroid hormone formed from vitamin D in the liver and kidneys. Its primary action is to increase calcium absorption from the intestine. Calcitonin, a calcium-lowering hormone secreted primarily by the thyroid gland, inhibits bone resorption. Although the role of calcitonin seems to be relatively minor, all three hormones probably operate in concert to maintain the constancy of the calcium level in the body fluids. Phosphate homeostasis is likewise critical to normal body function, particularly given its inclusion in adenosine triphosphate (ATP), its role as a biologic buffer, and its role as a modifier of proteins. Many of the systems that regulate calcium homeostasis also contribute to that of phosphate, albeit sometimes in a reciprocal fashion.

■ CALCIUM & PHOSPHORUS METABOLISM

CALCIUM

The body of a young adult human contains about 1100 g (27.5 moles) of calcium. Ninety-nine percent is in the skeleton. Plasma calcium, normally at a concentration of around 10 mg/dL (5 mEq/L, 2.5 mmol/L), is partly bound to protein and partly diffusible.

It is the free, ionized calcium (Ca^{2+}) in the body fluids that is a vital second messenger and is necessary for blood coagulation, muscle contraction, and nerve function. A decrease in extracellular Ca^{2+} exerts a net excitatory effect on nerve and muscle cells. The result is hypocalcemic tetany, characterized by extensive spasms of skeletal muscle, involving especially muscles of the extremities and the larynx. Laryngospasm can become so severe that the airway is obstructed and fatal asphyxia is produced.

Because the extent of Ca^{2+} binding by plasma proteins is proportional to the plasma protein level, it is important to know the plasma protein level when evaluating the total plasma calcium. Other electrolytes and pH also affect free Ca^{2+}. For example, symptoms of tetany appear at higher calcium levels if the patient hyperventilates, thereby increasing plasma pH. Plasma proteins are more ionized when the pH is high, providing more protein anions to bind with Ca^{2+}.

The calcium in bone is of two types: a readily exchangeable reservoir and a much larger pool of stable calcium that is only slowly exchangeable. Two independent but interacting homeostatic systems affect calcium in bone. One is the system that regulates plasma Ca^{2+}, providing for the movement of about 500 mmol of Ca^{2+} per day into and out of the readily exchangeable pool in the bone (**Figure 21–1**). The other system involves bone remodeling by the constant interplay of bone resorption and deposition (see following text). However, the Ca^{2+} interchange between plasma and this stable pool of bone calcium is only about 7.5 mmol/day.

Ca^{2+} is transported across the brush border of intestinal epithelial cells via transient receptor potential vanilloid type 6 channels (TRPV6) and binds to an intracellular protein known as calbindin-D9k. Calbindin-D9k sequesters the absorbed calcium so that it does not disturb epithelial signaling processes. The absorbed Ca^{2+} is delivered to the basolateral membrane of the epithelial cell, from where it can be transported into the bloodstream by either a Na^+/Ca^{2+} exchanger (NCX1) or a Ca^{2+}-dependent ATPase. The overall transport process is regulated by 1,25-dihydroxycholecalciferol (see below). As Ca^{2+} uptake rises, 1,25-dihydroxycholecalciferol levels fall in response to increased plasma Ca^{2+}.

Plasma Ca^{2+} is filtered in the kidneys, but 98–99% of the filtered Ca^{2+} is reabsorbed. About 60% of the reabsorption occurs in the proximal tubules and the remainder in the ascending limb of the loop of Henle and the distal tubule. Distal tubular reabsorption depends on the TRPV5 channel, which is related to TRPV6, and whose expression is regulated by PTH.

PHOSPHORUS

Total body phosphorus is 500–800 g (16.1–25.8 moles), 85–90% of which is in the skeleton. Total plasma phosphorus is about 12 mg/dL, with two-thirds of this total in organic compounds and the remaining inorganic phosphorus (Pi) mostly in, HPO_4^{2-}, and $H_2PO_4^-$. The amount of phosphorus normally entering bone is about 3 mg (97 μmol)/kg/day, with an equal amount leaving via reabsorption.

Pi in the plasma is filtered in the glomeruli, and 85–90% of the filtered Pi is reabsorbed. Active transport in the proximal tubule accounts for most of the reabsorption and involves two related sodium-dependent Pi cotransporters, NaPi-IIa and NaPi-IIc. NaPi-IIa is powerfully inhibited by PTH, causing a reduction in renal Pi reabsorption (see below).

Pi is absorbed in the duodenum and small intestine. Uptake occurs by a transporter related to those in the kidney, NaPi-IIb. However, the pathway by which Pi exits into the bloodstream is not known. Many stimuli that increase Ca^{2+} absorption, including 1,25-dihydroxycholecalciferol, also increase Pi absorption via increased NaPi-IIb activity.

■ VITAMIN D & THE HYDROXYCHOLECALCIFEROLS

CHEMISTRY

The term "**vitamin D**" refers to a group of closely related sterols produced from certain provitamins. Vitamin D_3, which is also called cholecalciferol, is produced in the skin from 7-dehydrocholesterol

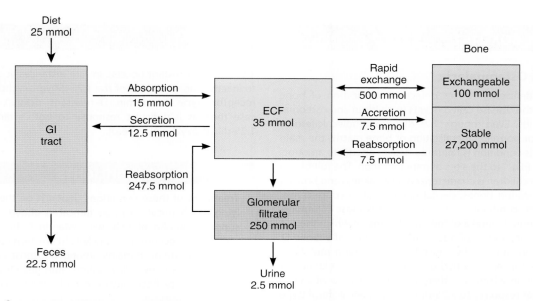

FIGURE 21–1 Calcium metabolism in an adult human. A typical daily dietary intake of 25 mmol Ca^{2+} (1000 mg) moves through many body compartments. Note that the majority of body calcium is in bones, in a pool that is only slowly exchangeable with the extracellular fluid (ECF).

by the action of sunlight. Vitamin D_3 and its hydroxylated derivatives are transported in the plasma bound to a globulin, vitamin D–binding protein (DBP). Vitamin D_3 is also ingested in the diet.

Vitamin D_3 is metabolized by cytochrome P450 (CYP) enzymes. In the liver, vitamin D_3 is converted to 25-hydroxycholecalciferol (calcidiol, 25-OHD$_3$). 25-Hydroxycholecalciferol is converted in the proximal tubules of the kidneys to the more active metabolite 1,25-dihydroxycholecalciferol (calcitriol or 1,25-(OH)$_2$D$_3$). The normal plasma level of 25-hydroxycholecalciferol is about 30 ng/mL, and that of 1,25-dihydroxycholecalciferol is about 0.03 ng/mL (approximately 100 pmol/L). The less active metabolite 24,25-dihydroxycholecalciferol is also formed in the kidneys.

MECHANISM OF ACTION

1,25-Dihydroxycholecalciferol stimulates the expression of genes involved in Ca^{2+} transport and handling via its receptor, which is a transcriptional regulator in its ligand-bound form. One target is the family of **calbindin-D** proteins that are found in human intestine, brain, and kidneys. 1,25-Dihydroxycholecalciferol also increases the expression of Ca^{2+}–ATPase and TRPV6 in intestinal cells, and thus, the capacity for calcium absorption.

In addition to increasing Ca^{2+} absorption from the intestine, 1,25-dihydroxycholecalciferol facilitates renal Ca^{2+} reabsorption via increased TRPV5 expression, increases the synthetic activity of osteoblasts, and is necessary for normal calcification of matrix (Clinical Box 21–1).

REGULATION OF SYNTHESIS

Formation of 25-hydroxycholecalciferol does not appear to be stringently regulated. However, the formation of 1,25-dihydroxycholecalciferol in the kidneys is regulated in a feedback fashion by plasma Ca^{2+} and PO_4^{3+} (**Figure 21–2**). When the plasma Ca^{2+} level is high, little 1,25-dihydroxycholecalciferol is produced, and the kidneys produce 24,25-dihydroxycholecalciferol instead. Conversely, expression of 1α-hydroxylase is stimulated by PTH, and when the plasma Ca^{2+} level is low, PTH secretion is increased. The production of 1,25-dihydroxycholecalciferol is also increased by low plasma PO_4^{3-} levels and high PO_4^{3-} levels directly inhibit the 1α-hydroxylase. Additional control of 1,25-dihydroxycholecalciferol formation results from its direct negative feedback effect on 1α-hydroxylase, a positive feedback action on the formation of 24,25-dihydroxycholecalciferol, and a direct action on the parathyroid gland to inhibit PTH expression.

An "anti-aging" protein called α-Klotho also plays important roles in calcium and phosphate homeostasis, in part by reciprocal effects on 1,25-dihydroxycholecalciferol levels. Mice deficient in α-Klotho display accelerated aging, decreased bone mineral density, calcifications, and hypercalcemia and hyperphosphatemia. α-Klotho stabilizes TRPV5 and Na, K ATPase. Likewise, it enhances the activity of fibroblast growth factor 23 (FGF23) at its receptor. FGF23 decreases renal NaPi-IIa and NaPi-IIc expression and inhibits the production of 1α-hydroxylase, reducing levels of 1,25-dihydroxycholecalciferol.

■ THE PARATHYROID GLANDS

ANATOMY

Humans usually have four parathyroid glands embedded in the poles of the thyroid gland. Each parathyroid gland is a richly vascularized disk, about $3 \times 6 \times 2$ mm, containing two distinct types of cells. The abundant **chief cells** synthesize and secrete **PTH.**

CLINICAL BOX 21–1

Rickets & Osteomalacia

Vitamin D deficiency causes defective calcification of bone matrix and the disease called rickets in children and osteomalacia in adults. Even though 1,25-dihydroxycholecalciferol is necessary for normal mineralization of bone matrix, the main defect in this condition is failure to deliver adequate amounts of Ca^{2+} and PO_4^{3-} to the sites of mineralization. The full-blown condition in children is characterized by weakness and bowing of weight-bearing bones, dental defects, and hypocalcemia. In adults, the condition is less obvious. It is most commonly due to inadequate intake of the provitamins on which the sun acts in the skin, and responds to administration of vitamin D. The condition can also be caused by inactivating mutations of the gene for renal 1α-hydroxylase, or in severe kidney or liver diseases, in which case there is no response to vitamin D but a normal response to 1,25-dihydroxycholecalciferol (type

1 vitamin D–resistant rickets). In rare instances, it can be due to inactivating mutations of the 1,25-dihydroxycholecalciferol receptor (type 2 vitamin D–resistant rickets), in which case there is a deficient response to both vitamin D and 1,25-dihydroxycholecalciferol.

THERAPEUTIC HIGHLIGHTS

Treatment of these conditions depends on the underlying biochemical basis, as indicated above. Routine supplementation of milk with vitamin D has greatly reduced the occurrence of rickets in Western countries, but the condition remains among the most common childhood diseases in developing countries. Orthopedic surgery may be necessary in severely affected children.

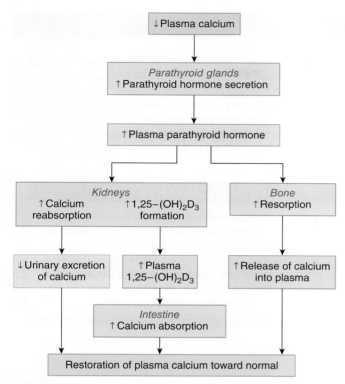

FIGURE 21–2 Effects of PTH and 1,25-dihydroxycholecalciferol on whole body calcium homeostasis. A reduction in plasma calcium stimulates parathyroid hormone secretion. PTH in turn causes calcium conservation and production of 1,25-dihydroxycholecalciferol in the kidneys, the latter of which increases calcium uptake in the intestine. PTH also releases calcium from the readily exchangeable pool in the bone. All of these actions act to restore normal plasma calcium. (Reproduced with permission from Vander A, Sherman J, Lueiano D: *Vander's Human Physiology*, 8th ed. McGraw-Hill, 2001.)

The less abundant and larger **oxyphil cells** contain oxyphil granules. In humans, few oxyphil cells are seen before puberty, and thereafter they increase in number with age. Their function is unknown. Consequences of loss of the parathyroid glands are discussed in **Clinical Box 21–2.**

SYNTHESIS & METABOLISM OF PTH

Human PTH is a linear 84 amino acid polypeptide. It is synthesized as part of a larger molecule (**preproPTH**). On entry of preproPTH into the endoplasmic reticulum, a leader sequence is removed from the amino terminal to form **proPTH.** Six additional amino acid residues are removed from the amino terminal of proPTH in the Golgi apparatus, and the resulting PTH is packaged in secretory granules and secreted as the main product of the chief cells.

The normal plasma level of PTH is 10–55 pg/mL. The half-life of PTH is approximately 10 min, and the polypeptide is

---

CLINICAL BOX 21–2

Effects of Parathyroidectomy

Occasionally, inadvertent parathyroidectomy occurs in humans during thyroid surgery. This can have serious consequences as PTH is essential for life. After parathyroidectomy, there is a steady decline in plasma Ca^{2+}. Signs of neuromuscular hyperexcitability appear, followed by full-blown tetany. Plasma phosphate levels usually rise as the plasma Ca^{2+} level falls. The signs of tetany in humans include Chvostek sign, a quick contraction of the ipsilateral facial muscles elicited by tapping over the facial nerve at the angle of the jaw, and Trousseau sign, a spasm of the muscles of the upper extremity that causes flexion of the wrist and thumb with extension of the fingers. In individuals with mild tetany in whom spasm is not yet evident, Trousseau sign can sometimes be produced by occluding the circulation for a few minutes with a blood pressure cuff.

THERAPEUTIC HIGHLIGHTS

Treatment centers around replacing the PTH that would normally be produced by the missing glands. Injections of Ca^{2+} salts can also give temporary relief.

---

rapidly cleaved by Kupffer cells in the liver. PTH and its fragments are then cleared by the kidneys.

PTH acts directly on bone to increase bone resorption and mobilize Ca^{2+}. In addition to increasing plasma Ca^{2+}, PTH increases phosphate excretion in the urine and thereby depresses plasma phosphate levels. This phosphaturic action is due to a decrease in reabsorption of phosphate via effects on NaPi-IIa in the proximal tubules. PTH also increases reabsorption of Ca^{2+} in the distal tubules, although Ca^{2+} excretion in the urine is often increased in hyperparathyroidism because the increase in the load of filtered calcium overwhelms the effect on reabsorption (**Clinical Box 21–3**). PTH also increases the formation of 1,25-dihydroxycholecalciferol, and this increases Ca^{2+} absorption from the intestine. On a longer time scale, PTH stimulates both osteoblasts and osteoclasts.

MECHANISM OF ACTION

There are at least three different PTH receptors. One also binds parathyroid hormone–related protein (PTHrP; see below) and is known as the hPTH/PTHrP receptor. A second receptor, PTH2 (hPTH2-R), does not bind PTHrP and is found in the brain, placenta, and pancreas. In addition, there is evidence for a third receptor, CPTH, which reacts with the carboxyl terminal rather than the amino terminal of PTH. The first two receptors are coupled to Gs and increase intracellular

CLINICAL BOX 21–3

Diseases of Parathyroid Excess

Hyperparathyroidism due to hypersecretion from a functioning parathyroid tumor in humans is characterized by hypercalcemia and hypophosphatemia. Humans with PTH-secreting adenomas are usually asymptomatic, with the condition detected when plasma Ca^{2+} is measured in conjunction with a routine physical examination. However, there may be minor changes in personality, and calcium-containing kidney stones occasionally form. In conditions such as chronic kidney disease and rickets, in which the plasma Ca^{2+} level is chronically low, stimulation of the parathyroid glands causes compensatory parathyroid hypertrophy and secondary hyperparathyroidism. The plasma Ca^{2+} level is low in chronic kidney disease primarily because the diseased kidneys lose the ability to form 1,25-dihydroxycholecalciferol. Finally, mutations in the Ca^{2+}-sensing receptor gene CaSR cause predictable long-term changes in plasma Ca^{2+}. Individuals heterozygous for inactivating mutations have familial benign hypocalciuric hypercalcemia, a condition in which there is a chronic moderate elevation in plasma Ca^{2+} because feedback inhibition of PTH secretion is reduced. Plasma PTH levels are normal or even elevated. However, children who are homozygous for inactivating mutations develop severe primary hyperparathyroidism. Conversely, individuals with gain-of-function mutations in the CASR gene develop familial hypercalciuric hypocalcemia due to increased sensitivity of the parathyroid glands to plasma Ca^{2+}.

THERAPEUTIC HIGHLIGHTS

Subtotal parathyroidectomy is sometimes necessary in patients in whom parathyroid adenoma or hyperplasia with associated hypercalcemia and resulting symptoms develops. However, because parathyroid disease is often benign or only slowly progressing, surgery and is typically reserved for those who have experienced life-threatening complications of hypercalcemia.

---

cAMP. The hPTH/PTHrP receptor also activates PLC via Gq, increasing intracellular Ca^{2+} concentrations and activating protein kinase C.

In the disease called pseudohypoparathyroidism, the signs and symptoms of hypoparathyroidism develop but the circulating level of PTH is normal or even elevated. There are two forms. In the more common form, a congenital 50% reduction of the activity of Gs occurs and PTH fails to produce a normal increase in cAMP concentration. In a different, less common form, the cAMP response is normal but the phosphaturic action of the hormone is defective.

REGULATION OF SECRETION

Circulating Ca^{2+} acts directly on the parathyroid glands in a negative feedback fashion to regulate the secretion of PTH. The key to this regulation is a cell membrane Ca^{2+} sensing receptor (CaSR). In the parathyroid, its activation inhibits PTH secretion. When plasma Ca^{2+} is high, PTH secretion is inhibited and Ca^{2+} is deposited in the bones. When it is low, secretion is increased and Ca^{2+} is mobilized from the bones.

1,25-Dihydroxycholecalciferol acts on the parathyroid glands to decrease preproPTH mRNA. Increased plasma phosphate stimulates PTH secretion by lowering plasma levels of free Ca^{2+} and inhibiting the formation of 1,25-dihydroxycholecalciferol. Magnesium is required to maintain normal parathyroid secretory responses. Impaired PTH release along with diminished target organ responses to PTH account for the hypocalcemia that occasionally occurs in magnesium deficiency.

PTHrP

Parathyroid hormone–related protein (PTHrP), another protein with PTH activity, is produced by many different tissues in the body. PTHrP and PTH have marked homology at their amino terminal ends and they both bind to the hPTH/PTHrP receptor, yet their physiologic effects are very different. PTHrP is primarily a paracrine factor, acting close to where it is produced. It may be that circulating PTH cannot reach at least some of these sites. Second, subtle conformational differences may be produced by binding of PTH versus PTHrP to their receptor. Another possibility is action of one or the other hormone on additional, more selective receptors.

PTHrP has a marked effect on the growth and development of cartilage in utero. PTHrP is also expressed in the brain, where it inhibits excitotoxic damage to developing neurons. In addition, there is evidence that it is involved in Ca^{2+} transport in the placenta. PTHrP is also found in keratinocytes in the skin, in smooth muscle, and in the teeth, where it is present in the enamel epithelium that caps each tooth. In the absence of PTHrP, teeth cannot erupt.

HYPERCALCEMIA OF MALIGNANCY

Hypercalcemia is a common metabolic complication of cancer. About 20% of hypercalcemic patients have bone metastases that produce hypercalcemia by eroding bone (**local osteolytic hypercalcemia**). In the remaining 80% of the patients, circulating PTHrP is elevated (**humoral hypercalcemia of malignancy**).

The tumors responsible for this hypersecretion include cancers of the breast, kidney, ovary, and skin.

CALCITONIN

ORIGIN

In dogs, perfusion of the thyroparathyroid region with solutions containing high concentrations of Ca^{2+} leads to a fall in peripheral plasma Ca^{2+}, and after damage to this region, Ca^{2+} infusions cause a greater increase in plasma Ca^{2+} than they do in control animals. The Ca^{2+}-lowering hormone responsible is **calcitonin.** It is produced by the **parafollicular cells** of the thyroid gland, also known as the clear or C cells.

SECRETION & METABOLISM

Human calcitonin has a molecular weight of 3500 and contains 32 amino acid residues. Its secretion is increased when the thyroid gland is exposed to a plasma calcium level of approximately 9.5 mg/dL. β-Adrenergic agonists, dopamine, and estrogens also stimulate calcitonin secretion. The actions of calcitonin are short lived because it has a half-life of less than 10 min in humans.

ACTIONS

Receptors for calcitonin are found in bones and the kidneys. Calcitonin lowers circulating calcium and phosphate levels. It exerts its calcium-lowering effect by inhibiting the activity of osteoclasts and by increasing Ca^{2+} excretion in the urine.

The exact physiologic role of calcitonin is uncertain. The calcitonin content of the human thyroid is low, and after thyroidectomy, bone density and plasma Ca^{2+} level are normal as long as the parathyroid glands are intact. In addition, after thyroidectomy, there are only transient abnormalities of Ca^{2+} homeostasis when a Ca^{2+} load is injected. This may be explained in part by secretion of calcitonin from tissues other than the thyroid. However, there is general agreement that the hormone has little long-term effect on the plasma Ca^{2+} level in adult animals and humans. Further, unlike PTH and 1,25-dihydroxycholecalciferol, calcitonin does not appear to be directly involved in phosphate homeostasis. Moreover, patients with medullary carcinoma of the thyroid have a very high circulating calcitonin level but no symptoms directly attributable to the hormone, and their bones are essentially normal. No syndrome due to calcitonin deficiency has been described. More hormone is secreted in young individuals, and it may play a role in skeletal development. In addition, it may protect the bones of the mother from excess calcium loss during pregnancy. Bone formation in the infant and lactation are major drains on Ca^{2+} stores, and plasma concentrations of 1,25-dihydroxycholecalciferol are elevated in pregnancy. They would cause bone loss in the mother if bone resorption were not simultaneously inhibited by an increase in plasma calcitonin.

EFFECTS OF OTHER HORMONES & HUMORAL AGENTS ON CALCIUM METABOLISM

Calcium metabolism is affected by various hormones in addition to 1,25-dihydroxycholecalciferol, PTH, and calcitonin. **Glucocorticoids** lower plasma Ca^{2+} levels by inhibiting osteoclast formation and activity, but over long periods they cause osteoporosis by decreasing bone formation and increasing bone resorption. They decrease bone formation by inhibiting protein synthesis in osteoblasts. They also decrease the absorption of Ca^{2+} and PO_4^{3-} from the intestine and increase their renal excretion. The decrease in plasma Ca^{2+} concentration also increases the secretion of PTH, and bone resorption is facilitated. **Growth hormone** increases Ca^{2+} excretion in the urine, but it also increases intestinal absorption of Ca^{2+}, and this effect may be greater than the effect on excretion, with a resultant positive calcium balance. Insulin-like growth factor I (IGF-I) stimulates protein synthesis in bone. **Thyroid hormones** may cause hypercalcemia, hypercalciuria, and, in some instances, osteoporosis. **Estrogens** prevent osteoporosis by inhibiting the stimulatory effects of certain cytokines on osteoclasts. **Insulin** increases bone formation, and there is significant bone loss in untreated diabetes.

BONE PHYSIOLOGY

Bone is a special form of connective tissue with a collagen framework impregnated with Ca^{2+} and PO_4^{3-} salts, particularly **hydroxyapatites,** which have the general formula $Ca_{10}(PO_4)_6(OH)_2$. Bone is also involved in overall Ca^{2+} and PO_4^{3-} homeostasis. It protects vital organs, and the rigidity it provides permits locomotion and the support of loads against gravity. Old bone is constantly being resorbed and new bone formed, permitting remodeling that allows it to respond to the stresses and strains that are put upon it. It is a living tissue that is well vascularized and has a total blood flow of 200–400 mL/min in adult humans.

STRUCTURE

There are two types of bone: **compact** or **cortical bone,** which makes up the outer layer of most bones (**Figure 21–3**) and accounts for 80% of the bone in the body; and **trabecular** or **spongy bone** inside the cortical bone, which makes up the remaining 20% of bone in the body. In compact bone, the surface-to-volume ratio is low, and bone cells lie in lacunae. They receive nutrients by way of canaliculi that ramify throughout the compact bone (Figure 21–3). Trabecular bone is made up of spicules or plates, with a high surface to volume ratio and many cells sitting on the surface of the plates. Nutrients diffuse from bone extracellular fluid (ECF) into the trabeculae, but in compact bone, nutrients are provided via **haversian canals** (Figure 21–3), which contain blood vessels. Around each haversian canal, collagen is arranged in concentric layers, forming cylinders called **osteons** or **haversian systems.** The protein in bone

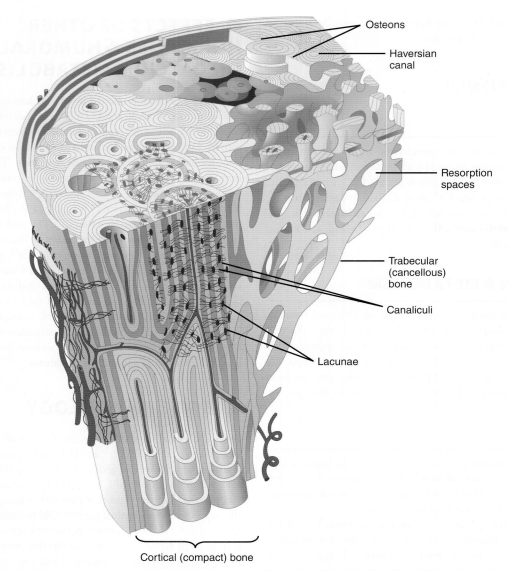

FIGURE 21–3 Structure of compact and trabecular bone. The compact bone is shown in horizontal section (top) and vertical section (bottom). (Reproduced with permission from Standring E: *Gray's Anatomy*, 40th ed. Churchill Livingstone/Elsevier, 2008.)

matrix is over 90% type 1 collagen, which is also the major structural protein in tendons and skin.

BONE GROWTH

During fetal development, most bones are modeled in cartilage and then transformed into bone by ossification **(enchondral bone formation).** The exceptions are the clavicles, the mandibles, and certain bones of the skull in which mesenchymal cells form bone directly **(intramembranous bone formation).**

During growth, specialized areas at the ends of each long bone (epiphyses) are separated from the shaft of the bone by a plate of actively proliferating cartilage, the epiphysial plate **(Figure 21–4)**. The bone increases in length as this plate lays down new bone on the end of the shaft. The width of the epiphysial plate is proportional to the rate of growth. Linear bone growth can occur as long as the epiphyses are separated from the shaft of the bone, but such growth ceases after the epiphyses unite with the shaft (epiphysial closure). The epiphyses of the various bones close in an orderly temporal sequence, the last epiphyses closing after puberty. The normal age at which each of the epiphyses closes is known, and the "bone age" of a young individual can be determined by radiographing the skeleton and noting which epiphyses are open and which are closed.

The periosteum is a dense fibrous, vascular, and innervated membrane that covers the surface of bones. This layer consists of an outer layer of collagenous tissue and an inner layer of fine elastic fibers that can include cells that have the potential to contribute to bone growth. The periosteum covers all surfaces of the bone except for those capped with cartilage (eg, at the joints) and serves as a site of attachment of ligaments and tendons. As one

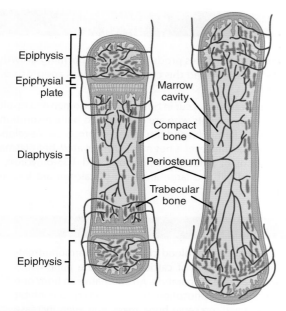

FIGURE 21–4 **Structure of a typical long bone before (left) and after (right) epiphysial closure.** Note the rearrangement of cells and growth of the bone as the epiphysial plate closes (see text for details).

ages, the periosteum becomes thinner and loses some of its vasculature. This renders bones more susceptible to injury and disease.

BONE FORMATION & RESORPTION

The cells responsible for bone formation are **osteoblasts** and the cells responsible for bone resorption are **osteoclasts.**

Osteoblasts are modified fibroblasts. Normal osteoblasts are able to lay down type 1 collagen and form new bone. Osteoclasts, on the other hand, are members of the monocyte family. Osteoclasts erode and absorb previously formed bone. They become attached to bone via integrins in a membrane extension called the sealing zone. This creates an isolated area between the bone and a portion of the osteoclast. Proton pumps (ie, H+-dependent ATPases) then move from endosomes into the cell membrane apposed to the isolated area, and they acidify the area to approximately pH 4.0. The acidic pH dissolves hydroxyapatite, and acid proteases secreted by the cell break down collagen, forming a shallow depression in the bone. The products of digestion are then endocytosed and move across the osteoclast by transcytosis, with release into the interstitial fluid.

Throughout life, bone is being constantly resorbed and new bone is being formed. The calcium in bone turns over at a rate of 100% per year in infants and 18% per year in adults. Bone remodeling is mainly a local process carried out in small areas by populations of cells called bone-remodeling units. First, osteoclasts resorb bone, and then osteoblasts lay down new bone in the same general area. This cycle takes about 100 days. Modeling drifts also occur in which the shapes of bones change as bone is

resorbed in one location and added in another. Osteoclasts tunnel into cortical bone followed by osteoblasts, whereas trabecular bone remodeling occurs on the surface of the trabeculae. About 5% of the bone mass is being remodeled by about 2 million bone-remodeling units in the human skeleton at any one time. The renewal rate for bone is about 4% per year for compact bone and 20% per year for trabecular bone. The remodeling is related in part to the stresses and strains imposed on the skeleton by gravity.

The bone remodeling process is primarily under endocrine control. Not surprisingly, hormonal control of bone metabolism can be quite complex, and this can be illustrated by examining effects of the weight-associated hormone leptin on bone metabolism. When administered intracerebroventricularly, leptin decreases bone formation. This is thought to occur via release of various substances from the hypothalamus that can reduce osteoblast function. However, circulating leptin can increase bone mass through osteoblast and pre-osteoblast cell signaling pathways. More generally, PTH accelerates bone resorption, and estrogens slow bone resorption by inhibiting the production of bone-eroding cytokines.

BONE DISEASE

In **osteopetrosis,** a rare and often severe disease, the osteoclasts are defective and are unable to resorb bone in their usual fashion so the osteoblasts operate unopposed. The result is a steady increase in bone density, neurologic defects due to narrowing and distortion of foramina through which nerves normally pass, and hematologic abnormalities due to crowding out of the marrow cavities.

On the other hand, osteoporosis is caused by a relative excess of osteoclastic function. Loss of bone matrix in this condition is marked, and the incidence of fractures is increased. Fractures are particularly common in the distal forearm (Colles fracture), vertebral body, and hip. All of these areas have a high content of trabecular bone, and because trabecular bone is more active metabolically, it is lost more rapidly. Fractures of the vertebrae with compression cause kyphosis, with the production of a typical "widow's hump" that is common in elderly women with osteoporosis. Fractures of the hip in elderly individuals are associated with a mortality rate of 12–20%, and half of those who survive require prolonged expensive care.

Osteoporosis has multiple causes, but by far the most common form is involutional osteoporosis. Humans normally gain bone during growth early in life. After a plateau, they begin to lose bone as they grow older. When this loss is accelerated or exaggerated, it leads to osteoporosis (**Clinical Box 21–4**). Increased intake of calcium, particularly from natural sources such as milk, and moderate exercise may help prevent or slow the progress of osteoporosis, although their effects are not great. Bisphosphonates such as etidronate, which inhibit osteoclastic activity, increase the mineral content of bone and decrease the rate of new vertebral fractures when administered in a cyclical fashion.

CLINICAL BOX 21-4

Osteoporosis

Adult women have less bone mass than adult men, and after menopause they initially lose it more rapidly than men of comparable age. Consequently, they are more prone to development of serious osteoporosis. The cause of bone loss after menopause is primarily estrogen deficiency, and estrogen treatment arrests the progress of the disease. Estrogens inhibit secretion of cytokines such as interleukin-1 (IL-1), IL-6, and tumor necrosis factor-alpha (TNF-α), cytokines that otherwise foster the development of osteoclasts.

Estrogen also stimulates production of transforming growth factor-beta (TGF-β), and this cytokine increases apoptosis of osteoclasts.

Bone loss can also occur in both men and women as a result of inactivity. In patients who are immobilized bone resorption exceeds bone formation and disuse osteoporosis can develop. The plasma calcium level is not markedly elevated, but plasma concentrations of parathyroid hormone and 1,25-dihydroxycholecalciferol fall and large amounts of calcium are lost in the urine.

THERAPEUTIC HIGHLIGHTS

Hormone therapy has traditionally been used to offset osteoporosis. Estrogen replacement therapy begun shortly after menopause can help maintain bone density. However, it appears that even small doses of estrogens may increase the incidence of uterine and breast cancer, and in carefully controlled studies, estrogens do not protect against cardiovascular disease. Therefore, treatment of a postmenopausal woman with estrogens is no longer used as a primary option. Raloxifene is a selective estrogen receptor modulator that can mimic the beneficial effects of estrogen on bone density in postmenopausal women without some of the risks associated with estrogen. However, this too carries risk of side effects (eg, blood clots). Other hormone treatments include the use of calcitonin and the parathyroid hormone analogue teriparatide. An alternative to hormone treatments is the bisphosphonates. These drugs can inhibit bone breakdown, preserve bone mass, and even increase bone density in the spine and hip to reduce the risk of fractures. Unfortunately, these drugs also can cause mild to serious side effects and require monitoring for patient suitability. In addition to hormones and medications listed above, physical therapy to increase appropriate mechanical load and improve balance and muscle strength can significantly improve quality of life.

CHAPTER SUMMARY

- Circulating levels of calcium and phosphate ions are controlled by cells that sense the levels of these electrolytes and release hormones, and these hormones influence mobilization of the minerals from the bones, intestinal absorption, and/or renal wasting.
- The majority of the calcium in the body is stored in the bones but it is the free, ionized calcium in the cells and extracellular fluids that fulfills physiologic roles.
- Phosphate is likewise predominantly stored in the bones and regulated by many of the same factors that influence calcium levels, sometimes reciprocally.
- The two major hormones regulating calcium and phosphate homeostasis are 1,25-dihydroxycholecalciferol (a derivative of vitamin D) and parathyroid hormone; calcitonin is also capable of regulating levels of these ions, but its physiologic contribution is unclear.
- 1,25-Dihydroxycholecalciferol elevates plasma calcium and phosphate by predominantly transcriptional mechanisms, whereas parathyroid hormone elevates calcium but decreases phosphate by increasing the latter's renal excretion. Calcitonin lowers both calcium and phosphate levels.
- Deficiencies of 1,25-dihydroxycholecalciferol activity lead to decreases in circulating calcium, defective calcification of the bones, and bone weakness. Disease states also result from either deficiencies or overproduction of parathyroid hormone.

- Bone is a highly structured mass with outer cortical and inner trabecular layers. The larger cortical layer has a high surface to volume layer with haversian canals that provide nutrients and gaps (lacunae) inhabited by bone cells that are connected by a canaliculi network. The smaller trabecular layer has a much higher surface to volume layer that relies on diffusion for nutrients supply.
- Regulated bone growth through puberty occurs through epiphysial plates. These plates are located near the end of the bone shaft and fuse with the shaft of the bone to cease linear bone growth.
- Bone is constantly remodeled by osteoclasts, which erode and absorb bone, and osteoblasts, which lay down new bone.

MULTIPLE-CHOICE QUESTIONS

For all questions, select the single best answer unless otherwise directed.

1. 10 days after thyroid surgery, a patient returns to his physician complaining of problems that have gradually developed in the intervening period. It is determined that he has parathyroid deficiency due to inadvertent damage to the parathyroid glands because his signs and symptoms include
   A. low plasma phosphate and Ca^{2+} levels and tetany.
   B. low plasma phosphate and Ca^{2+} levels and tetanus.
   C. a low plasma Ca^{2+} level, increased muscular excitability, and spasm of the muscles of the upper extremity (Trousseau sign).

D. high plasma phosphate and Ca²⁺ levels and bone demineralization.

E. increased muscular excitability, a high plasma Ca²⁺ level, and bone demineralization.

2. In an experiment, a rat is infused with a small volume of a calcium chloride solution, or sodium chloride as a control. Compared to the control condition, which of the following would result from the calcium load?
A. Bone demineralization
B. Increased formation of 1,25-dihydroxycholecalciferol
C. Decreased secretion of calcitonin
D. Decreased blood coagulability
E. Increased formation of 24,25-dihydroxycholecalciferol

3. A 50-year-old man comes to his primary care physician complaining of muscle spasms and a blood test reveals that he is hypocalcemic. His disease signs and symptoms could be reflective of underlying disease in any of the following organs *except*?
A. Kidneys
B. Skin
C. Liver
D. Lungs
E. Intestine

4. A scientist interested in the physiology of intestinal calcium absorption treats an intestinal epithelial cell line with 1,25-dihydroxycholecalciferol and measures the uptake of radioactive Ca²⁺ that results. The increase in calcium uptake that is observed would be reversed by an inhibitor of which biological process?
A. Gene transcription
B. Adenylyl cyclase activity
C. Cell proliferation
D. Protein degradation
E. Endocytosis

5. At a routine employment physical, a 30-year-old man is found to be mildly hypocalcemic, although he denies any symptoms. He does reveal that he has markedly reduced his consumption of dairy products and leafy greens over the past two months, citing gastrointestinal distress when these items were previously consumed. Analysis of his blood or an intestinal biopsy would be expected to reveal which of the following?
A. Increased formation of 24,25-dihydroxycholecalciferol
B. Decreased amounts of calcium-binding protein in intestinal epithelial cells
C. Increased parathyroid hormone secretion
D. A high plasma calcitonin concentration
E. Increased plasma phosphate

6. A mouse is engineered to lack a transcription factor necessary for the normal development of osteoclasts. Compared to normal littermate mice, which of the following would be reduced in the knock-out animals?
A. Phosphate deposition in trabecular bone
B. Hydroxyapatite levels in bone
C. Osteoblast proliferation
D. Secretion of acid proteases
E. Bone collagen

7. Two siblings have come to the clinic for general physicals so they could participate in sports. One is a college-aged male and he brought with him his 7-year-old brother. Using novel equipment, you had the opportunity to fully compare detailed features of the siblings' skeletons. Which of the following features might you find in the 7-year-old that would not be a standard feature in the college-aged male?
A. Merging of cortical bone and trabecular bone
B. Differentiation of osteoclasts and osteoblasts
C. The presence of a periosteum on a typical bone
D. A meeting of the lacunae with the trabecular bone
E. Ephyses that are united with the bone shaft

8. A mother brings her 5-year-old son to the pediatrician because she is concerned that his legs are becoming progressively bowed. She reports that he plays outside frequently and that his diet includes large quantities of dairy products. Therapeutic trials of vitamin D supplements and 1,25-dihydroxycholecalciferol fail to halt the progression of his skeletal changes. The child's condition is most likely attributable to a primary defect in
A. TRPV6.
B. vitamin D receptor (VDR).
C. renal 1α-hydroxylase.
D. TRPV5.
E. PTH.

9. A 50-year-old woman suffering from chronic kidney disease is referred to an endocrinologist for evaluation of worsening muscle spasms over a period of several months. Blood and urine tests in this patient would be expected to reveal which of the following patterns of changes compared to a healthy individual?

	Plasma calcium	Urinary calcium	Plasma PTH
A.	Unchanged	Increased	Increased
B.	Increased	Decreased	Increased
C.	Decreased	Increased	Decreased
D.	Increased	Decreased	Decreased
E.	Decreased	Increased	Increased

10. A family is identified in which some individuals are heterozygous for an inactivating mutation of the calcium-sensing receptor, CaSR. These individuals are asymptomatic, but compared to their unaffected relatives, which of the following will be decreased?
A. Plasma calcium
B. Plasma PTH
C. Exocytotic activity in chief cells of the parathyroid glands
D. Urinary calcium
E. Bone resorption

ANSWERS

1. The correct answer is **C**. The lack of PTH results in a steady decline in the levels of circulating Ca²⁺, in part due to a lack of mobilization of calcium from the bones (rules out options **D** and **E**). The reduction in circulating calcium exerts a net excitatory effect on muscle (and nerves), eventually progressing to spasm/tetany. However, phosphate levels increase reciprocally as calcium levels fall (rules out options **A** and **B**). One should also distinguish between tetanus (the normal summation of contractile responses, without relaxation, when a muscle receives multiple inputs at high frequency, see Chapter 5) and the pathological condition of tetany, an involuntary contraction of muscle fibers due to their heightened sensitivity.

2. The correct answer is **E.** Circulating calcium acts directly on the parathyroid glands via binding to CaSR to inhibit secretion of PTH. Thus, the key to understanding this question is to recognize that circulating levels of PTH will be reduced in the experimental animal compared to the control. PTH normally acts on the kidney, via an increase in the expression of 1α-hydroxylase, to trigger the production of 1,25-dihydroxycholecalciferol. When calcium levels are high, therefore, 1,25-dihydroxycholecalciferol synthesis is reduced and the less active metabolite 24,25-dihydroxy-cholecalciferol is produced instead (rules out option **B**). PTH also acts on the bone to trigger calcium mobilization (rules out option **A**). Further, while calcitonin is thought to play only an accessory role in calcium homeostasis, its secretion from the thyroid gland is increased rather than decreased by an increase in plasma calcium because it functions to lower circulating calcium levels (rules out option **C**). Finally, plasma calcium is required for the clotting reaction, so an increase in circulating calcium would be expected to increase, rather than decrease, the coagulability of the blood (rules out option **D**).

3. The correct answer is **D.** The skin is involved in regulating calcium homeostasis because it is the site in which 7-dehydrocholesterol is converted into vitamin D_3 by the action of sunlight (rules out option **B**). Vitamin D_3 is converted to 25-hydroxycholecalciferol by the 25-hydroxylase in the liver, and the product of this reaction is **further** converted to 1,25-dihydroxycholecalciferol when circulating Ca^{2+} is low by the 1α-hydroxylase that is predominantly expressed by cells of the proximal tubule of the kidney (rules out options **A** and **C**). The intestine is a key target of 1,25-dihydroxycholecalciferol, where it acts to increase calcium absorption from the diet (rules out option **E**). On the other hand, the lungs have no significant role in calcium homeostasis beyond that of any other tissue in the body.

4. The correct answer is **A.** 1,25-dihydroxycholecalciferol exerts its biological effects by binding to the vitamin D receptor (VDR), a member of the family of nuclear hormone receptors that bind to DNA and are thereby direct regulators of gene transcription when ligand-bound. While PTH, a trigger of 1,25-dihydroxycholecalciferol production in vivo, binds to a receptor linked to G_s and thus activates adenylyl cyclase, in this in vitro experiment 1,25-dihydroxy-cholecalciferol was added directly without a requirement for PTH (rules out option **B**). 1,25-dihydroxycholecalciferol increases calcium absorption by enterocytes by stimulating the production of proteins involved in membrane transport of the cation (as well as its intracellular handling), a process that is independent of cell proliferation (rules out option **C**). Inhibiting the turnover of these newly synthesized proteins would, if anything, be expected to enhance rather than reduce calcium uptake (rules out option **D**). Finally, the stimulated uptake of calcium occurs via TRPV6 channels in the enterocyte apical membrane, rather than by endocytosis (rules out option **E**).

5. The correct answer is **C.** Dairy products and leafy greens are important dietary sources of calcium. Reduced dietary intake of calcium will result in a suppression of the levels of calcium circulating in the blood, and thereby trigger homeostatic responses designed to upregulate intestinal capacity for calcium absorption. These responses include PTH secretion, which triggers the expression of 1α-hydroxylase in the kidney and thus the production of 1,25-dihydroxycholecalciferol at the expense of 24,25-dihydroxycholecalcferol (rules out option **A**). 1,25-Dihydroxycholecalciferol acts on the intestine to increase expression of the calbindin-D class of calcium-binding proteins (rules out option **B**). Calcitonin is released from the thyroid gland when circulating plasma levels of calcium rise, and thus would not be elevated here (rules out option **D**). Finally, while 1,25-dihydroxycholecalciferol increases the absorption of phosphate from the diet, PTH powerfully inhibits the NaPi-IIa transporter in the kidney that normally contributes significantly to phosphate reabsorption, and so phosphate will also be lost to the urine in increased amounts. This phosphaturic effect means that it is unlikely that plasma phosphate levels will rise (rules out option **E**).

6. The correct answer is **D.** Osteoclasts are the major cells that break down the bone for remodeling. Phosphates, hydroxyapatite and collagen all represent components that make up bone and thus, targets for reduction by osteoclasts. Since the mouse would be deficient in osteoclasts, these components would not be reduced in the knock-out animal (ruling out **A, B,** and **E,** respectively). Osteoclasts, derived from a monocyte **lineage,** and osteoblasts, which are modified fibroblasts, do not share transcription factors in their differentiation pathways, eliminating **C**. Osteoclasts function to erode and absorb previously derived bone. They do this in part by secretion of acid proteases.

7. The answer is **E.** The basic structure of bone is quite similar in both youths and adults, and thus would include cortical bone next to trabecular bone, established lacunae, and a **periosteum**, eliminating **A, C,** and **D.** Likewise, remodeling of bone occurs throughout life so the presence of mature cells that contribute to remodeling (osteoclasts and osteoblasts) as well as proliferating cartilage would be present, eliminating **B** and **C**. Epiphyses are common in young people undergoing rapid bone growth. These structures eventually merge with the bone shaft and bone elongation is halted. Thus, epiphyses would be prominent in the 7-year-old boy's bone, but not in the college-aged male's bone.

8. The correct answer is **B.** The child's presentation is consistent with rickets despite adequate sun exposure as well as calcium and vitamin D in the diet. His failure to respond to either vitamin D or 1,25-dihydroxycholecalciferol given therapeutically further implies that he has type 2 vitamin D–resistant rickets, a rare condition that results from inactivating mutations in the VDR. PTH acts upstream of 1,25-dihydroxycholecalciferol, and also acts to mobilize calcium from bone, so a defect in this hormone would not produce the picture seen (ruling out option **E**). 1,25-Dihydroxycholecalciferol stimulates the expression of TRPV5 and TRPV6, increasing both intestinal absorption and renal retention of calcium, but they would not be the primary cause of disease in this patient (rules out options **A** and **D**). Finally, a patient lacking the renal 1α-dehydroxylase would be unable to synthesize 1,25-dihydroxycholecalciferol, but rickets caused by this defect can successfully be treated by administration of 1,25-dihydroxy-cholecalciferol (rules out option **C**).

9. The correct answer is **E.** The patient is exhibiting symptoms of hypocalcemia. In the setting of kidney disease, these most likely arise because the kidneys have reduced capacity to synthesize 1,25-dihydroxycholecalciferol as nephrons are injured. 1,25-Dihydroxycholecalciferol normally stimulates expression of TRPV6 and other proteins involved in the absorption

of dietary calcium by the intestine, as well as expression of TRPV5 in the proximal tubule that participates in the reabsorption of filtered calcium by the kidney. Finally, the trigger for PTH release is a decrease in plasma calcium.

10. The correct answer is **D.** CaSR is expressed in the parathyroid gland, where it mediates feedback inhibition of PTH secretion as levels of circulating calcium rise. In an individual harboring a heterozygous inactivating mutation of CaSR, PTH secretion from parathyroid chief cells will persist even as calcium levels rise (rules out option **B** and **C**) and will continue to trigger mechanisms that increase plasma calcium, such as resorption of bone (rules out options **A** and **E**). On the other hand, urinary calcium will fall as PTH and 1,25-dihydroxycholecalciferol produced in response to PTH induce expression of transporters responsible for the reabsorption of filtered calcium.

Reproductive Development & Function of the Female Reproductive System

O B J E C T I V E S

After studying this chapter, you should be able to:

- Name the key hormones secreted by Leydig cells and Sertoli cells of the testes and by Graafian follicles and corpora lutea of the ovaries.
- Outline the role of chromosomes, hormones, and related factors in sex determination and development.
- Summarize the hormonal changes that occur at puberty in males and females.
- Outline the hormonal changes and their physiologic effects during perimenopause and menopause.
- Describe the physiologic changes that occur in the female reproductive organs during the menstrual cycle.
- Know the general structures of 17β-estradiol and progesterone, and describe their biosynthesis, transport, metabolism, and actions.
- Describe the roles of the pituitary and the hypothalamus in the regulation of ovarian function, and the role of feedback loops in this process.
- Describe the hormonal changes that accompany pregnancy and parturition.
- Outline the processes involved in lactation.

■ SEX DIFFERENTIATION & DEVELOPMENT

CHROMOSOMAL SEX

The Sex Chromosomes

Sex is determined genetically by two chromosomes, called the **sex chromosomes,** to distinguish them from the **somatic chromosomes (autosomes).** Sex chromosomes are called X and Y. The Y chromosome is necessary and sufficient for the production of testes, and the testis-determining gene product is called **SRY** (for sex-determining region of the Y chromosome). SRY is a DNA-binding regulatory protein. SRY is a transcription factor that initiates transcription of genes necessary for testicular differentiation, including the gene for **müllerian inhibiting substance (MIS;** see further). Diploid male cells contain an X and a Y chromosome (XY pattern), whereas female cells contain two X chromosomes (XX pattern). As a consequence of meiosis during gametogenesis, each normal ovum contains a single X chromosome, but half of the normal sperm contain an X chromosome and half contain a Y chromosome. When a sperm containing a Y chromosome fertilizes an ovum, an XY pattern results and the zygote develops into a **genetic male.** When fertilization occurs with an X-containing sperm, an XX pattern and a **genetic female** results.

PUBERTY

Puberty is the period when the endocrine and gametogenic functions of the gonads have developed to the point where reproduction is possible. In girls, the first event is **thelarche,** the development of breasts, followed by **pubarche,** the development of axillary and pubic hair, and then by **menarche,** the first menstrual period. Initial menstrual periods are generally anovulatory, and regular ovulation appears about a year later. In the United States in recent years, puberty generally occurs between the ages of 8 and 13. The pulsatile secretion of GnRH brings on puberty.

■ THE FEMALE REPRODUCTIVE SYSTEM

THE MENSTRUAL CYCLE

The reproductive system of women **(Figure 22–1)**, unlike that of men, shows regular cyclic changes that teleologically may be regarded as periodic preparations for fertilization and pregnancy. The cycle is a **menstrual cycle,** and is composed of an **ovarian cycle** and an **endometrial cycle.** The most conspicuous feature of the menstrual cycle is the periodic vaginal bleeding that occurs with the shedding of the endometrial mucosa **(menstruation).** The length of the cycle is variable in women, but 28 days from the start of one menstrual period to the start of the next is the average. The **follicular phase** that includes menstruation averages 15 days, the **ovulatory phase** is 1–3 days and culminates with ovulation, and the **luteal phase** averages 13 days and is less variable in length than the follicular phase.

Ovarian Cycle

From the time of birth, there are many **primordial follicles** under the ovarian capsule. Each contains an immature ovum that is stopped in prophase of the first meiosis (Figure 22–1). At the start of each cycle, several of these follicles enlarge, and a cavity forms around the ovum **(antrum formation).** This cavity is filled with follicular fluid. One of the follicles in one ovary starts to grow rapidly and becomes the **dominant follicle,** while the others regress, forming **atretic follicles.**

The structure of a maturing ovarian **(graafian)** follicle is shown in Figure 22–1. The primary source of circulating estrogen is the **granulosa cells** of the ovaries; however, the cells of the **theca interna** of the follicle are necessary for the production of

estrogen as they secrete androgens that are aromatized to estrogen by the granulosa cells. Granulosa cells contain no desmolase, so they produce progesterone, but not androgens. Thecal cells contain desmolase and can produce androgens, but not aromatase so cannot produce estrogens.

At about the 14th day of the cycle, the distended follicle ruptures, and the ovum is extruded into the abdominal cavity. This is the process of **ovulation.** The ovum is picked up by the fimbriated ends of the **fallopian tubes** (oviducts), transported to the uterus, and, if it is fertilized, is implanted into the endometrium. If fertilization does not occur, the ovum moves out through the vagina.

The follicle that ruptures at the time of ovulation promptly fills with blood. The granulosa and theca cells of the follicle lining promptly begin to proliferate, and the clotted blood is rapidly replaced with yellowish, lipid-rich **luteal cells,** forming the **corpus luteum.** This initiates the **luteal phase** of the menstrual cycle, during which the luteal cells secrete **estrogen and progesterone.**

If pregnancy occurs, the corpus luteum persists as a source of progesterone to maintain the early pregnancy until chorionic gonadotropin is made. If pregnancy does not occur, the corpus luteum begins to degenerate about 4 days before the next menses and is eventually replaced by scar tissue, the **corpus albicans.**

No new ova are formed after birth. During fetal development, the ovaries contain over 7 million primordial follicles, many undergo atresia before birth and others are lost after birth. At the time of birth, there are 2 million ova, 50% are atretic. The million that are normal undergo the first part of the first meiotic division at about this time and enter a stage of arrest in prophase in which those that survive persist until adulthood. Atresia continues during development, and the number of ova in both of the ovaries at the time of puberty is less than 300,000. Only one of these ova per cycle (or about 500 in the course of a normal reproductive life) normally reaches maturity; the remainder degenerate.

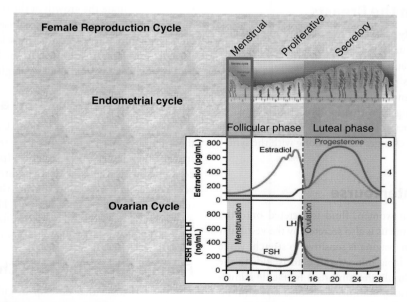

FIGURE 22–1 **Hormonal changes during normal reproductive cycle.** (Adapted with permission from Hall JE: Guyton and Hall Textbook of Medical Physiology, 13th ed. Philadelphia: Elsevier; 2016.)

Just before ovulation, the first meiotic division is completed. One of the daughter cells, the **secondary oocyte,** receives most of the cytoplasm, while the other, the **first polar body,** fragments and disappears. The secondary oocyte immediately begins the second meiotic division, but this division stops at metaphase and is completed only when a sperm penetrates the oocyte. At that time, the **second polar body** is cast off and the fertilized ovum proceeds to form a new individual.

Endometrial (Uterine) Cycle

At the end of menstruation, all but the deep layers of the endometrium have sloughed. A new endometrium then regrows under the influence of estrogens from the developing follicle. The endometrium increases rapidly in thickness from the 5th to the 14th days of the menstrual cycle. These endometrial changes are called proliferative, and this part of the menstrual cycle is sometimes called the **proliferative phase** (see Figure 22–1), or follicular phase. After ovulation, the endometrium becomes more highly vascularized and slightly edematous under the influence of estrogen and progesterone from the corpus luteum. Consequently, this phase of the cycle is called the **secretory** or **luteal phase.** At the end of the luteal phase if there is no fertilization, there is a precipitous drop in progesterone and estradiol that leads to menstruation.

Cyclical Changes in the Uterine Cervix

Although it is continuous with the body of the uterus, the cervix of the uterus is different in a number of ways. The mucosa of the cervix does not undergo cyclical desquamation, but there are regular changes in the cervical mucus. Estrogen makes the mucus thinner and more alkaline, changes that promote the survival and transport of sperm. The mucus is thinnest at the time of ovulation. Progesterone makes it thick, tenacious, and cellular.

Cyclical Changes in the Breasts

Although lactation normally does not occur until the end of pregnancy, cyclical changes take place in the breasts during the menstrual cycle. Estrogens cause proliferation of mammary ducts, whereas progesterone causes growth of lobules and alveoli. The breast swelling, tenderness, and pain experienced by many women during the 10 days preceding menstruation are probably due to distension of the ducts, hyperemia, and edema of the interstitial tissue of the breast. All these changes regress, along with the symptoms, during menstruation.

Changes During Intercourse

During sexual excitement in women, fluid is secreted onto the vaginal walls. A lubricating mucus is also secreted by the vestibular glands. The upper part of the vagina is sensitive to stretch, while tactile stimulation from the labia minora and clitoris adds to the sexual excitement. These stimuli are reinforced by tactile stimuli from the breasts, and by visual, auditory, and olfactory stimuli, which may build to the crescendo known as **orgasm.** During orgasm, autonomically mediated rhythmic contractions occur in the vaginal walls. Impulses also travel via the pudendal nerves and produce rhythmic contraction of the bulbocavernosus and ischiocavernosus muscles. The vaginal contractions may aid sperm transport but are not essential for it, since fertilization of the ovum is not dependent on female orgasm.

OVARIAN HORMONES

Chemistry, Biosynthesis, & Metabolism of Estrogens

The naturally occurring estrogens are **17β-estradiol, estrone,** and **estriol.** They are secreted primarily by the granulosa cells of the ovarian follicles, the corpus luteum, and the placenta. Their biosynthesis depends on the enzyme **aromatase** (CYP19), which converts testosterone to estradiol and androstenedione to estrone. The latter reaction also occurs in fat, liver, muscle, and the brain.

Theca interna cells have many LH receptors, and LH acts via cAMP to increase conversion of cholesterol to androstenedione. The theca interna cells supply androstenedione to the granulosa cells. The granulosa cells make estradiol when provided with androgens. Mature granulosa cells also acquire LH receptors, and LH also stimulates estradiol production.

Two percent of the circulating estradiol is free and is most bioactive, and the remainder is bound to protein: 60% to albumin and 38% to **steroid hormone–binding globulin** (SHBG) that binds testosterone.

In the liver, estradiol, estrone, and estriol are converted to glucuronide and sulfate conjugates that along with other metabolites, are mainly excreted in the urine.

Estrogen Effects on the Female Genitalia and Breasts

Estrogens facilitate the growth of the ovarian follicles, increase the motility of the fallopian tubes, increase uterine blood flow and increase the amount of uterine muscle and contractile proteins. Estrogens produce duct growth in the breasts and are responsible for breast enlargement at puberty in girls.

Estrogen Effects on FSH and LH

Estrogens decrease FSH secretion. Under some circumstances, they inhibit LH secretion (negative feedback); in other circumstances, they increase LH secretion (positive feedback). Women are sometimes given large doses of estrogens for 4–6 days to prevent conception after coitus during the fertile period (postcoital or "morning-after" contraception). However, in this instance, pregnancy is probably prevented by interference with implantation of the ovum rather than changes in gonadotropin secretion.

Female Secondary Sex Characteristics

The body changes that develop in girls at puberty—in addition to enlargement of breasts, uterus, and vagina—are due in part to estrogens, which are the "feminizing hormones," and in part simply to the absence of testicular androgens. Women have narrow shoulders and broad hips, thighs that converge, and arms that diverge. In women, the larynx retains its prepubertal proportions and the voice stays high-pitched. Women have less body hair and more scalp hair, and the pubic hair generally has a characteristic flat-topped pattern (female escutcheon). However, growth of pubic and axillary hair in both sexes is due primarily to androgens rather than estrogens.

Other Actions of Estrogens

Normal women retain salt and water just before menstruation, in part due to estrogens. However, aldosterone secretion is slightly elevated in the luteal phase, and this also contributes to the premenstrual fluid retention.

Estrogens have a significant plasma cholesterol-lowering action, and they rapidly produce vasodilation by increasing local production of nitric oxide.

Estrogen Mechanism of Action

There are two principal types of nuclear estrogen receptors: **estrogen receptor** α (ERα) and **estrogen receptor** β (ERβ). Both are members of the nuclear receptor super-family (see Chapter 2). After binding estrogen, they form homodimers and bind to DNA, altering transcription. Some tissues contain one type or the other, but overlap also occurs, with some tissues containing both ERα and ERβ. ERα is found primarily in the uterus, kidneys, liver, and heart, whereas ERβ is found primarily in the ovaries, prostate, lungs, gastrointestinal tract, hemopoietic system, and central nervous system (CNS). ERα and ERβ can also form heterodimers. There is also a **G-protein–coupled estrogen receptor** located in plasma membranes (GPER) that may be responsible for rapid, nongenomic actions in tissues.

Synthetic Estrogens—SERMs

Because natural estrogens have undesirable as well as desirable effects (eg, they preserve bone in osteoporosis but can cause uterine and breast cancer), **selective estrogen receptor modulators** (SERMs), have been developed to have selective effects. Tamoxifen is used in treatment of breast cancer since it does not stimulate the breast, and raloxifene does not stimulate the breast or uterus. Neither combats the symptoms of menopause, but both have the bone-preserving effects of estradiol.

Progesterone

Progesterone is secreted by the corpus luteum, the placenta, and (in small amounts) the follicle. It is an important intermediate in steroid biosynthesis in all tissues that secrete steroid hormones, and small amounts enter the circulation from the testes and adrenal cortex. Progesterone has a short half-life and is converted in the liver to pregnanediol, which is conjugated to glucuronic acid and excreted in the urine. The stimulating effect of LH on progesterone secretion by the corpus luteum is due to activation of adenylyl cyclase and involves a subsequent step that is dependent on protein synthesis.

Actions of Progesterone

The principal target organs of progesterone are the uterus, the breasts, and the brain. Progesterone is responsible for the luteal changes in the endometrium and the cyclical changes in the cervix and vagina described above. It has an antiestrogenic effect on the myometrial cells, decreasing their excitability, their sensitivity to oxytocin, and their spontaneous electrical activity while increasing their membrane potential. It also decreases the number of estrogen receptors in the endometrium and increases the rate of conversion of 17β-estradiol to less active estrogens.

In the breast, progesterone stimulates the development of lobules and alveoli. It induces differentiation of estrogen-prepared ductal tissue and supports the secretory function of the breast during lactation.

The feedback effects of progesterone are complex and are exerted at both the hypothalamic and pituitary levels. Large doses of progesterone inhibit LH secretion and potentiate the inhibitory effect of estrogens, preventing ovulation.

Progesterone is thermogenic and is probably responsible for the rise in basal body temperature at the time of ovulation. It stimulates respiration, and the alveolar P_{CO_2} (see Chapter 34) in women during the luteal phase of the menstrual cycle is lower than that in men. In pregnancy, the P_{CO_2} falls as progesterone secretion rises. However, the physiologic significance of this respiratory response is unknown.

Large doses of progesterone produce natriuresis, probably by blocking the action of aldosterone on the kidney. The hormone does not have a significant anabolic effect.

Progesterone Mechanism of Action

The progesterone receptor is a transcription factor that is bound to a heat shock protein in the absence of the steroid, and progesterone binding releases the heat shock protein, exposing the DNA-binding domain of the receptor. The synthetic steroid **mifepristone (RU 486)** binds to the receptor but does not release the heat shock protein, and it blocks the binding of progesterone. Because the maintenance of early pregnancy depends on the stimulatory effect of progesterone on endometrial growth and its inhibition of uterine contractility, mifepristone combined with a prostaglandin can be used to produce elective abortions.

There are two isoforms of the progesterone receptor—PR_A and PR_B—that are produced by differential processing from a single gene. PR_A is a truncated form, but it is likely that both isoforms mediate unique subsets of progesterone action.

Substances that mimic the action of progesterone are sometimes called **progestational agents, gestagens,** or **progestins.** They are used along with synthetic estrogens as oral contraceptive agents.

Relaxin

Relaxin is a polypeptide hormone that is produced in the corpus luteum, uterus, placenta, and mammary glands in women and in the prostate gland in men. During pregnancy, it relaxes the pubic symphysis and other pelvic joints and softens and dilates the uterine cervix. Thus, it facilitates delivery. It also inhibits uterine contractions and may play a role in the development of the mammary glands. In nonpregnant women, relaxin is found in the corpus luteum and the endometrium during the secretory but not the proliferative phase of the menstrual cycle. Its function in nonpregnant women is unknown. In men, it is found in semen, where it may help maintain sperm motility and aid in sperm penetration of the ovum.

CONTROL OF OVARIAN FUNCTION

Hypothalamic Components

The hypothalamus occupies a key position in the control of gonadotropin secretion. Hypothalamic control is exerted by GnRH secreted into the portal hypophysial vessels. GnRH stimulates the secretion of FSH and LH.

GnRH is normally secreted in episodic bursts, and these bursts produce the peaks of LH secretion. Frequency of GnRH bursts is increased by estrogens and decreased by progesterone and testosterone. The frequency increases late in the follicular phase of the cycle, culminating in the LH surge. During the luteal phase, the frequency decreases as a result of the action of progesterone (Figure 22–1), but when estrogen and progesterone secretion decrease at the end of the cycle, the frequency once again increases.

Feedback Effects

Changes in plasma LH, FSH, sex steroids, and inhibin during the menstrual cycle are shown in Figure 22–1. During the early part of the follicular phase, inhibin B is low and FSH is modestly elevated, fostering follicular growth. LH secretion is held in check by the negative feedback effect of the rising plasma estrogen level. At 36–48 h before ovulation, the estrogen feedback effect becomes positive, and this initiates the burst of LH secretion (LH surge) that produces ovulation. Ovulation occurs about 9 h after the LH peak. FSH secretion also peaks, despite a small rise in inhibin. During the luteal phase, the secretion of LH and FSH is low because of the elevated levels of estrogen, progesterone, and inhibin. Once regression of the corpus luteum (**luteolysis**) begins, estrogen and progesterone levels fall and the secretion of FSH and LH increases. A new crop of follicles develops, and a single dominant follicle matures as a result of the action of FSH and LH. Near midcycle, estrogen secretion from the follicle rises augmenting GnRH-mediated LH surge.

Contraception

There are numerous methods of contraception including pharmaceutical methods (discussed further), barrier methods (condoms, femidoms), and "natural" methods in which the vaginal mucus is monitored along with body temperature to determine ovulation. This method is easier now with the advent of home tests that determine ovulation. Once conception has occurred, abortion can be produced by progesterone antagonists such as mifepristone (**RU 486**). Intrauterine implantation of pieces of metal or plastic

(**intrauterine devices [IUDs]**) typically do not affect normal menstrual cycle, but may have a spermicidal effect if they contain copper appear. They also cause thickening cervical mucus so that entry of sperm into the uterus is impeded.

Large doses of estrogen prevent ovulation, likely due to depressed FSH levels and irregular bursts of LH secretion. Women treated with similar doses of estrogen plus a progestational agent do not ovulate because the secretion of both gonadotropins is suppressed. In addition, the progestin makes the cervical mucus thick and unfavorable to sperm migration, and it may also interfere with implantation. For contraception, an orally active estrogen such as ethinyl estradiol is often combined with a synthetic progestin such as norethindrone. The pills are administered for 21 days, then withdrawn for 5–7 days to permit menstrual flow, and started again. Like ethinyl estradiol, norethindrone has an ethinyl group on position 17 of the steroid nucleus, so it is resistant to hepatic metabolism and consequently is effective by mouth. In addition to being a progestin, it is partly metabolized to ethinyl estradiol, and for this reason it also has estrogenic activity. Small as well as large doses of estrogen are effective.

Implants of progestins such as levonorgestrel can be inserted under the skin and can prevent pregnancy for up to 5 years. They often produce amenorrhea, but otherwise they appear to be effective and well tolerated.

MENOPAUSE

The human ovaries become unresponsive to gonadotropins with advancing age, and their function declines, so that sexual cycles disappear (**menopause**). The ovaries no longer secrete progesterone and estrogen is formed only in small amounts by aromatization of androstenedione in peripheral tissues. As the negative feedback effect of estrogens and progesterone is reduced, secretion of FSH is increased, and plasma FSH and LH increases to high levels. The uterus and the vagina gradually become atrophic. During perimenopause FSH levels increase before an increase in LH due to a decrease in estrogen, progesterone, and inhibins, and menses become irregular. This usually occurs between the ages of 45 and 55. The average age at onset of the menopause is 52 years.

Loss of ovarian function causes symptoms such as night sweats and sensations of warmth spreading from the trunk to the face (hot flushes; also called hot flashes) that occur in 75% of menopausal women and may continue intermittently for as long as 40 years.

ABNORMALITIES OF OVARIAN FUNCTION

Menstrual Abnormalities

Some women who are infertile have **anovulatory cycles;** they fail to ovulate but have menstrual periods at fairly regular intervals. **Amenorrhea** is the absence of menstrual periods. If menstrual bleeding has never occurred, the condition is called **primary amenorrhea.** Some women with primary amenorrhea have small breasts and other signs of failure to mature sexually.

Cessation of cycles in a woman with previously normal periods is called **secondary amenorrhea.** The most common cause of secondary amenorrhea is pregnancy. Other causes of amenorrhea include emotional stimuli and changes in the environment, extreme exercise, hypothalamic diseases, pituitary disorders, primary ovarian disorders, and various systemic diseases.

The terms **hypomenorrhea** and **menorrhagia** refer to scanty and abnormally profuse flow, respectively, during regular periods. **Metrorrhagia** is bleeding from the uterus between periods, and **oligomenorrhea** is reduced frequency of periods. **Dysmenorrhea** is painful menstruation. The severe menstrual cramps that are common in young women quite often disappear after the first pregnancy. Most of the symptoms of dysmenorrhea are due to accumulation of prostaglandins in the uterus, and symptomatic relief has been obtained by treatment with inhibitors of prostaglandin synthesis.

Some women develop symptoms such as irritability, bloating, edema, decreased ability to concentrate, depression, headache, and constipation during the last 7–10 days of their menstrual cycles. These symptoms of the **premenstrual syndrome (PMS)** have been attributed to salt and water retention.

PREGNANCY

Fertilization & Implantation

In humans, **fertilization** of the ovum by the sperm (see Chapter 23) usually occurs in the ampulla of the fallopian tube. Fertilization involves (1) chemoattraction of the sperm to the ovum by substances produced by the ovum; (2) adherence to the **zona pellucida,** the membranous structure surrounding the ovum; (3) penetration of the zona pellucida and the acrosome reaction; and (4) adherence of the sperm head to the cell membrane of the ovum, with breakdown of the area of fusion and release of the sperm nucleus into the cytoplasm of the ovum. Millions of sperm are deposited in the vagina during intercourse. Eventually, 50–100 sperm reach the ovum, and many of them contact the **zona pellucida.** Sperm bind to a receptor in the zona, and this is followed by the **acrosomal reaction,** the breakdown of the **acrosome,** the lysosome-like organelle on the head of the sperm that releases various enzymes required for the penetration of the sperm through the zona pellucida. When one sperm reaches the membrane of the ovum, fusion to the ovum membrane is mediated by **fertilin.** The fusion sets off an increase in intracellular calcium that causes a reduction in the membrane potential of the ovum that prevents polyspermy, the fertilization of the ovum by more than one sperm. This transient potential change is followed by a "hardening" in the zona pellucida that provides protection against polyspermy on a more long-term basis.

The developing embryo, now called a **blastocyst,** moves down the tube into the uterus, a journey taking about 3 days, during which the blastocyst reaches the 8- or 16-cell stage. Once in contact with the endometrium, the blastocyst becomes surrounded by an outer layer of **syncytiotrophoblast,** a multi-nucleate mass with no discernible cell boundaries, and an inner layer of **cytotrophoblasts** made up of individual cells. The syncytiotrophoblast erodes the endometrium, and the blastocyst burrows into it **(implantation).** The implantation site is usually on the dorsal wall of the uterus. The cytotrophoblasts then burrow into the spiral arteries of the uterus developing the blood perfusion for the chorionic villus of the placenta. Lack of adequate cytotrophoblast invasion and thus low blood supply to the developing fetus is thought to be the major cause of **preeclampsia,** that is new onset hypertension, edema and proteinuria, that is responsible for the highest incidence of mortality of fetus and mother.

Endocrine Changes

The corpus luteum in the ovary at the time of fertilization fails to regress and instead enlarges in response to stimulation by gonadotropic hormones secreted by the placenta. The placental gonadotropin is called **human chorionic gonadotropin (hCG),** is produced by the syncytiotrophoblast, and its presence in the urine is used as the basis of pregnancy tests since it can be detected as early as 14 days after fertilization. hCG, a glycoprotein-containing galactose and hexosamine, is made up of α and β subunits. hCG-α is identical to the α subunit of LH, FSH, and TSH, and works through the LH receptor. hCG is primarily luteinizing and luteotropic, and has little FSH activity.

The enlarged **corpus luteum of pregnancy** secretes estrogens, progesterone, and relaxin. Progesterone and relaxin help maintain pregnancy by inhibiting myometrial contractions. After the sixth week of pregnancy the placenta produces sufficient estrogen and progesterone from maternal and fetal precursors to take over the function of the corpus luteum. The function of the corpus luteum begins to decline after 8 weeks of pregnancy, but it persists throughout pregnancy. hCG secretion decreases after an initial marked rise, but estrogen and progesterone secretion increases until just before parturition.

Human Chorionic Somatomammotropin

The syncytiotrophoblast also secretes large amounts of **human chorionic somatomammotropin (hCS),** a protein hormone that is lactogenic and has a small amount of growth-stimulating activity. Large quantities of hCS are found in maternal blood, but very little reaches the fetus. hCS functions as a "maternal growth hormone of pregnancy" to bring about the nitrogen, potassium, and calcium retention, lipolysis, and decreased glucose utilization seen in pregnancy. These latter two actions divert glucose to the fetus. The amount of hCS secreted is proportional to the size of the placenta, which normally weighs about one-sixth as much as the fetus. Low hCS levels are a sign of placental insufficiency.

Production of Steroids by the Fetoplacental Unit

The fetus and the placenta interact in the formation of steroid hormones (**Figure 22–2**). The placenta synthesizes pregnenolone and progesterone from cholesterol, but cannot metabolize progesterone to produce estrogens. The fetus cannot make progesterone, so progesterone from the placenta enters the fetal circulation,

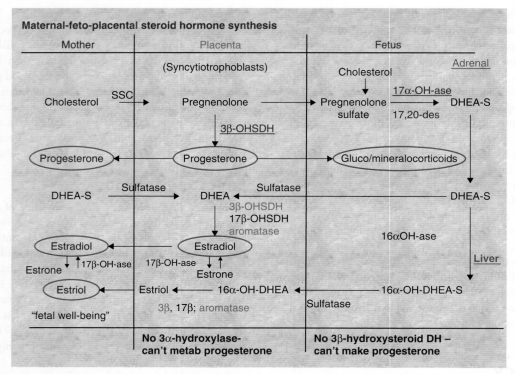

FIGURE 22–2 Differences in synthesis of hormones produced during pregnancy by the fetus, the placenta and the mother.

and provides the substrate for the formation of cortisol and corticosterone in the fetal adrenal glands. Pregnenolone enters the fetus from the placenta and is the substrate for the formation of dehydroepiandrosterone sulfate (DHEAS) and 16-hydroxydehydroepiandrosterone sulfate (16-OHDHEAS) in the fetal adrenal. DHEAS and 16-OHDHEAS are transported back to the placenta, where DHEAS forms estradiol and 16-OHDHEAS forms estriol. The principal estrogen formed is estriol, and since fetal 16-OHDHEAS is the principal substrate for the estrogens, the urinary estriol excretion of the mother can be monitored as an index of fetal well-being.

Parturition

The duration of pregnancy averages 270 days from fertilization (284 days from the first day of the menstrual period preceding conception). The mechanism(s) responsible for the onset of parturition are unknown.

At the time of delivery, the cervix softens and dilates, and the body of the uterus contracts and expels the fetus. Once labor is started, the uterine contractions dilate the cervix, and this dilation in turn sets up signals in afferent nerves that increase oxytocin secretion. Plasma oxytocin level rises and more oxytocin becomes available to act on the uterus, thus setting up a positive feedback loop that aids in delivery and expulsion of the placenta. Oxytocin increases uterine contractions in two ways: (1) It acts directly on uterine smooth muscle cells to make them contract and (2) it stimulates the formation of prostaglandins in the decidua. The prostaglandins enhance the oxytocin-induced contractions.

LACTATION

Estrogens are primarily responsible for proliferation of the mammary ducts and progesterone for the development of the lobules. The breasts enlarge during pregnancy in response to high circulating levels of estrogens, progesterone, prolactin, and possibly hCG. During pregnancy, prolactin levels increase steadily until term, producing full lobuloalveolar development and milk production. Ejection of milk from the alveoli into the ducts is caused by oxytocin-mediated contraction of the myoepithelial cells lining the duct walls. Suckling not only evokes reflex oxytocin release and milk ejection, it also maintains and augments the secretion of milk because of the stimulation of prolactin secretion it produces (**Figure 22–3**).

CHAPTER SUMMARY

■ Differences between males and females depend primarily on a single chromosome (the Y chromosome) and a single pair of endocrine structures (the gonads); testes in the male and ovaries in the female.

■ The gonads have a dual function: the production of germ cells (gametogenesis) and the secretion of sex hormones. The testes secrete large amounts of androgens, principally testosterone, but they also secrete small amounts of estrogens. The ovaries secrete large amounts of estrogens and small amounts of androgens.

■ The reproductive system of women has regular cyclical changes that can be thought of as periodic preparations for fertilization

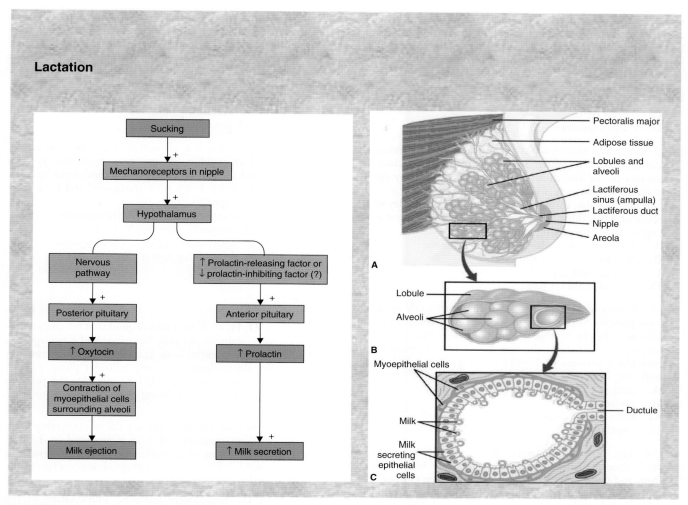

FIGURE 22–3 **Mechanisms for lactation and milk secretion.** (Adapted with permission from Hall JE: Guyton and Hall Textbook of Medical Physiology, 13th ed. Philadelphia: Elsevier; 2016.)

and pregnancy. In humans and other primates, the cycle is a **menstrual** cycle, and features the periodic vaginal bleeding that occurs with the shedding of the uterine mucosa **(menstruation).**

■ Ovaries also secrete progesterone, a steroid that has special functions in preparing the uterus for pregnancy. During pregnancy, the ovaries secrete relaxin, which facilitates the delivery of the fetus. In both sexes, the gonads secrete other polypeptides, including inhibin B, a polypeptide that inhibits FSH secretion.

■ In women, a period called perimenopause precedes menopause, and can last up to 10 years; during this time, the menstrual cycles become irregular and the level of inhibins decrease.

■ Once in menopause, the ovaries no longer secrete progesterone and 17β-estradiol and estrogen is formed only in small amounts by aromatization of androstenedione in peripheral tissues.

■ The naturally occurring estrogens are **17β-estradiol, estrone, and estriol.** They are secreted primarily by the granulosa cells of the ovarian follicles, the corpus luteum, and the placenta. Their biosynthesis depends on the enzyme **aromatase** (CYP19), which converts testosterone to estradiol and androstenedione to estrone. The latter reaction also occurs in fat, liver, muscle, and the brain.

MULTIPLE-CHOICE QUESTIONS

For all questions, select the single best answer unless otherwise directed.

1. A 29-year-old woman takes a home pregnancy test 8 weeks after her last menstrual period. The test is positive that she is pregnant. What hormone in the urine is the test measuring?
   A. Estradiol
   B. Progesterone
   C. Luteinizing hormone
   D. Human chorionic gonadotropin

2. A 28-year-old woman comes to see her physician with symptoms of weight gain and nausea. The physician diagnoses her as being at 24 weeks gestation. Her circulating estradiol is elevated due to its production by the placenta. Estradiol cannot be synthesized by the fetal adrenal gland due to its inability to produce what steroid hormone? The fetus is not capable of synthesizing what steroid hormone?
   A. Progesterone
   B. Pregnenolone
   C. DHEAS
   D. Cholesterol

3. A 35-year-old woman takes a home pregnancy test 4 weeks after her last menstrual period and the test is positive. At this time immediately following fertilization and early after implantation into the endometrium, nutrition of the blastocyst is due to what structure?
   A. Placenta
   B. Decidua
   C. Thecal cells
   D. Corpus luteum

4. A 30-year-old woman wants to go back to work 3 weeks after delivery of her daughter. She is able to do this because her mother-in-law lives close by and take care of the baby during the day. The women is planning to nurse the baby at night but not planning to pump her breasts during the day while she is at work. What is the consequence of intermittent nursing of the neonate by the mother?
   A. An increase in prolactin releasing hormone
   B. An increase in oxytocin
   C. Lack of birth control
   D. Lack of prolactin surge

5. A 23-year-old woman who is in the 24th week of gestation presents to the emergency department complaining of dizziness, headache, and swelling of hands and feet. Upon physical examination, she was found to have proteinuria and blood pressure of 168/98 mm Hg. This lady is likely suffering from
   A. anxiety.
   B. preterm labor.
   C. spontaneous abortion or miscarriage.
   D. preeclampsia.

6. An obese 30-year-old woman presents to her gynecologist with abnormal menstrual periods, increases in dark facial hair, and upon examination has elevated urine glucose. The physician measures her plasma testosterone level and finds it increased about fivefold compared to normal. The physician makes the diagnosis of polycystic ovary syndrome. In order to control the levels of testosterone and provide some relief to the women, the physician prescribes:
   A. estrogen.
   B. GnRH inhibitors.
   C. progesterone.
   D. growth hormone.

7. A 25-year-woman who reports normal menstrual cycle, would have what pattern of circulating sex steroids on day 19 (day 1 is first day of menstrual period)?

	estradiol	progesterone	FSH	LH	inhibin
A.	↑	↓	↓	↓	↑
B.	↑	↑	↓	↓	↑
C.	↓	↑	↓	↓	↑
D.	↑	↑	↑	↓	↓

8. In contrast to the young woman above, a 60-year-old woman would be expected to have what levels of circulating hormones?

	estradiol	progesterone	FSH	LH	inhibin
A.	↓	↓	↓	↓	↑
B.	↓	↑	↓	↓	↑
C.	↓	↓	↑	↑	↓
D.	↓	↑	↑	⇔	↓

9. A 32-year-old woman enters your OB clinic after taking an over-the-counter pregnancy test that was positive. Your physical examination suggests that she is pregnant. She has type 1 diabetes. In order to verify your physical findings, you order a blood test for pregnancy that measures which hormone?
   A. Gonadotropin releasing hormone
   B. Luteinizing hormone
   C. Follicular stimulating hormone
   D. Chorionic gonadotropin

10. A baby is born that is a phenotypic male, but has an XX genotype. Transposition of one gene from one paternal chromosome has occurred during sperm production to create this situation. What is the gene transposed and from what chromosomal origin?
    A. TSPY (testis specific protein); X chromosome
    B. TSPY (testis specific protein); Y chromosome
    C. SRY (sex determining region); X chromosome
    D. SRY (sex determining region); Y chromosome

ANSWERS

1. Answer is **D**. HCG is the nutrient produced by syncytiotrophoblasts to maintain the early blastocyst and downregulates GnRH release. Estradiol levels are beginning to increase but would also do so during the early follicular phase, so can't be used as a pregnancy test. LH is only elevated prior to ovulation and is decreased during pregnancy due to negative feedback on GnRH.

2. Answer is **A**. Fetal adrenal is not capable of converting pregnenolone to progesterone. DHEAS is produced in the fetal adrenal by conversion of pregnenolone sulfate. Cholesterol is not a steroid but is converted to pregnenolone sulfate in the fetal adrenal gland.

3. Answer is **D**. Immediately following implantation of the blastocyst, there is no placenta developed yet. Similarly, there is no decidua developed yet. Thecal cells are on the outside of the follicle and remain there following ovulation. The corpus luteum is maintained at first by progesterone and then later by human chorionic gonadotropin.

4. Answer is **D**. Failure to nurse the baby causes a lack of prolactin surge, and loss of milk production in the lobules of the breast, and thus a *reduction* in prolactin releasing hormone, not an increase. Failure to nurse also causes a *reduction* in oxytocin and thus failure of the milk to be secreted from the breast. Breast feeding is not a method of preventing subsequent pregnancy.

5. Answer is **D**. Anxiety alone won't cause proteinuria or swelling of extremities (peripheral edema). Similarly preterm labor or spontaneous abortion rarely is accompanied with such a high blood pressure especially diastolic.

6. Answer is **B**. None of the others, estrogen, progesterone or growth hormone, can be given at high enough doses to downregulate GnRH to prevent synthesis of LH and FSH to reduce androgen levels without causing unwanted side effects. GnRH inhibitors will down regulate LH, FSH, prevent androgen synthesis, but will also prevent pregnancy, although with fivefold increase in androgens, she is not cycling normally.

7. Answer is **B**. Day 19 is in the luteal phase when the corpus luteum is involuting. It is characterized by elevated estradiol

and progesterone. As such FSH and LH are low. Inhibin attenuates synthesis of FSH and its levels would be high.

8. **Answer is C.** Menopause occurs at approximately 51 years of age. Thus estradiol and progesterone levels are low. There is no negative feedback on GnRH, so LH and FSH are high. Because FSH is high, inhibin is low.

9. **Answer is D.** GnRH is not measured since it may be variable or even low with a new pregnancy. LH is also low with a new pregnancy since progesterone and estradiol levels are elevated and thus have a negative feedback on GnRH so reduced LH. Same with FSH.

10. **Answer is D.** A phenotypic male will develop only in the presence of an SRY gene, so the answer can't be TSPY. Therefore, if SRY from the father's chromosome Y is transposed to the father's X chromosome, the offspring could have an XX genotype but a male phenotype.

Function of the Male Reproductive System

CHAPTER

23

OBJECTIVES

After studying this chapter, you should be able to:

- Name the key hormones secreted by Leydig cells and Sertoli cells of the testes.
- Outline the steps involved in spermatogenesis.
- Outline the mechanisms that produce erection and ejaculation.
- Know the general structure of testosterone, and describe its biosynthesis, transport, metabolism, and actions.
- Describe the processes involved in regulation of testosterone secretion.

STRUCTURE

The testes are made up of loops of convoluted **seminiferous tubules,** in the walls of which the spermatozoa are formed from the primitive germ cells **(spermatogenesis).** Both ends of each loop drain into a network of ducts in the head of the **epididymis.** From there, spermatozoa pass through the tail of the epididymis into the **vas deferens.** They enter through the **ejaculatory ducts** into the urethra in the body of the **prostate** at the time of ejaculation. Between the tubules in the testes are nests of cells containing lipid granules, the **interstitial cells of Leydig** (Leydig cells), which secrete testosterone into the bloodstream. The walls of the seminiferous tubules are lined by primitive germ cells and **Sertoli cells,** large, complex glycogen-containing cells that stretch from the basal lamina of the tubule to the lumen. The fluid in the lumen of the seminiferous tubules contains very little protein and glucose but is rich in androgens, estrogens, K^+, inositol, and glutamic and aspartic acids.

Spermatogenesis

Spermatogonia, the primitive germ cells next to the basal lamina of the seminiferous tubules, mature into **primary spermatocytes** beginning during adolescence **(Figure 23–1).** The primary spermatocytes undergo meiotic division, reducing the number of chromosomes. In this two-stage process, they divide into **secondary spermatocytes** and then into **spermatids,** which contain the haploid number of 23 chromosomes. The spermatids mature into **spermatozoa (sperm).** As a single spermatogonium divides and matures, its descendants remain tied together by cytoplasmic bridges until the late spermatid stage. The formation of a mature sperm from a primitive germ cell by spermatogenesis takes approximately 74 days.

Each sperm is made up of a head of chromosomal material and a flagellum tail for motility **(Figure 23–2).** Covering the head like a cap is the **acrosome,** a lysosome-like organelle rich in enzymes involved in sperm penetration of the ovum. The motile tail of the sperm is wrapped in its proximal portion by a sheath holding numerous mitochondria.

Spermatids mature into spermatozoa in the cytoplasm of Sertoli cells. Mature spermatozoa are released from the Sertoli cells and become free in the lumen of the tubules. The Sertoli cells secrete **androgen-binding protein (ABP), inhibin,** and **MIS.** They do not synthesize androgens, but they contain **aromatase (CYP19),** the enzyme responsible for conversion of androgens to estrogens, and they can produce estrogens. ABP probably functions to maintain a high, stable supply of androgen in the tubular fluid. Inhibin inhibits follicle-stimulating hormone (FSH) secretion. FSH and androgens maintain the gametogenic function of the testis.

Spermatozoa continue their maturation and acquire motility during their passage through the epididymis. Ejaculation of the spermatozoon involves contractions of the vas deferens. Once ejaculated into the female, the spermatozoa move up the uterus to the isthmus of the fallopian tubes, where they slow down and undergo capacitation in preparation for fertilization.

Spermatogenesis requires a temperature considerably lower than that of the interior of the body. The testes are normally

292

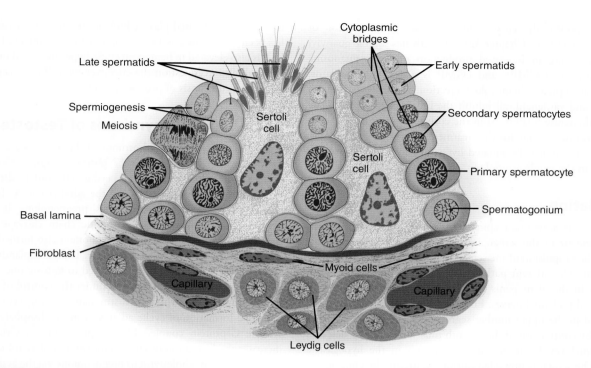

FIGURE 23–1 **Seminiferous epithelium.** Note that maturing germ cells remain connected by cytoplasmic bridges through the early spermatid stage and that these cells are closely invested by Sertoli cell cytoplasm as they move from the basal lamina to the lumen. (Reproduced with permission from Junqueira LC, Carneiro J: Basic Histology: Text & Atlas, 10th ed. New York, NY: McGraw-Hill; 2003.)

maintained at a temperature of about 32°C, kept cool by air circulating around the scrotum and likely by heat exchange in a countercurrent manner between the spermatic arteries and veins.

Semen

The fluid that is ejaculated at the time of orgasm, the **semen,** contains sperm and the secretions of the seminal vesicles, prostate, Cowper glands, and urethral glands. An average volume per ejaculate is 2.5–3.5 mL after several days of abstinence from sexual activity. Each milliliter of semen contains about 100 million sperm. Reduction in sperm production is associated with infertility: 50% of men with counts of 20–40 million/mL and essentially all of those with counts under 20 million/mL are sterile. The presence of many morphologically abnormal or immotile spermatozoa also correlates with infertility. Human sperm move at a speed of about 3 mm/min through the female genital tract. Sperm reach the uterine tubes

30–60 min after copulation. Contractions of the female organs may facilitate the transport of the sperm to the uterine tubes.

Erection

Erection is initiated by dilation of the arterioles of the penis. As the erectile tissue of the penis fills with blood, the veins are compressed, blocking outflow and adding to the turgor of the organ. The integrating centers in the lumbar segments of the spinal cord are activated by impulses in afferents from the genitalia and descending tracts that mediate erection in response to erotic psychological stimuli. The efferent parasympathetic fibers are in the pelvic splanchnic nerves **(nervi erigentes).** The fibers presumably release acetylcholine and the vasodilator vasoactive intestinal polypeptide (VIP) as cotransmitters (see Chapter 7).

Nonadrenergic noncholinergic fibers are also present in the nervi erigentes, and these contain large amounts of **nitric oxide**

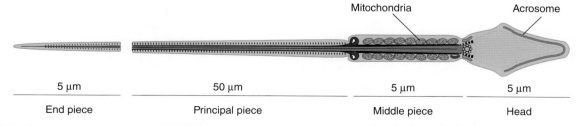

FIGURE 23–2 **Human spermatozoon, profile view.** Note the acrosome, an organelle that covers half the sperm head inside the plasma membrane of the sperm. (Reproduced with permission from Junqueira LC, Carneiro J: Basic Histology: Text & Atlas, 11th ed. New York, NY: McGraw-Hill; 2005.)

synthase (NOS), the enzyme that catalyzes the formation of nitric oxide (NO; see Chapter 32). NO activates soluble guanylyl cyclase, resulting in increased production of cyclic guanosine monophosphate (cGMP), and cGMP is a potent vasodilator, thus playing a predominant role in erection. The drugs, sildenafil, tadalafil, and vardenafil, all inhibit the breakdown of cGMP by phosphodiesterase 5 (PDE-5) in the corpora cavernosa, and have gained worldwide fame for the treatment of erectile dysfunction. Normally, erection is terminated by sympathetic vasoconstrictor impulses to the penile arterioles.

Ejaculation

Ejaculation is a two-part spinal reflex that involves **emission,** the movement of the semen into the urethra; and **ejaculation** proper, the propulsion of the semen out of the urethra at the time of orgasm. The afferent pathways are mostly fibers from touch receptors in the glans penis that reach the spinal cord through the internal pudendal nerves. Emission is a sympathetic response, integrated in the upper lumbar segments of the spinal cord and affected by contraction of the smooth muscle of the vasa deferens and seminal vesicles in response to stimuli in the hypogastric nerves. The semen is propelled out of the urethra by contraction of the bulbocavernosus muscle, a skeletal muscle. The spinal reflex centers for this part of the reflex are in the upper sacral and lowest lumbar segments of the spinal cord, and the motor pathways traverse the first to third sacral roots and the internal pudendal nerves.

Prostate-Specific Antigen

The prostate produces and secretes into the semen and the bloodstream a 30-kDa serine protease generally called **prostate-specific antigen (PSA).** The gene for PSA has two androgen response elements. PSA hydrolyzes the sperm motility inhibitor semenogelin

in semen. An elevated plasma PSA occurs in prostate cancer and has been widely used as a screening test for this disease. However, PSA is also elevated in benign prostatic hyperplasia and prostatitis, thus calling into question the effectiveness of PSA screening as a sole tool in diagnosis of prostate cancer.

Chemistry & Biosynthesis of Testosterone

Testosterone, the principal hormone of the testes, is a C_{19} steroid with a hydroxyl group in the 17 position (**Figure 23–3**). It is synthesized from cholesterol in Leydig cells and is also formed from androstenedione secreted by the adrenal cortex. In Leydig cells, 17α-hydroxylase hydroxylates pregnenolone in the 17 position that is then subjected to side chain cleavage to form dehydroepiandrosterone. Androstenedione is also formed via progesterone and 17-hydroxyprogesterone. Dehydroepiandrosterone and androstenedione are then converted to testosterone.

The secretion of testosterone is under the control of LH, and the mechanism by which LH stimulates Leydig cells involves increased formation of cyclic adenosine monophosphate (cAMP) via the G-protein–coupled LH receptor and G_s. Cyclic AMP increases the formation of cholesterol from cholesterol esters and the conversion of cholesterol to pregnenolone via the activation of protein kinase A.

Ninety-eight percent of the testosterone in plasma is bound to protein: 65% is bound to a β-globulin called **sex hormone binding globulin (SHBG),** and 33% to albumin.

Secondary Sex Characteristics

The widespread changes in hair distribution, body configuration, and genital size that develop in boys at puberty—the male **secondary sex characteristics**. The prostate and seminal vesicles enlarge, and the seminal vesicles begin to secrete fructose. This sugar appears to function as the main nutritional supply for the

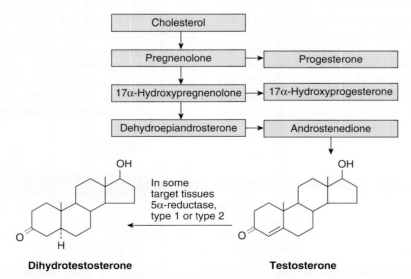

FIGURE 23–3 Biosynthesis of testosterone. Although the main secretory product of the Leydig cells is testosterone, some of the precursors also enter the circulation.

spermatozoa. The effects of androgens and estrogens on sexual behavior are considered in detail in Chapter 15. Although body hair is increased by androgens, scalp hair is decreased.

Anabolic Effects

Androgens increase the synthesis and decrease the breakdown of protein, leading to an increase in the rate of growth. Secondary to their anabolic effects, androgens cause moderate Na^+, K^+, H_2O, Ca^{2+}, SO_4^-, and PO_4^- retention; and they also increase the size of the kidneys. Doses of exogenous testosterone that exert significant anabolic effects are also masculinizing and increase libido, which limits the usefulness of the hormone as an anabolic agent in patients with wasting diseases.

Mechanism of Action

Like other steroids, testosterone binds to an intracellular receptor, and the receptor/steroid complex then binds to DNA in the nucleus, facilitating transcription of various genes. In addition, testosterone is converted to **DHT** by 5α-reductase in some target cells, and DHT binds to the same intracellular receptor as testosterone. DHT also circulates, with a plasma level that is about 10% of the testosterone level. Testosterone–receptor complexes are less stable than DHT–receptor complexes in target cells, and they conform less well to the DNA-binding state. Thus, DHT formation is a way of amplifying the action of testosterone in target tissues.

Testosterone–receptor complexes are responsible for the maturation of Wolffian duct structures and consequently for the formation of male internal genitalia during development, but DHT–receptor complexes are needed to form male external genitalia. DHT–receptor complexes are also primarily responsible for enlargement of the prostate and the penis at the time of puberty, as well as for the facial hair, the acne, and the temporal recession of the hairline. On the other hand, the increase in muscle mass and the development of male sex drive and libido depend primarily on testosterone rather than DHT.

CONTROL OF TESTICULAR FUNCTION

FSH is tropic for Sertoli cells, and FSH and androgens maintain the gametogenic function of the testes. FSH also stimulates the secretion of ABP and inhibin to inhibit FSH secretion. LH is tropic for Leydig cells and stimulates the secretion of testosterone, which in turn feeds back to inhibit LH secretion.

Inhibins

Testosterone reduces plasma LH but has no effect on plasma FSH. Plasma FSH is elevated in patients who have atrophy of the seminiferous tubules but normal levels of testosterone and LH secretion. Inhibin inhibits FSH secretion by a direct action on the pituitary, although it appears that it is inhibin B that is the FSH-regulating inhibin in adult men and women. Inhibins are produced by Sertoli cells in males and granulosa cells in females.

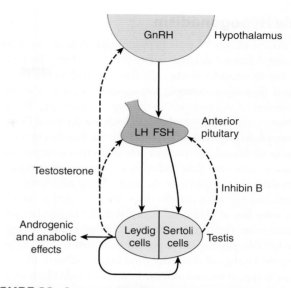

FIGURE 23–4 **The hypothalamus, pituitary and testes interact via signaling molecules.** Postulated signaling pathways between the hypothalamus, anterior pituitary and testis are shown. Solid arrows indicate excitatory effects, whereas dashed arrows indicate inhibitory effects.

Steroid Feedback

A current "working hypothesis" of the way the functions of the testes are regulated by steroids is shown in **Figure 23–4**. Testosterone inhibits LH secretion by acting directly on the anterior pituitary and by inhibiting the secretion of gonadotropin-releasing hormone (GnRH) from the hypothalamus. Inhibin acts directly on the anterior pituitary to inhibit FSH secretion. In response to LH, some of the testosterone secreted from the Leydig cells bathes the seminiferous epithelium and provides the high local concentration of androgen to the Sertoli cells that is necessary for normal spermatogenesis.

ABNORMALITIES OF TESTICULAR FUNCTION

Cryptorchidism

The testes develop in the abdominal cavity and normally migrate to the scrotum during fetal development. **Testicular descent** to the inguinal region depends on MIS, and descent from the inguinal region to the scrotum depends on other factors. Descent is incomplete on one or, less commonly, both sides in 10% of newborn males, with the testes remaining in the abdominal cavity or inguinal canal. The incidence of boys with undescended testes (**cryptorchidism**) falls to 2% at age 1 year and 0.3% after puberty. However, early treatment with either gonadotropic hormone treatment or by surgical correction is recommended since the incidence of malignant tumors is higher in undescended than in scrotal testes and because after puberty the higher temperature in the abdomen eventually causes irreversible damage to the spermatogenic epithelium.

Male Hypogonadism

The clinical picture of male hypogonadism depends on whether testicular deficiency develops before or after puberty. In adults, if it is due to testicular disease, circulating gonadotropin levels are elevated (**hypergonadotropic hypogonadism**); if it is secondary to disorders of the pituitary or the hypothalamus (eg, Kallmann syndrome), circulating gonadotropin levels are depressed (**hypogonadotropic hypogonadism**). If the endocrine function of the testes is lost in adulthood, the secondary sex characteristics regress slowly because it takes very little androgen to maintain them once they are established. The growth of the larynx during adolescence is permanent, and the voice remains deep. Men castrated in adulthood suffer some loss of libido, although the ability to copulate persists for some time. They occasionally have hot flushes and are generally more irritable, passive, and depressed than men with intact testes. When the Leydig cell deficiency dates from childhood, the clinical picture is that of **eunuchoidism.** Eunuchoid individuals over the age of 20 are characteristically tall, although not as tall as hyperpituitary giants. They have narrow shoulders and small muscles, a body configuration resembling that of the adult female. The genitalia are small and the voice high pitched. Pubic hair and axillary hair are present because of adrenocortical androgen secretion. However, the hair is sparse, and the pubic hair has the female "triangle with the base up" distribution rather than the "triangle with the base down" pattern (male escutcheon) seen in normal males.

CHAPTER SUMMARY

- The gonads have a dual function: the production of germ cells (gametogenesis) and the secretion of sex hormones. The testes secrete large amounts of androgens, principally testosterone, but they also secrete small amounts of estrogens.
- Spermatogonia develop into mature spermatozoa in the seminiferous tubules via a process called spermatogenesis. This is a multistep process that includes maturation of spermatogonia into primary spermatocytes, which undergo meiotic division, resulting in haploid secondary spermatocytes. Several further divisions result in spermatids. Each cell division from a spermatogonium to a spermatid is incomplete, with cells remaining connected via cytoplasmic bridges. Spermatids eventually mature into motile spermatozoa to complete spermatogenesis; this last part of maturation is called spermiogenesis.
- Testosterone is the principal hormone of the testis. It is synthesized from cholesterol in Leydig cells. The secretion of testosterone from Leydig cells is under control of luteinizing hormone at a rate of 4–9 mg/day in adult males. Most testosterone is bound to albumin or to gonadal steroid–binding globulin in the plasma. Testosterone plays an important role in the development and maintenance of male secondary sex characteristics, as well as other defined functions.

MULTIPLE-CHOICE QUESTIONS

For all questions, select the single best answer unless otherwise directed.

1. Mr Smith visits his primary care physician complaining of being tired. His BMI is 35 and his blood pressure is 145/90.

The physician decides to measure his serum testosterone levels since testosterone levels are reduced with chronic diseases and obesity. Testosterone is produced mainly by the
   A. Leydig cells.
   B. Sertoli cells.
   C. seminiferous tubules.
   D. epididymis.
   E. vas deferens.

2. A 46-year-old obese man visits his primary care provider for his yearly checkup. While there, the physician asks about his sex life and mentions that he is having trouble getting and maintaining an erection. What drug will the physician prescribe for the man?
   A. Nitric synthase inhibitors
   B. Tamoxifen
   C. Phosphodiesterase-5 inhibitors
   D. 5-alpha-reductase inhibitors

3. A 45-year-old man is prescribed 5-alpha-reductase inhibitor, finasteride, for benign prostatic hypertrophy. His physician mentions potential side effects of the drug that include
   A. gynecomastia.
   B. increases in prostatic serum antigen (PSA).
   C. eunuchism.
   D. impotence.

4. A 60-year-old man comes to see his physician for his yearly checkup. His physician measures his serum prostatic antigen levels and finds that they are elevated. What is the potential diagnosis for this man?
   A. Breast cancer
   B. Skin cancer
   C. Benign prostatic hypertrophy
   D. Prostate cancer

5. Although the man has been having some difficulty with urinating, the physician decides to wait 6 months to retest and provide the man with an antibiotic. The physician did this because
   A. the man is too old for surgery.
   B. the man is taking finasteride, the reductase inhibitor.
   C. the man has just returned from vacation to a ranch where he rode horses.
   D. the man has type 2 diabetes.

6. A 25-year-old man is diagnosed with atrophy of the seminiferous tubules. When is circulating reproductive hormones are measured what was the result?

	FSH	LH	testosterone	inhibin
A.	↑	↑	↓	↓
B.	WNL	↑	↓	WNL
C.	↑	WNL	WNL	↓
D.	↓	↓	↓	↑

7. A 45-year-old man who has five children has a vasectomy. As a result the sperm he produces will no longer be present in which part of his reproductive system?
   A. Epididymis
   B. Seminiferous tubules
   C. Ejaculatory ducts
   D. Vas deferens

8. A weight lifter seeks help from his physician after he has been disqualified for chronic anabolic steroid use. The physician

decides to have lab work done in order to evaluate his current reproductive hormone levels. What abnormalities of GnRH, FSH, and LH would you expect to find?
   A. Decreased FSH, decreased LH, decreased GnRH
   B. Decreased FSH, decreased LH, increased GnRH
   C. Increased FSH, decreased LH, increased GnRH
   D. Increased FSH, increased LH, decreased GnRH
   E. WNL FSH, WNL LH, WNL GnRH

9. A 40-year-old man develops a benign pituitary tumor and undergoes a complete hypophysectomy. The surgeon counsels him that he will need hormone replacement therapy. Without hormone replacement therapy, which hormone would be found in the patient's blood?
   A. Increased GnRH
   B. Increased androgen binding protein
   C. Increased inhibin
   D. Increased testosterone

10. An XY male is born with female external genitalia, and is diagnosed with 5α-reductase deficiency. If there is no intervention, what development is likely to take place as this individual matures?
   A. Development of male pattern facial hair
   B. Deepening of the voice
   C. Development of a menstrual cycle
   D. Development of a male sex drive

ANSWERS

1. Answer is **A.** Testosterone is produced in Leydig cells. Sertoli cells are required for spermatogenesis and production of ABP and aromatization of estrogens. Seminiferous tubules are where spermatozoa are produced. The epididymis is where sperm is matured. The vas deferens is where sperm are stored and connects the epididymis with ejaculatory duct and the urethra for ejaculation.

2. Answer is **C.** NO causes erection thus would not give NOS inhibitors. Tamoxifen is a SERM that is given for breast cancer. 5-Alpha-reductase inhibitors prevent conversion of testosterone to 5-alpha-dihydrotestosterone.

3. Answer is **A.** Gynecomastia is caused by dihydrotestosterone (DHT). Thus blocking the synthesis of DHT will cause more aromatase activity and increases in estradiol. Estradiol causes increase in breast development, or gynecomastia, in men. DHT or its inhibition has no effect on PSA. Eunuchism is lack of production of all androgens. Reductions in DHT do not cause impotence because there is still testosterone to increase libido and performance.

4. Answer is **D.** PSA is not a biomarker for either breast cancer or skin cancer. PSA is also a marker for benign prostatic hypertrophy, and would not be elevated unless there was inflammation accompanying the BPH.

5. Answer is **C.** Inflammation, such as with horse back riding, can increase PSA without there being a tumor. Neither type 2 diabetes nor finasteride should affect PSA.

6. Answer is **C.** Seminiferous tubules contain Sertoli cells. Therefore, the Leydig cells are not affected by the atrophy of the tubules. So testosterone levels produced by Leydig cells are normal, LH is normal. FSH is increased and so inhibin would be decreased.

7. Answer is **C.** The ejaculatory ducts are distal to the vas deferens and thus will no longer carry sperm. The other structures will not be affected.

8. Answer is **A.** Anabolic steroids will cause a downregulation of GnRH, causing a reduction in synthesis of both LH and FSH.

9. Answer is **A.** GnRH is produced in the hypothalamus, and in response to low levels of LH, FSH, and testosterone due to the lack of a pituitary, the GnRH levels would be elevated. Androgen binding protein is not a hormone.

10. Answer is **D.** Developmental changes such as increase in facial hair, deepening of the voice, lengthening of the penis and hairline recession is mainly due to dihydrotestosterone. Testosterone is responsible for the male sex drive (increase in libido) and development of muscle mass. Testosterone is also important in libido of females.

Endocrine Functions of the Pancreas & Regulation of Carbohydrate Metabolism

OBJECTIVES

After studying this chapter, you should be able to:

- List the hormones that affect the plasma glucose concentration and briefly describe the action of each.

- Describe the structure of the pancreatic islets and name the hormones secreted by each of the cell types in the islets.

- Describe the structure of insulin and outline the steps involved in its biosynthesis and release into the bloodstream.

- List the consequences of insulin deficiency and explain how each of these abnormalities is produced.

- Describe insulin receptors, the way they mediate the effects of insulin, and the way they are regulated.

- Describe the types of glucose transporters found in the body and the function of each.

- List the major factors that affect the secretion of insulin.

- Describe the structure of glucagon and other physiologically active peptides produced from its precursor.

- List the physiologically significant effects of glucagon and the factors that regulate glucagon secretion.

- Describe the physiologic effects of somatostatin in the pancreas.

- Outline the mechanisms by which thyroid hormones, adrenal glucocorticoids, catecholamines, and growth hormone affect carbohydrate metabolism.

- Understand the major differences between type 1 and type 2 diabetes.

INTRODUCTION

At least four polypeptides with regulatory activity are secreted by the islets of Langerhans in the pancreas. Two of these, **insulin** and **glucagon,** are hormones and have important functions in the regulation of the intermediary metabolism of carbohydrates, proteins, and fats. The third polypeptide, **somatostatin,** plays a role in the regulation of islet cell secretion, and the fourth, **pancreatic polypeptide,** is probably concerned primarily with the regulation of ion transport in the intestine. Glucagon, somatostatin, and possibly pancreatic polypeptide are also secreted by cells in the mucosa of the gastrointestinal tract.

Insulin is anabolic, increasing the storage of glucose, fatty acids, and amino acids. Glucagon is catabolic, mobilizing glucose, fatty acids, and the amino acids from stores into the bloodstream. The two hormones are thus reciprocal in their overall action and are reciprocally secreted in most circumstances. Insulin excess causes hypoglycemia, which leads to convulsions and coma. Insulin deficiency, either absolute or relative, causes **diabetes mellitus** (chronic elevated blood glucose), a complex and debilitating disease that if untreated is eventually fatal. Glucagon deficiency can cause hypoglycemia, and glucagon excess makes diabetes worse. Excess pancreatic production of somatostatin causes hyperglycemia and other manifestations of diabetes.

■ ISLET CELL STRUCTURE

The islets of Langerhans are ovoid, 76 × 175-μm collections of cells. The islets are scattered throughout the pancreas, although they are more plentiful in the tail than in the body and head. β-Islets make up about 2% of the volume of the gland, whereas the exocrine portion of the pancreas (see Chapter 25) makes up 80%, and ducts and blood vessels make up the remainder. Humans have 1–2 million islets. Each has a copious blood supply; blood from the islets, like that from the gastrointestinal tract (but unlike that from any other endocrine organs) drains into the hepatic portal vein.

The cells in the islets can be divided into types on the basis of their staining properties and morphology. Humans have at least four distinct cell types: A, B, D, and F cells. A, B, and D cells are also called α, β, and δ cells. However, this leads to confusion in view of the use of Greek letters to refer to other structures in the body, particularly adrenergic receptors (see Chapter 7). The A cells secrete glucagon, the B cells secrete insulin, the D cells secrete somatostatin, and the F cells secrete pancreatic polypeptide. The B cells, which are the most common and account for 60–75% of the cells in the islets, are generally located in the center of each islet. They tend to be surrounded by the A cells, which make up 20% of the total, and the less common D and F cells. The islets in the tail, the body, and the anterior and superior part of the head of the human pancreas have many A cells and few if any F cells in the outer rim, whereas in rats and probably in humans, the islets in the posterior part of the head of the pancreas have a relatively large number of F cells and few A cells. The A-cell-rich (glucagon-rich) islets arise embryologically from the dorsal pancreatic bud, and the F-cell-rich (pancreatic polypeptide-rich) islets arise from the ventral pancreatic bud. These buds arise separately from the duodenum.

The B-cell granules are packets of insulin in the cell cytoplasm. The shape of the packets varies from species to species; in humans, some are round whereas others are rectangular. In the B cells, the insulin molecule forms polymers and also complexes with zinc. The differences in the shape of the packets are probably due to differences in the size of polymers or zinc aggregates of insulin. The A granules, which contain glucagon, are relatively uniform from species to species **(Figure 24–1)**. The D cells also contain large numbers of relatively homogeneous granules.

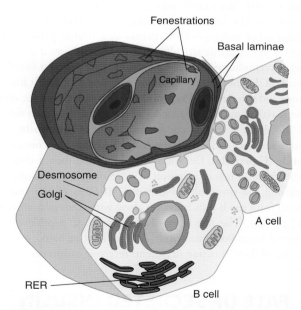

FIGURE 24–1 A and B cells, showing their relation to a blood vessel. Insulin from the B cell and glucagon from the A cell are secreted by exocytosis and cross the basal lamina of the cell and the basal lamina of the capillary before entering the lumen of the fenestrated capillary. RER, rough endoplasmic reticulum. (Reproduced with permission from Junqueira IC, Carneiro J: *Basic Histology: Text and Atlas,* 10th ed. New York, NY: McGraw-Hill; 2003.)

■ STRUCTURE, BIOSYNTHESIS, & SECRETION OF INSULIN

STRUCTURE & SPECIES SPECIFICITY

Insulin is a polypeptide, containing two chains of amino acids linked by disulfide bridges. Minor differences occur in the amino acid composition of the molecule from species to species. The differences are generally not sufficient to affect the biologic activity of a particular insulin in heterologous species but are sufficient to make the insulin antigenic. If insulin of one species is injected for a prolonged period into another species, the anti-insulin antibodies formed inhibit the injected insulin. Almost all humans who have received commercial bovine insulin for more than 2 months have antibodies against bovine insulin, but the titer is usually low. Porcine insulin differs from human insulin by only one amino acid residue and has low antigenicity. Human insulin produced in bacteria by recombinant DNA technology is now widely used to avoid antibody formation.

BIOSYNTHESIS & SECRETION

Insulin is synthesized in the rough endoplasmic reticulum of the B cells. It is then transported to the Golgi apparatus, where it is packaged into membrane-bound granules. These granules move to the plasma membrane by a process involving microtubules, and their contents are expelled by exocytosis (see Chapters 2 and 16). The insulin then crosses the basal lamina of the B cell and a neighboring capillary and the fenestrated endothelium of the capillary to reach the bloodstream. The fenestrations are discussed in detail in Chapter 31.

Like other polypeptide hormones and related proteins that enter the endoplasmic reticulum, insulin is synthesized as part of a larger preprohormone (see Chapter 1). The gene for insulin is located on the short arm of chromosome 11 in humans. It has two introns and three exons. **Preproinsulin** originates from the endoplasmic reticulum. The remainder of the molecule is then folded, and the disulfide bonds are formed to make **proinsulin.** The peptide segment connecting the A and B chains, the **connecting peptide (C peptide),** facilitates the folding and then is detached in the granules before secretion. Two proteases are involved in processing the proinsulin. Normally, 90–97% of the product released from the B cells is insulin along with equimolar amounts of C peptide. The rest is mostly proinsulin. C peptide can be measured by radioimmunoassay, and its level in blood provides an index of B cell function in patients receiving exogenous insulin.

■ FATE OF SECRETED INSULIN

INSULIN & INSULIN-LIKE ACTIVITY IN BLOOD

Plasma contains a number of substances with insulin-like activity in addition to insulin. The activity that is not suppressed by anti-insulin antibodies has been called nonsuppressible insulin-like activity (NSILA). Most, if not all, of this activity persists after pancreatectomy and is due to the insulin-like growth factors **IGF-I** and **IGF-II** (see Chapter 18). These IGFs are polypeptides. Small amounts are free in the plasma (low-molecular-weight fraction), but large amounts are bound to proteins (high-molecular-weight fraction).

One may well ask why pancreatectomy causes diabetes mellitus when NSILA persists in the plasma. However, the insulin-like activities of IGF-I and IGF-II are weak compared to that of insulin and likely subserve other specific functions.

METABOLISM

The half-life of insulin in the circulation in humans is about 5 min. Insulin binds to insulin receptors, and some is internalized. It is destroyed by proteases in the endosomes formed by the endocytotic process.

EFFECTS OF INSULIN

The physiologic effects of insulin are far-reaching and complex. They are conveniently divided into rapid, intermediate, and delayed actions (Table 24–1). The best known is the hypoglycemic effect, but there are additional effects on amino acid and electrolyte transport, many enzymes, and growth. The net effect of the hormone is storage of carbohydrate, protein, and fat. Therefore, insulin is appropriately called the "hormone of abundance."

The actions of insulin on adipose tissue; skeletal, cardiac, and smooth muscle; and the liver are summarized in Table 24–2.

GLUCOSE TRANSPORTERS

Glucose enters cells by **facilitated diffusion** (see Chapter 1) or, in the intestine and kidneys, by secondary active transport with Na^+. In muscle, adipose, and some other tissues, insulin stimulates glucose entry into cells by increasing the number of glucose transporters (GLUTs) in the cell membranes.

TABLE 24–1　Principal actions of insulin.

Rapid (seconds)
Increased transport of glucose, amino acids, and K^+ into insulin-sensitive cells
Intermediate (minutes)
Stimulation of protein synthesis
Inhibition of protein degradation
Activation of glycolytic enzymes and glycogen synthase
Inhibition of phosphorylase and gluconeogenic enzymes
Delayed (hours)
Increase in mRNAs for lipogenic and other enzymes

Used with permission from ID Goldfine

TABLE 24–2 Effects of insulin on various tissues.

Adipose tissue

   Increased glucose entry

   Increased fatty acid synthesis

   Increased glycerol phosphate synthesis

   Increased triglyceride deposition

   Activation of lipoprotein lipase

   Inhibition of hormone-sensitive lipase

   Increased K^+ uptake

Muscle

   Increased glucose entry

   Increased glycogen synthesis

   Increased amino acid uptake

   Increased protein synthesis in ribosomes

   Decreased protein catabolism

   Decreased release of gluconeogenic amino acids

   Increased ketone uptake

   Increased K^+ uptake

Liver

   Decreased ketogenesis

   Increased protein synthesis

   Increased lipid synthesis

   Decreased glucose output due to decreased gluconeogenesis, increased glycogen synthesis, and increased glycolysis

General

   Increased cell growth

The GLUTs that are responsible for facilitated diffusion of glucose across cell membranes are a family of closely related proteins that span the cell membrane 12 times and have their amino and carboxyl terminals inside the cell. They differ from and have no homology with the sodium-glucose linked transporters (SGLT-1 and SGLT-2), which are responsible for the secondary active transport of glucose in the intestine (see Chapter 26) and renal tubules (see Chapter 38), although the SGLTs also have 12 transmembrane domains.

Seven different GLUTs, named GLUT 1–7 in order of discovery, have been characterized. They contain 492–524 amino acid residues and their affinity for glucose varies. Each transporter appears to have evolved for special tasks. **GLUT-4** is the transporter in muscle and adipose tissue that is stimulated by insulin. A pool of GLUT-4 molecules is maintained within vesicles in the cytoplasm of insulin-sensitive cells. When insulin receptors of these cells are activated, the vesicles move rapidly to the cell membrane and fuse with it, inserting the transporters into the cell membrane. When insulin action ceases, the transporter-containing patches of membrane are endocytosed and the vesicles are ready for the next exposure to insulin. Activation of the insulin receptor brings about the movement of the vesicles to the cell membrane by activating phosphatidylinositol 3-kinase.

In the tissues in which insulin increases the number of GLUTs in cell membranes, the rate of phosphorylation of the glucose, once it has entered the cells, is regulated by other hormones and is rate-limiting in B cells only.

Insulin also increases the entry of glucose into liver cells, but it does not exert this effect by increasing the number of GLUT-4 transporters in the cell membranes. Instead, it induces glucokinase, and this increases the phosphorylation of glucose, so that the intracellular free glucose concentration stays low, facilitating the entry of glucose into the cell.

Insulin-sensitive tissues also contain a population of GLUT-4 vesicles that move into the cell membrane in response to exercise, a process that occurs independent of the action of insulin. This is why exercise lowers blood sugar. A 5′-adenosine monophosphate (AMP)–activated kinase may trigger the insertion of these vesicles into the cell membrane.

INSULIN PREPARATIONS

The maximal decline in plasma glucose occurs 30 min after intravenous injection of insulin. After subcutaneous administration, the maximal fall occurs in 2–3 h. A wide variety of insulin preparations are now available commercially. These include insulins that have been complexed with protamine and other polypeptides to delay absorption and degradation, and synthetic insulins in which there have been changes in amino acid residues. In general, they fall into three categories: rapid, intermediate acting, and long acting (24–36 h).

RELATION TO POTASSIUM

Insulin causes K^+ to enter cells, with a resultant lowering of the extracellular K^+ concentration. Infusions of insulin and glucose significantly lower the plasma K^+ level in normal individuals and are very effective for the temporary relief of hyperkalemia in patients with renal failure. **Hypokalemia** often develops when patients with diabetic acidosis are treated with insulin. The reason for the intracellular migration of K^+ is still uncertain. However, insulin increases the activity of Na, K ATPase in cell membranes, so that more K^+ is pumped into cells.

OTHER ACTIONS

The hypoglycemic and other effects of insulin are summarized in temporal terms in Table 24–1, and the net effects on various tissues are summarized in Table 24–2. The action on glycogen synthase fosters glycogen storage, and the actions on glycolytic enzymes favor glucose metabolism to two carbon fragments (see Chapter 1), with resulting promotion of lipogenesis. Stimulation of protein synthesis from amino acids entering the cells and inhibition of protein degradation foster growth.

The anabolic effect of insulin is aided by the protein-sparing action of adequate intracellular glucose supplies. Failure to grow is a symptom of diabetes in children, and insulin stimulates the growth of immature hypophysectomized rats to almost the same degree as growth hormone.

■ MECHANISM OF ACTION

INSULIN RECEPTORS

Insulin receptors are found on many different cells in the body, including cells in which insulin does not increase glucose uptake. The insulin receptor is a tetramer made up of two α and two β glycoprotein subunits. The α subunits bind insulin and are extracellular, whereas the β subunits span the membrane. The intracellular portions of the β subunits have tyrosine kinase activity. The α and β subunits are both glycosylated, with sugar residues extending into the interstitial fluid.

Binding of insulin triggers tyrosine kinase activity of the β subunits, producing autophosphorylation of the β subunits on tyrosine residues. The autophosphorylation, which is necessary for insulin to exert its biologic effects, triggers phosphorylation of some cytoplasmic proteins and dephosphorylation of others, mostly on serine and threonine residues. Insulin receptor substrate (IRS-1) mediates some of the effects in humans but there are other effector systems as well. The growth-promoting protein anabolic effects of insulin are mediated via **phosphatidylinositol 3-kinase (PI3K).**

When insulin binds to its receptors, they aggregate in patches and are taken up into the cell by receptor-mediated endocytosis (see Chapter 2). Eventually, the insulin–receptor complexes enter lysosomes, where the receptors are broken down or recycled. The half-life of the insulin receptor is about 7 h.

■ CONSEQUENCES OF INSULIN DEFICIENCY

GLUCOSE TOLERANCE

In diabetes, glucose piles up in the bloodstream, especially after meals. If a glucose load is given to a diabetic, the plasma glucose rises higher and returns to the baseline more slowly than it does in normal individuals. The response to a standard oral test dose of glucose, the **oral glucose tolerance test,** is used in the clinical diagnosis of diabetes.

Impaired glucose tolerance in diabetes is due in part to reduced entry of glucose into cells **(decreased peripheral utilization).** In the absence of insulin, the entry of glucose into skeletal, cardiac, and smooth muscle and other tissues is decreased (Figure 24–2). Glucose uptake by the liver is also reduced, but the effect is indirect. Intestinal absorption of glucose is unaffected, as is its reabsorption from the urine by the cells of the proximal tubules of the kidneys. Glucose uptake by most of the brain and the red blood cells is also normal.

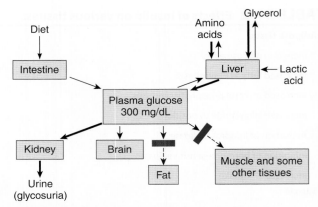

FIGURE 24–2 Disordered plasma glucose homeostasis in insulin deficiency. The heavy arrows indicate reactions that are accentuated. The rectangles across arrows indicate reactions that are blocked.

The second and the major cause of hyperglycemia in diabetes is derangement of the glucostatic function of the liver (see Chapter 28). The liver takes up glucose from the bloodstream and stores it as glycogen, but because the liver contains glucose-6-phosphatase it also discharges glucose into the bloodstream. Insulin facilitates glycogen synthesis and inhibits hepatic glucose output. When the plasma glucose is high, insulin secretion is normally increased and hepatic glucogenesis is decreased. This response does not occur in type 1 diabetes mellitus (as insulin is absent) and in type 2 diabetes mellitus (as tissues are insulin resistant). Glucagon can contribute to hyperglycemia as it stimulates gluconeogenesis. Glucose output by the liver can be stimulated by catecholamines, cortisol, and growth hormone (ie, during a stress response).

EFFECTS OF HYPERGLYCEMIA

Hyperglycemia by itself can cause symptoms resulting from the hyperosmolality of the blood. In addition, there is glycosuria because the renal capacity for glucose reabsorption is exceeded (Figure 24-2). Excretion of the osmotically active glucose molecules entails the loss of large amounts of water (osmotic diuresis; see Chapter 38). The resultant dehydration activates the mechanisms regulating water intake, leading to polydipsia. There is an appreciable urinary loss of Na^+ and K^+ as well. When plasma glucose is episodically elevated over time, small amounts of hemoglobin A are nonenzymatically glycated to form **HbA$_{1c}$** (see Chapter 31). Careful control of diabetes with insulin reduces the amount formed and consequently HbA$_{1c}$ concentration is measured clinically as an integrated index of diabetic control for the 4–6 weeks period before the measurement.

EFFECTS OF INTRACELLULAR GLUCOSE DEFICIENCY

Glucose catabolism is normally a major source of energy for cellular processes, and in diabetes energy requirements can be met only by drawing on protein and fat reserves. Mechanisms are activated that greatly increase the catabolism of protein and fat, and one of the consequences of increased fat catabolism is ketosis.

Deficient glucose utilization and deficient hormone sensing (insulin, leptin, CCK) in the cells of the hypothalamus that regulate satiety are the probable causes of hyperphagia in diabetes. The feeding area of the hypothalamus is not inhibited and thus satiety is not sensed so food intake is increased.

Glycogen depletion is a common consequence of intracellular glucose deficit, and the glycogen content of liver and skeletal muscle in diabetic animals is usually reduced.

CHANGES IN PROTEIN METABOLISM

In diabetes, the rate at which amino acids are catabolized to CO_2 and H_2O is increased. In addition, more amino acids are converted to glucose in the liver. The increased gluconeogenesis has many causes. Glucagon stimulates gluconeogenesis, and hyperglucagonemia is generally present in diabetes. Adrenal glucocorticoids also contribute to increased gluconeogenesis when they are elevated in severely ill diabetics. The supply of amino acids is increased for gluconeogenesis because, in the absence of insulin, less protein synthesis occurs in muscle and hence blood amino acid levels rise. Alanine is particularly easily converted to glucose. In addition, the activity of the enzymes that catalyze the conversion of pyruvate and other two-carbon metabolic fragments to glucose is increased. These include phosphoenolpyruvate carboxykinase, which facilitates the conversion of oxaloacetate to phosphoenolpyruvate (see Chapter 1). They also include fructose 1,6-diphosphatase, which catalyzes the conversion of fructose diphosphate to fructose 6-phosphate, and glucose 6-phosphatase, which controls the entry of glucose into the circulation from the liver. Increased acetyl-CoA increases pyruvate carboxylase activity, and insulin deficiency increases the supply of acetyl-CoA because lipogenesis is decreased. Pyruvate carboxylase catalyzes the conversion of pyruvate to oxaloacetate (see Figure 1–22).

In diabetes, the net effect of accelerated protein conversion to CO_2, H_2O, and glucose, plus diminished protein synthesis, is protein depletion and wasting. Protein depletion from any cause is associated with poor "resistance" to infections.

FAT METABOLISM IN DIABETES

The principal abnormalities of fat metabolism in diabetes are accelerated lipid catabolism, with increased formation of ketone bodies, and decreased synthesis of fatty acids and triglycerides. The manifestations of the disordered lipid metabolism are so prominent that diabetes has been called "more a disease of lipid than of carbohydrate metabolism."

Fifty percent of an ingested glucose load is normally burned to CO_2 and H_2O; 5% is converted to glycogen; and 30–40% is converted to fat in the fat depots. In diabetes, less than 5% of ingested glucose is converted to fat, despite a decrease in the amount burned to CO_2 and H_2O, and no change in the amount converted to glycogen. Therefore, glucose accumulates in the bloodstream and spills over into the urine.

The role of lipoprotein lipase and hormone-sensitive lipase in the regulation of the metabolism of fat depots is discussed in Chapter 1. In diabetes, conversion of glucose to fatty acids in the depots is decreased because of the intracellular glucose deficiency. Insulin inhibits the hormone-sensitive lipase in adipose tissue, and, in the absence of this hormone, the plasma level of **free fatty acids** (NEFA, UFA, FFA) is more than doubled. The increased glucagon also contributes to the mobilization of FFA. Thus, the FFA level parallels the plasma glucose level in diabetes and in some ways is a better indicator of the severity of the diabetic state. In the liver and other tissues, the fatty acids are catabolized to acetyl-CoA. Some of the acetyl-CoA is burned along with amino acid residues to yield CO_2 and H_2O in the citric acid cycle. However, the supply exceeds the capacity of the tissues to catabolize the acetyl-CoA.

In addition to the previously mentioned increase in gluconeogenesis and marked outpouring of glucose into the circulation, the conversion of acetyl-CoA to malonyl-CoA and thence to fatty acids is markedly impaired. This is due to a deficiency of acetyl-CoA carboxylase, the enzyme that catalyzes the conversion. The excess acetyl-CoA is converted to ketone bodies.

In uncontrolled diabetes, the plasma concentration of triglycerides and chylomicrons as well as FFA is increased, and the plasma is often lipemic. The rise in these constituents is mainly due to decreased removal of triglycerides into the fat depots. The decreased activity of lipoprotein lipase contributes to this decreased removal.

ACIDOSIS

As noted in Chapter 1, acetoacetate and β-hydroxybutyrate are anions of the fairly strong acids acetoacetic acid and β-hydroxybutyric acids. The hydrogen ions from these acids are buffered, but the buffering capacity is soon exceeded if production is increased. The resulting acidosis stimulates respiration, producing the rapid, deep respiration described by Kussmaul as "air hunger" and named (for him) **Kussmaul breathing.** The urine becomes acidic. However, when the ability of the kidneys to replace the plasma cations accompanying the organic anions with H^+ and NH_4^+ is exceeded, Na^+ and K^+ are lost in the urine. The electrolyte and water losses lead to dehydration, hypovolemia, and hypotension. Finally, the acidosis and dehydration depress consciousness to the point of coma. Diabetic acidosis is a medical emergency. Now that the infections that used to complicate the disease can be controlled with antibiotics, acidosis is the most common cause of early death in persons with clinical diabetes.

In severe acidosis, total body Na^+ is markedly depleted, and when Na^+ loss exceeds water loss, plasma Na^+ may also be low. Total body K^+ is also low, but the plasma K^+ is usually normal, partly because extracellular fluid (ECF) volume is reduced and partly because K^+ moves from cells to ECF when the ECF H^+ concentration is high. Another factor tending to maintain the plasma K^+ is the lack of insulin-induced entry of K^+ into cells.

COMA

Coma in diabetes can be due to acidosis and dehydration. However, the plasma glucose can be elevated to such a degree that independent of plasma pH, the hyperosmolarity of the plasma causes unconsciousness (**hyperosmolar coma**). Accumulation of lactate in the blood (**lactic acidosis**) may also complicate diabetic ketoacidosis if the tissues become hypoxic, and lactic acidosis may itself cause coma. Brain edema occurs in about 1% of children with ketoacidosis, and it can cause coma. Its cause is unsettled, but it is a serious complication, with a mortality rate of about 25%.

CHOLESTEROL METABOLISM

In diabetes, the plasma cholesterol level is usually elevated and this plays a role in the accelerated development of the atherosclerotic vascular disease that is a major long-term complication of diabetes in humans. The rise in plasma cholesterol level is due to an increase in the plasma concentration of very low-density lipoprotein (VLDL) and low-density lipoprotein (LDL) (see Chapter 1). These in turn may be due to increased hepatic production of VLDL or decreased removal of VLDL and LDL from the circulation.

SUMMARY

Because of the complexities of the metabolic abnormalities in diabetes, a summary is in order. One of the key features of insulin deficiency (**Figure 24–3**) is decreased entry of glucose into many tissues (decreased peripheral utilization). Also, the net release of glucose from the liver is increased (increased production), due in part to glucagon excess. The resultant hyperglycemia leads to glycosuria

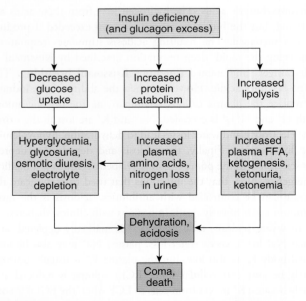

FIGURE 24–3 Effects of insulin deficiency. (Used with permission of RJ Havel.)

and a dehydrating osmotic diuresis. Dehydration leads to polydipsia. In the face of intracellular glucose deficiency, appetite is stimulated, glucose is formed from protein (gluconeogenesis), and energy supplies are maintained by metabolism of proteins and fats. Weight loss, debilitating protein deficiency, and inanition are the result.

Fat catabolism is increased and the system is flooded with triglycerides and FFA. Fat synthesis is inhibited and the overloaded catabolic pathways cannot handle the excess acetyl-CoA that is formed. In the liver, the acetyl-CoA is converted to ketone bodies. Two of these are organic acids, and metabolic acidosis develops as ketones accumulate. Na^+ and K^+ depletion is added to the acidosis because these plasma cations are excreted with the organic anions not covered by the H^+ and NH_4^+ secreted by the kidneys. Finally, the acidotic, hypovolemic, hypotensive, depleted animal or patient becomes comatose because of the toxic effects of acidosis, dehydration, and hyperosmolarity on the nervous system and dies if treatment is not instituted.

All of these abnormalities are corrected by administration of insulin. Although emergency treatment of acidosis also includes administration of alkali to combat the acidosis as well as parenteral water, Na^+, and K^+ to replenish body stores, only insulin repairs the fundamental defects in a way that permits a return to normal.

■ INSULIN EXCESS

SYMPTOMS

All the known consequences of insulin excess are manifestations, directly or indirectly, of the effects of hypoglycemia on the nervous system. Except in individuals who have been fasting for some time, glucose is the only fuel used in appreciable quantities by the brain. The carbohydrate reserves in neural tissue are very limited and normal function depends on a continuous glucose supply. As the plasma glucose level falls, the first symptoms are palpitations, sweating, and nervousness due to autonomic discharge. At lower plasma glucose levels, so-called **neuroglycopenic symptoms** begin to appear. These include hunger as well as confusion and the other cognitive abnormalities. At even lower plasma glucose levels, lethargy, coma, convulsions, and eventually death occur.

COMPENSATORY MECHANISMS

One important compensation for hypoglycemia is cessation of the insulin secretion. Inhibition of insulin secretion is complete at a plasma glucose level of about 80 mg/dL. In addition, hypoglycemia triggers increased secretion of at least four counterregulatory hormones: glucagon, epinephrine, growth hormone, and cortisol. Glucagon and epinephrine increase the hepatic output of glucose by increasing glycogenolysis. Growth hormone decreases the utilization of glucose in various peripheral tissues, and cortisol has a similar action. The keys to counterregulation appear to be epinephrine and glucagon: if the plasma concentration of either increases, the decline in the plasma glucose level is reversed; but if both fail to increase, there is little if any compensatory rise in the plasma glucose level. The actions of the other hormones are supplementary.

■ REGULATION OF INSULIN SECRETION

Factors that stimulate and inhibit insulin secretion are summarized in Table 24–3.

EFFECTS OF THE PLASMA GLUCOSE LEVEL

It has been known for many years that glucose acts directly on pancreatic B cells to increase insulin secretion. The response to glucose is biphasic; there is a rapid but short-lived increase in insulin secretion followed by a more slowly developing prolonged increase.

Glucose enters the B cells via GLUT-2 transporters and is phosphorylated by glucokinase then metabolized to pyruvate in the cytoplasm. The pyruvate enters the mitochondria and is metabolized to CO_2 and H_2O via the citric acid cycle with the formation of ATP by oxidative phosphorylation. The ATP enters the cytoplasm, where it inhibits ATP-sensitive K^+ channels, reducing K^+ efflux. This depolarizes the B cell, and Ca^{2+} enters the cell via voltage-gated Ca^{2+} channels. The Ca^{2+} influx causes exocytosis of a readily releasable pool of insulin-containing secretory granules, producing the initial spike of insulin secretion.

Metabolism of pyruvate via the citric acid cycle also causes an increase in intracellular glutamate. The glutamate appears to act on a second pool of secretory granules, committing them to the

TABLE 24–3 Factors affecting insulin secretion.

Stimulators	Inhibitors
Glucose	Somatostatin
Mannose	2-Deoxyglucose
Amino acids (leucine, arginine, others)	Mannoheptulose
Intestinal hormones (GIP, GLP-1 [7–36], gastrin, secretin, CCK; others?)	α-Adrenergic stimulators (norepinephrine, epinephrine)
β-Keto acids	β-Adrenergic blockers (propranolol)
Acetylcholine	
Glucagon	Galanin
Cyclic AMP and various cAMP-generating substances	Diazoxide
	Thiazide diuretics
β-Adrenergic stimulators	K^+ depletion
Theophylline	Phenytoin
Sulfonylureas	Alloxan
	Microtubule inhibitors
	Insulin

releasable form. The action of glutamate may be to decrease the pH in the secretory granules, a necessary step in their maturation. The release of these granules then produces the prolonged second phase of the insulin response to glucose. Thus, glutamate appears to act as an intracellular second messenger that primes insulin secretory granules for secretion.

The feedback control of plasma glucose on insulin secretion normally operates with great precision so that plasma glucose and insulin levels parallel each other with remarkable consistency.

PROTEIN & FAT DERIVATIVES

Insulin stimulates the incorporation of amino acids into proteins and combats fat catabolism that produces the β-keto acids. Therefore, it is not surprising that arginine, leucine, and certain other amino acids stimulate insulin secretion, as do β-keto acids such as acetoacetate. Like glucose, these compounds generate ATP when metabolized, and this closes ATP-sensitive K^+ channels in the B cells. In addition, L-arginine is the precursor of NO, and NO stimulates insulin secretion.

ORAL HYPOGLYCEMIC AGENTS

Tolbutamide and other sulfonylurea derivatives such as acetohexamide, tolazamide, glipizide, and glyburide are orally active hypoglycemic agents that lower blood glucose by increasing the secretion of insulin. They only work in patients with some remaining B cells. They bind to the ATP-inhibited K^+ channels in the B cell membranes and inhibit channel activity, depolarizing the B cell membrane and increasing Ca^{2+} influx and hence insulin release, independent of increases in plasma glucose.

Persistent hyperinsulinemic hypoglycemia of infancy is a condition in which plasma insulin is elevated despite the hypoglycemia. The condition is caused by mutations in the genes for various enzymes in B cells that decrease K^+ efflux via the ATP-sensitive K^+ channels. Treatment consists of administration of diazoxide, a drug that increases the activity of the K^+ channels or, in more severe cases, subtotal pancreatectomy.

The biguanide **metformin** is an oral hypoglycemic agent that acts in the absence of insulin. Metformin acts primarily by reducing gluconeogenesis and therefore decreasing hepatic glucose output. It is sometimes combined with a sulfonylurea in the treatment of type 2 diabetes. Metformin can cause lactic acidosis, but the incidence is usually low.

Troglitazone (Rezulin) and related **thiazolidinediones** are also used in the treatment of diabetes because they increase insulin-mediated peripheral glucose disposal, thus reducing insulin resistance. They bind to and activate peroxisome proliferator-activated receptor γ (PPARγ) in the nucleus of cells. Activation of this receptor, which is a member of the superfamily of hormone-sensitive nuclear transcription factors, has a unique ability to normalize a variety of metabolic functions.

CYCLIC AMP & INSULIN SECRETION

Stimuli that increase cAMP levels in B cells increase insulin secretion, including β-adrenergic agonists, glucagon, and phosphodiesterase inhibitors such as theophylline.

Catecholamines have a dual effect on insulin secretion; they inhibit insulin secretion via α_2-adrenergic receptors and stimulate insulin secretion via β-adrenergic receptors. The net effect of epinephrine and norepinephrine is usually inhibition. However, if catecholamines are infused after administration of α-adrenergic blocking drugs, the inhibition is converted to stimulation.

EFFECT OF AUTONOMIC NERVES

Branches of the right vagus nerve innervate the pancreatic islets, and stimulation of this parasympathetic pathway causes increased insulin secretion via M_4 receptors. Atropine blocks the response and acetylcholine stimulates insulin secretion. The effect of acetylcholine, like that of glucose, is due to increased cytoplasmic Ca^{2+}, but acetylcholine activates phospholipase C, with the released IP_3 releasing the Ca^{2+} from the endoplasmic reticulum.

Stimulation of the sympathetic nerves to the pancreas inhibits insulin secretion. The inhibition is produced by released norepinephrine acting on α_2-adrenergic receptors. However, if α-adrenergic receptors are blocked, stimulation of the sympathetic nerves causes increased insulin secretion mediated by β_2-adrenergic receptors. The polypeptide galanin is found in some of the autonomic nerves innervating the islets, and galanin inhibits insulin secretion by activating the K^+ channels that are inhibited by ATP. Thus, although the denervated pancreas responds to glucose, the autonomic innervation of the pancreas is involved in the overall regulation of insulin secretion.

INTESTINAL HORMONES

Orally administered glucose exerts a greater insulin-stimulating effect than intravenously administered glucose, and orally administered amino acids also produce a greater insulin response than intravenous amino acids. These observations led to exploration of the possibility that a substance secreted by the gastrointestinal mucosa stimulated insulin secretion. Glucagon, glucagon derivatives, secretin, cholecystokinin (CCK), gastrin, and gastric inhibitory peptide (GIP) all have such an action (see Chapter 25), and CCK potentiates the insulin-stimulating effects of amino acids. However, GIP is the only one of these peptides that produces stimulation when administered in doses that reflect blood GIP levels produced by an oral glucose load.

Recently, attention has focused on glucagon-like polypeptide 1 (7–36) (GLP-1 [7–36]) as an additional gut factor that stimulates insulin secretion. This polypeptide is a product of preproglucagon. B cells have GLP-1 (7–36) receptors as well as GIP receptors, and GLP-1 (7–36) is a more potent insulinotropic hormone than GIP. GIP and GLP-1 (7–36) both appear to act by increasing Ca^{2+} influx through voltage-gated Ca^{2+} channels.

LONG-TERM CHANGES IN B-CELL RESPONSES

The magnitude of the insulin response to a given stimulus is determined in part by the secretory history of the B cells. Individuals fed a high-carbohydrate diet for several weeks not only have higher fasting plasma insulin levels but also show a greater secretory response to a glucose load than individuals fed an isocaloric low-carbohydrate diet.

Although B cells respond to stimulation with hypertrophy like other endocrine cells, they become exhausted and stop secreting (**B-cell exhaustion**) when the stimulation is marked or prolonged.

■ GLUCAGON

CHEMISTRY

Human glucagon is produced by A cells of the pancreatic islets and the upper gastrointestinal tract. It contains 29 amino acid residues. Preproglucagon is a 179-amino-acid protein that is found in pancreatic A cells, in L cells in the lower gastrointestinal tract, and in the brain. In A cells, it is processed primarily to glucagon and major proglucagon fragment (MPGF). In L cells, it is processed primarily to **glicentin,** a polypeptide that consists of glucagon extended by additional amino acid residues at either end, plus **glucagon-like polypeptides 1 and 2 (GLP-1 and GLP-2).** GLP-1 is processed further by removal of its amino-terminal amino acid residues and the product, **GLP-1 (7–36),** is a potent stimulator of insulin secretion that also increases glucose utilization (see earlier). GLP-1 and GLP-2 are also produced in the brain. The function of GLP-1 in this location is uncertain, but GLP-2 appears to be the mediator in a pathway from the nucleus tractus solitarius (NTS) to the dorsomedial nuclei of the hypothalamus, and injection of GLP-2 lowers food intake.

ACTION & METABOLISM & SECRETION

Glucagon is glycogenolytic, gluconeogenic, lipolytic, and ketogenic. It acts on G-protein–coupled receptors. **In the liver,** it acts via G_s to activate adenylyl cyclase and increase intracellular cAMP. This leads via protein kinase A to activation of phosphorylase and increased breakdown of glycogen and increase in plasma glucose. However, glucagon acts on different glucagon receptors located on the same hepatic cells to activate phospholipase C, resulting in increase in cytoplasmic Ca^{2+} that also stimulates **glycogenolysis.** Protein kinase A also decreases the metabolism of glucose-6-phosphate by inhibiting the conversion of phosphoenolpyruvate to pyruvate. It also decreases the concentration of fructose 2,6-diphosphate and this in turn inhibits the conversion of fructose 6-phosphate to fructose 1,6-diphosphate. The resultant buildup of glucose-6-phosphate leads to increased glucose synthesis and release.

In **muscle** glucagon increases **gluconeogenesis** from available amino acids from the liver and elevates the metabolic rate. It increases ketone body formation by decreasing malonyl-CoA levels in the liver. Its lipolytic activity, which leads in turn to increased **ketogenesis.** Glucagon also stimulates the secretion of growth hormone, insulin, and pancreatic somatostatin.

Glucagon has a half-life in the circulation of 5–10 min. It is degraded by many tissues but particularly by the liver. Because glucagon is secreted into the portal vein and reaches the liver before it reaches the peripheral circulation, peripheral blood levels are relatively low. The rise in peripheral blood glucagon levels produced by excitatory stimuli is exaggerated in patients with cirrhosis, presumably because of decreased hepatic degradation of the hormone.

Secretion of glucagon is increased by hypoglycemia and decreased by a rise in plasma glucose. Pancreatic B cells contain GABA, and with hyperglycemia, GABA is released and acts on the A cells to inhibit glucagon secretion by activating GABA$_A$ receptors (**Table 24–4**).

Secretion is also increased by stimulation of sympathetic nerves to the pancreas, which is mediated via β-adrenergic receptors and cAMP. A cells are like the B cells in that stimulation of β-adrenergic receptors increases secretion and stimulation of α-adrenergic receptors inhibits secretion. However, the effect of β-receptors predominates in the glucagon-secreting cells. Vagal stimulation also increases glucagon secretion.

A protein meal and infusion of amino acids increase glucagon secretion with glucogenic amino acids being particularly potent, since these are the amino acids that are converted to glucose in the liver under the influence of glucagon. The increase in glucagon secretion following a protein meal is also valuable, since the amino acids stimulate insulin secretion and the secreted glucagon prevents the development of hypoglycemia while the insulin promotes storage of the absorbed carbohydrates and lipids. The glucagon response to oral administration of amino acids is greater than the response to intravenous infusion of amino acids, suggesting that a glucagon-stimulating factor is secreted from the gastrointestinal mucosa. CCK and gastrin increase glucagon secretion, whereas

secretin inhibits it. Because CCK and gastrin secretion are both increased by a protein meal, either hormone could be the gastrointestinal mediator of the glucagon response.

Glucagon secretion increases during starvation. It reaches a peak on the third day of a fast, at the time of maximal gluconeogenesis. Thereafter, the plasma glucagon level declines as fatty acids and ketones become the major sources of energy.

During exercise, there is an increase in glucose utilization that is balanced by an increase in glucose production caused by an increase in circulating glucagon levels.

Glucagon secretion is also inhibited by FFA and ketones, but this inhibition can be overridden, since plasma glucagon levels are high in diabetic ketoacidosis.

INSULIN–GLUCAGON MOLAR RATIOS

Insulin is glycogenic, antigluconeogenic, antilipolytic, and antiketotic in its actions. It thus favors storage of absorbed nutrients and is a "hormone of energy storage." Glucagon, on the other hand, is glycogenolytic, gluconeogenetic, lipolytic, and ketogenic. It mobilizes energy stores and is a "hormone of energy release." Because they have opposite effects, blood levels of both hormones must be considered in any given situation. It is convenient to think in terms of the molar ratios of these hormones.

The insulin–glucagon molar ratios fluctuate markedly because the secretions of glucagon and insulin are both modified by conditions that preceded the application of any given stimulus. Thus, for example, the insulin–glucagon molar ratio on a balanced diet is approximately 2.3. An infusion of arginine increases the secretion of both hormones and raises the ratio to 3.0. After 3 days of starvation, the ratio falls to 0.4, and an infusion of arginine in this state lowers the ratio to 0.3. Conversely, the ratio is 25 in individuals receiving a constant infusion of glucose and rises to 170 on ingestion of a protein meal during the infusion. When energy is needed during starvation, the insulin–glucagon molar ratio is low, favoring glycogen breakdown and gluconeogenesis; conversely, when the need for energy mobilization is low, the ratio is high, favoring the deposition of glycogen, protein, and fat.

SOMATOSTATIN

Somatostatin and its receptors are discussed in Chapter 7. Somatostatin inhibits the secretion of insulin, glucagon, and pancreatic polypeptide. Insulin in turn inhibits the secretion of glucagon; and glucagon stimulates the secretion of insulin and somatostatin. The secretion of pancreatic somatostatin is increased by glucose and amino acids, particularly arginine and leucine, and CCK. Somatostatin is released from the pancreas and the gastrointestinal tract into the peripheral blood. Patients with somatostatin-secreting pancreatic tumors (**somatostatinomas**) develop hyperglycemia and other manifestations of diabetes that disappear when the tumor is removed.

TABLE 24–4 Factors affecting glucagon secretion.

Stimulators	Inhibitors
Amino acids (particularly the glucogenic amino acids: alanine, serine, glycine, cysteine, and threonine)	Glucose
CCK, gastrin	Somatostatin
Cortisol	Secretin
Exercise	FFA
Infections	Ketones
Other stresses	Insulin
β-Adrenergic stimulators	Phenytoin
Theophylline	α-Adrenergic stimulators
Acetylcholine	GABA

■ EFFECTS OF OTHER HORMONES & EXERCISE ON CARBOHYDRATE METABOLISM

EXERCISE

The entry of glucose into skeletal muscle is increased during exercise in the absence of insulin by causing an insulin-independent increase in the number of GLUT-4 transporters in muscle cell membranes. This increase in glucose entry persists for several hours after exercise, and regular exercise training can also produce prolonged increases in insulin sensitivity.

CATECHOLAMINES

The activation of phosphorylase in liver by catecholamines occurs via β-adrenergic receptors, that increase intracellular cAMP and α-adrenergic receptors to increase intracellular Ca^{2+}. Hepatic glucose output is increased, producing hyperglycemia. In muscle, phosphorylase is also activated via cAMP and Ca^{2+}, but the glucose-6-phosphate formed can be catabolized only to pyruvate because of the absence of glucose-6-phosphatase. Large amounts of pyruvate are converted to lactate, which diffuses from the muscle into the circulation. Lactate is oxidized in the liver to pyruvate and converted to glycogen. Therefore, the response to an injection of epinephrine is an initial glycogenolysis followed by a rise in hepatic glycogen content.

THYROID HORMONES

The principal diabetogenic effect of thyroid hormones is to increase absorption of glucose from the intestine, but the hormones also cause some degree of hepatic glycogen depletion. Glycogen-depleted liver cells are easily damaged which will cause a diabetic glucose tolerance curve because the liver takes up less of the absorbed glucose. Thyroid hormones may also accelerate the degradation of insulin. All these actions have a hyperglycemic effect and, if the pancreatic reserve is low, may lead to B-cell exhaustion.

ADRENAL GLUCOCORTICOIDS

Glucocorticoids from the adrenal cortex elevate blood glucose and produce a diabetic type of glucose tolerance curve, but may occur only in individuals with a genetic predisposition to diabetes. Glucocorticoids are necessary for glucagon to exert its gluconeogenic action during fasting. In adrenal insufficiency, blood glucose is normal as long as food intake is maintained, but fasting precipitates hypoglycemia and collapse. The plasma-glucose-lowering effect of insulin is greatly enhanced in patients with adrenal insufficiency. The major diabetogenic effects are an increase in protein catabolism with increased gluconeogenesis in the liver; increased hepatic glycogenesis and ketogenesis; and a decrease in peripheral glucose utilization relative to the blood insulin level that may be due to inhibition of glucose phosphorylation.

GROWTH HORMONE

Human growth hormone makes clinical diabetes worse, and 25% of patients with growth hormone–secreting tumors of the anterior pituitary have diabetes. Hypophysectomy ameliorates diabetes and decreases insulin resistance even more than adrenalectomy, whereas growth hormone treatment increases insulin resistance.

■ HYPOGLYCEMIA & DIABETES MELLITUS

HYPOGLYCEMIA

Hypoglycemic episodes, often called "insulin reactions," are common in type 1 diabetics and is often a consequence of tight glycemic control. The autonomic discharge caused by lowered blood glucose that produces shakiness, sweating, anxiety, and hunger normally occurs at plasma glucose levels that are higher than the glucose levels that cause cognitive dysfunction, thereby serving as a warning to ingest sugar.

However, in some individuals, these warning symptoms fail to occur, and this **hypoglycemia unawareness** is potentially dangerous. The condition also occurs in patients with insulinomas and in diabetics receiving intensive insulin therapy, so it appears that repeated bouts of hypoglycemia cause the eventual development of hypoglycemia unawareness. If blood sugar rises again for some time, the warning symptoms again appear at a higher plasma glucose level than cognitive abnormalities and coma.

Symptomatic hypoglycemia also occurs in nondiabetics as well. Chronic mild hypoglycemia can cause incoordination and slurred speech, and the condition can be mistaken for drunkenness. Mental aberrations and convulsions in the absence of frank coma also occur. When the level of insulin secretion is chronically elevated by an **insulinoma,** a rare, insulin-secreting tumor of the pancreas, symptoms are most common in the morning.

In liver disease, the glucose tolerance curve is diabetic but the fasting plasma glucose level is low. In **functional hypoglycemia,** the plasma glucose rise is normal after a test dose of glucose, but the subsequent fall overshoots to hypoglycemic levels, producing symptoms 3–4 h after meals. This pattern is sometimes seen in prediabetic individuals in whom diabetes develops later.

DIABETES MELLITUS

The cause of clinical diabetes mellitus (DM) is always a deficiency of the effects of insulin at the tissue level, but the deficiency may be relative. One of the common forms, **type 1,** or **insulin-dependent diabetes mellitus (IDDM),** is due to insulin deficiency caused by autoimmune destruction of the β cells in the pancreatic islets. The second common form, **type 2 diabetes,** is characterized by insulin resistance, often accompanied by obesity and other characteristics of metabolic syndrome.

Type 1 DM usually develops before the age of 40 and is often called **juvenile diabetes.** Patients with this disease are not obese, and have a high incidence of ketosis and acidosis. Various anti-β cell antibodies are present in plasma, but the current thinking is that type 1 DM is primarily a T lymphocyte–mediated disease. Immunosuppression with drugs such as cyclosporine ameliorate type 1 diabetes if given early in the disease before all islet β cells are lost. β-cell transplant is becoming more common for individuals with type 1 DM and studies show the earlier in the disease the transplant is done, the better.

Type 2 is the most common type of DM and is usually associated with obesity. It usually develops after age 40, but may be present in obese children, and is associated with insulin resistance and increased insulin levels until later in the disease when the β cells become exhausted and fail to secrete insulin. It is rarely associated with ketosis.

OBESITY, THE METABOLIC SYNDROME, & TYPE 2 DIABETES

Obesity is increasing in incidence. As body weight increases, insulin resistance increases, such that there is decreased ability of insulin to move glucose into fat and muscle and to shut off glucose release from the liver. Weight reduction attenuates insulin resistance. Associated with obesity, there is hyperinsulinemia, dyslipidemia (characterized by high circulating triglycerides and low HDL), and accelerated development of atherosclerosis. This combination of findings is commonly called the **metabolic syndrome.** Some of the patients with the metabolic syndrome are prediabetic, that is, have hyperinsulinemia, but normal plasma glucose, whereas others have frank T2DM.

One possible signal for T2DM is the circulating level of FFAs, which is elevated in many insulin-resistant states. Other possibilities are peptides and proteins secreted by fat cells. White adipose tissue is an endocrine organ that secretes not only leptin, an antiorexigenic, but also other hormones that affect fat metabolism, known as **adipokines** as they are *cytokines* secreted by *adipose tissue.* Known adipokines are leptin, adiponectin, and resistin. Some adipokines decrease, rather than increase, insulin resistance. Leptin and adiponectin, for example, decrease insulin resistance, whereas resistin increases insulin resistance.

CHAPTER SUMMARY

- Four polypeptides with hormonal activity are secreted by the pancreas: insulin, glucagon, somatostatin, and pancreatic polypeptide.
- Insulin increases the entry of glucose into cells. In skeletal muscle cell it increases the number of GLUT-4 transporters in the cell membranes. In liver it induces glucokinase, which increases the phosphorylation of glucose, facilitating the entry of glucose into the cell.

- Insulin causes K^+ to enter cells, with a resultant lowering of the extracellular K^+ concentration. Insulin increases the activity of Na, K ATPase in cell membranes, so that more K^+ is pumped into cells. Hypokalemia often develops when patients with diabetic acidosis are treated with insulin.
- Insulin receptors are found on many different cells in the body and have two subunits, α and β. Binding of insulin to its receptor triggers a signaling pathway that involves autophosphorylation of the β subunits on tyrosine residues. This triggers phosphorylation of some cytoplasmic proteins and dephosphorylation of others, mostly on serine and threonine residues.
- The constellation of abnormalities caused by insulin deficiency is called diabetes mellitus. Type 1 diabetes is due to insulin deficiency caused by autoimmune destruction of the B cells in the pancreatic islets. Type 2 diabetes is characterized by the dysregulation of insulin release from the B cells, along with insulin resistance in peripheral tissues such as skeletal muscle, brain, and liver.

MULTIPLE-CHOICE QUESTIONS

For all questions, select the single best answer unless otherwise directed.

1. A 48-year-old man with type 1 diabetes mellitus injects himself with insulin. Insulin increases the entry of glucose into what tissues?
   A. Renal tubular cells
   B. Mucosa of the small intestine
   C. Skeletal muscle
   D. All of the above

2. A meal rich in proteins containing the amino acids that stimulate insulin secretion but low in carbohydrates does not cause hypoglycemia because
   A. the meal causes a compensatory increase in T_4 secretion.
   B. cortisol in the circulation prevents glucose from entering muscle.
   C. glucagon secretion is also stimulated by the meal.
   D. the amino acids in the meal are promptly converted to glucose.
   E. insulin does not bind to insulin receptors if the plasma concentration of amino acids is elevated.

3. A 20-year-old man with known type 1 DM visits his physician because he was feeling unwell. On physical examination, he was found have deep, rapid respirations, and he was immediately sent to the ED. What abnormality did the physician correctly identify from the physical symptoms?
   A. Metabolic alkalosis
   B. Metabolic acidosis
   C. Pulmonary congestion
   D. Hypercapnia
   E. Hypoxia

4. A diabetic checks his blood glucose before and after exercise and find a significant reduction in the glucose levels. What type of cells in the body mostly responsible for this responsible and what cell membrane glucose transporter do they express?
   A. Muscle; GLUT-2
   B. Liver; GLUT-2
   C. Muscle; GLUT-4
   D. Liver; GLUT-4
   E. Brain; GLUT-4
   F. Adipose; GLUT-1

5. A 32-year-old woman who has type 2 diabetes and is in the 34th week of gestation is brought to the ED with premature contractions. She has not been taking any medications since the beginning of her pregnancy except prenatal vitamins. Vaginal delivery is done and the neonate's length is more than 80 percentile and weight is more than 95 percentile. What condition is the neonate most likely at risk for in the next few days after delivery?
   A. Hypoglycemia
   B. Necrotizing enterocolitis
   C. Glaucoma
   D. Hyperglycemia
   E. Intracranial hemorrhage

6. A 40-year-old man is complaining of right upper quadrant abdominal pain and fullness is diagnosed with somatostatinoma. What would her lab work look like upon diagnosis?
   A. Increased insulin; decreased glucagon; decreased glucose
   B. Increased insulin; increased glucagon; decreased glucose
   C. Decreased insulin; decreased glucagon; increased glucose
   D. Increased insulin; increased glucagon; increased glucose
   E. Decreased insulin; increased glucagon; increased glucose
   F. Decreased insulin; decreased glucagon; decreased glucose

7. A 45-year-old mechanic was found caught under a car that fell on him in his workshop and suffered from crush injuries. While hospitalized, he developed acute kidney injury. His lab work shows he has an increase creatine kinase and an abnormal ECG along with other abnormalities. The man is started on insulin in order to help treat which complication expected to result from his condition?
   A. Hyperglycemia
   B. Myoglobinemia
   C. Acute kidney injury
   D. Hyperkalemia

8. A 50-year-old man is brought to the ED in a coma. Several of his lab values are abnormal. Which of the following would reduce insulin secretion from β cells of the pancreas thus worsening his condition?
   A. Hyperglycemia
   B. Acidosis
   C. Hypokalemia
   D. Hyperglucagonemia

9. A 10-year-old boy is diagnosed with type 1 diabetes. What cell types will maintain normal glucose uptake in his body?
   A. RBCs
   B. Adipocytes
   C. Skeletal muscle cells
   D. Smooth muscle cells
   E. Liver cells

10. A physician decides to switch his diabetic patients to a new sulfonylurea that has just come on the market. Which of the following patients would have no effect from the drug?
   A. A 60-year-old man with type 2 diabetes
   B. A 15-year-old girl with type 2 diabetes
   C. A 65-year-old woman with type 2 diabetes and a partial pancreatectomy
   D. A 30-year-old man with type 1 diabetes

ANSWERS

1. Answer is **D.** Insulin causes glucose uptake in most tissues via GLUT-4 transporter, with the exceptions of liver and brain. In the kidney, the SGLT transporters are responsible for glucose uptake in tubules.

2. Answer is **C.** A high-protein meal increases both insulin and glucagon so that blood sugar remains stable.

3. Answer is **B.** The man has diabetic ketoacidosis. The increased respiratory rate an attempt to blow off the CO_2 that was associated with elevated glucose and acidosis.

4. Answer is **C.** Muscle cells contain GLUT-4 transporters that localize to the cell surface in response to insulin. Exercise can also activate GLUT-4 transporters in skeletal muscles via AMP-protein kinase causing an increase in uptake of glucose and decrease in blood glucose.

5. Answer is **A.** The baby has macrosomia due to elevated blood glucose from his mother. This will cause hyperinsulinemia in the neonate to compensate and without the elevated glucose continuing after delivery, the elevated insulin will cause hypoglycemia.

6. Answer is **C.** Somatostatin causes increase in glucose release and inhibits both insulin and glucagon release. These consequences would cause hyperglycemia.

7. Answer is **D.** The man has developed rhabdomyolysis as a result of muscle damage from his traumatic injuries. As renal function is compromised, the kidneys lose the ability to modulate potassium excretion and increased plasma potassium can occur which would first be detected by abnormal ECG. Insulin causes potassium to be reabsorbed into cells and thus cause a reduction in plasma potassium and prevent arrhythmias.

8. Answer is **C.** Potassium depletion inhibits insulin release from β cells. Hyperglycemia would stimulate insulin secretion. Acidosis is a consequence of low insulin and hyperglycemia and would stimulate insulin secretion. Hyperglucagonemia would also stimulate insulin secretion in an attempt to normalize insulin-glucagon molarities.

9. Answer is **A.** RBCs are insulin independent and glucose uptake remains normal even with no insulin produced. Glucose transport in RBCs is via GLUT-1 rather than the typical GLUT-4.

10. Answer is **D.** Sulfonylureas activate KATP channels in pancreatic β cells to depolarize the cell membranes cause opening of voltage-gated Ca^{++} channels increasing insulin secretion by exocytosis. This process doesn't work in type 1 diabetics since their β cells do not synthesize insulin.

SECTION IV GASTROINTESTINAL PHYSIOLOGY

For unicellular organisms, nutritional requirements can be satisfied by membrane transport proteins that permit the uptake of specific molecules. However, for multicellular organisms, the challenges of delivering nutrients to appropriate sites in the body are significantly greater. Further, most of the food we eat is in the form of macromolecules, and even when these are digested, most of the end products are water-soluble and do not readily cross cell membranes. Thus, the gastrointestinal system has evolved to permit nutrient acquisition and assimilation into the body, while prohibiting the uptake of undesirable substances.

The intestine is a continuous tube that extends from mouth to anus and is formally contiguous with the external environment. A single layer of epithelial cells comprises the semipermeable barrier across which controlled uptake of nutrients takes place. Various glandular structures empty into the intestinal lumen along its length, providing for digestion of food components, signaling to distal segments, and regulation of the intestinal microbiota. Motility functions move the intestinal contents and resulting waste products along the length of the gut, and a rich innervation regulates motility, secretion, and nutrient uptake, in many cases independent of the central nervous system. There are also many endocrine cells that release hormones that work together with neurotransmitters to coordinate overall regulation of the gastrointestinal system. In general, there is considerable redundancy of control systems as well as excess capacity for nutrient digestion and uptake. This served humans well in ancient times but may now contribute to the modern epidemic of obesity.

The liver, while playing important roles in whole body metabolism, is usually considered a part of the gastrointestinal system for two main reasons. First, it provides for excretion from the body of lipid-soluble waste products that cannot enter the urine. Second, the blood flow draining the intestine is arranged such that substances that are absorbed pass first through the liver, allowing for the removal and metabolism of any toxins that have been taken up, as well as clearance of particulates, such as small numbers of enteric bacteria.

In this section, the function of the gastrointestinal system and liver will be considered, and the ways in which the various segments communicate to provide an integrated response to a meal. The relevance of gastrointestinal physiology for the development of digestive diseases will also be considered. Digestive diseases represent a substantial burden in terms of morbidity and lost productivity. A 2009 report of the US National Institutes of Diabetes, Digestive and Kidney Diseases found that on an annual basis, for every 100 US residents, there were 35 ambulatory care visits and nearly five overnight hospital stays that involved a gastrointestinal diagnosis. Digestive diseases also appear to be increasing in this population (although mortality, principally from cancers, is thankfully in decline). On the other hand, digestive diseases, and in particular infectious diarrhea, remain important causes of mortality in developing countries where clean sources of food and water cannot be ensured.

Overview of Gastrointestinal Function & Regulation

OBJECTIVES

After studying this chapter, you should be able to:

- Understand the functional significance of the gastrointestinal system, and in particular, its roles in nutrient assimilation, excretion, and immunity.
- Describe the structure of the gastrointestinal tract, the glands that drain into it, and its subdivision into functional segments.
- List the major gastrointestinal secretions, their components, and the stimuli that regulate their production.
- Describe water balance in the gastrointestinal tract and explain how the level of luminal fluidity is adjusted.
- Identify the major hormones, other peptides, and key neurotransmitters of the gastrointestinal system.
- Describe the special features of the enteric nervous system and the splanchnic circulation.

INTRODUCTION

The primary function of the gastrointestinal tract is to serve as a portal whereby nutrients and water can be absorbed into the body. In fulfilling this function, the meal is mixed with a variety of secretions from the gastrointestinal tract itself and organs that drain into it, such as the pancreas, gallbladder, and salivary glands. Likewise, the intestine displays motility patterns that mix the meal with digestive secretions and move it along the length of the gastrointestinal tract. Ultimately, residues of the meal that cannot be absorbed, along with cellular debris, are expelled from the body. All of these functions are tightly regulated via mechanisms that act both locally and over long distances to coordinate the function of the gut and the organs that drain into it.

STRUCTURAL CONSIDERATIONS

The parts of the gastrointestinal tract that are encountered by the meal or its residues include, in order, the mouth, esophagus, stomach, duodenum, jejunum, ileum, cecum, colon, rectum, and anus. Throughout the length of the intestine, glandular structures deliver secretions into the lumen. Also important in the process of digestion are secretions from the pancreas and the biliary system of the liver. The intestine has a very substantial surface area, which is important for its absorptive function. The intestinal tract is functionally divided into segments by means of muscle rings known as **sphincters,** which restrict the flow of intestinal contents to optimize digestion and absorption. These sphincters include the upper and lower esophageal sphincters, the pylorus that retards emptying of the stomach, the ileocecal valve that retains colonic contents in the large intestine, and the inner and outer anal sphincters.

The intestine is composed of functional layers. Immediately adjacent to nutrients in the lumen is a single layer of columnar epithelial cells. Below the epithelium is a layer of loose connective tissue known as the lamina propria, which in turn is surrounded by circular and longitudinal muscle layers. The intestine is also amply supplied with blood vessels, nerve endings, and lymphatics.

The epithelium of the intestine is also further specialized in a way that maximizes its surface area. Throughout the small intestine, it is folded into fingerlike projections called villi. Between the villi are infoldings known as crypts. Stem cells that give rise to both crypt and villus epithelial cells reside toward the base of the crypts and are responsible for renewing the epithelium every few days. Daughter cells undergo several rounds of cell division in the crypts then migrate out onto the villi, where they are eventually shed and lost in the stool. Villus epithelial cells are also notable for the extensive microvilli that characterize their apical membranes. These microvilli are endowed with a dense glycocalyx (the brush border) that probably protects the cells to some extent from the effects of digestive enzymes. Some digestive enzymes are membrane-bound proteins. These so-called "brush border hydrolases" perform the final steps of digestion for specific nutrients.

■ GASTROINTESTINAL SECRETIONS

SALIVARY SECRETION

The first secretion encountered when food is ingested is saliva. Saliva is produced by three pairs of salivary glands that drain into the oral cavity. It has a number of organic constituents that serve to initiate digestion and protect the oral cavity from bacteria. Saliva also serves to lubricate the food bolus. Saliva is hypotonic compared to plasma and alkaline; the latter feature is important to neutralize any gastric secretions that reflux into the esophagus.

The salivary glands consist of acini that produce a secretion containing the organic constituents dissolved in a fluid that is essentially identical to plasma in terms of its electrolyte content. The salivary glands can secrete their own weight in saliva every minute. To accomplish this, they are richly endowed with surrounding blood vessels that dilate when secretion is initiated. The composition of the saliva is modified as it flows from the acini out into ducts that eventually coalesce and deliver the saliva into the mouth. Na^+ and Cl^- are extracted and K^+ and bicarbonate are added. Because the ducts are relatively impermeable to water, the loss of NaCl renders the saliva hypotonic, particularly at low secretion rates. As the rate of secretion increases, there is less time for NaCl to be extracted and the tonicity of the saliva rises, but it always stays somewhat hypotonic. Overall, the salivary glands supply 1000–1500 mL of saliva per day.

Salivary secretion is primarily controlled by parasympathetic neural influences (Figure 25–1). Sympathetic input slightly increases proteinaceous content of saliva but has little influence on volume. Secretion is triggered by reflexes that are stimulated by chewing, but is actually initiated even before the meal is taken into the mouth via central triggers that are prompted by thinking about, seeing, or smelling food. Salivary secretion is also prompted by nausea but inhibited by fear or during sleep.

Saliva performs a number of important functions: it facilitates swallowing, keeps the mouth moist, serves as a solvent for the molecules that stimulate the taste buds, aids speech, and keeps the mouth and teeth clean. Saliva also has some antibacterial action, and patients with deficient salivation (**xerostomia**) have an increased incidence of dental caries.

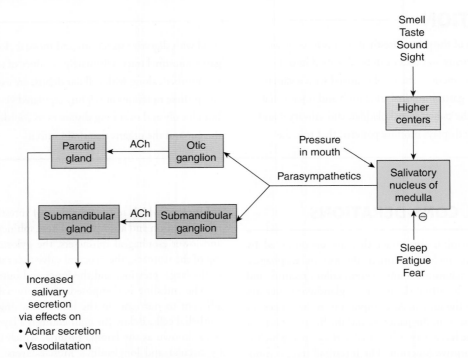

FIGURE 25–1 **Regulation of salivary secretion by the parasympathetic nervous system.** ACh, acetylcholine. Saliva is also produced by the sublingual glands (not depicted), but these are a minor contributor to both resting and stimulated salivary flows. (Adapted with permission from Barrett KE: *Gastrointestinal Physiology*. New York: McGraw-Hill; 2006.)

GASTRIC SECRETION

Food is stored in the stomach; mixed with acid, mucus, and pepsin; and released at a controlled, steady rate into the duodenum (Clinical Box 25–1).

ANATOMIC CONSIDERATIONS

The gross anatomy of the stomach is shown in Figure 25–2. The gastric mucosa contains many deep glands. In the cardia and the pyloric region, the glands secrete mucus. In the body of the stomach, including the fundus, the glands also contain **parietal cells,** which secrete hydrochloric acid and intrinsic factor, and **chief cells,** which secrete pepsinogens. These secretions mix with mucus secreted by the cells in the necks of the glands. Several of the glands open onto a **gastric pit** that opens in turn onto the surface of the mucosa. Mucus is also secreted along with HCO_3^- by mucus cells on the surface of the epithelium between glands.

The stomach has a very rich blood and lymphatic supply. Its parasympathetic nerve supply comes from the vagi and its sympathetic supply from the celiac plexus.

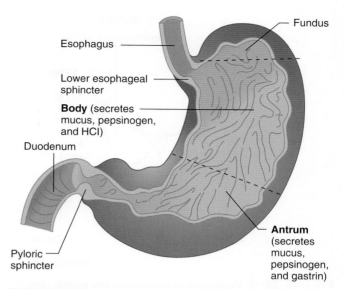

FIGURE 25–2 Anatomy of the stomach. The principal secretions of the body and antrum are listed in parentheses. (Reproduced with permission from Widmaier EP, Raff H, Strang KT: *Vander's Human Physiology: The Mechanisms of Body Function,* 11th ed. McGraw-Hill, 2008.)

CLINICAL BOX 25–1

Peptic Ulcer Disease

Gastric and duodenal ulceration in humans is related primarily to a breakdown of the barrier that normally prevents irritation and autodigestion of the mucosa by the gastric secretions. Infection with the bacterium *Helicobacter pylori* disrupts this barrier, as do aspirin and other nonsteroidal anti-inflammatory drugs (NSAIDs), which inhibit the production of prostaglandins and consequently decrease mucus and HCO_3^- secretion. An additional cause of ulceration is prolonged excess secretion of acid. An example of this is the ulcers that occur in **Zollinger–Ellison syndrome.** This syndrome is seen in patients with gastrinomas. The gastrin causes prolonged hypersecretion of acid, and severe ulcers are produced.

THERAPEUTIC HIGHLIGHTS

Gastric and duodenal ulcers can be given a chance to heal by inhibition of acid secretion with drugs such as omeprazole that inhibit H^+–K^+ ATPase ("proton pump inhibitors"). If present, *H. pylori* can be eradicated with antibiotics, and NSAID-induced ulcers can be treated by stopping the NSAID or, when this is not advisable, by treatment with the prostaglandin agonist misoprostol. Gastrinomas can sometimes be removed surgically.

ORIGIN & REGULATION OF GASTRIC SECRETION

The stomach adds a significant volume of digestive juices to the meal. Like salivary secretion, the stomach readies itself to receive the meal before it is actually taken in, during the so-called cephalic phase that can be influenced by food preferences. Subsequently, there is a gastric phase of secretion that is quantitatively the most significant, and finally an intestinal phase once the meal has left the stomach. Each phase is closely regulated by both local and distant triggers.

The gastric secretions arise from the glands and also from the surface cells that secrete mucus and bicarbonate to protect the stomach from digesting itself, as well as trefoil peptides that stabilize the mucus-bicarbonate layer. The glandular secretions of the stomach differ in different regions. The most characteristic secretions derive from the glands in the fundus or body of the stomach. The acid secreted by parietal cells serves to sterilize the meal and also begins hydrolysis of dietary macromolecules. Intrinsic factor is important for the later absorption of vitamin B_{12}, or cobalamin. Pepsinogen is the precursor of pepsin, which initiates protein digestion. Lipase similarly begins the digestion of dietary fats.

There are three primary stimuli of gastric secretion (Figure 25–3). Gastrin is a hormone released by G cells in the antrum in response to a specific neurotransmitter released from enteric nerve endings known as gastrin-releasing peptide (GRP) or bombesin, and also in response to oligopeptides in the gastric lumen. Gastrin is carried through the bloodstream to the fundic glands, where it binds to receptors on parietal and chief cells to activate secretion, but also on so-called enterochromaffin-like cells (ECL cells) located in the gland, which release histamine.

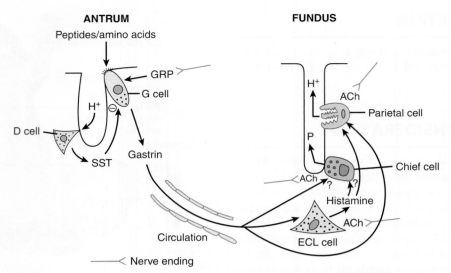

FIGURE 25-3 **Regulation of gastric acid and pepsin secretion by soluble mediators and neural input.** Gastrin is released from G cells in the antrum in response to gastrin-releasing peptide (GRP) and travels through the circulation to influence the activity of enterochromaffin-like (ECL) cells and parietal cells. ECL cells release histamine, which also acts on parietal cells. Acetylcholine (ACh), released from nerves, is an agonist for ECL cells, chief cells, and parietal cells. Other specific agonists of the chief cell are not well understood. Gastrin release is negatively regulated by luminal acidity via the release of somatostatin from antral D cells. P, pepsinogen. (Adapted with permission from Barrett KE: *Gastrointestinal Physiology.* New York: McGraw-Hill; 2006.)

Histamine also triggers parietal cell secretion, via H_2-receptors. Finally, parietal and chief cells can also be stimulated by acetylcholine, released from enteric nerve endings.

Gastric secretion during the cephalic phase is activated predominantly by vagal input from the brain region known as the dorsal vagal complex, which coordinates input from higher centers. Vagal outflow to the stomach then releases GRP and acetylcholine, initiating secretory function. However, before the meal enters the stomach, there are few additional triggers and secretion is limited. Once the meal is swallowed, its constituents trigger substantial release of gastrin and its physical presence also distends the stomach and activates stretch receptors, which provoke a "vago-vagal" as well as local reflexes that further amplify secretion during the gastric phase. The presence of the meal also buffers gastric acidity that would otherwise feedback to shut off secretion secondary to the release of somatostatin (**Figure 25–3**). The latter probably represents a key mechanism whereby gastric secretion is terminated after the meal moves into the small intestine.

Gastric parietal cells are highly specialized for their task of secreting acid. They are packed with mitochondria that supply energy to drive the apical H^+, K^+-ATPase that moves H^+ ions out of the parietal cell. At rest, the proton pumps are sequestered within membrane compartments known as tubulovesicles. When the cell begins to secrete, these vesicles fuse with invaginations of the apical membrane known as canaliculi, thereby amplifying the apical membrane area and positioning the proton pumps to begin acid secretion. The apical membrane also contains potassium and chloride channels. The secretion of protons is accompanied by the release of equivalent numbers of bicarbonate ions into the bloodstream, which are later used to neutralize gastric acidity once its function is complete.

Gastrin, histamine, and acetylcholine bind to distinct receptors on the parietal cell basolateral membrane. Gastrin and acetylcholine promote secretion via cytosolic calcium, whereas histamine increases intracellular cyclic adenosine 3′,5′-monophosphate (cAMP). These two distinct pathways for cell activation are synergistic, with a greater than additive effect on secretion rates when histamine plus gastrin or acetylcholine, or all three, are present simultaneously. Thus, high rates of secretion can be stimulated with relatively small changes in each of the stimuli. Synergism is also therapeutically significant because secretion can be markedly inhibited by blocking the action of only one of the triggers.

Gastric secretion adds about 2.5 L/day to the intestinal contents. However, despite their substantial volume and fine control, gastric secretions are dispensable for the full digestion and absorption of a meal, with the exception of cobalamin absorption. However, if gastric secretion is chronically reduced, individuals may display increased susceptibility to infection via the oral route.

PANCREATIC SECRETION

Pancreatic juice contains enzymes that are of major importance in digestion (**Table 25–1**). Its secretion is controlled by both reflexes and the hormones secretin and cholecystokinin (CCK).

ANATOMIC CONSIDERATIONS

The portion of the pancreas that secretes pancreatic juice resembles the salivary glands. Granules containing digestive enzymes (**zymogen granules**) are formed in acinar cells and discharged by exocytosis into the pancreatic ducts. The common duct opens

TABLE 25–1 Principal digestive enzymes.[a]

Source	Enzyme	Activator	Substrate	Catalytic Function or Products
Salivary glands	Salivary α-amylase	Cl⁻	Starch	Hydrolyzes 1:4α linkages, producing α-limit dextrins, maltotriose, and maltose
Stomach	Pepsins (pepsinogens)	HCl	Proteins and polypeptides	Cleave peptide bonds adjacent to aromatic amino acids
	Gastric lipase		Triglycerides	Fatty acids, monoglycerides and glycerol
Exocrine pancreas	Trypsin (trypsinogen)	Enteropeptidase	Proteins and polypeptides	Cleave peptide bonds on carboxyl side of basic amino acids (arginine or lysine)
	Chymotrypsins (chymotrypsinogens)	Trypsin	Proteins and polypeptides	Cleave peptide bonds on carboxyl side of aromatic amino acids
	Elastase (proelastase)	Trypsin	Elastin, some other proteins	Cleaves bonds on carboxyl side of aliphatic amino acids
	Carboxypeptidase A (procarboxypeptidase A)	Trypsin	Proteins and polypeptides	Cleave carboxyl terminal amino acids that have aromatic or branched aliphatic side chains
	Carboxypeptidase B (procarboxypeptidase B)	Trypsin	Proteins and polypeptides	Cleave carboxyl terminal amino acids that have basic side chains
	Colipase (procolipase)	Trypsin	Fat droplets	Binds pancreatic lipase to oil droplet in the presence of bile acids
	Pancreatic lipase	…	Triglycerides	Monoglycerides and fatty acids
	Cholesteryl ester hydrolase	…	Cholesteryl esters	Cholesterol
	Pancreatic α-amylase	Cl⁻	Starch	Same as salivary α-amylase
	Ribonuclease	…	RNA	Nucleotides
	Deoxyribonuclease	…	DNA	Nucleotides
	Phospholipase A₂ (prophospholipase A₂)	Trypsin	Phospholipids	Fatty acids, lysophospholipids
Intestinal mucosa	Enteropeptidase	…	Trypsinogen	Trypsin
	Aminopeptidases	…	Polypeptides	Cleave amino terminal amino acid from peptide
	Carboxypeptidases	…	Polypeptides	Cleave carboxyl terminal amino acid from peptide
	Endopeptidases	…	Polypeptides	Cleave between residues in midportion of peptide
	Dipeptidases	…	Dipeptides	Two amino acids
	Maltase	…	Maltose, maltotriose	Glucose
	Lactase	…	Lactose	Galactose and glucose
	Sucrase[b]	…	Sucrose; also maltotriose and maltose	Fructose and glucose
	Isomaltase[b]	…	α-Limit dextrins, maltose, maltotriose	Glucose
	Nuclease and related enzymes	…	Nucleic acids	Pentoses and purine and pyrimidine bases
Cytoplasm of mucosal cells	Various peptidases	…	Di-, tri-, and tetrapeptides	Amino acids

[a]Corresponding proenzymes, where relevant, are shown in parentheses.

[b]Sucrase and isomaltase are separate subunits of a single protein.

through the duodenal papilla, and its orifice is encircled by the sphincter of Oddi.

COMPOSITION OF PANCREATIC JUICE

The pancreatic juice is alkaline and has a high HCO_3^- content (approximately 113 mEq/L vs 24 mEq/L in plasma). About 1500 mL of pancreatic juice are secreted per day. Bile and intestinal juices are also neutral or alkaline, and these three secretions neutralize the gastric acid, raising the pH of the duodenal contents to 6.0–7.0. By the time the chyme reaches the jejunum, its pH is nearly neutral.

The pancreatic juice also contains digestive enzymes that are mostly released in inactive forms and only activated when they reach the intestinal lumen (see Chapter 26). They are activated following proteolytic cleavage by trypsin, itself a pancreatic protease released as an inactive precursor (trypsinogen). Release of a small amount of trypsin into the pancreas would be dangerous; the resulting chain reaction could produce active enzymes that digest the pancreas. Another enzyme activated by trypsin is phospholipase A_2. This enzyme splits a fatty acid off phosphatidylcholine (PC), forming lyso-PC that can damage cell membranes. The pancreas thus also normally secretes a trypsin inhibitor.

Small amounts of pancreatic enzymes normally leak into the circulation, but in acute pancreatitis, their circulating levels rise markedly. Measurement of plasma amylase or lipase is therefore of value in diagnosing the disease.

REGULATION OF THE SECRETION OF PANCREATIC JUICE

Pancreatic secretion is primarily under hormonal control. Secretin acts on the ducts to cause copious secretion of a very alkaline juice that is poor in enzymes. The effect on duct cells is via cAMP. Secretin also stimulates bile secretion. CCK acts on the acinar cells to release zymogen granules and produce pancreatic juice rich in enzymes but low in volume. Its effect is mediated by calcium (see Chapter 2).

As the volume of pancreatic secretion increases in response to secretin, its Cl^- concentration falls and its HCO_3^- concentration increases. Although HCO_3^- is secreted in the small ducts, it is reabsorbed in the large ducts in exchange for Cl^-. The magnitude of the exchange is inversely proportional to the rate of flow.

Like CCK, acetylcholine acts on acinar cells via phospholipase C to cause discharge of zymogen granules, and stimulation of the vagi causes secretion of a small amount of pancreatic juice rich in enzymes. Vagally mediated reflex secretion of pancreatic juice may occur in response to the sight or smell of food.

BILIARY SECRETION

Bile arises from the liver, and the bile acids it contains are important in the digestion and absorption of fats. Bile also serves as a critical excretory fluid to dispose of lipid-soluble end products of metabolism, and xenobiotics. Bile is also the only route by which the body can dispose of cholesterol.

Bile

Bile is made up of the bile acids, bile pigments, and other substances in an alkaline solution that resembles pancreatic juice. About 500 mL is secreted per day. Some of the components of the bile are reabsorbed in the intestine and then excreted again by the liver (**enterohepatic circulation).**

The glucuronides of the **bile pigments,** bilirubin and biliverdin, are responsible for the golden yellow color of bile. The formation of these is discussed in Chapter 28.

When considering bile as a digestive secretion, **bile acids** are the most important components. They are synthesized from cholesterol and secreted into the bile conjugated to glycine or taurine. The four major bile acids found in humans are listed

| | Group at position | | | Percent in |
	3	7	12	human bile
Cholic acid	OH	OH	OH	50
Chenodeoxycholic acid	OH	OH	H	30
Deoxycholic acid	OH	H	OH	15
Lithocholic acid	OH	H	H	5

FIGURE 25–4   Human bile acids. The numbers in the formula for cholic acid refer to the positions in the steroid ring.

in **Figure 25–4.** Bile acids contain the steroid nucleus (see Chapter 20). The two primary bile acids formed in the liver are cholic acid and chenodeoxycholic acid. In the colon, bacteria convert them to the secondary bile acids deoxycholic acid and lithocholic acid, respectively. In addition, small quantities of ursodeoxycholic acid are formed from chenodeoxycholic acid.

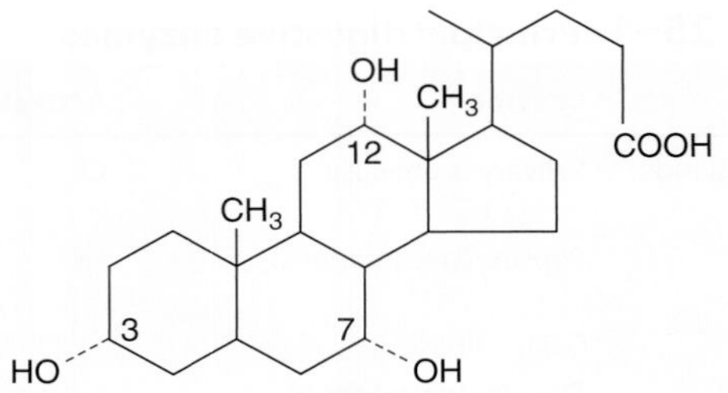

Bile acids have a number of important actions: they reduce surface tension and, in conjunction with phospholipids and monoglycerides, are responsible for the emulsification of fat preparatory to its digestion and absorption (see Chapter 26). They are **amphipathic,** that is, they have both hydrophilic and hydrophobic domains. Therefore, the bile acids tend to form cylindrical disks called **micelles** where the hydrophilic portions face out and the hydrophobic portions face in. Above the **critical micelle concentration,** all bile salts added to a solution form micelles. Ninety to 95% of the bile acids are absorbed from the small intestine. Once they are deconjugated, they can be absorbed by nonionic diffusion, but most are absorbed in their conjugated forms from the terminal ileum (**Figure 25–5**) by a Na^+–bile salt cotransport system (ABST). The remaining 5–10% of the bile salts enter the colon and are converted to deoxycholic acid and lithocholic acid. Lithocholate is relatively insoluble and is mostly excreted in the stools; only 1% is absorbed. However, deoxycholate is absorbed. The absorbed bile acids are transported back to the liver in the portal vein and re-excreted in the bile (Figure 25–5). Those lost in the stool are replaced by synthesis; the normal rate of synthesis is 0.2–0.4 g/day. The total bile acid pool of approximately 3.5 g recycles repeatedly, likely twice per meal and 6–8 times per day.

INTESTINAL FLUID & ELECTROLYTE TRANSPORT

The intestine itself also supplies a fluid environment in which the processes of digestion and absorption can occur. Then, when the meal has been assimilated, the fluid used is reclaimed by transport

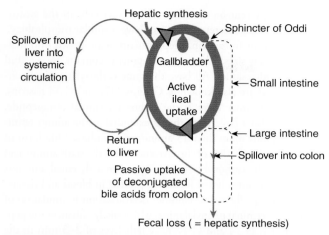

FIGURE 25–5 Quantitative aspects of the circulation of bile acids. The majority of the bile acid pool circulates between the small intestine and liver. A minority of the bile acid pool is in the systemic circulation (due to incomplete hepatocyte uptake from the portal blood) or spills over into the colon and is lost to the stool. Fecal loss must be equivalent to hepatic synthesis of bile acids at steady state. (Adapted with permission from Barrett KE: *Gastrointestinal Physiology.* New York: McGraw-Hill; 2006.)

back across the epithelium to avoid dehydration. Water moves passively into and out of the gastrointestinal lumen, driven by electrochemical gradients established by the active transport of ions and other solutes. The intestines are presented each day with about 2000 mL of ingested fluid plus 7000 mL of secretions from the mucosa of the gastrointestinal tract and associated glands. Ninety-eight percent of this fluid is reabsorbed, with a daily fluid loss of only 200 mL in the stools.

In the small intestine, secondary active transport of Na^+ is important in bringing about absorption of glucose, some amino acids, and other substances such as bile acids (see above). Conversely, the presence of glucose in the intestinal lumen facilitates the reabsorption of Na^+. In the period between meals, when nutrients are not present, sodium and chloride are absorbed together from the lumen by the coupled activity of a sodium/ hydrogen exchanger (NHE) and chloride/bicarbonate exchanger in the apical membrane, in a so-called electroneutral mechanism. Water follows to maintain osmotic balance. In the colon, an additional electrogenic mechanism for sodium absorption is expressed, particularly in the distal colon. In this mechanism, sodium enters across the apical membrane via epithelial sodium channels (ENaC). This underpins the ability of the colon to desiccate the stool and ensure that only a small portion of the fluid load used daily is lost from the body.

Despite the predominance of absorptive mechanisms, secretion also takes place continuously throughout the small intestine and colon to adjust the local fluidity of the intestinal contents as needed. Cl^- normally enters enterocytes from the interstitial fluid via Na^+–K^+–$2Cl^-$ cotransporters in their basolateral membranes, and the Cl^- is secreted into the intestinal lumen via channels that are regulated by various protein kinases. The cystic fibrosis

transmembrane conductance regulator (CFTR) channel is quantitatively most important, and is activated by protein kinase A and hence by cAMP (Clinical Box 25–2).

Water moves into or out of the intestine until the osmotic pressure of the intestinal contents equals that of the plasma. The osmolality of the duodenal contents may be hypertonic or hypotonic, depending on the meal ingested, but by the time the meal enters the jejunum, its osmolality is close to that of plasma. This osmolality is maintained throughout the rest of the small intestine. In the colon, Na^+ is pumped out and water moves passively with it, again along the osmotic gradient.

CLINICAL BOX 25–2

Cholera

Cholera is a severe secretory diarrheal disease that often occurs in epidemics associated with natural disasters. Along with other secretory diarrheal illnesses produced by bacteria and viruses, cholera causes a significant amount of morbidity and mortality. The cAMP concentration in intestinal epithelial cells is increased in cholera. The cholera bacillus stays in the intestinal lumen, but it produces a toxin that binds to GM-1 ganglioside receptors on the apical membrane of intestinal epithelial cells, and this permits part of the A subunit (A[1] peptide) of the toxin to enter the cell. The A[1] peptide binds adenosine diphosphate ribose to the α subunit of G_s, inhibiting its GTPase activity (see Chapter 2). Therefore, the constitutively activated G-protein produces a prolonged increase in intracellular cAMP. In addition to increased Cl^- secretion, the function of the mucosal NHE transporter for Na^+ is reduced, thus reducing NaCl absorption. The resultant increase in electrolyte and water content of the intestinal contents causes the diarrhea. However, Na, K ATPase, and the Na^+/glucose cotransporter are unaffected, so coupled reabsorption of glucose and Na^+ bypasses the defect.

THERAPEUTIC HIGHLIGHTS

Treatment for cholera is mostly supportive, since the infection will eventually clear. The most important therapeutic approach is to ensure that the large amounts of fluid and electrolytes lost to the stool are replaced. When sterile supplies are available, fluids and electrolytes can most conveniently be replaced intravenously. However, this is often not possible in the setting of an epidemic. Instead, the persistent activity of the Na^+/glucose cotransporter provides a physiologic basis for the treatment of Na^+ and water loss by oral administration of solutions containing NaCl and glucose. Oral rehydration solution, a pre-packaged mixture of sugar and salt to be dissolved in water, is a simple remedy that has dramatically reduced mortality in epidemics of cholera and other diarrheal diseases.

Some K^+ is secreted into the intestinal lumen via K^+ channels, especially as a component of mucus. The accumulation of K^+ in the colon is partially offset by H^+–K^+ ATPase in the luminal membrane of cells in the distal colon, with resulting active transport of K^+ into the cells. Nevertheless, loss of ileal or colonic fluids in chronic diarrhea can lead to severe hypokalemia.

GASTROINTESTINAL REGULATION

The various functions of the gastrointestinal tract, including secretion, digestion, and absorption (Chapter 26), and motility (Chapter 27), must be regulated in an integrated way to ensure efficient assimilation of nutrients. There are three main modalities for gastrointestinal regulation that operate in a complementary fashion. First, **endocrine** regulation is mediated by the release of hormones. These hormones travel through the bloodstream to change the activity of a distant segment of the gastrointestinal tract, an organ draining into it (eg, the pancreas), or both. Second, some mediators are not sufficiently stable to persist in the bloodstream, but instead alter the function of cells in the local area where they are released, in a **paracrine** fashion. Finally, the intestinal system is endowed with extensive neural connections. These include connections to the central nervous system (**extrinsic innervation),** but also the activity of the **enteric nervous system.** The enteric nervous system integrates central input to the gut but can also regulate gut function independently.

HORMONES/PARACRINES

Biologically active polypeptides act in a paracrine fashion, but may also enter the circulation. Measurement of their concentrations in blood after a meal has shed light on the roles these **gastrointestinal hormones** play in the regulation of gastrointestinal function.

The physiologic effects of these hormones appear to be relatively discrete. On the basis of structural similarity and, to a degree, similarity of function, the key hormones fall into two families: the gastrin family, the primary members of which are gastrin and CCK; and the secretin family, the primary members of which are secretin, glucagon, vasoactive intestinal peptide (VIP; actually a neurotransmitter, or neurocrine), and gastric inhibitory polypeptide (also known as glucose-dependent insulinotropic peptide, or GIP).

ENTEROENDOCRINE CELLS

More than 15 types of hormone-secreting **enteroendocrine cells** have been identified in the mucosa of the stomach, small intestine, and colon. Many of these secrete only one hormone and are identified by letters (G cells, S cells, etc). Others manufacture serotonin or histamine and are called **ECL cells,** respectively.

GASTRIN

Gastrin is produced by G cells in the antral portion of the gastric mucosa. Microvilli project from the apical end of G cells into the lumen. Receptors mediating gastrin responses to changes in gastric contents are present on the microvilli. Other cells in the gastrointestinal tract that secrete hormones have a similar morphology.

The precursor for gastrin, preprogastrin, is processed into fragments of various sizes. Three main fragments contain 34, 17, and 14 amino acid residues. All have the same carboxyl terminal configuration, and are also known as G 34, G 17, and G 14 gastrins, respectively. Another form is the carboxyl terminal tetrapeptide, and there is also a large form that is extended at the amino terminal and contains more than 45 amino acid residues. One form of derivatization is sulfation of the tyrosine that is the sixth amino acid residue from the carboxyl terminal. Approximately equal amounts of nonsulfated and sulfated forms are present in blood and tissues, and they are equally active. Another derivatization is amidation of the carboxyl terminal phenylalanine, which likely enhances the peptide's stability. G 14 and G 17 have half-lives of 2–3 min in the circulation, whereas G 34 has a half-life of 15 min. Gastrins are inactivated primarily in the kidney and small intestine.

The principal physiologic actions of gastrin are stimulation of gastric acid and pepsin secretion and stimulation of the growth of the mucosa of the stomach and small and large intestines (**trophic action).** Gastrin secretion is affected by the contents of the stomach, the rate of discharge of the vagus nerves, and bloodborne factors. Atropine does not inhibit the gastrin response to a test meal in humans, because the transmitter secreted by the vagal fibers that innervate G cells is GRP (see further) rather than acetylcholine. Gastrin secretion is also increased by amino acids in the stomach, which act directly on the G cells. Phenylalanine and tryptophan are particularly effective. Gastrin acts via a receptor (CCK-B) that is related to the primary receptor (CCK-A) for CCK (see further). This likely reflects the structural similarity of the two hormones, and may result in some overlapping actions if excessive quantities of either hormone are present (eg, in the case of a gastrinoma).

Acid in the antrum inhibits gastrin secretion, partly by a direct action on G cells and partly by release of somatostatin. In conditions such as pernicious anemia in which the acid-secreting cells of the stomach are damaged, gastrin secretion is chronically elevated.

CHOLECYSTOKININ

CCK is secreted by I cells in the mucosa of the upper small intestine. It has a plethora of actions in the gastrointestinal system, but the most important appear to be the stimulation of pancreatic enzyme secretion; contraction of the gallbladder (the action for which it was named); and relaxation of the sphincter of Oddi, which allows both bile and pancreatic juice to flow into the intestinal lumen.

Like gastrin, CCK is produced from a larger precursor, prepro-CCK, which is processed into many fragments. A large CCK contains 58 amino acid residues (CCK 58). In addition, there are CCK peptides that contain 39 (CCK 39) and 33 amino acid residues (CCK 33), several forms that contain 12 (CCK 12), and a form that contains eight amino acid residues (CCK 8). All of these forms have the same five amino acids at the carboxyl terminal as gastrin. The carboxyl terminal tetrapeptide (CCK 4) also exists in tissues. The carboxyl terminal is amidated, and the tyrosine that is the seventh amino acid residue from the carboxyl terminal is sulfated. Unlike gastrin, the nonsulfated form of CCK has not been found in tissues. The half-life of circulating CCK is about 5 min, but little is known about its metabolism.

In addition to its secretion by I cells, CCK is found in nerves in the distal ileum and colon. It is also found in neurons in the brain, especially the cerebral cortex, and in nerves in many parts of the body. In the brain, it may be involved in the regulation of food intake, and it appears to be related to the production of anxiety and analgesia.

In addition to its primary actions, CCK augments the action of secretin in producing secretion of an alkaline pancreatic juice. It also inhibits gastric emptying, exerts a trophic effect on the pancreas, increases the synthesis of enterokinase, and may enhance the motility of the small intestine and colon. Two CCK receptors have been identified. CCK-A receptors are primarily located in the periphery, whereas both CCK-A and CCK-B (gastrin) receptors are found in the brain. Both activate PLC.

The secretion of CCK is increased by products of digestion, particularly peptides and amino acids, and also by fatty acids containing more than 10 carbon atoms. There are also two protein releasing factors, known as CCK-releasing peptide and monitor peptide, which derive from the intestinal mucosa and pancreas, respectively. Because the bile and pancreatic juice that enter the duodenum in response to CCK enhance the digestion of protein and fat, and the products of this digestion stimulate further CCK secretion, a sort of positive feedback operates in the control of CCK secretion. However, the positive feedback is terminated when the products of digestion move on to the lower portions of the gastrointestinal tract, and also because CCK-releasing peptide and monitor peptide are degraded by proteolytic enzymes once these are no longer occupied in digesting dietary proteins.

SECRETIN

Secretin occupies a unique position in the history of physiology. In 1902, Bayliss and Starling first demonstrated that the excitatory effect of duodenal stimulation on pancreatic secretion was due to a bloodborne factor. Their research led to the identification of the first hormone, secretin. They also suggested that many chemical agents might be secreted by cells in the body and pass in the circulation to affect organs some distance away. Starling introduced the term **hormone** to categorize such "chemical messengers."

Secretin is secreted by S cells located deep in the glands of the mucosa of the upper portion of the small intestine. The structure of secretin is different from that of CCK and gastrin, but very similar to that of GIP, glucagon, and VIP. Only one active form of secretin has been isolated. Its half-life is about 5 min, but little is known about its metabolism.

Secretin increases the secretion of bicarbonate by duct cells of the pancreas and biliary tract. Its action is mediated via cAMP. It also augments the action of CCK in producing pancreatic secretion of digestive enzymes. It decreases gastric acid secretion and may cause contraction of the pyloric sphincter.

The secretion of secretin is increased by the products of protein digestion and by acid in the lumen of the upper small intestine. The release of secretin by acid is another example of feedback control.

GIP

GIP contains 42 amino acid residues and is produced by K cells in the mucosa of the duodenum and jejunum. Its secretion is stimulated by glucose and fat in the duodenum, and because in large doses it inhibits gastric secretion and motility, it was named gastric inhibitory peptide. However, it now appears that it does not have significant gastric inhibiting activity when administered in amounts comparable to those seen after a meal. In the meantime, it was found that GIP stimulates insulin secretion. For this reason, it is often called **glucose-dependent insulinotropic peptide.**

The integrated action of gastrin, CCK, secretin, and GIP in facilitating digestion and utilization of absorbed nutrients is summarized in **Figure 25–6.**

VIP

VIP contains 28 amino acid residues. It is found in nerves in the gastrointestinal tract and thus is not itself a hormone, despite similarities to secretin. VIP is, however, found in blood, in which it has a half-life of about 2 min. In the intestine, it markedly stimulates

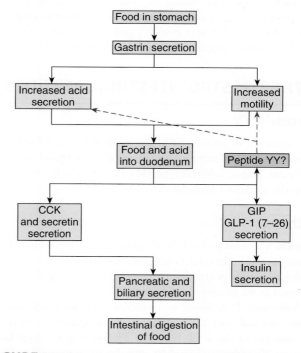

FIGURE 25–6 Integrated action of gastrointestinal hormones in regulating digestion and utilization of absorbed nutrients. The dashed arrows indicate inhibition. The exact identity of the hormonal factor or factors from the intestine that inhibit(s) gastric acid secretion and motility is unsettled, but it may be peptide YY.

intestinal secretion of electrolytes. Its other actions include relaxation of intestinal smooth muscle, including sphincters; dilation of peripheral blood vessels; and inhibition of gastric acid secretion. It is also found in the brain and many autonomic nerves, where it often occurs in the same neurons as acetylcholine. It potentiates the action of acetylcholine in salivary glands. However, VIP and acetylcholine do not coexist in neurons that innervate other parts of the gastrointestinal tract. VIP-secreting tumors (VIPomas) have been described in patients with severe diarrhea.

MOTILIN

Motilin is a polypeptide containing 22 amino acid residues that is secreted by enterochromaffin cells and Mo cells in the stomach, small intestine, and colon. It acts on G-protein-coupled receptors on enteric neurons in the duodenum and colon and produces contraction of smooth muscle in the stomach and intestines in the period between meals (see Chapter 27).

SOMATOSTATIN

Somatostatin is secreted as a paracrine by D cells in the pancreatic islets (see Chapter 24) and by similar D cells in the gastrointestinal mucosa. It exists in tissues in two forms, somatostatin 14 and somatostatin 28, and both are secreted. Somatostatin inhibits the secretion of gastrin, VIP, GIP, secretin, and motilin. Its secretion is stimulated by acid in the lumen, and it probably acts in a paracrine fashion to mediate the inhibition of gastrin secretion produced by acid. It also inhibits pancreatic exocrine secretion; gastric acid secretion and motility; gallbladder contraction; and the absorption of glucose, amino acids, and triglycerides.

OTHER GASTROINTESTINAL PEPTIDES

Peptide YY

The structure of peptide YY is discussed in Chapter 24. It also inhibits gastric acid secretion and motility and is a good candidate to be the gastric inhibitory peptide (**Figure 25–6**). Its release from the jejunum is stimulated by fat.

Others

Ghrelin is secreted primarily by the stomach and appears to play an important role in the central control of food intake (see Chapter 26). It also stimulates growth hormone secretion by acting directly on receptors in the pituitary (see Chapter 18).

Substance P is found in endocrine and nerve cells in the gastrointestinal tract and may enter the circulation. It increases the motility of the small intestine. The neurotransmitter **GRP** contains 27 amino acid residues, and the 10 amino acid residues at its carboxyl terminal are almost identical to those of amphibian **bombesin.** It is present in the vagal nerve endings that terminate on G cells and is the neurotransmitter producing vagally-mediated increases in gastrin secretion. **Glucagon** from the gastrointestinal

tract may be responsible (at least in part) for the hyperglycemia seen after pancreatectomy.

Guanylin is a gastrointestinal polypeptide that binds to guanylyl cyclase. It is made up of 15 amino acid residues and is secreted by cells of the intestinal mucosa. Stimulation of guanylyl cyclase increases the concentration of intracellular cyclic 3′,5′-guanosine monophosphate (cGMP), and this in turn causes increased secretion of Cl⁻ into the intestinal lumen. Guanylin appears to act predominantly in a paracrine fashion. In an interesting example of molecular mimicry, the heat-stable enterotoxin of certain diarrhea-producing strains of *Escherichia coli* has a structure very similar to guanylin and activates guanylin receptors in the intestine. Guanylin receptors are also found in the kidneys, and guanylin may act to integrate the actions of the intestine and kidneys.

■ THE ENTERIC NERVOUS SYSTEM

Two major networks of nerve fibers are intrinsic to the gastrointestinal tract: the **myenteric plexus** (Auerbach plexus), between the outer longitudinal and middle circular muscle layers, and the **submucous plexus** (Meissner plexus), between the middle circular layer and the mucosa. Collectively, these neurons constitute the **enteric nervous system.** The system contains about 100 million sensory neurons, interneurons, and motor neurons in humans—as many as are found in the whole spinal cord. It is sometimes referred to as the "little brain." It is connected to the CNS by parasympathetic and sympathetic fibers but can function autonomously without these connections (see further). The myenteric plexus innervates the longitudinal and circular smooth muscle layers and is concerned primarily with motor control, whereas the submucous plexus innervates the glandular epithelium, intestinal endocrine cells, and submucosal blood vessels and is primarily involved in the control of intestinal secretion. The neurotransmitters in the system include acetylcholine, norepinephrine, serotonin, γ-aminobutyrate (GABA), adenosine triphosphate (ATP), the gases NO and CO, and many different peptides and polypeptides.

EXTRINSIC INNERVATION

Parasympathetic cholinergic activity from the autonomic nervous system generally increases the activity of intestinal smooth muscle and sympathetic noradrenergic activity generally decreases it, while causing sphincters to contract. The preganglionic parasympathetic fibers generally end on cholinergic nerve cells of the myenteric and submucous plexuses. The sympathetic fibers are postganglionic, but many of them end on postganglionic cholinergic neurons, where the norepinephrine they secrete inhibits acetylcholine secretion by activating α₂ presynaptic receptors. Other sympathetic fibers appear to end directly on intestinal smooth muscle cells. Still other fibers innervate blood vessels, where they produce vasoconstriction. It appears that intestinal blood vessels have a dual innervation: they have an extrinsic noradrenergic innervation and an intrinsic innervation by fibers of the enteric nervous system. VIP and NO are among the mediators in the intrinsic innervation, which seems, among other things, to be responsible for the increase in local blood flow (**hyperemia**) that accompanies digestion of food.

■ GASTROINTESTINAL (MUCOSAL) IMMUNE SYSTEM

The mucosal immune system was mentioned in Chapter 3, but it bears repeating here that the gastrointestinal system is an important portal for infection. Similarly, the intestine benefits from interactions with the microbiota, a complex community of commensal (ie, nonpathogenic) bacteria that provide beneficial metabolic functions as well as likely increasing resistance to pathogens. In the face of this constant microbial stimulation, it is not surprising that the intestine has a sophisticated set of both innate and adaptive immune mechanisms to distinguish friend from foe. Indeed, the intestinal mucosa contains more lymphocytes than are found in the circulation, as well as large numbers of inflammatory cells that rapidly defend the mucosa if epithelial defenses are breached. It is likely that immune cells, and their products, also impact the physiologic function of the epithelium, endocrine cells, nerves, and smooth muscle, particularly at times of infection and if inappropriate immune responses are perpetuated, such as in inflammatory bowel diseases (see Chapter 3).

■ GASTROINTESTINAL (SPLANCHNIC) CIRCULATION

The gastrointestinal tract has unusual circulatory features. The blood flow to the stomach, intestines, pancreas, and liver is arranged in a series of parallel circuits, with all the blood from the intestines and pancreas draining via the portal vein to the liver (**Figure 25–7**). The blood from the intestines, pancreas, and spleen drains via the hepatic portal vein to the liver and from the liver via the hepatic veins to the inferior vena cava. The viscera and the liver receive about 30% of the cardiac output via the celiac, superior mesenteric, and inferior mesenteric arteries. The liver receives about 1300 mL/min from the portal vein and 500 mL/min from the hepatic artery during fasting, and the portal supply increases still further after meals.

CHAPTER SUMMARY

■ The gastrointestinal system evolved to permit controlled nutrient uptake in multicellular organisms. It is functionally continuous with the outside environment.

■ Digestive secretions alter the components of meals (particularly macromolecules) such that their constituents can be

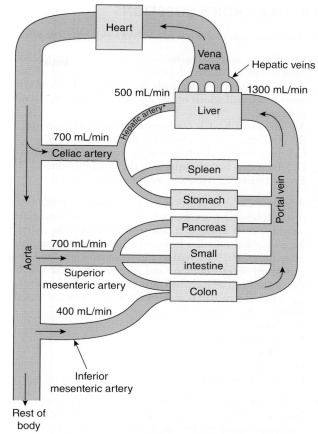

*Branches of the hepatic artery also supply the stomach, pancreas and small intestine.

FIGURE 25–7   Schematic of the splanchnic circulation under fasting conditions. Note that even during fasting, the liver receives the majority of its blood supply via the portal vein.

absorbed. Meal components are acted on sequentially by saliva, gastric juice, pancreatic juice, and bile.

■ The intestine and the organs that drain into it secrete about 8 L of fluid per day, which is added to water consumed in food and beverages. Most of this fluid is reabsorbed, leaving only approximately 200 mL to be lost to the stool. Fluid secretion and absorption are both dependent on the active epithelial transport of ions, nutrients, or both.

■ Gastrointestinal functions are regulated in an integrated fashion by endocrine, paracrine, and neurocrine mechanisms. Hormones and paracrine factors are released from enteroendocrine cells in response to signals coincident with meals.

■ The enteric nervous system conveys information from the central nervous system to the gastrointestinal tract, but also often can activate secretion and motility in an autonomous fashion.

■ The intestine harbors an extensive mucosal immune system that regulates responses to the complex microbiota normally resident in the lumen, as well as defending the body against pathogens.

■ The intestine has an unusual circulation, in that the majority of its venous outflow does not return directly to the heart, but rather is directed initially to the liver via the portal vein.

MULTIPLE-CHOICE QUESTIONS

For all questions, select the single best answer unless otherwise directed.

1. Following a natural disaster in Haiti, there is an outbreak of cholera among displaced persons living in a tent encampment. The affected individuals display severe diarrheal symptoms because of which of the following changes in intestinal transport?
   A. Increased K^+–Cl^- cotransport in the small intestine
   B. Decreased K^+ secretion into the colon
   C. Increased K^+ absorption in the crypts of Lieberkühn
   D. Increased Na^+ absorption in the small intestine
   E. Increased Cl^- secretion into the intestinal lumen

2. A 50-year-old man comes to see his clinician complaining of severe epigastric pain, frequent heartburn, and unexplained weight loss of 20 lb over a 6-month period. He claims to have obtained no relief from over-the-counter H_2 antihistamine drugs. He is referred to a gastroenterologist, and upper endoscopy reveals erosions and ulcerations in the proximal duodenum and an increased output of gastric acid in the fasting state. The patient is most likely to have a tumor secreting which of the following hormones?
   A. Secretin
   B. Somatostatin
   C. Motilin
   D. Gastrin
   E. Cholecystokinin

3. A 60-year-old woman undergoes total pancreatectomy because of the presence of a tumor. Which of the following outcomes would *not* be expected after she recovers from the operation?
   A. Steatorrhea
   B. Hyperglycemia
   C. Metabolic alkalosis
   D. Ongoing weight gain
   E. Decreased absorption of amino acids

4. In a study of the secretion of gastrointestinal hormones, portal concentrations are measured in a rat during luminal perfusion of buffered salt solutions at various pH levels. Which of the following hormones will increase during perfusion with a buffered solution at pH 3.0?
   A. Cholecystokinin
   B. Gastrin
   C. Glucose-dependent isulinotropic peptide
   D. Motilin
   E. Secretin

5. In an experiment in mice, a scientist infuses PYY intravenously. Compared with controls, these animals would be expected to display an increase in which of the following?
   A. Time taken to initiate the next meal
   B. Gastric emptying
   C. Lipid concentrations in the jejunal lumen
   D. Hydrogen ion concentrations in the gastric lumen
   E. Pancreatic secretion

6. A patient suffering from anemia comes to his physician complaining of frequent bouts of gastroenteritis. A blood test reveals the presence of antibodies directed against gastric parietal cells. The anemia in this patient is attributable to the hyposecretion of which gastric product?

   A. Histamine
   B. Gastrin
   C. Pepsinogen
   D. Intrinsic factor
   E. Hydrochloric acid

7. Two medical students studying for their physiology final decide to take a break for a lunchtime hamburger. Before reaching the cafeteria, nervous impulses from the dorsal vagal complex will initiate gastric acid secretion by triggering release of which neurotransmitter from the enteric nervous system?
   A. Norepinephrine
   B. Vasoactive intestinal polypeptide
   C. Substance P
   D. Gastrin-releasing peptide
   E. Nitric oxide

8. A 4-year-old boy is brought to his pediatrician for an evaluation because of failure to thrive and frequent diarrhea characterized by pale, bulky, foul-smelling stools. Sweat chloride concentrations are measured and found to be elevated. Diminished secretion of which pancreatic product is most likely to be the primary cause of the patient's apparent fat malabsorption?
   A. Lipase
   B. Procolipase
   C. Monitor peptide
   D. Cholecystokinin
   E. Bicarbonate

9. A researcher conducts a study of the regulation of salivary secretion in a group of normal volunteers under various conditions. Which of the following conditions would be expected to be associated with the lowest rates of secretion?
   A. Chewing gum
   B. Undergoing a mock dental exam
   C. Sleep
   D. Exposure to a nauseating odor
   E. Resting control conditions

10. A 50-year-old female patient who has suffered for several years from severe dryness of her eyes due to inadequate tear production is referred to a gastroenterologist for evaluation of chronic heartburn. Endoscopic evaluation reveals erosions and scarring of the distal esophagus. Reduced production of which salivary product most likely contributed to this tissue injury?
    A. Bicarbonate
    B. Lactoferrin
    C. IgA
    D. Mucus
    E. Amylase

ANSWERS

1. The correct answer is **E.** The active **(A)** subunit of cholera toxin is internalized by intestinal epithelial cells and causes an irreversible increase in intracellular cAMP, which in turn activates intestinal chloride secretion driving fluid accumulation in the lumen. cAMP also activates ENaC activity thereby stimulating Na^+ absorption, but this mechanism only exists in the distal colon; furthermore, electroneutral NaCl absorption

in the small intestine is inhibited rather than stimulated by cAMP (rules out option **D**). Similarly, basolateral K⁺–Cl⁻ cotransport contributes to electroneutral NaCl absorption, but would be reduced rather than increased in the setting of cholera (rules out option **A**). Finally, neither secretion nor absorption of K⁺ ions is of large enough magnitude to account for the marked fluid loss seen in cholera, nor are the direction of effects stated consistent with luminal fluid accumulation and thus diarrhea (rules out options **B** and **C**).

2. The correct answer is **D**. Zollinger–Ellison syndrome, with increased gastric acid secretion even in the absence of signals triggered by ingestion of a meal, is caused by a secreting gastrinoma. The uncontrolled increase in circulating gastrin markedly upregulates gastric secretion, which overcomes normal defensive mechanisms and leads to mucosal injury. Somatostatin inhibits rather than stimulates gastric secretion, and thus the clinical picture is not consistent with a somatostatinoma (rules out option **B**). The primary biological effect of secretin is to increase bicarbonate secretion, which would be expected to protect against duodenal injury and would not increase acid secretion (rules out option **A**). A tumor secreting motilin would not be expected to alter gastric secretion since its primary effect is to trigger phase III of the migrating motor complex during fasting (rules out option **C**). Finally, while high levels of CCK such as might be produced by a tumor could increase gastric secretion via nonspecific activation of CCK-B receptors, this would be countermanded by the ability of CCK to trigger or augment the secretion of alkaline bile and pancreatic juice (rules out option **E**).

3. The correct answer is **D**. The patient can be expected to have a profound decrease in the luminal availability of all pancreatic enzymes, and these are needed for the digestion of macromolecular nutrients into forms that the intestine can absorb. Thus, adequate nutrition is unlikely, along with any weight gain. On the other hand, malabsorption of lipids and the products of protein digestion are likely to occur (rules out options **A** and **E**). Pancreatectomy will also remove the endocrine portion of the pancreas, ablating the capacity for insulin secretion in response to rising blood glucose levels, resulting in hyperglycemia (rules out option **B**). Finally, because ductular secretion from the pancreas supplies a great deal of the bicarbonate that normally neutralizes gastric acid, bicarbonate will accumulate in the bloodstream (rules out option **C**).

4. The correct answer is **E**. The biologic function of secretin is to increase the secretion of bicarbonate from pancreatic and biliary duct cells, thereby neutralizing acid coming from the stomach and returning the pH in the intestinal lumen towards neutrality. In keeping with this biological function, secretin is released from S cells when the pH in the intestinal lumen declines. On the other hand, the function of gastrin is to increase acid secretion, and its release is decreased rather than increased by a fall in luminal pH (rules out option **B**). Cholecystokinin augments secretin-induced bicarbonate secretion, but is released in response to peptide-releasing factors and dietary components such as specific amino acids (rules out option **A**). Glucose-dependent insulinotropic peptide is released in response to carbohydrate, and motilin is released cyclically during fasting by an unknown mechanism, but perhaps in response to an alkaline pH in the lumen (rules out options **C** and **D**).

5. The correct answer is **A**. Peptide YY has been described as a "brake" that is released in response to nutrients (especially fat)

in the distal small intestine and whose role is to slow the delivery of nutrients from more proximal segments to allow adequate time for digestion and absorption. It is also believed to act centrally to signal satiety. Peptide YY also acts by inhibiting gastric emptying and secretion (rules out options **B** and **D**); it may also suppress pancreatic secretion (rules out option **E**). Finally, while peptide YY is released in response to elevated lipid concentrations, its exogenous administration should decrease the concentration of lipid in the jejunum by slowing the delivery of these nutrients (rules out option **C**).

6. The correct answer is **D**. Parietal cells secrete intrinsic factor, which binds to and allows the absorption of cobalamin (vitamin B₁₂), which is required in turn for the production of red blood cells. Autoimmune destruction of parietal cells can lead to anemia secondary to an inability to secrete intrinsic factor (pernicious anemia). Such patients will also have a reduction in gastric acid secretion, but this does not account for the anemia, whereas pepsinogen secretion from chief cells should be unaffected (rules out options **C** and **E**). If anything, gastrin and histamine levels should be increased due to a lack of negative feedback signals in response to gastric acidity (rules out options **A** and **B**).

7. The correct answer is **D**. The cephalic phase of the gastric secretory response is initiated by the release of gastrin-releasing peptide from enteric nerve endings adjacent to G cells in the antrum of the stomach. Gastric secretion during the cephalic phase, in common with most intestinal secretory responses, is not normally triggered by sympathetic nerve activity, nor is norepinephrine a transmitter expressed by the enteric nervous system (rules out option **A**). The remaining enteric neurotransmitters listed are predominantly involved in causing the contraction (substance P) or relaxation (vasoactive intestinal polypeptide, nitric oxide) of gastrointestinal smooth muscle (rules out options **B, C,** and **E**).

8. The correct answer is **A**. The patient appears to be suffering from cystic fibrosis with associated pancreatic insufficiency. While the production of all pancreatic products is likely to be impaired, the loss of lipase will be most significant for fat digestion and absorption. Notably, the nutritional consequences of cystic fibrosis can be treated, at least in part, by providing oral supplements of pancreatic enzymes. Procolipase will be less important in the patient because lipase activity should not be as significantly inhibited by bile acids as seen in a healthy individual since cystic fibrosis also impairs biliary secretion (rules out option **B**). Similarly, while a failure to neutralize gastric acid may impede lipase activity, this is not relevant if there is no lipase to inhibit (rules out option **E**). Finally, while pancreatic monitor peptide is also likely to be reduced, it is the overall lack of pancreatic enzymes, rather than a decreased ability to trigger cholecystokinin release or the response to this hormone, that accounts for fat malabsorption; cholecystokinin is also not a pancreatic product (rules out options **C** and **D**).

9. The correct answer is **C**. Sleep signals through the salivatory nucleus of the medulla to inhibit the secretion of saliva compared to resting control conditions (rules out option **E**). On the other hand, pressure in the mouth stimulates the salivatory nucleus to trigger secretion via parasympathetic pathways (rules out options **A** and **B**). Nausea also triggers pro-secretory signals via the salivatory nucleus, presumably in an effort to protect the oral mucosa and esophagus from the damaging effects of vomited gastric acid (rules out option **D**).

10. The correct answer is **A.** The patient is most likely suffering from Sjögren's syndrome, which involves autoimmune destruction of the salivary and tear glands. Saliva is normally alkaline, and serves to neutralize gastric acid that may reflux into the esophagus; when salivary secretion is reduced, this acid cannot be washed away and causes tissue injury and pain. Lactoferrin, IgA, and mucus are also present in saliva and protect against pathogens and physical damage to the oral mucosa, but do not neutralize the gastric acid that is injurious in this patient (rules out options **B, C,** and **D**). Finally, while salivary amylase will also be reduced in this patient, this is unlikely to be of physiological significance for digestion unless she also has pancreatic dysfunction, and in any event would be unrelated to her esophageal erosions (rules out option **E**).

Digestion, Absorption, & Nutritional Principles

OBJECTIVES

After studying this chapter, you should be able to:

- Understand how nutrients are delivered to the body and the chemical processes needed to convert them to a form suitable for absorption.

- List the major dietary carbohydrates and define the processes that produce absorbable monosaccharides as well as the transport mechanisms that provide for uptake of these hydrophilic molecules.

- Understand the process of protein assimilation and the ways in which it is comparable to, or converges from, that used for carbohydrates.

- Define the stepwise processes of lipid digestion and absorption, the role of bile acids in solubilizing the products of lipolysis, and the consequences of fat malabsorption.

- Identify the source and functions of short-chain fatty acids in the colon.

- Delineate the mechanisms of uptake for vitamins and minerals.

- Understand basic principles of energy metabolism and nutrition.

INTRODUCTION

The gastrointestinal system is the portal through which nutritive substances, vitamins, minerals, and fluids enter the body. Proteins, fats, and complex carbohydrates are broken down into absorbable units **(digested),** principally in the small intestine. The products of digestion and the vitamins, minerals, and water cross the mucosa and enter the lymph or the blood **(absorption).**

Digestion of the major foodstuffs is an orderly process involving the action of a large number of **digestive enzymes** discussed in the previous chapter. Enzymes from the salivary glands attack carbohydrates (and fats in some species); enzymes from the stomach attack proteins and fats; and enzymes from the exocrine portion of the pancreas attack carbohydrates, proteins, lipids, DNA, and RNA. Other enzymes that complete the digestive process are found in the luminal membranes and the cytoplasm of the cells that line the small intestine. The action of the enzymes is aided by acid and bile secreted by the stomach and liver, respectively.

■ DIGESTION & ABSORPTION: CARBOHYDRATES

DIGESTION

The principal dietary carbohydrates are polysaccharides, disaccharides, and monosaccharides. Starches (glucose polymers) and their derivatives are the only polysaccharides that are digested to any degree in the human gastrointestinal tract by human enzymes. Amylopectin, which typically constitutes around 75% of dietary starch, is a branched molecule, whereas amylose is a straight chain with only 1:4α linkages. The disaccharides **lactose** (milk sugar) and **sucrose** (table sugar) are also ingested, along with the monosaccharides fructose and glucose.

In the mouth, starch is attacked by salivary α-amylase. The optimal pH for this enzyme is 6.7. However, it remains partially active even once it moves into the stomach, despite the acidic gastric juice, because the active site is protected by the presence of substrate. In the small intestine, both the salivary and the pancreatic α-amylase also act on the ingested polysaccharides. Both enzymes hydrolyze internal 1:4α linkages but spare 1:6α linkages and terminal 1:4α linkages. Consequently, the end products of α-amylase digestion are oligosaccharides: the disaccharide **maltose;** the trisaccharide **maltotriose;** and α-limit dextrins, polymers of glucose containing an average of about eight glucose molecules with 1:6α linkages.

The oligosaccharidases responsible for the further digestion of the starch derivatives are located in the brush border of small intestinal epithelial cells. Some of these enzymes have more than one substrate. **Isomaltase** is mainly responsible for hydrolysis of 1:6α linkages. Along with **maltase and sucrase,** it also breaks down maltotriose and maltose. Sucrase hydrolyzes sucrose into a molecule of glucose and a molecule of fructose. In addition, **lactase** hydrolyzes lactose to glucose and galactose.

Deficiency of one or more of the brush border oligosaccharidases may cause diarrhea, bloating, and flatulence after ingestion of sugar (**Clinical Box 26–1**). The diarrhea is due to the increased number of osmotically active oligosaccharide molecules that remain in the intestinal lumen, causing the volume of the intestinal contents to increase. In the colon, bacteria break down some of the oligosaccharides, further increasing the number of osmotically active particles. The bloating and flatulence are due to the production of gas (CO_2 and H_2) from disaccharide residues in the lower small intestine and colon.

CLINICAL BOX 26–1

Lactose Intolerance

In most mammals and in many races of humans, intestinal lactase activity is high at birth, then declines to low levels during adulthood. The low lactase levels are associated with intolerance to milk (**lactose intolerance**). Most Europeans and their American descendants retain sufficient intestinal lactase activity in adulthood. However, 70–100% of blacks, American Indians, Asians, and Mediterranean populations are lactose intolerant. When such individuals ingest dairy products, they are unable to digest lactose sufficiently, and so symptoms such as bloating, pain, gas, and diarrhea are produced.

THERAPEUTIC HIGHLIGHTS

The simplest treatment for lactose intolerance is to avoid dairy products in the diet, but this can sometimes be challenging. Symptoms can be ameliorated by administration of commercial lactase preparations, but this is expensive. Yogurt is better tolerated than milk in intolerant individuals because it contains its own bacterial lactase.

ABSORPTION

Hexoses are rapidly absorbed across the wall of the small intestine. Essentially all the hexoses are removed before the remains of a meal reach the terminal part of the ileum. The sugar molecules pass from the mucosal cells to the blood in the capillaries draining into the portal vein.

The transport of glucose and galactose depends on Na^+ in the intestinal lumen. This is because these sugars and Na^+ share the same **cotransporter,** the **sodium-dependent glucose transporter** (SGLT, Na^+ glucose cotransporter) (**Figure 26–1**). SGLT-1 is responsible for uptake of dietary glucose from the gut. The related transporter, SGLT-2, is responsible for glucose transport out of the renal tubules (see Chapter 37).

Because the intracellular Na^+ concentration is low, Na^+ moves into the epithelial cell along its concentration gradient. Glucose moves with the Na^+ and is released in the cell (Figure 26–1). Glucose is then transported by GLUT2 into the interstitium and thence to the capillaries. When the Na^+/glucose cotransporter is congenitally defective, the resulting **glucose/galactose malabsorption** causes severe diarrhea that is often fatal if glucose and galactose are not promptly removed from the diet. Glucose and its polymers can also be used to retain Na^+ in diarrheal disease, as was discussed in Chapter 25.

As indicated, SGLT-1 also transports galactose, but fructose utilizes a different mechanism. Its absorption is independent of Na^+ or the transport of glucose and galactose; it is transported instead by facilitated diffusion from the intestinal lumen into the enterocytes by GLUT5 and out of the enterocytes by GLUT2. Some fructose is converted to glucose in the mucosal cells.

■ PROTEINS & NUCLEIC ACIDS

PROTEIN DIGESTION

Protein digestion begins in the stomach, where pepsins cleave some of the peptide linkages. Like many of the other enzymes concerned with protein digestion, pepsins are secreted in the form of inactive precursors (**proenzymes**). The pepsin precursors are called pepsinogens and are activated by gastric acid. Pepsins hydrolyze the bonds between aromatic amino acids such as phenylalanine or tyrosine and a second amino acid, so the products of peptic digestion are polypeptides of diverse sizes. Because pepsins have a pH optimum of 1.6–3.2, their action is terminated when the gastric contents are mixed with the alkaline pancreatic juice in the duodenum and jejunum. The pH of the intestinal contents in the duodenal bulb is 3.0–4.0, but rapidly rises; in the rest of the duodenum it is about 6.5.

In the small intestine, the polypeptides formed by digestion in the stomach are further digested by the powerful proteolytic enzymes of the pancreas and intestinal mucosa. Trypsin, the chymotrypsins, and elastase act at interior peptide bonds in the peptide molecules and are called **endopeptidases.** The formation of the active endopeptidases from their inactive precursors occurs only when they have reached their site of action, secondary to the action of the brush border hydrolase, **enterokinase.**

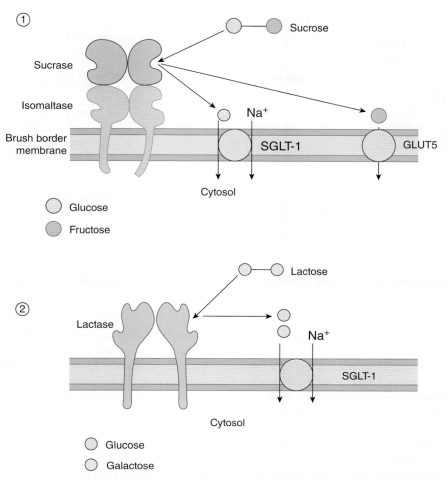

FIGURE 26–1 **Brush border digestion and assimilation of the disaccharides sucrose (panel 1) and lactose (panel 2).** Uptake of glucose and galactose is driven secondarily by the low intracellular sodium concentration established by the basolateral Na$^+$, K$^+$ ATPase (not shown). SGLT-1, sodium-glucose cotransporter-1.

Trypsinogen is converted to the active enzyme trypsin by enterokinase. Trypsin converts chymotrypsinogens into chymotrypsins and other proenzymes into active enzymes. Trypsin can also activate trypsinogen; therefore, once some trypsin is formed, there is an auto-catalytic chain reaction. Enterokinase deficiency occurs as a congenital abnormality and leads to protein malnutrition.

The carboxypeptidases of the pancreas are **exopeptidases** that hydrolyze the amino acids at the carboxyl ends of the polypeptides **(Figure 26–2).** Some free amino acids are liberated in the intestinal lumen, but others are liberated at the cell surface by the aminopeptidases, carboxypeptidases, endopeptidases, and dipeptidases in the brush border. Some dipeptides and tripeptides are actively transported into the intestinal cells and hydrolyzed by intracellular peptidases, with the amino acids entering the bloodstream.

ABSORPTION

At least seven different transport systems transport amino acids into enterocytes. Five of these require Na$^+$ and cotransport amino acids and Na$^+$ in a fashion similar to the cotransport of Na$^+$ and

glucose. Two of these five also require Cl$^-$. In two systems, transport is independent of Na$^+$.

Di- and tripeptides are transported into enterocytes by a system known as PepT1 (or peptide transporter 1) that requires H$^+$ instead of Na$^+$. There is very little absorption of larger peptides. In the enterocytes, amino acids released from the peptides by intracellular hydrolysis plus the amino acids absorbed from the intestinal lumen and brush border are transported out of the enterocytes along their basolateral borders by at least five transport systems. From there, they enter the hepatic portal blood.

Absorption of amino acids is rapid in the duodenum and jejunum. There is little absorption in the ileum in health, because the majority of the free amino acids have already been assimilated. Approximately 50% of the digested protein comes from ingested food, 25% from proteins in digestive juices, and 25% from desquamated mucosal cells. Only 2–5% of the protein in the small intestine escapes digestion and absorption. Some of this is eventually digested by bacteria in the colon. Almost all of the protein in the stools comes from bacteria and cellular debris. Evidence suggests that the peptidase activities of the brush border and the mucosal cell cytoplasm are increased by resection of part of the ileum and that they are independently altered

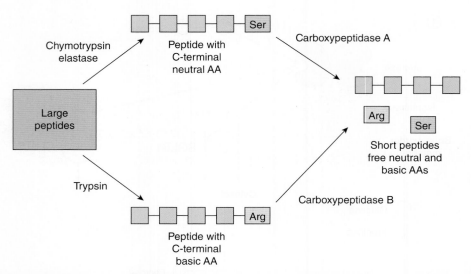

FIGURE 26–2 **Luminal digestion of peptides by pancreatic endopeptidases and exopeptidases.** Individual amino acids (AAs) are shown as squares.

in starvation. Thus, these enzymes appear to be subject to homeostatic regulation. In humans, a congenital defect in the mechanism that transports neutral amino acids in the intestine and renal tubules causes **Hartnup disease.** A congenital defect in the transport of basic amino acids causes **cystinuria.** However, most patients do not experience nutritional deficiencies of these amino acids because peptide transport compensates.

In infants, moderate amounts of undigested proteins are also absorbed. The protein antibodies in maternal colostrum are largely secretory immunoglobulins (IgAs), the production of which is increased in the breast in late pregnancy. They cross the mammary epithelium by transcytosis and enter the circulation of the infant from the intestine, providing passive immunity against infections. Absorption of intact proteins declines sharply after weaning, but adults still absorb small quantities. Foreign proteins that enter the circulation provoke the formation of antibodies, and the antigen–antibody reaction occurring on subsequent entry of more of the same protein may cause allergic symptoms. However, in most individuals food allergies do not occur, and there is evidence for a genetic component in susceptibility.

Absorption of protein antigens, particularly bacterial and viral proteins, takes place in large **microfold cells** or **M cells,** specialized intestinal epithelial cells that overlie aggregates of lymphoid tissue (Peyer patches). These cells pass the antigens to the lymphoid cells, and lymphocytes are activated. The activated lymphoblasts enter the circulation, but they later return to the intestinal mucosa and other epithelia, where they secrete IgA in response to subsequent exposures to the same antigen. This **secretory immunity** is an important defense mechanism (see Chapter 3).

NUCLEIC ACIDS

Nucleic acids are split into nucleotides in the intestine by the pancreatic nucleases, and the nucleotides are split into nucleosides and phosphoric acid by enzymes on the luminal surfaces of the

mucosal cells. The nucleosides are then split into their constituent sugars and purine and pyrimidine bases. The bases are absorbed by active transport. Families of equilibrative (ie, passive) and concentrative (ie, secondary active) nucleoside transporters have recently been identified on the apical membrane of enterocytes.

■ LIPIDS

FAT DIGESTION

A lingual lipase is secreted by Ebner glands on the dorsal surface of the tongue in some species, and the stomach also secretes a lipase. They are of little quantitative significance for lipid digestion other than in the setting of pancreatic insufficiency, but they may generate free fatty acids that signal to more distal parts of the gastrointestinal tract (eg, causing the release of CCK; see Chapter 25).

Most fat digestion begins in the duodenum, pancreatic lipase being one of the most important enzymes involved. This enzyme hydrolyzes the 1- and 3-bonds of the triglycerides (triacylglycerols) with relative ease but acts on the 2-bonds at a very low rate, so the principal products of its action are free fatty acids and 2-monoglycerides (2-monoacylglycerols). It acts on fats that have been emulsified (see further). **Colipase,** a protein that enhances the action of lipase, is also secreted in the pancreatic juice. Colipase is secreted in an inactive proform (Table 26–1) and is activated in the intestinal lumen by trypsin. Colipase allows lipase to remain associated with droplets of dietary lipid even in the presence of bile acids.

Cholesterol esterase represents about 4% of the total protein in pancreatic juice. In adults, pancreatic lipase is 10–60 times more active, but unlike pancreatic lipase, cholesterol esterase catalyzes the hydrolysis of cholesterol esters, esters of fat-soluble vitamins, and phospholipids, as well as triglycerides. A very similar enzyme is found in human milk.

TABLE 26–1 Normal transport of substances by the intestine and location of maximum absorption or secretion.[a]

Absorption of	Small Intestine			Colon
	Upper[b]	Mid	Lower	
Sugars (glucose, galactose, etc.)	++	+++	++	0
Amino acids	++	++	++	0
Water-soluble and fat-soluble vitamins except vitamin B_{12}	+++	++	0	0
Betaine, dimethylglycine, sarcosine	+	++	++	?
Antibodies in newborns	+	++	+++	?
Pyrimidines (thymine and uracil)	+	+	?	?
Long-chain fatty acid absorption and conversion to triglyceride	+++	++	+	0
Bile acids	+	+	+++	
Vitamin B_{12}	0	+	+++	0
Na^+	+++	++	+++	+++
K^+	+	+	+	Sec
Ca^{2+}	+++	++	+	?
Fe^{2+}	+++	+	+	?
Cl^-	+++	++	+	+
SO_4^{2-}	++	+	0	?

[a]Amount of absorption is graded + to +++. Sec, secreted when luminal K^+ is low.

[b]Upper small intestine refers primarily to jejunum, although the duodenum is similar in most cases studied (with the notable exception that the duodenum secretes HCO_3^- and shows little net absorption or secretion of NaCl).

Fats are relatively insoluble, which limits their ability to cross the unstirred layer and reach the surface of the mucosal cells. However, they are finely emulsified in the small intestine by the detergent action of bile acids, phosphatidylcholine, and monoglycerides. When the concentration of bile acids in the intestine is high, lipids and bile acids interact spontaneously to form **micelles.** These cylindrical aggregates take up lipids, and although their lipid concentration varies, they generally contain fatty acids, monoglycerides, and cholesterol in their hydrophobic centers. Micellar formation further solubilizes the lipids and provides a mechanism for their transport to the enterocytes. The lipids diffuse out of the micelles, maintaining a saturated aqueous solution of the lipids in contact with the brush border.

STEATORRHEA

Pancreatectomized animals and patients with diseases that destroy the exocrine portion of the pancreas have fatty, bulky, clay-colored stools (**steatorrhea**) because of the impaired digestion and absorption of fat. The steatorrhea is mostly due to lipase deficiency. The lack of alkaline secretion from the pancreas also contributes by lowering the pH of the intestine contents. In some cases, hypersecretion of gastric acid can cause steatorrhea. Another cause of steatorrhea is defective reabsorption of bile acids in the distal ileum (see Chapter 28).

When bile is excluded from the intestine, up to 50% of ingested fat appears in the feces. A severe malabsorption of fat-soluble vitamins also results. When bile acid reabsorption is prevented by resection of the terminal ileum or by disease in this portion of the small intestine, the amount of fat in the stools is also increased because when the enterohepatic circulation is interrupted, the liver cannot increase the rate of bile acid production to a sufficient degree to compensate.

FAT ABSORPTION

Traditionally, lipids were thought to enter enterocytes by passive diffusion, but some evidence now suggests that carriers are involved. Inside the cells, lipids are rapidly esterified, maintaining a favorable concentration gradient from the lumen into the cells (Figure 26–3). There are also carriers that export certain lipids back into the lumen, thereby limiting their oral availability. This is the case for plant sterols as well as cholesterol.

The fate of the fatty acids in enterocytes depends on their size. Fatty acids containing less than 10–12 carbon atoms are water-soluble enough that they pass through the enterocyte unmodified and are actively transported into the portal blood. Fatty acids containing more than 10–12 carbon atoms are too insoluble for this. They are reesterified to triglycerides in the enterocytes. In addition, some of the absorbed cholesterol is esterified. The triglycerides and cholesterol esters are then coated with a layer of protein, cholesterol, and phospholipid to form chylomicrons. These leave the cell and enter the lymphatics, because they are too large to pass through the junctions between capillary endothelial cells (Figure 26–3).

In mucosal cells, most of the triglyceride is formed by the acylation of the absorbed 2-monoglycerides, primarily in the smooth endoplasmic reticulum. The formation of lipoproteins occurs in the

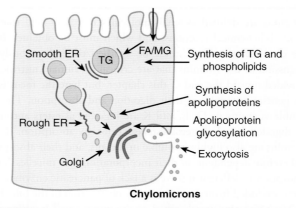

FIGURE 26–3 Intracellular handling of the products of lipid digestion. Absorbed fatty acids (FA) and monoglycerides (MG) are reesterified to form triglyceride (TG) in the smooth endoplasmic reticulum (ER). Apoproteins synthesized in the rough ER are coated around lipid cores, and the resulting chylomicrons are secreted from the basolateral pole of epithelial cells by exocytosis.

rough endoplasmic reticulum. Carbohydrate moieties are added to the proteins in the Golgi apparatus, and the finished chylomicrons are extruded by exocytosis from the basolateral aspect of the cell.

Absorption of long-chain fatty acids is greatest in the upper parts of the small intestine, but appreciable amounts are also absorbed in the ileum. On a moderate fat intake, 95% or more of the ingested fat is absorbed. The processes involved in fat absorption are not fully mature at birth, and infants fail to absorb 10–15% of ingested fat. Thus, they are more susceptible to the ill effects of disease processes that reduce fat absorption.

SHORT-CHAIN FATTY ACIDS IN THE COLON

Increasing attention is being focused on short-chain fatty acids (SCFAs) that are produced in the colon and absorbed from it. SCFAs are 2–5-carbon weak acids that have an average normal concentration of about 80 mmol/L in the lumen. About 60% of this total is acetate, 25% propionate, and 15% butyrate. They are formed by the action of colonic bacteria on undigested complex carbohydrates, resistant starches, and other components of the dietary fiber.

Absorbed SCFAs are metabolized and make a significant contribution to the total caloric intake. In addition, they exert a trophic effect on the colonic epithelial cells; combat inflammation; and are absorbed in part by exchange for H^+, helping maintain acid-base equilibrium. SCFAs are absorbed by specific transporters present in colonic epithelial cells. SCFAs also promote the absorption of Na^+, although the exact mechanism for coupled Na^+–SCFA absorption is unsettled.

■ ABSORPTION OF VITAMINS & MINERALS

VITAMINS

Vitamins are defined as small molecules that play vital roles in bodily biochemical reactions, and which must be obtained from the diet because they cannot be synthesized endogenously. A discussion of the vitamins that are critical for human nutrition is provided toward the end of this chapter, but here the focus is on the general principles of their digestion and absorption. The fat-soluble vitamins A, D, E, and K are ingested as esters and must be digested by cholesterol esterase prior to absorption. These vitamins are also highly insoluble in the gut, and their absorption is therefore dependent on their incorporation into micelles. Their absorption is deficient if there is a lack of pancreatic enzymes or if bile is excluded from the intestine by obstruction of the bile duct.

Most vitamins are absorbed in the upper small intestine, but vitamin B_{12} is absorbed in the ileum. This vitamin binds to intrinsic factor, a protein secreted by the parietal cells of the stomach, and the complex is absorbed across the ileal mucosa.

Vitamin B_{12} absorption and folate absorption are Na^+-independent, but all seven of the remaining water-soluble vitamins—thiamin, riboflavin, niacin, pyridoxine, pantothenate, biotin, and ascorbic acid—are absorbed by carriers that are Na^+ cotransporters.

CALCIUM

A total of 30–80% of ingested calcium is absorbed. The absorptive process and its relation to 1,25-dihydroxycholecalciferol are discussed in Chapter 21. Through this vitamin D derivative, Ca^{2+} absorption is adjusted to body needs; absorption is increased in the presence of Ca^{2+} deficiency and decreased in the presence of Ca^{2+} excess. Ca^{2+} absorption is also inhibited by phosphates and oxalates because these anions form insoluble salts with Ca^{2+} in the intestine.

IRON

In adults, total body stores of iron are regulated by changes in the rate at which it is absorbed from the intestine. Men lose about 0.6 mg/day, largely in the stools. Premenopausal women have a variable, larger loss averaging about twice this value because of the additional iron lost during menstruation. The average daily iron intake in the United States and Europe is about 20 mg, but the amount absorbed is equal only to the losses.

Most of the iron in the diet is in the ferric (Fe^{3+}) form, whereas it is the ferrous (Fe^{2+}) form that is absorbed. Fe^{3+} reductase activity is associated with the iron transporter in the brush borders of the enterocytes. Gastric secretions dissolve the iron and permit it to form soluble complexes with ascorbic acid and other substances that aid its reduction to the Fe^{2+} form.

Almost all iron absorption occurs in the duodenum. Transport of Fe^{2+} into the enterocytes occurs via divalent metal transporter 1 (**DMT1**). Some is stored in ferritin, and the remainder is transported out of the enterocytes by a basolateral transporter named **ferroportin 1.** A protein called **hephaestin (Hp)** is associated with ferroportin 1. It is not a transporter itself, but it facilitates basolateral transport. In the plasma, Fe^{2+} is converted to Fe^{3+} and bound to the iron transport protein **transferrin.** Normally, transferrin is about 35% saturated with iron, and the normal plasma iron level is about 130 μg/dL (23 μmol/L) in men and 110 μg/dL (19 μmol/L) in women.

Heme (see Chapter 31) binds to an apical transport protein in enterocytes and is carried into the cytoplasm. In the cytoplasm, HO-2, a subtype of heme oxygenase, removes Fe^{2+} from the porphyrin and adds it to the intracellular Fe^{2+} pool.

Seventy percent of the iron in the body is in hemoglobin, 3% in myoglobin, and the rest in ferritin, which is present not only in enterocytes, but also in many other cells. Ferritin is readily visible under the electron microscope and has been used as a tracer in studies of phagocytosis and related phenomena.

Intestinal absorption of iron is regulated by three factors: recent dietary intake of iron, the state of the iron stores in the body, and the state of erythropoiesis in the bone marrow. The normal operation of the factors that maintain iron balance is essential for health (**Clinical Box 26–2**).

CLINICAL BOX 26-2

Disorders of Iron Uptake

Iron deficiency causes anemia. Conversely, iron overload causes **hemosiderin** to accumulate in the tissues, producing **hemosiderosis.** Large amounts of hemosiderin can damage tissues, such as is seen in the common genetic disorder of hemochromatosis. This syndrome is characterized by pigmentation of the skin, pancreatic damage with diabetes ("bronze diabetes"), cirrhosis of the liver, a high incidence of hepatic carcinoma, and gonadal atrophy. Hemochromatosis may be hereditary or acquired. The most common cause of the hereditary forms is a mutated *HFE* gene that is common in the white population. It is still unknown precisely how mutations in *HFE* cause hemochromatosis, but individuals who are homogenous for *HFE* mutations absorb excess amounts of iron because

HFE normally inhibits expression of the duodenal transporters that participate in iron uptake. Acquired hemochromatosis occurs when the iron-regulating system is overwhelmed by excess iron loads due to chronic destruction of red blood cells, liver disease, or repeated transfusions in diseases such as intractable anemia.

THERAPEUTIC HIGHLIGHTS

If hereditary hemochromatosis is diagnosed before excessive amounts of iron accumulate in the tissues, life expectancy can be prolonged substantially by repeated withdrawal of blood.

■ CONTROL OF FOOD INTAKE

The intake of nutrients is under complex control involving signals from both the periphery and the central nervous system. Complicating the picture, higher functions also modulate the response to both central and peripheral cues that either trigger or inhibit food intake. Thus, food preferences, emotions, environment, lifestyle, and circadian rhythms may all have profound effects on whether food is sought, and the type of food that is ingested.

Many of the hormones and other factors that are released coincident with a meal, and may play other important roles in digestion and absorption (see Chapter 25) are also involved in the regulation of feeding behavior (Figure 26–4). For example, CCK inhibits food intake and thus is defined as a **satiety factor**

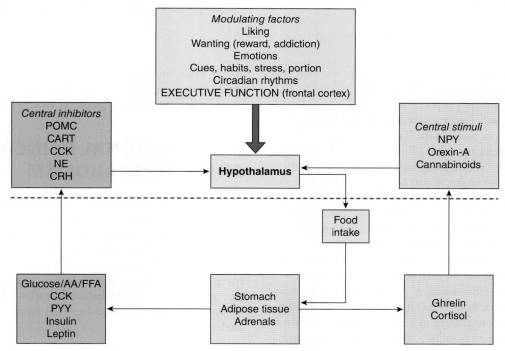

FIGURE 26–4 Summary of mechanisms controlling food intake. Peripheral stimuli and inhibitors, released in anticipation of, or in response to, food intake, cross the blood–brain barrier (indicated by the broken red line) and activate the release and/or synthesis of central factors in the hypothalamus that either increase or decrease subsequent food intake. Food intake can also be modulated by signals from higher centers, as shown. Not shown, peripheral orexins can reduce production of central inhibitors, and vice versa. Abbreviations are defined in the text. (Based on a figure kindly provided by Dr Samuel Klein, Washington University.)

CLINICAL BOX 26–3

Obesity

Obesity is the most common and expensive nutritional problem in the United States. A convenient and reliable indicator of body fat is the **body mass index (BMI),** which is body weight (in kilograms) divided by the square of height (in meters). Values above 25 are abnormal. Individuals with values of 25–30 are considered overweight, and those with values greater than 30 are obese. In the United States, 34% of the population is overweight and 34% is obese. The incidence of obesity is also increasing in other countries. Indeed, although starvation continues to be a problem in many parts of the world, the number of overweight people is now as great as the number of underfed. Obesity is a problem because of its complications, such as accelerated atherosclerosis and an increased incidence of gallbladder and other diseases. Its association with type 2 diabetes is especially striking. As weight increases, insulin resistance increases and frank diabetes appears. At least in some cases, glucose tolerance is restored when weight is lost. In addition, the mortality rates from many kinds of cancer are increased in obese individuals. The causes of the high incidence of obesity in the general population are probably multiple. Studies of twins raised apart show a definite genetic component. It has been pointed out that through much of human evolution, famines were common, and mechanisms that permitted increased energy storage as fat had survival value. Now, however, the ability to gain and retain fat has become a liability. The fundamental cause of obesity is an excess of energy intake over energy expenditure. If human volunteers are fed a fixed high-calorie diet, some gain weight more rapidly than others, but the slower weight gain is due to increased energy expenditure in the form of small, fidgety movements **(nonexercise activity thermogenesis; NEAT).** Body weight generally increases at a slow but steady rate throughout adult life. Decreased physical activity is undoubtedly a factor, but decreased sensitivity to leptin may also play a role.

THERAPEUTIC HIGHLIGHTS

Obesity is such a vexing medical and public health problem because its effective treatment depends so dramatically on lifestyle changes. Long-term weight loss can only be achieved with decreased food intake, increased energy expenditure, or, ideally, some combination of both. Exercise alone is rarely sufficient because it typically induces the patient to ingest more calories. For those who are seriously obese and who have developed serious health complications, surgical approaches can reduce the size of the stomach reservoir and/or bypass it altogether. These surgical maneuvers are intended to reduce the size of meals that can be tolerated, but also have dramatic metabolic effects even before significant weight loss occurs, perhaps as a result of reduced production of peripheral orexins. Pharmaceutical companies are also actively exploring the science of orexins and anorexins to develop drugs that might act centrally to modify food intake (Figure 26–4).

or **anorexin.** CCK and other similar factors have attracted great interest as aids to combat obesity (Clinical Box 26–3).

Leptin and ghrelin are peripheral factors that act reciprocally on food intake. Both activate signaling in the hypothalamus leading to changes in food intake. Leptin is produced by adipose tissue, and signals the status of the fat stores. As adipocytes increase in size, they release greater quantities of leptin and this tends to decrease food intake, in part by increasing the expression of other anorexigenic factors in the hypothalamus such as proopiomelanocortin (POMC), cocaine- and amphetamine-regulated transcript (CART), neurotensin, and corticotropin-releasing hormone (CRH). Leptin also stimulates the metabolic rate. Animal studies have shown that resistance to leptin can allow food intake to persist despite adequate (or even growing) adipose stores.

Ghrelin, on the other hand, is predominantly a fast-acting **orexin** that stimulates food intake. It is produced mainly by the stomach in responses to changes in nutritional status—circulating ghrelin levels increase preprandially, then decrease after a meal. It is believed to be involved primarily in meal initiation, unlike the longer-term effects of leptin. Like leptin, however, the effects of ghrelin are produced mostly via actions in the hypothalamus. It increases synthesis and/or release of central orexins, including neuropeptide Y and cannabinoids, and suppresses the ability of leptin to stimulate the anorexigenic factors discussed above. Loss of the activity of ghrelin may account in part for the effectiveness of gastric bypass procedures for obesity. Its secretion may also be inhibited by leptin, underscoring the reciprocity of these hormones.

■ NUTRITIONAL PRINCIPLES & ENERGY METABOLISM

Humans oxidize carbohydrates, proteins, and fats, producing principally CO_2, H_2O, and the energy necessary for life processes (Clinical Box 26–3). Oxidation occurs via a complex, slow, stepwise process called **catabolism,** which liberates energy in small, usable amounts. Energy can be stored in the body in the form of energy-rich phosphate compounds and in the form of proteins, fats, and complex carbohydrates. Formation of these substances by processes that take up rather than liberate energy is called **anabolism.**

METABOLIC RATE

The amount of energy liberated by catabolism is the same as the amount liberated when food is burned outside the body. The energy liberated by catabolic processes in the body is used for maintaining body functions. It appears as external work, heat, and energy storage:

$$\text{Energy output} = \text{External work} + \text{Energy storage} + \text{Heat}$$

The amount of energy liberated per unit of time is the **metabolic rate.** Isotonic muscle contractions perform work at a peak efficiency approximating 50%:

$$\text{Efficiency} = \frac{\text{Work done}}{\text{Total energy expended}}$$

Essentially all of the energy of isometric contractions appears as heat, because little or no external work is done (see Chapter 5). Energy is stored by forming energy-rich compounds. The amount of energy storage varies, but in fasting individuals it is zero or negative. Therefore, in an adult individual who has not eaten recently and who is not moving (or growing, reproducing, or lactating), all of the energy output appears as heat.

CALORIES

The standard unit of heat energy is the **calorie (cal),** defined as the amount of energy necessary to raise the temperature of 1 g of water by 1°. This unit is also called the gram calorie, small calorie, or standard calorie. The unit commonly used in physiology and medicine is the **Calorie (kilocalorie; kcal),** which equals 1000 cal.

The caloric values of the common foodstuffs, as measured in a bomb calorimeter, are 4.1 kcal/g of carbohydrate, 9.3 kcal/g of fat, and 5.3 kcal/g of protein. In the body, similar values are obtained for carbohydrate and fat, but the oxidation of protein is incomplete. Therefore, the caloric value of protein in the body is only 4.1 kcal/g.

RESPIRATORY QUOTIENT

The **respiratory quotient (RQ)** is the ratio of the steady-state volume of CO_2 produced to the volume of O_2 consumed per unit of time. It should be distinguished from the **respiratory exchange ratio (R),** which is the ratio of CO_2 to O_2 at any given time whether or not equilibrium has been reached. R is affected by factors other than metabolism. RQ and R can be calculated for reactions outside the body, for individual organs and tissues, and for the whole body. The RQ of carbohydrate is 1.00, and that of fat is about 0.70. This is because H and O are present in carbohydrate in the same proportions as in water, whereas in the various fats, extra O_2 is necessary for the formation of H_2O.

Determining the RQ of protein in the body is a complex process, but an average value of 0.82 has been calculated. The approximate amounts of carbohydrate, protein, and fat being oxidized at any given time can be calculated from the RQ and urinary nitrogen excretion. RQ and R for the whole body differ in various conditions. For example, during hyperventilation, R rises because CO_2 is being blown off. During strenuous exercise, R may reach 2.00 because CO_2 is being blown off and lactic acid is being converted to CO_2 (see further). After exercise, R may fall for a while to 0.50 or less. In metabolic acidosis, R rises because respiratory compensation for the acidosis causes the amount of CO_2 expired

to rise (see Chapter 34). In severe acidosis, R may be greater than 1.00. In metabolic alkalosis, R falls.

The O_2 consumption and CO_2 production of an organ can be calculated at equilibrium by multiplying its blood flow per unit of time by the arteriovenous differences for O_2 and CO_2 across the organ, and the RQ can then be calculated. Data on the RQ of individual organs are of interest in drawing inferences about metabolic processes. For example, the RQ of the brain is regularly 0.97–0.99, indicating that its principal fuel is carbohydrate.

FACTORS AFFECTING THE METABOLIC RATE

The metabolic rate is affected by many factors (Table 26–2). The most important is muscular exertion. O_2 consumption is elevated not only during exertion but also for as long afterward as is necessary to repay the O_2 debt (see Chapter 5). Recently ingested foods also increase the metabolic rate because of their **specific dynamic action (SDA).** The SDA of a food is the obligatory energy expenditure for its assimilation. It takes 30 kcal to assimilate the amount of protein sufficient to raise the metabolic rate 100 kcal; 6 kcal to assimilate a similar amount of carbohydrate; and 5 kcal to assimilate a similar amount of fat.

Another factor that stimulates metabolism is the environmental temperature. The curve relating the metabolic rate to the environmental temperature is U-shaped. When the environmental temperature is lower than body temperature, heat-producing mechanisms are activated and the metabolic rate rises. When the temperature is high enough to raise the body temperature, metabolic processes generally accelerate, and the metabolic rate rises about 14% for each degree Celsius of elevation.

The metabolic rate determined at rest in a room at a comfortable temperature in the thermoneutral zone 12–14 h after the last meal is called the **basal metabolic rate (BMR).** This value falls about 10% during sleep and up to 40% during prolonged starvation. The **maximum metabolic rate** reached during exercise is often said to be 10 times the BMR, but trained athletes can increase their metabolic rate as much as 20-fold.

The BMR of a man of average size is about 2000 kcal/day. Large animals have higher absolute BMRs, but the ratio of BMR

TABLE 26–2 Factors affecting the metabolic rate.

Muscular exertion during or just before measurement
Recent ingestion of food
High or low environmental temperature
Height, weight, and surface area
Sex
Age
Growth
Reproduction
Lactation
Emotional state
Body temperature
Circulating levels of thyroid hormones
Circulating epinephrine and norepinephrine levels

to body weight in small animals is much greater. One variable that correlates well with the metabolic rate in different species is the body surface area. This would be expected, since heat exchange occurs at the body surface.

For clinical use, the BMR is usually expressed as a percentage increase or decrease above or below a set of generally used standard normal values. Thus, a value of +65 means that the individual's BMR is 65% above the standard for their age and sex.

The decrease in metabolic rate related to a decrease in body weight is part of the explanation of why, when an individual is trying to lose weight, weight loss is initially rapid and then slows down.

ENERGY BALANCE

The first law of thermodynamics, the principle that states that energy is neither created nor destroyed when it is converted from one form to another, applies to living organisms as well as inanimate systems. One may therefore speak of an **energy balance** between caloric intake and energy output. If the caloric content of food is less than the energy output, that is, if the balance is negative, endogenous stores are utilized. Glycogen, body protein, and fat are catabolized, and the individual loses weight.

If the caloric value of the food intake exceeds energy loss, that is, if the balance is positive, energy is stored, and the individual gains weight.

■ NUTRITION

The aim of the science of nutrition is the determination of the kinds and amounts of foods that promote health and well-being. This includes not only the problems of undernutrition but those of overnutrition, taste, and availability (**Clinical Box 26–4**). However, certain substances are essential constituents of any human diet. Many of these compounds have been mentioned in previous sections of this chapter, and a brief summary of the essential and desirable dietary components is presented next.

ESSENTIAL DIETARY COMPONENTS

An optimal diet includes, in addition to sufficient water (see Chapter 37), adequate calories, protein, fat, minerals, and vitamins.

The distribution of the calories among carbohydrate, protein, and fat is determined partly by physiologic factors and partly

---

CLINICAL BOX 26–4

The Malabsorption Syndrome

The digestive and absorptive functions of the small intestine are essential for life. However, the digestive and absorptive capacity of the intestine is larger than needed for normal function (the **anatomic reserve**). Removal of short segments of the jejunum or ileum generally does not cause severe symptoms, and compensatory hypertrophy and hyperplasia of the remaining mucosa occur. However, when more than 50% of the small intestine is resected or bypassed (**short gut syndrome**), absorption of nutrients and vitamins is so compromised that it is difficult to prevent malnutrition and wasting (**malabsorption**). Resection of the terminal ileum also prevents the absorption of bile acids, and this leads to deficient fat absorption. It also causes diarrhea because the unabsorbed bile acids enter the colon, where they activate chloride secretion (see Chapter 25). Other complications of intestinal resection or bypass include hypocalcemia, arthritis, and possibly fatty infiltration of the liver, followed by cirrhosis. Various disease processes can also impair absorption without a loss of intestinal length. The pattern of deficiencies is sometimes called the **malabsorption syndrome**. This pattern varies somewhat with the cause, but it can include deficient absorption of amino acids, with marked body wasting and, eventually, hypoproteinemia and edema. Carbohydrate and fat absorption are also depressed. Because of defective fat absorption, the fat-soluble vitamins (vitamins A, D, E, and K) are not absorbed in adequate amounts. One of the most interesting conditions causing the malabsorption syndrome

is the autoimmune disease **celiac disease**. This disease occurs in genetically predisposed individuals in whom gluten and closely related proteins cause intestinal T cells to mount an inappropriate immune response that damages the intestinal epithelial cells and results in a loss of villi and a flattening of the mucosa. The proteins are found in wheat, rye, barley, and to a lesser extent in oats—but not in rice or corn. When grains containing gluten are omitted from the diet, bowel function is generally restored to normal.

THERAPEUTIC HIGHLIGHTS

Treatment of malabsorption depends on the underlying cause. In celiac disease, foods containing gluten should be strictly excluded from the diet, although this may be difficult to achieve. The diarrhea that accompanies bile acid malabsorption can be treated with a resin (cholestyramine) that binds bile acids in the lumen and prevents their secretory action. Patients deficient in fat-soluble vitamins may be given these compounds as water-soluble derivatives. For serious cases of short bowel syndrome, it may be necessary to supply nutrients parenterally. There is hope that small bowel transplantation may eventually become routine, but of course transplantation carries its own long-term disadvantages and also requires a reliable supply of donor tissues.

by taste and economic considerations. A daily protein intake of 1 g/kg body weight to supply essential amino acids and other amino acids is desirable. The source of the protein is also important. **Grade I proteins,** the animal proteins of meat, fish, dairy products, and eggs, contain amino acids in approximately the proportions required for protein synthesis and other uses. Some plant proteins are also grade I, but most are **grade II** because they supply different proportions of amino acid and some lack one or more of the essential amino acids. Protein needs can be met with a mixture of grade II proteins, but intake must be large because of the amino acid wastage.

Fat is the most compact form of food, since it supplies 9.3 kcal/g. Western diets have typically contained large amounts (100 g/day or more). In Central and South American Indian communities where corn (carbohydrate) is the dietary staple, adults live without ill effects for years on a very low-fat intake. Therefore, provided that the needs for essential fatty acids are met, a low-fat intake does not seem to be harmful, and a diet low in saturated fats is desirable.

Carbohydrate is the cheapest source of calories and provides 50% or more of the calories in most diets. In the average American diet, approximately 50% of the calories come from carbohydrate, 15% from protein, and 35% from fat. When calculating dietary needs, it is usual to meet the protein requirement first and then split the remaining calories between fat and carbohydrate, depending on taste, income, and other factors. For example, a 65-kg man who is moderately active needs about 2800 kcal/day. He should eat at least 65 g of protein daily, supplying 267 (65 × 4.1) kcal. Some of this should be grade I protein. A reasonable figure for fat intake is 50–60 g. The rest of the caloric requirement can be met by supplying carbohydrate.

MINERAL REQUIREMENTS

A number of minerals must be ingested daily for the maintenance of health. Trace elements are defined as elements found in tissues in minute amounts. Those believed to be essential for life, at least in experimental animals, are listed in Table 26–3. In humans, iron deficiency causes anemia. Cobalt is part of the vitamin B_{12} molecule, and vitamin B_{12} deficiency leads to anemia (see Chapter 31). Iodine deficiency causes thyroid disorders (see Chapter 19). Zinc deficiency causes skin ulcers, depressed immune responses, and hypogonadal dwarfism. Copper deficiency causes anemia and changes in ossification. Chromium

TABLE 26–3 Trace elements believed essential for life.

Arsenic	Manganese
Chromium	Molybdenum
Cobalt	Nickel
Copper	Selenium
Fluorine	Silicon
Iodine	Vanadium
Iron	Zinc

deficiency causes insulin resistance. Fluorine deficiency increases the incidence of dental caries.

Some minerals can be toxic in excess. For example, severe iron overload with toxic effects is seen in hemochromatosis (Clinical Box 26–2). Similarly, copper excess causes brain damage (Wilson disease). Sodium and potassium are also essential minerals, but it is very difficult to prepare a sodium-free or potassium-free diet. A low-salt diet is, however, well tolerated because of compensatory mechanisms that conserve Na^+.

VITAMINS

Vitamins were discovered when it was observed that certain diets otherwise adequate in calories, essential amino acids, fats, and minerals failed to maintain health (eg, in sailors engaged in long voyages without access to fresh fruits and vegetables). The term **vitamin** has now come to refer to any organic dietary constituent necessary for life, health, and growth that does not function by supplying energy.

Most vitamins have important functions in intermediary metabolism or the special metabolism of the various organ systems. Those that are water soluble (vitamin B complex, vitamin C) are easily absorbed, but the fat-soluble vitamins (vitamins A, D, E, and K) are poorly absorbed in the absence of bile and/or pancreatic enzymes. Some dietary fat intake is necessary for their absorption, and in obstructive jaundice or disease of the exocrine pancreas, deficiencies can develop. Vitamin A and vitamin D are bound to transfer proteins in the circulation. The α-tocopherol form of vitamin E is normally bound to chylomicrons. In the liver, it is transferred to very low-density lipoprotein (VLDL) and distributed to tissues by an α-tocopherol transfer protein. When this protein is abnormal due to mutation of its gene, there is cellular deficiency of vitamin E and the development of a condition resembling Friedreich ataxia.

It is also worth remembering that very large doses of the fat-soluble vitamins are definitely toxic. **Hypervitaminosis A** is characterized by anorexia, headache, hepatosplenomegaly, irritability, scaly dermatitis, patchy loss of hair, bone pain, and hyperostosis. **Hypervitaminosis D** is associated with weight loss, calcification of many soft tissues, and acute kidney injury. **Hypervitaminosis K** is characterized by gastrointestinal disturbances and anemia. Large doses of water-soluble vitamins have been thought to be less likely to cause problems because they can be rapidly cleared from the body. However, it has been demonstrated that ingestion of megadoses of pyridoxine (vitamin B_6) can produce peripheral neuropathy.

CHAPTER SUMMARY

■ A typical mixed meal consists of carbohydrates, proteins, and lipids (the latter largely as triglycerides). Each must be digested to allow its uptake into the body. Specific transporters carry the products of digestion into the body.

■ The epithelium can only transport carbohydrate monomers, whereas short peptides can be absorbed in addition to amino acids.

- The proteases in pancreatic juice are not activated until they reach their substrates in the small intestinal lumen. This is accomplished by the restricted localization of an activating enzyme, enterokinase.

- Lipids face special challenges to assimilation given their hydrophobicity. Bile acids solubilize the products of lipolysis in micelles and accelerate their diffusion to the epithelial surface. The assimilation of cholesterol and fat-soluble vitamins absolutely requires this mechanism.

- The catabolism of nutrients provides energy to the body in a controlled fashion. The caloric value of dietary intake must be approximately equal to energy expenditure for homeostasis.

- A balanced diet is important for health, and certain dietary substances are essential.

MULTIPLE-CHOICE QUESTIONS

For all questions, select the single best answer unless otherwise directed.

1. A premenopausal woman who is physically active seeks advice from her primary care clinician regarding measures she can take to ensure adequate availability of dietary calcium to ensure bone health later in life. Which of the following dietary components should enhance calcium uptake?
   A. Protein
   B. Oxalates
   C. Iron
   D. Vitamin D
   E. Sodium

2. A child is brought to his pediatrician for an investigation of his failure to thrive. Genetic tests reveal a congenital absence of enterokinase. A decrease in which of the following is expected in this patient?
   A. Incidence of pancreatitis
   B. Carbohydrate assimilation
   C. Bile acid reabsorption
   D. Gastric pH
   E. Protein assimilation

3. A healthy individual who decides to have his DNA sequenced learns that he has a mutation in a protein responsible from the transport of neutral amino acids consistent with a diagnosis of Hartnup disease. The fact that he has experienced no nutritional consequence of this mutation is directly attributable to the presence of which of the following?
   A. PepT1
   B. brush border peptidases
   C. Na+, K+ ATPase
   D. Cystic fibrosis transmembrane conductance regulator (CFTR)
   E. Trypsin

4. A newborn baby is brought to the pediatrician suffering from severe diarrhea that worsens after feeding. The symptoms diminish when nutrients are delivered intravenously. The child most likely has a mutation in which of the following intestinal transporters?
   A. Na$^+$, K$^+$ ATPase
   B. NHE3
   C. SGLT-1
   D. H$^+$, K$^+$ ATPase
   E. NKCC1

5. An infant who was previously healthy but is displaying symptoms of acute diarrhea and dehydration after an infection is given an oral solution of glucose and electrolytes (Pedialyte). What membrane protein accounts for the ability of this solution to provide rapid hydration?
   A. Sucrase-isomaltase
   B. SGLT-1
   C. CFTR
   D. Chloride-bicarbonate exchanger
   E. Lactose-phlorizin hydrolase

6. In the situation described in Question 5, the child's mother does not have any Pedialyte available, and so gives her baby some boiled water in which she has dissolved salt and table sugar. Activity of which enzyme, in addition to SGLT-1, will be needed for this to be effective in rehydrating her baby?
   A. Salivary amylase
   B. Pancreatic amylase
   C. Glucoamylase
   D. Lactose-phlorizin hydrolase
   E. Sucrase-isomaltase

7. A child is brought to her pediatrician exhibiting signs of malnutrition, diarrhea, and edema of the extremities. Duodenal aspirates are obtained at endoscopy after intravenous administration of cholecystokinin, and are found to be incapable of protein hydrolysis at neutral pH unless a trace amount of trypsin is added that by itself would not result in appreciable hydrolysis. The patient is most likely suffering from a deficiency in which of the following?
   A. Pepsinogen
   B. PepT1
   C. Trypsinogen
   D. Carboxypeptidases
   E. Enterokinase

8. A patient with obstructive jaundice who is scheduled for gallbladder surgery is found to have an elevated prothrombin time. This laboratory finding is most likely due to malabsorption of which of the following vitamins?
   A. A
   B. C
   C. B$_{12}$
   D. K
   E. E

9. A patient is treated with cholestyramine, a bile-acid binding resin, for hypercholesterolemia. Absorption of which of the following is likely to be abnormal in this patient?
   A. Long-chain triglyceride
   B. Medium-chain triglyceride
   C. Starch
   D. Vitamin D
   E. Vitamin B$_6$

10. A 20-year-old man with a history of mild cystic fibrosis notices that his stools are becoming bulky, pale-colored and oily. Laboratory tests confirm steatorrhea. Which of the following would not be involved in his apparent decrease in fat assimilation?
    A. Lipase inactivation
    B. Decreased pancreatic lipase output
    C. Reduced pancreatic bicarbonate secretion
    D. Loss of the anatomic reserve
    E. Decreased colipase synthesis

ANSWERS

1. The correct answer is **D.** Calcium is absorbed across the brush border of intestinal epithelial cells via TRPV6 channels and sequestered in the cytosol by calcium-binding proteins (see Chapter 21). Vitamin D increases expression of these proteins as well as those mediating calcium export across the basolateral membrane. Dietary iron and oxalate can chelate calcium, potentially reducing its absorption (note that kidney stones are most commonly made up of calcium oxalate) (rules out options **B** and **C**). Adequate protein intake is important for bone health, but this effect is related to the synthesis of bone matrix proteins rather than an influence on calcium absorption (rules out option **A**). Finally, the mechanism for apical calcium uptake from the diet is via a channel rather than a Na$^+$/Ca^{++} exchanger, so dietary sodium should not influence calcium uptake. Na$^+$/Ca^{++} exchange may contribute to basolateral calcium export, but this process would be inhibited rather than stimulated by an increase in cytosolic sodium ions (rules out option **E**).

2. The correct answer is **E.** Enterokinase, localized to the intestinal brush border, is responsible for activating pancreatic trypsin in the gut lumen, which in turn activates the remaining pancreatic proteases. In the absence of protease activation, dietary proteins will not be digested to forms that can be assimilated. Absorption of carbohydrates should be unaffected because amylase is released by the pancreas in active form (rules out option **B**). The incidence of pancreatitis should be unaltered since the defect is in the intestine (rules out option **A**). Active bile acid reabsorption takes place in the terminal ileum via a sodium-coupled pathway and should not be affected by a lack of enterokinase (rules out option **C**). Finally, excessive acid secretion by the stomach can inactivate pancreatic enzymes, but would not be expected in this patient in the absence of other pathologies (rules out option **D**).

3. The correct answer is **A.** Patients with Hartnup disease can be asymptomatic, particularly if their diet is high in protein. Although they lack the ability to absorb certain amino acids (and particularly tryptophan) in a sodium-dependent manner, the required amino acids can instead be assimilated in the form of short peptides via PepT1, with the amino acids subsequently liberated by cytosolic peptidases. The presence of brush border peptidases is not protective—if anything, these can exacerbate the transport defect by cleaving short peptides in the lumen (rules out option **B**). Also, PepT1 is a proton-coupled transporter, rather than sodium-coupled, so its activity is not dependent on that of the Na$^+$, K$^+$ ATPase (rules out option **C**). The chloride channel, CFTR, is not involved at all in protein assimilation (rules out option **D**). Finally, while trypsin generates short peptides from dietary protein, it is not the only protease/peptidase involved, and thus is not directly required to maintain health in this patient (rules out option **E**).

4. The correct answer is **C.** Glucose-galactose malabsorption is a congenital disorder caused by a variety of mutations in SGLT-1. Children with this disorder tolerate diets containing either sugar poorly, and manifest with osmotic diarrhea. Lactose in milk is a disaccharide comprised of glucose and galactose, accounting for the postprandial symptoms. SGLT-1 is sodium-coupled, so in theory the symptoms would be consistent with a defect in Na$^+$, K$^+$ ATPase, but the ubiquitous nature of this transporter means that mutations are

likely incompatible with life, and would anyway result in the failure to absorb electrolytes in addition to nutrients (rules out option **A**). A mutation in NHE3 would impair the electroneutral NaCl absorption mechanism, and could result in diarrhea, but this would not be in keeping with the postprandial worsening of diarrhea because the transport mechanism is predominantly responsible for NaCl uptake in the period between meals (rules out option **B**). Defects in H$^+$, K$^+$ ATPase and NKCC1 would impair gastric acid secretion and intestinal chloride secretion, respectively, but neither would be expected to lead to diarrhea and the latter might even reduce it (rules out options **D** and **E**).

5. The correct answer is **B.** Sodium uptake can be driven by providing its transport partner, glucose, and taking advantage of the low intracellular sodium concentration in the intestinal epithelium. SGLT-1 activity is typically spared in acute infectious diarrhea. Because the solution contains monomeric glucose, its carbohydrate component does not require digestion by brush border hydrolases prior to assimilation (rules out options **A** and **E**). Further, CFTR is often activated in diarrheal illness and accounts for fluid and electrolyte loss from the body (rules out option **C**). Similarly, intestinal chloride-bicarbonate exchangers contribute to NaCl uptake but are not driven by glucose availability; they are also downregulated by the signals that activate chloride secretion and thus worsen diarrhea (rules out option **D**).

6. The correct answer is **C.** Table sugar is the common name for sucrose, a dimer of glucose and fructose. It is not digested luminally, but rather at the level of the brush-border by the sucrase activity of sucrase-isomaltase. Sucrose is not a substrate for the luminal amylase enzymes that digest starch to glucose oligomers and alpha-limit dextrins (rules out options **A** and **B**). Nor is it a substrate for the brush border hydrolases glucoamylase and lactose-phlorizin hydrolase, which act on glucose oligomers and lactose, respectively (rules out options **C** and **D**).

7. The correct answer is **E.** Enterokinase, localized to the intestinal brush border, acts on pancreatic trypsinogen to form active trypsin, which in turn activates the remaining pancreatic proteases. Because the duodenal aspirates can hydrolyse proteins when a trace amount of trypsin is supplied exogenously, they presumably contain adequate concentrations of the inactive precursors of the pancreatic proteases and peptidases (rules out options **C** and **D**). Gastric pepsinogen is also dispensable for protein digestion and assimilation since it produces mostly long oligopeptides that are too large to be absorbed (rules out option **A**). Finally, an isolated deficiency in PepT1 might result in deficiencies of specific amino acids that are absorbed poorly by amino acid transporters, but would not be expected to result in generalized hypoproteinemia and edema (rules out option **B**).

8. The correct answer is **D.** The fat-soluble vitamin, vitamin K, is required for the post-translational modification of several clotting factors to allow them to bind calcium ions, which is required for the formation of a blood clot. In the absence of bile acids, micelles cannot form in the intestinal contents and the absorption of all fat-soluble vitamins is dramatically impaired. Vitamins A and E are also fat-soluble vitamins that will be absorbed poorly in this patient, but they are not involved in the clotting mechanism (rules out options **A** and **E**). Vitamins C and B$_{12}$, on the other hand, are water-soluble vitamins that are taken up by specific transporters and do not

depend on bile acids or micelles for their absorption (rules out options **B** and **C**).

9. The correct answer is **D.** Vitamin D is a fat-soluble vitamin whose uptake is entirely dependent on micelles. Cholestyramine will reduce the concentration of free bile acids in the intestinal lumen, likely below the critical micellar concentration such that micelles will not form. Absorption of the products of digestion of both long- and medium chain triglycerides is accelerated by the presence of micelles, but these products also have appreciable aqueous solubility. Coupled with the anatomic reserve, there is likely to be adequate time for their absorption to avoid steatorrhea. Medium chain fatty acids are also absorbed paracellularly due to their even greater aqueous solubility (rules out options **A** and **B**). Finally, starch and vitamin B_6 are water-soluble nutrients whose digestion/ assimilation is completely independent of micelles (rules out options **C** and **E**).

10. The correct answer is **D.** The intestinal surface area available for lipid absorption should not be altered in this patient. Cystic fibrosis, arising from mutations in CFTR, results in a decrease in the ability of the pancreatic ducts to secrete bicarbonate (rules out option **C**). Those with mild mutations can retain some level of pancreatic function into adulthood, but the decreased flow of pancreatic juice results in retention of pancreatic enzymes and injury to the pancreatic acinar cells, reducing their ability to synthesize proteins, including those involved in fat digestion (rules out options **B** and **E**). Further, the lack of bicarbonate secretion means that the pH in the duodenal lumen will fall, inactivating any remaining lipase, which is more sensitive to acidic pH than other digestive enzymes (rules out option **A**).

Gastrointestinal Motility

- List the major forms of motility in the gastrointestinal tract and their roles.
- Distinguish between peristalsis and segmentation.
- Explain the electrical basis of gastrointestinal contractions and the role of basic electrical activity in governing motility patterns.
- Describe how gastrointestinal motility changes during fasting.
- Understand how food is swallowed.
- Define the factors that govern gastric emptying and the abnormal response of vomiting.
- Define how the motility patterns of the colon help to desiccate and evacuate the stool.

INTRODUCTION

Digestion and absorption depend on a variety of mechanisms that soften the food, propel it through the length of the gastrointestinal tract, and mix it with bile and digestive enzymes. Some of these mechanisms depend on intrinsic properties of the intestinal smooth muscle. Others involve the operation of reflexes involving the neurons intrinsic to the gut, reflexes involving the central nervous system (CNS), paracrine effects of chemical messengers, and gastrointestinal hormones.

◼ GENERAL PATTERNS OF MOTILITY

PERISTALSIS

Peristalsis is a reflex response that is initiated when the gut wall is stretched, and occurs in all parts of the gastrointestinal tract. The stretch initiates a circular contraction behind the stimulus and an area of relaxation in front of it (Figure 27–1). The wave of contraction then moves in an oral-to-caudal direction, propelling the contents forward. Peristalsis can be increased or decreased by autonomic input, but its occurrence is independent of extrinsic innervation. It is an excellent example of the integrated activity of the enteric nervous system. Local stretch releases serotonin, which activates sensory neurons that activate the myenteric plexus. Cholinergic neurons in this plexus passing in a retrograde direction activate neurons that release substance P and acetylcholine,

causing smooth muscle contraction behind the bolus. At the same time, cholinergic neurons passing in an anterograde direction activate neurons that secrete NO and vasoactive intestinal polypeptide (VIP), producing the relaxation ahead of the stimulus.

SEGMENTATION & MIXING

When the meal is present, a motility pattern known as segmentation occurs that is designed to retard the movement of the intestinal contents to provide time for digestion and absorption (Figure 27–1). A segment of bowel contracts at both ends, and then a second contraction occurs in the center of the segment to force the contents (chyme) both backward and forward. Unlike peristalsis, retrograde movement of the chyme occurs routinely in the setting of segmentation. This mixing pattern persists for as long as nutrients remain in the lumen. It reflects programmed activity of the enteric nervous system.

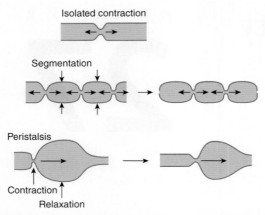

FIGURE 27–1 Patterns of gastrointestinal motility and propulsion. An isolated contraction moves contents orally and aborally. Segmentation mixes contents over a short stretch of intestine, as indicated by the time sequence from left to right. In the diagram on the left, the vertical arrows indicate the sites of subsequent contraction. Peristalsis involves both contraction and relaxation, and moves contents aborally.

BASIC ELECTRICAL ACTIVITY & REGULATION OF MOTILITY

Except in the esophagus and the proximal stomach, the smooth muscle of the gastrointestinal tract has spontaneous rhythmic fluctuations in membrane potential between about –65 and –45 mV.

This **basic electrical rhythm (BER)** is initiated by the **interstitial cells of Cajal,** pacemaker cells with smooth muscle-like features that send long branched processes into the intestinal smooth muscle.

The BER itself rarely causes muscle contraction, but **spike potentials** superimposed on the most depolarizing portions of the BER waves do increase muscle tension. The depolarizing portion of each spike is due to Ca^{2+} influx, and the repolarizing portion is due to K^+ efflux. Acetylcholine increases the number of spikes and the tension of the smooth muscle, whereas epinephrine decreases the number of spikes and the tension. The rate of the BER is about 4/min in the stomach. It is about 12/min in the duodenum and falls to about 8/min in the distal ileum. In the colon, the BER rate rises from about 2/min at the cecum to about 6/min at the sigmoid. The function of the BER is to coordinate peristaltic and other motor activity, such as setting the rhythm of segmentation.

MIGRATING MOTOR COMPLEX

During fasting, the pattern of motor activity in gastrointestinal smooth muscle becomes modified so that cycles migrate from the stomach to the distal ileum. Each cycle, or **migrating motor complex (MMC),** starts with a quiescent period (phase I), continues with a period of irregular electrical and mechanical activity (phase II), and ends with a burst of regular activity (phase III) **(Figure 27–2).** The MMCs are initiated by motilin, which increases at intervals of approximately 100 min in the interdigestive state. The contractions migrate aborally at a rate of about 5 cm/min. Gastric secretion, bile flow, and pancreatic secretion

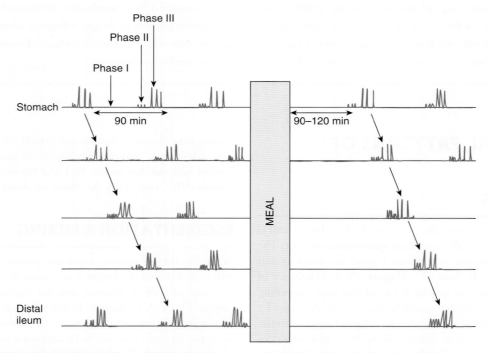

FIGURE 27–2 Migrating motor complexes (MMCs). The three phases include a quiescent phase (phase I); a phase consisting of small, irregular contractions that do not propagate (phase II); and a phase of regular activity lasting about 5 min (phase III), which sweeps along the length of the intestine. The entire cycle repeats every 90–100 min under fasting conditions. Note that the complexes are completely inhibited by a meal and resume 90–120 min later.

increase during each MMC, to clear the stomach and small intestine of luminal contents in preparation for the next meal.

Conversely, when a meal is ingested, secretion of motilin is suppressed, and the MMC is abolished until digestion and absorption are complete. The antibiotic erythromycin binds to motilin receptors, and its derivatives may be of value in treating patients with decreased gastrointestinal motility.

■ SEGMENT-SPECIFIC PATTERNS OF MOTILITY

■ MOUTH & ESOPHAGUS

In the mouth, food is mixed with saliva and propelled into the esophagus. Peristaltic waves in the esophagus move the food into the stomach.

MASTICATION

Chewing (**mastication**) breaks up large food particles and mixes the food with saliva. This wetting and homogenizing action aids swallowing and digestion. Large food particles cause strong and often painful contractions of the esophageal musculature. Edentulous patients are generally restricted to a soft diet and have difficulty eating dry food.

SWALLOWING

Swallowing (**deglutition**) is a reflex response that is triggered by afferent impulses in the trigeminal, glossopharyngeal, and vagus nerves (Figure 27–3). These impulses are integrated in the nucleus of the tractus solitarius and the nucleus ambiguus. Swallowing is initiated by the voluntary action of collecting the oral contents on the tongue and propelling them backward into the pharynx. This starts a wave of involuntary contraction that pushes the material into the esophagus. Inhibition of respiration and glottic closure are part of the reflex response. A peristaltic ring contraction of the esophageal muscle forms behind the material, which is then swept down the esophagus. If any food remains in the esophagus, it is cleared by a second wave of peristalsis.

LOWER ESOPHAGEAL SPHINCTER

Unlike the rest of the esophagus, the musculature of the gastroesophageal junction (**lower esophageal sphincter [LES]**) is tonically active but relaxes on swallowing. The tonic activity of the LES prevents reflux of gastric contents and is under neural control. Release of acetylcholine from vagal endings causes the sphincter to contract, and release of NO and VIP from interneurons innervated by other vagal fibers causes it to relax. Thus, the sphincter operates to permit orderly flow of food into the stomach (Clinical Box 27–1).

AEROPHAGIA & INTESTINAL GAS

Some air is unavoidably swallowed in the process of eating and drinking (**aerophagia**). Some of the swallowed air is regurgitated (belching), and some of the gases it contains are absorbed, but much of it passes on to the colon. Here, some of the oxygen is absorbed, and hydrogen, hydrogen sulfide, carbon dioxide, and methane formed by the colonic bacteria from carbohydrates and other substances are added to it. It is then expelled as **flatus**. The smell is largely due to sulfides. In some individuals, gas in the

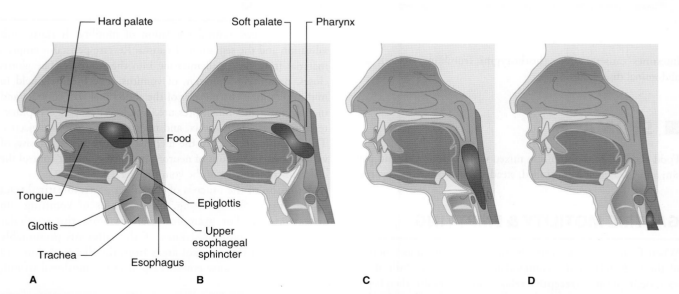

FIGURE 27–3 Movement of food through the pharynx and upper esophagus during swallowing. (A) The tongue pushes the food bolus to the back of the mouth. **(B)** The soft palate elevates to prevent food from entering the nasal passages. **(C)** The epiglottis covers the glottis to prevent food from entering the trachea and the upper esophageal sphincter relaxes. **(D)** Food descends into the esophagus.

Motor Disorders of the Esophagus

Achalasia (literally, failure to relax) is a condition in which food accumulates in the esophagus and the organ can become massively dilated. It is due to increased resting LES tone and incomplete relaxation on swallowing. The myenteric plexus of the esophagus is deficient at the LES in this condition and the release of NO and VIP is defective. The opposite condition is LES incompetence, which permits reflux of acid gastric contents into the esophagus **(gastroesophageal reflux disease)**. This common condition is the most frequent digestive disorder causing patients to seek care from a clinician. It causes heartburn and esophagitis and can lead to ulceration and stricture of the esophagus due to scarring. Most cases are caused by intermittent periods of poorly understood decreases in the neural drive to the sphincter.

THERAPEUTIC HIGHLIGHTS

Achalasia can be treated by pneumatic dilation of the sphincter or incision of the esophageal muscle (myotomy). Inhibition of acetylcholine release by injection of botulinum toxin into the LES is also effective and produces relief that lasts for several months. Gastroesophageal reflux disease can be treated by inhibition of acid secretion with H_2-receptor blockers or proton pump inhibitors (see Chapter 25). Surgical treatment in which a portion of the fundus of the stomach is wrapped around the lower esophagus so that the LES is inside a short tunnel of stomach **(fundoplication)** can also be tried, although in many patients who undergo this procedure the symptoms eventually return.

intestines causes cramps, **borborygmi** (rumbling noises), and abdominal discomfort.

■ STOMACH

Food is stored in the stomach; mixed with acid, mucus, and pepsin; and released at a controlled, steady rate into the duodenum.

GASTRIC MOTILITY & EMPTYING

When food enters the stomach, the fundus and upper portion of the body relax and accommodate the food with little if any increase in pressure **(receptive relaxation)**. Peristalsis then begins in the lower portion of the body, mixing and grinding the food and permitting small, semiliquid portions of it to pass through the pylorus and enter the duodenum.

Receptive relaxation is, in part, vagally mediated and triggered by movement of the pharynx and esophagus. Intrinsic reflexes also lead to relaxation as the stomach wall is stretched. Peristaltic waves sweep toward the pylorus. The contraction of the distal stomach caused by each wave is sometimes called **antral systole** and can last up to 10 s.

In the regulation of gastric emptying, contraction of the antrum is followed by sequential contraction of the pyloric region and the duodenum. In the antrum, partial contraction ahead of the advancing gastric contents prevents solid masses from entering the duodenum, and they are mixed and crushed instead. The more liquid gastric contents are squirted a bit at a time into the small intestine. Normally, regurgitation from the duodenum does not occur, in part because cholecystokinin (CCK) and secretin stimulate contraction of the pyloric sphincter.

REGULATION OF GASTRIC MOTILITY & EMPTYING

The rate at which the stomach empties depends on the type of food ingested. Food rich in carbohydrate leaves the stomach in a few hours. Protein-rich food leaves more slowly, and emptying is slowest after a meal containing fat. The rate of emptying also depends on the osmotic pressure of the material entering the duodenum. Hyperosmolality is sensed by "duodenal osmoreceptors" that decrease gastric emptying.

Fats, carbohydrates, and acid in the duodenum inhibit gastric acid and pepsin secretion and gastric motility via neural and hormonal mechanisms. The messenger involved is probably peptide YY. CCK has also been implicated as an inhibitor of gastric emptying (**Clinical Box 27–2**).

VOMITING

Vomiting reflects central regulation of motility. It starts with salivation and the sensation of nausea. Reverse peristalsis empties material from the small intestine into the stomach. The glottis closes, preventing aspiration of vomitus. The breath is held in mid inspiration. The muscles of the abdominal wall contract and increase intra-abdominal pressure. The lower esophageal sphincter and the esophagus relax, and the gastric contents are ejected. The "vomiting center" in the medulla (**Figure 27–4**) consists of various scattered groups of neurons in this region that control the different components of the vomiting act.

Irritation of the mucosa of the upper gastrointestinal tract is one trigger for vomiting. Other causes of vomiting can arise centrally. For example, afferents from the vestibular nuclei mediate motion sickness. Other afferents presumably reach the vomiting control areas from the diencephalon and limbic system, because emetic responses to emotional stimuli also occur.

Chemoreceptor cells in the medulla can also initiate vomiting when stimulated by certain chemicals. The **chemoreceptor trigger zone** (Figure 27–4) is in the **area postrema.** This structure

CLINICAL BOX 27-2

Consequences of Gastric Bypass Surgery

Patients who are morbidly obese may undergo surgery in which the stomach is stapled so that most of it is bypassed, losing its reservoir function. As a result, such patients must eat frequent small meals. If larger meals are eaten, because of rapid absorption of glucose from the intestine and the resultant hyperglycemia and abrupt rise in insulin secretion, hypoglycemic symptoms sometimes develop. Weakness, dizziness, and sweating after meals, due in part to hypoglycemia, are part of the **"dumping syndrome"** that also develops in patients in whom portions of the stomach have been removed or the jejunum has been anastomosed to the stomach. Another cause of the symptoms is rapid entry of hypertonic meals into the intestine; this provokes the movement of so much water into the gut that hypovolemia and hypotension are produced.

THERAPEUTIC HIGHLIGHTS

There are no treatments, per se, for the dumping syndrome, other than avoiding large meals. Indeed, it may contribute to the success of bypass surgery in reducing food intake.

is one of the circumventricular organs (see Chapter 33) and is not protected by the blood–brain barrier. Lesions of the area postrema have little effect on the vomiting response to gastrointestinal irritation or motion sickness, but abolish the vomiting that follows injection of emetic drugs.

Serotonin (5-HT) released from enterochromaffin cells appears to initiate impulses via 5-HT$_3$ receptors that trigger vomiting. In addition, there are dopamine D$_2$ receptors and 5-HT$_3$ receptors in the area postrema and adjacent nucleus of the solitary tract. 5-HT$_3$ antagonists and D$_2$ antagonists are effective antiemetic agents.

■ SMALL INTESTINE

In the small intestine, the intestinal contents are mixed with the digestive secretions.

INTESTINAL MOTILITY

In the small intestine, there are three types of smooth muscle contractions: peristaltic waves, segmentation contractions, and tonic contractions. **Peristalsis** is described above. It propels the chyme

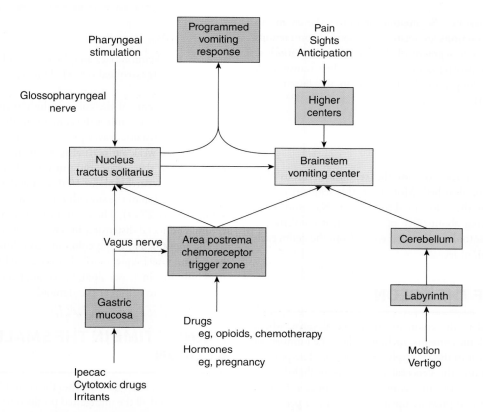

FIGURE 27–4 Neural pathways leading to the initiation of vomiting in response to various stimuli.

Ileus

When the intestines are traumatized, there is a direct inhibition of smooth muscle, which causes a decrease in motility. It is due in part to activation of opioid receptors. When the peritoneum is irritated, reflex inhibition occurs due to increased discharge of noradrenergic fibers in the splanchnic nerves. Both types of inhibition operate to cause **paralytic (adynamic) ileus** after abdominal surgeries. Because of the diffuse decrease in peristaltic activity in the small intestine, its contents are not propelled into the colon, and it becomes irregularly distended by pockets of gas and fluid. Intestinal peristalsis returns in 6–8 h, followed by gastric peristalsis, but colonic activity takes 2–3 days to return.

THERAPEUTIC HIGHLIGHTS

Ileus can be relieved by passing a tube through the nose down to the small intestine and aspirating the fluid and gas until peristalsis returns. The occurrence of ileus has been reduced by more widespread use of minimally invasive surgery. Postsurgical regimens also encourage early ambulation, which tends to enhance intestinal motility. There are also ongoing trials of specific opioid antagonists in this condition.

Hirschsprung Disease

Some children have a genetically determined condition of abnormal colonic motility known as Hirschsprung disease or **aganglionic megacolon,** which is characterized by abdominal distension, anorexia, and lassitude. The disease is typically diagnosed in infancy. It is due to a congenital absence of ganglion cells in both the myenteric and submucous plexuses of a segment of the distal colon, as a result of failure of the normal migration of neural crest cells during development. The action of endothelins on the endothelin B receptor (see Chapter 7) is necessary for normal migration of certain neural crest cells; megacolon developed in knockout mice lacking endothelin B receptors. In addition, one cause of congenital aganglionic megacolon in humans appears to be a mutation in the endothelin B receptor gene. The absence of peristalsis in patients with this disorder causes feces to pass the aganglionic region with difficulty, and children with the disease may defecate as infrequently as once every 3 weeks.

THERAPEUTIC HIGHLIGHTS

The symptoms of Hirschsprung disease can be relieved completely if the aganglionic portion of the colon is resected. However, this is not possible if an extensive segment is involved. In this case, patients may require a colectomy.

toward the large intestines. **Segmentation** moves the chyme to and fro. **Tonic contractions** are relatively prolonged contractions that in effect isolate one segment of the intestine from another. Note that these last two types of contractions slow transit such that transit time is longer in the fed than in the fasted state (**Clinical Box 27–3**).

■ COLON

The colon serves as a reservoir for the residues of meals that cannot be digested or absorbed. Motility in this segment is likewise slowed to allow the colon to absorb water, Na^+, and other minerals. By removing about 90% of the fluid, it converts the 1000–2000 mL of isotonic chyme that enters from the ileum each day to about 200 mL of feces.

MOTILITY OF THE COLON

The ileum is linked to the colon by the ileocecal valve, which restricts reflux of colonic contents, including the large numbers of commensal bacteria, into the relatively sterile ileum. The portion of the ileum containing the ileocecal valve projects slightly into the cecum, so that increases in colonic pressure squeeze it shut, whereas increases in ileal pressure open it. Each time a peristaltic wave reaches the valve, it opens briefly. When food leaves the stomach, the cecum relaxes and the passage of chyme through the valve increases **(gastroileal reflex).** This is presumably a vagovagal reflex.

The movements of the colon include segmentation and peristalsis. Segmentation mixes the contents of the colon and facilitate absorption. Peristaltic waves propel the contents toward the rectum, although weak antiperistalsis is sometimes seen. A third type of contraction that occurs only in the colon is the **mass action contraction,** occurring about 10 times per day, involving simultaneous contraction of the smooth muscle over large confluent areas (**Clinical Box 27–4**). These contractions move material into the rectum, and rectal distension initiates the defecation reflex.

The movements of the colon are coordinated by the BER of the colon. The frequency of this wave, unlike the wave in the small intestine, increases along the colon, from about 2/min at the ileocecal valve to 6/min at the sigmoid.

TRANSIT TIME IN THE SMALL INTESTINE & COLON

The first part of a test meal reaches the cecum in about 4 h in most individuals, and all the undigested portions have entered the colon in 8 or 9 h. On average, the first remnants of the meal traverse the first third of the colon in 6 h, the second third in 9 h, and reach the terminal part of the colon (the sigmoid colon) in 12 h. From the sigmoid colon to the anus, transport is much slower (**Clinical Box 27–5**).

DEFECATION

Distension of the rectum with feces initiates reflex contractions of its musculature and the desire to defecate. In humans, the sympathetic nerve supply to the internal (involuntary) anal sphincter is excitatory, whereas the parasympathetic supply is inhibitory. This sphincter relaxes when the rectum is distended. The nerve supply to the external anal sphincter, a skeletal muscle, comes from the pudendal nerve. The sphincter is maintained in a state of tonic contraction, and moderate distension of the rectum increases the force of its contraction. The urge to defecate first occurs when rectal pressure increases to about 18 mm Hg. When this pressure reaches 55 mm Hg, the external as well as the internal sphincter relaxes and there is reflex expulsion of the contents of the rectum. Before the pressure that relaxes the external anal sphincter is reached, voluntary defecation can be initiated by straining. Normally, the angle between the anus and the rectum is approximately 90°, and this plus contraction of the puborectalis muscle inhibits defecation. With straining, the abdominal muscles contract, the pelvic floor is lowered 1–3 cm, and the puborectalis muscle relaxes. The anorectal angle is reduced to 15° or less. This is combined with relaxation of the external anal sphincter and defecation occurs. Defecation is therefore a spinal reflex that can be voluntarily inhibited by keeping the external sphincter contracted or facilitated by relaxing the sphincter and contracting the abdominal muscles.

Distension of the stomach by food initiates contractions of the colon and rectum and, frequently, a desire to defecate. The response is called the **gastrocolic reflex,** and may be amplified by an action of gastrin on the colon.

CHAPTER SUMMARY

- The regulatory factors that govern gastrointestinal secretion also regulate its motility.
- Two major patterns of motility are peristalsis and segmentation, which propel or retard/mix the luminal contents, respectively.
- The membrane potential of the majority of gastrointestinal smooth muscle undergoes rhythmic fluctuations that sweep along the length of the gut. The rhythm is established by interstitial cells of Cajal. This basic electrical rhythm (BER) provides for sites of muscle contraction when stimuli superimpose spike potentials on the depolarizing portion of the BER waves.
- In the period between meals, the intestine is relatively quiescent, but every 100 min or so it is swept through by a large peristaltic wave triggered by the hormone motilin. This migrating motor complex presumably serves a "housekeeping" function.
- Swallowing is triggered centrally and is coordinated with a peristaltic wave along the length of the esophagus. Relaxation of the lower esophageal sphincter is timed to just precede the arrival of the bolus, thereby limiting reflux of the gastric contents. Nevertheless, gastroesophageal reflux disease is common.
- The stomach accommodates the meal by a process of receptive relaxation. This permits an increase in volume without a significant increase in pressure. The stomach then serves to mix the meal and to control its delivery to downstream segments.
- Luminal contents move slowly through the colon, which enhances water recovery. Distension of the rectum causes reflex contraction of the internal anal sphincter and the desire to defecate. After toilet training, defecation can be delayed until a convenient time via voluntary contraction of the external anal sphincter.

MULTIPLE-CHOICE QUESTIONS

For all questions, select the single best answer unless otherwise directed.

1. In infants, defecation often follows a meal. The cause of colonic contractions in this situation is
   A. histamine.
   B. increased circulating levels of CCK.
   C. the gastrocolic reflex.
   D. increased circulating levels of somatostatin.
   E. the enterogastric reflex.

2. A patient who has undergone a partial gastric resection to remove a tumor reports to his primary care physician that he has experienced several episodes of nausea, cramping, dizziness, sweating and a rapid heart rate after ingesting sugary beverages. His symptoms are caused in part by
   A. increased blood pressure.
   B. increased secretion of acid.

C. increased secretion of CCK.
D. hypoglycemia.
E. hyperglycemia.

3. For the patient in Question 2, what is the most likely diagnosis?
   A. Constipation-predominant irritable bowel syndrome (IBS-C)
   B. Hirschsprung disease
   C. Achalasia
   D. Peptic ulcer disease
   E. Dumping syndrome.

4. A scientist studies the regulation of gastric motility by placing a pressure sensor in the stomach of a mouse that remotely reports intragastric pressure over time. She notes that gastric pressures seldom rise above the levels that breach the lower esophageal sphincter, even when the stomach is filled with a meal and its volume is expanded considerably as a result. Which process is responsible for this finding?
   A. Peristalsis
   B. Gastroileal reflex
   C. Segmentation
   D. Stimulation of the vomiting center
   E. Receptive relaxation

5. The physiological gastric pressure response to feeding described in Question 4 could be partially inhibited experimentally by all of the following pharmacological agents except:
   A. cholinergic antagonist.
   B. nitric oxide synthase inhibitor.
   C. cholecystokinin antagonist.
   D. histamine antagonist.
   E. VIP antagonist.

6. A patient is referred to a gastroenterologist for evaluation of suspected small bowel bacterial overgrowth. Motility studies reveal slowed gastrointestinal transit during fasting. The patient's symptoms are most likely due to a deficit in which of the following substances?
   A. Motilin
   B. NO
   C. CCK
   D. VIP
   E. Secretin

7. A patient is referred to a gastroenterologist because of persistent difficulties with swallowing. Endoscopic examination reveals that the lower esophageal sphincter fails to fully open as the bolus reaches it, and a diagnosis of achalasia is made. During the examination, or in biopsies taken from the sphincter region, a decrease would be expected in which of the following?
   A. Esophageal peristalsis
   B. Expression of neuronal NO synthase
   C. Acetylcholine receptors
   D. Substance P release
   E. Contraction of the crural diaphragm

8. A bed-ridden, 90-year-old man is referred for endoscopy because of difficulty in swallowing that developed rapidly after he took medication with water the night before, when he was supine. Endoscopy reveals a pill lodged in his esophagus that has triggered an inflammatory reaction. Compared

to the upright position, a reduction in which of the following influences on esophageal motility likely contributed to the adverse outcome in this patient?
   A. Primary peristalsis
   B. Secondary peristalsis
   C. Nucleus ambiguus activity
   D. Pharyngeal contraction
   E. Gravity

9. A 50-year-old man who is markedly overweight comes to his primary care physician complaining of a nightly burning sensation in his chest, which is made worse if he has a snack before retiring. Which of the following would be the most effective treatment for this patient if his symptoms are not eliminated by weight loss and foregoing late-night meals?
   A. Cholinergic agonist
   B. Smooth muscle relaxant
   C. Nitric oxide donor
   D. Injection of Botox into the lower esophageal sphincter
   E. Proton pump inhibitor

10. Following a forceps delivery of her third child, a woman returns to her physician complaining of mild fecal incontinence when lifting her older children, without any urinary incontinence. Her symptoms are most likely attributable to dysfunction of which of the following?
   A. Anal sensory nerves
   B. Internal anal sphincter
   C. External anal sphincter
   D. Pudendal nerves
   E. Puborectalis muscle

ANSWERS

1. The correct answer is **C.** The gastrocolic reflex readies the colon for the contents of a new meal by triggering colonic and rectal contractions. It is triggered when the stomach is distended, and is assumed to be neutrally mediated, although it may be modified by humoral agents. CCK levels increase in the circulation after a meal but the hormone is not the cause of the reflex (rules out option **B**) whereas histamine and somatostatin released in the course of responding to a meal are paracrines, whose concentration in the circulation changes little, if at all (rules out options **A** and **D**). Somatostatin would in any case be expected to reduce motility. Finally, the enterogastric reflex slows gastric emptying when the meal is in the small intestine, rather than targeting the colon (rules out option **E**).

2. The correct answer is **D.** With gastric surgery, the ability to regulate the delivery of meal constituents from the stomach to the small intestine may be significantly impaired. Especially when large amounts of sweets are ingested, the sugar is delivered rapidly to the small intestine and the osmotic forces draw in large volumes of fluid from the interstitium, resulting in bowel distension, pain and nausea. The associated hypovolemia would result in low blood pressure (rules out option **A**) and tachycardia. The rapid absorption of simple sugars also markedly stimulates the release of insulin and inappropriately triggers glucose sequestration leading to hypoglycemia (rules out option **E**). Acid and CCK secretion are not markedly triggered by carbohydrates, and acid secretion would likely be reduced in this patient in any event since the gastric mucosal

area is reduced and the stomach empties rapidly (rules out options **B** and **C**).

3. The correct answer is **E**. Dumping syndrome occurs when liquids containing nutrients empty too rapidly from the stomach, due to a loss of its reservoir function and/or reduced function of the pylorus. IBS-C is associated with abdominal pain, but is unlikely to be accompanied by the other symptoms (rules out option **A**). Hirschsprung disease predominantly affects the colon, is typically diagnosed in childhood, and results in slowed rather than accelerated motility (rules out option **B**). Neither achalasia (impairs swallowing) or peptic ulcer disease (causes epigastric pain; impairs duodenal bicarbonate secretion) would cause the symptoms described either (rules out options **C** and **D**).

4. The correct answer is **E**. Local and vagovagal reflexes respond to stretch in the stomach wall and induce relaxation of the gastric smooth muscle via the release of nitric oxide and vasoactive intestinal polypeptide. Peristalsis would increase gastric pressures, whereas segmentation is restricted to the intestine (rules out options **A** and **C**). The gastroileal reflex occurs when the stomach is filled with food, but results in relaxation of the ileocecal valve and should not affect gastric pressures (rules out option **B**). Finally, stimulation of the vomiting center will activate retroperistalsis that will, by design, result in the movement of gastric contents through the lower esophageal sphincter and out into the esophagus. Further, simply filling the stomach with food should not activate the vomiting center in the brain, unless the meal contains toxic components (rules out option **D**).

5. The correct answer is **D**. Histamine, which acts in the stomach via H_2 receptors to activate secretory responses, is not known to play any role in gastric motility. On the other hand, vagal efferents release acetylcholine to activate enteric inhibitory neurons that utilize nitric oxide and VIP to relax gastric smooth muscle. Thus, inhibition of any of these neurotransmitters in the stomach should abrogate receptive relaxation (rules out options **A**, **B**, and **E**). Similarly, CCK is released from the small intestine in response to dietary components, and activates vagal afferents to trigger vagovagal reflexes to further promote gastric relaxation and delay gastric emptying (rules out option **C**).

6. The correct answer is **A**. Many cases of small bowel bacterial overgrowth have been associated with a reduction in phase III of the migrating motor complex (MMC), which serves to sweep the fasting gut free of food residues, and is triggered by motilin. Nitric oxide and VIP are involved in the aboral relaxation phase of the peristaltic reflex; their absence would be expected to increase intestinal contractility, and during the fed rather than the fasting period (rules out options **B** and **D**). CCK and secretin are also released during the fed phase; CCK feeds back to slow gastric emptying but does not affect the MMC, whereas secretin is not thought to influence motility directly (rules out options **C** and **E**).

7. The correct answer is **B**. Achalasia results from a failure of the lower esophageal sphincter to relax, a response that is mediated by nitric oxide. In this condition, secondary esophageal peristalsis might be expected to increase rather than decrease, in an effort to clear the bolus from the esophagus (rules out option **A**). Similarly, cholinergic and tachykinergic mechanisms are involved in the tonic closure of the esophageal sphincter, so a reduction in acetylcholine receptors or in substance P release would be expected to relax rather than close the sphincter (rules out options **C** and **D**). Finally, the crural diaphragm wraps around the esophageal sphincter and contraction of the diaphragm aids the sphincter's patency, so a reduction in the tone of the diaphragm would not result in sphincter closure but rather the opposite (rules out option **E**).

8. The correct answer is **E**. Pill esophagitis is a common affliction in the elderly, particularly those who are institutionalized and/or confined to bed. None of the other mechanisms listed, which all do contribute to clearing the esophagus of ingested substances, is altered significantly by body position; indeed, one can swallow while suspended upside down, if one is so inclined (rules out options **A, B, C,** and **D**).

9. The correct answer is **E**. The patient's symptoms are consistent with the diagnosis of gastroesophageal reflux disease, which is common in middle age, particularly at night when reflux of gastric contents is no longer constrained by gravity. The pain occurs when acid gastric contents contact the esophageal mucosa. If gastric acidity is reduced by a proton pump inhibitor, pain and mucosal injury should be reduced even in the face of ongoing reflux. Sphincter tone might be increased by a cholinergic agonist, but this would have many other nonspecific effects that likely would preclude its usage (rules out option **A**). A smooth muscle relaxant might further worsen sphincter patency, and a nitric oxide donor should relax it (rules out option **B** and **C**). Finally, while Botox may be an effective treatment for achalasia, it would worsen rather than improve reflux (rules out option **D**).

10. The correct answer is **C**. Reflexive contraction of the external anal sphincter is important in preventing the release of anal contents when the pressure in the abdominal cavity is increased abruptly, such as when lifting a heavy object. The sphincter is vulnerable to obstetric injuries. Dysfunction of the internal sphincter alone should not cause incontinence if the external sphincter is intact (rules out option **B**). The anal sampling mechanism, which is mediated by anal sensory nerves and identifies whether the anal canal is filled with solid, liquid, or gaseous contents, is not involved in continence, *per se* (rules out option **A**). Relaxation of the puborectalis muscle aids in voluntary defecation, but injury to this structure should not cause incontinence if the other mechanisms are intact (rules out option **E**). Finally, pudendal nerve dysfunction would be expected to result in urinary incontinence to stress as well as fecal incontinence (rules out option **D**).

Transport & Metabolic Functions of the Liver

- Describe liver functions of metabolism, detoxification, and excretion.
- Understand the functional anatomy of the liver.
- Define the characteristics of the hepatic circulation and its role.
- Identify plasma proteins synthesized by the liver.
- Describe the formation of bile and its role in the excretion of cholesterol and bilirubin.
- Outline hepatic contributions to whole-body ammonia homeostasis.
- Describe normal functioning of the gallbladder and the basis of gallstone disease.

INTRODUCTION

The liver is the largest gland in the body. It is essential for life because it conducts a vast array of biochemical and metabolic functions. It is also the first port of call for most absorbed nutrients, supplies most of the plasma proteins, and synthesizes bile.

■ THE LIVER

FUNCTIONAL ANATOMY

The liver serves as a filter between blood coming from the gastrointestinal tract and the blood in the rest of the body. Blood from the intestines reaches the liver via the portal vein. It percolates in sinusoids between plates of hepatic cells (hepatocytes) and eventually drains into the hepatic veins. During its passage through the hepatic plates, it is modified chemically. Bile is formed on the other side of each plate. Bile passes to the intestine via the hepatic duct (Figure 28–1).

The plates of hepatocytes are usually only one cell thick. Large gaps occur between the endothelial cells, allowing plasma to contact the hepatocytes. Hepatic artery blood also enters the sinusoids. The central veins coalesce to form the hepatic veins. The average transit time for blood from the portal venule to the central hepatic vein is about 8.4 s. **Kupffer cells** are anchored to the endothelium of the sinusoids and project into the lumen.

Each hepatocyte is also apposed to **bile canaliculi.** The canaliculi drain into bile ducts, and these coalesce to form the right and left hepatic ducts. These ducts join outside the liver to form the common hepatic duct. The cystic duct drains the gallbladder. The hepatic duct unites with the cystic duct to form the common bile duct. The common bile duct enters the duodenum at the duodenal papilla. Its orifice is surrounded by the **sphincter of Oddi.** The sphincter is usually closed, but when gastric contents enter the duodenum, cholecystokinin (CCK) is released and relaxes the sphincter and makes the gallbladder contract.

The extrahepatic biliary ducts and the gallbladder are lined by a layer of columnar cells with scattered mucous glands. In the gallbladder, the surface is extensively folded; this increases its surface area. The cystic duct is also folded to form spiral valves that increase the turbulence of bile as it flows out of the gallbladder, reducing the risk that it will precipitate and form gallstones.

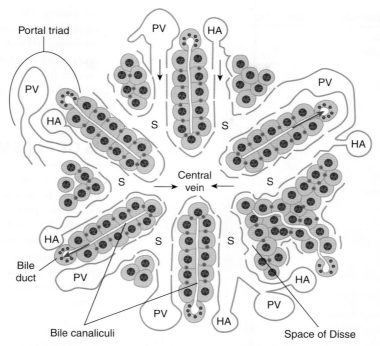

FIGURE 28–1 Schematic anatomy of the liver. Hepatocytes are arranged radially in plates surrounding a central vein. Blood is supplied to the liver by branches of the portal vein (PV) and hepatic artery (HA), which empty into sinusoids (S) surrounding the hepatocytes. The direction of blood flow is indicated with black arrows. The endothelial cells that line the sinusoids are fenestrated and thus provide little hindrance to the transfer of substances from the sinusoids to the space of Disse, which abuts the basolateral membrane of the hepatocytes. The apical membranes of adjacent hepatocytes form bile canaliculi, which transfer bile to the bile ducts lined by cholangiocytes. Bile flows in the opposite direction to blood (green arrows). The bile duct, portal vein and hepatic artery comprise the "portal triad." (Adapted with permission from Paulsen DF: *Histology and Cell Biology: Examination and Board Review.* 5th ed. McGraw-Hill, 2010.)

HEPATIC CIRCULATION

The functional unit of the liver is the acinus. The human liver contains about 100,000 acini. Each acinus is at the end of a vascular stalk containing terminal branches of portal veins, hepatic arteries, and bile ducts. Blood flows from the center of this unit to the terminal branches of the hepatic veins at the periphery. The central portion of the acinus, sometimes called zone 1, is well oxygenated, the intermediate zone (zone 2) is moderately well oxygenated, and the peripheral zone (zone 3) is least well oxygenated and most susceptible to anoxic injury.

Portal venous pressure is normally about 10 mm Hg in humans, and hepatic venous pressure is approximately 5 mm Hg. The mean pressure in the hepatic artery branches that converge on the sinusoids is about 90 mm Hg, but the pressure in the sinusoids is lower than the portal venous pressure, so a marked pressure drop occurs along the hepatic arterioles. Following a meal, portal flow to the liver increases considerably and "reserve" sinusoids are recruited. Thus, portal pressures do not increase linearly with portal flow until all sinusoids have been recruited. This may be important to prevent fluid loss from the highly permeable liver. Indeed, if hepatic pressures are increased in disease states, many liters of fluid can accumulate in the peritoneal cavity as **ascites**.

■ FUNCTIONS OF THE LIVER

The liver has many complex functions that are summarized in **Table 28–1**. Several will be touched upon briefly here.

METABOLISM & DETOXIFICATION

This chapter will focus on those aspects of liver metabolism most closely aligned to gastrointestinal physiology. First, the liver plays key roles in carbohydrate metabolism, including glycogen storage, conversion of galactose and fructose to glucose, and gluconeogenesis. The substrates for these reactions derive from the products of carbohydrate assimilation transported to the liver in the portal blood. The liver also plays a major role in maintaining the stability of blood glucose levels, removing excess glucose from the blood and returning it as needed—the so-called **glucose buffer function.** In liver failure, hypoglycemia is common. Similarly, the liver supports a high rate of fatty acid oxidation for energy supply. Amino acids and two carbon fragments derived from carbohydrates are also converted to fats for storage. The liver also synthesizes most of the lipoproteins and preserves cholesterol homeostasis by synthesizing this molecule and converting excess cholesterol to bile acids.

TABLE 28–1 Principal functions of the liver.

Formation and secretion of bile
Nutrient and vitamin metabolism
Glucose and other sugars
Amino acids
Lipids
Fatty acids
Cholesterol
Lipoproteins
Fat-soluble vitamins
Water-soluble vitamins
Inactivation of various substances
Toxins
Steroids
Other hormones
Synthesis of plasma proteins
Acute-phase proteins
Albumin
Clotting factors
Steroid-binding and other hormone-binding proteins
Immunity
Kupffer cells

The liver also detoxifies the blood of substances originating from the gut or elsewhere (Clinical Box 28–1). Bacteria and other particulates are trapped in and broken down by the Kupffer cells. Other toxins are metabolized by cytochrome P450 enzymes expressed in hepatocytes. These convert xenobiotics to inactive, less lipophilic metabolites. Detoxification reactions are divided into phase I (oxidation, hydroxylation, and other reactions mediated by cytochrome P450s) and phase II (esterification). Ultimately, metabolites are secreted into the bile for elimination. The liver is also responsible for metabolism of steroid hormones. Liver disease can therefore result in the apparent overactivity of the relevant hormone systems.

SYNTHESIS OF PLASMA PROTEINS

The principal proteins synthesized by the liver are listed in Table 28–1. Albumin is quantitatively the most significant, producing plasma oncotic pressure. There are also **acute-phase proteins,** synthesized and secreted on exposure to stressful stimuli. Others are proteins that transport steroids and other hormones in the plasma, and still others are clotting factors. Following blood loss, the liver replaces the plasma proteins in days to weeks. The only major class of plasma proteins not synthesized by the liver is the immunoglobulins.

BILE

Bile is made up of bile acids, bile pigments, and other substances dissolved in an alkaline solution that resembles pancreatic juice. Some of the components of the bile are reabsorbed in the intestine and then excreted again by the liver (**enterohepatic circulation**). In addition to its role in digestion and absorption of fats (Chapter 26), bile is the major excretory route for lipid-soluble waste products. The glucuronides of the **bile pigments,** bilirubin and biliverdin, are responsible for the yellow color of bile.

BILIRUBIN METABOLISM & EXCRETION

Most of the bilirubin in the body is formed in the tissues by the break down of hemoglobin (see Chapter 31). Bilirubin is bound to albumin in the circulation. Some of it is tightly bound, but most of it can dissociate in the liver, and free bilirubin enters liver cells via a member of the organic anion transporting polypeptide (OATP) family, and then becomes bound to cytoplasmic proteins. It is next conjugated to glucuronic acid in a reaction catalyzed by UDP-glucuronosyltransferase. Each bilirubin molecule reacts with two uridine diphosphoglucuronic acid (UDPGA) molecules to form bilirubin diglucuronide. This glucuronide, which is more water soluble than the free bilirubin, is then transported by multidrug resistance protein-2 (MRP-2) into the bile canaliculi. Most of the bilirubin glucuronide passes via the bile ducts to the intestine. A small amount escapes into the blood, where it is bound less tightly to albumin than is free bilirubin, and is excreted in the urine.

The intestinal mucosa is relatively impermeable to conjugated bilirubin but is permeable to unconjugated bilirubin and to urobilinogens, a series of colorless derivatives of bilirubin formed by bacteria. Consequently, some of the bile pigments and urobilinogens are reabsorbed in the portal circulation. Small amounts of urobilinogens enter the general circulation and are excreted in the urine.

CLINICAL BOX 28–1

Hepatic Encephalopathy

The clinical importance of hepatic ammonia metabolism is seen in liver failure, when increased levels of circulating ammonia cause the condition of hepatic encephalopathy. Initially, patients may seem merely confused, but if untreated, the condition can progress to coma. The disease results not only from the loss of functional hepatocytes, but also shunting of portal blood around the hardened liver, meaning that less ammonia is removed from the blood. Additional substances that are normally detoxified by the liver likely also contribute to the mental status changes.

THERAPEUTIC HIGHLIGHTS

The cognitive symptoms of advanced liver disease can be minimized by reducing the load of ammonia coming from the colon. However, in severe disease, the only truly effective treatment is to perform a liver transplant.

JAUNDICE

When free or conjugated bilirubin accumulates in the blood, the skin, scleras, and mucous membranes turn yellow. This yellowness is known as **jaundice** (icterus). Hyperbilirubinemia may be due to (1) excess production of bilirubin, (2) decreased uptake of bilirubin into hepatic cells, (3) disturbed intracellular protein binding or conjugation, (4) disturbed secretion of conjugated bilirubin into the bile canaliculi, or (5) intrahepatic or extrahepatic bile duct obstruction. When it is due to one of the first three processes, free bilirubin rises. When it is due to disturbed secretion of conjugated bilirubin or bile duct obstruction, bilirubin glucuronide regurgitates into the blood, and it is predominantly conjugated bilirubin in the plasma that is elevated.

OTHER SUBSTANCES EXCRETED IN THE BILE

Cholesterol and alkaline phosphatase are excreted in the bile. In patients with jaundice due to intrahepatic or extrahepatic obstruction of the bile duct, the blood levels of these two substances usually rise (Clinical Box 28-2). A smaller rise is seen when jaundice is due to nonobstructive hepatocellular disease. Adrenocortical and other steroid hormones and a number of drugs are excreted in the bile and subsequently reabsorbed (enterohepatic circulation).

AMMONIA METABOLISM & EXCRETION

The liver is critical for ammonia handling. Ammonia levels must be carefully controlled because it is toxic and can permeate across the blood–brain barrier. The liver is the only organ in which the complete urea cycle (also known as the Krebs–Henseleit cycle) is expressed. This converts circulating ammonia to urea, which can then be excreted in the urine.

Ammonia in the circulation comes primarily from the colon and kidneys with lesser amounts from the breakdown of red blood cells and metabolism in the muscles. Almost all circulating ammonia is normally cleared by the hepatocytes. It is converted to carbamoyl phosphate in the mitochondria, which reacts with ornithine to generate citrulline. Cytoplasmic reactions eventually produce arginine, which can be dehydrated to urea and ornithine. The latter returns to the mitochondria to begin another cycle, and urea diffuses readily back into the sinusoidal blood. It is then filtered in the kidneys and lost from the body in the urine.

■ THE BILIARY SYSTEM

BILE FORMATION

Bile contains substances that are actively secreted into it across the canalicular membrane, such as bile acids, phosphatidylcholine, conjugated bilirubin, cholesterol, and xenobiotics. Each enters the bile by means of a specific canalicular transporter. The active secretion of bile acids is the primary driving force for the initial formation of canalicular bile. Because they are osmotically active, the canalicular bile is transiently hypertonic. However, the tight junctions that join adjacent hepatocytes are relatively permeable allowing water, glucose, calcium, glutathione, amino acids, and urea to passively enter the bile from the plasma by diffusion.

Phosphatidylcholine in bile forms mixed micelles with bile acids and cholesterol. The ratio of bile acids:phosphatidylcholine: cholesterol in canalicular bile is approximately 10:3:1. Deviations from this ratio may cause cholesterol to precipitate, leading to one type of gallstones.

CLINICAL BOX 28-2

Gallstones

Cholelithiasis, that is, the presence of gallstones, is a common condition. In the United States, 20% of women and 5% of men between the ages of 50 and 65 have gallstones. The stones are of two types: calcium bilirubinate stones and, more commonly, cholesterol stones. Three factors appear to be involved in the formation of the latter. One is bile stasis. A second is supersaturation of the bile with cholesterol. Cholesterol is very insoluble in bile, and it is maintained in solution in micelles. If bile is supersaturated, it contains small crystals of cholesterol in addition to micelles. The third factor is a mix of nucleation factors that favors formation of stones from the supersaturated bile.

Gallstones that obstruct bile outflow can result in **obstructive jaundice**. If the flow of bile out of the liver is completely blocked, substances normally excreted in the bile accumulate in the bloodstream. The interruption of the enterohepatic circulation also induces the liver to synthesize bile acids at a greater rate. Some of these bile acids can be excreted by the kidney, and thus represent a mechanism for indirect excretion of at least a portion of cholesterol. However, retained biliary constituents may also cause liver toxicity.

THERAPEUTIC HIGHLIGHTS

The treatment of gallstones depends on their nature, and the severity of any symptoms. Many may be asymptomatic. Larger stones that cause obstruction may need to be removed surgically or endoscopically. Oral dissolution agents may dissolve small cholesterol stones, but the effect is slow and stones often return. A definitive cure for patients with symptomatic cholelithiasis is gallbladder removal.

The bile is transferred to progressively larger bile ductules and ducts, where it is modified. The bile ductules are lined by cholangiocytes. Their tight junctions are less permeable than those of the hepatocytes, although they remain freely permeable to water and thus bile remains isotonic. The ductules scavenge plasma constituents, such as glucose and amino acids, and return them to the circulation. Glutathione is also hydrolyzed to its constituent amino acids by an enzyme, gamma glutamyltranspeptidase (GGT), expressed on the cholangiocyte apical membrane. Removal of glucose and amino acids is likely important to prevent bacterial overgrowth. The ductules also secrete bicarbonate in response to secretin, as well as IgA and mucus for protection.

FUNCTIONS OF THE GALLBLADDER

In normal individuals, bile flows into the gallbladder when the sphincter of Oddi is closed. There it is concentrated by absorption of water. However, because bile acids form a micellar solution, the micelles simply become larger and bile remains isotonic. However, bile becomes slightly acidic as sodium ions are exchanged for protons.

REGULATION OF BILIARY SECRETION

When food enters the mouth, the resistance of the sphincter of Oddi decreases (Figure 28–2). Nutrients in the duodenum release CCK, which causes gallbladder contraction.

The production of bile is increased by stimulation of the vagus nerves and by secretin, which increases the water and HCO_3^- content of bile. Substances that increase the secretion of bile are

known as **choleretics.** Bile acids themselves are among the most important physiologic choleretics.

The periodic discharge of bile from the gallbladder aids digestion but is not essential. Cholecystectomized patients maintain good health with a constant slow discharge of bile into the duodenum, although eventually the bile duct becomes somewhat dilated, and more bile tends to enter the duodenum after meals than at other times.

CHAPTER SUMMARY

- The liver conducts a huge number of metabolic reactions and detoxifies and disposes of many exogenous substances, as well as endogenous metabolites.
- The liver filters large volumes of blood and removes even hydrophobic substances that are protein-bound due to its fenestrated endothelium. The liver also receives essentially all venous blood from the intestine.
- The liver buffers blood glucose, synthesizes the majority of plasma proteins, contributes to lipid metabolism, and preserves cholesterol homeostasis.
- Bilirubin is glucuronidated by the liver to permit its excretion in bile.
- The liver removes ammonia from the blood and converts it to urea for renal excretion. An accumulation of ammonia causes hepatic encephalopathy in liver failure.
- Bile contains substances actively secreted across the canalicular membrane by hepatocytes; notably bile acids, phosphatidylcholine, and cholesterol. The composition of bile is modified as it passes through the bile ducts and is stored in the gallbladder. Gallbladder contraction coordinates bile availability with the timing of meals.

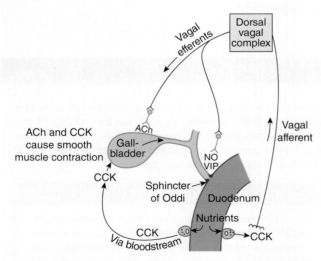

FIGURE 28–2 Neurohumoral control of gallbladder contraction and biliary secretion. Endocrine release of cholecystokinin (CCK) in response to nutrients causes gallbladder contraction. CCK also activates vagal afferents to trigger a vagovagal reflex that reinforces gallbladder contraction (via acetylcholine [ACh]) and relaxation of the sphincter of Oddi to permit bile outflow (via NO and vasoactive intestinal polypeptide [VIP]).

MULTIPLE-CHOICE QUESTIONS

For all questions, select the single best answer unless otherwise directed.

1. A patient suffering from severe ulcerative colitis undergoes a total colectomy with formation of a stoma. After a full recovery from surgery, and compared to his condition prior to surgery, which of the following would be expected to be decreased?
   A. Ability to absorb lipids
   B. Ability to clot the blood
   C. Circulating levels of conjugated bile acids
   D. Circulating bilirubin
   E. Urinary urobilinogen

2. A surgeon is studying new methods of liver transplantation. She performs a complete hepatectomy in an experimental animal. Before the donor liver is grafted, a rise in the blood level of which of the following would be expected?
   A. Glucose
   B. Fibrinogen
   C. 25-Hydroxycholecalciferol
   D. Conjugated bilirubin
   E. Estrogens

3. A scientist uses genetic approaches to selectively ablate the functions of the various cell types in the liver of mice. He finds that when a certain cell type is disabled, the mice show

increased levels of sepsis when the barrier function of the intestine is reduced by instillation of ethanol. Ablation of which hepatic cell type would account for this finding?
  A. Hepatic stellate cell
  B. Cholangiocyte
  C. Kupffer cell
  D. Hepatocyte
  E. Gallbladder epithelial cell

4. In the study described in Question 3, another set of mice with a different defect is created in which behavioral defects are observed consistent with encephalopathy. The function of which of the following cell types has likely been abrogated in this second group of animals?
  A. Hepatic stellate cell
  B. Cholangiocyte
  C. Kupffer cell
  D. Hepatocyte
  E. Gallbladder epithelial cell

5. A 40-year-old woman comes to her primary care clinician complaining of severe, episodic abdominal pain that is particularly intense after she ingests a fatty meal. An imaging procedure reveals that her gallbladder is acutely dilated, and a diagnosis of cholelithiasis is made. A gallstone lodged in which location will also increase her risk of pancreatitis?
  A. Left hepatic duct
  B. Right hepatic duct
  C. Cystic duct
  D. Common bile duct
  E. Sphincter of Oddi

6. In an animal study of biliary secretion, the common hepatic duct of a rat is cannulated under anesthesia and a sample of bile is collected. Bile is also collected from the gallbladder. Compared to hepatic bile, the gallbladder bile would be expected to contain a reduced concentration of which of the following?
  A. Bile acids
  B. Chloride ions
  C. Protons
  D. Glucose
  E. Calcium ions

7. An imaging study shows that a patient has a gallstone lodged in her biliary system, although her ability to assimilate fat-soluble vitamins is normal. In which location would the stone need to be lodged to increase bile acid flux through the left side of the liver?
  A. Cystic duct
  B. Common hepatic duct
  C. Right hepatic duct
  D. Left hepatic duct
  E. Common bile duct

8. A 60-year-old man comes to his physician complaining of a progressive increase in girth despite attempts to diet. He is also jaundiced and complains of nausea and malaise. When a large needle is inserted into his abdomen, several liters of tan fluid drain out. An increase in which of the following is not involved in this fluid accumulation?
  A. Portal pressure
  B. Hepatic collagen
  C. Plasma albumin
  D. Stellate cell activity
  E. Plasma transudation

9. A 45-year-old woman is brought to the emergency room complaining of a 3-day history of colicky epigastric pain that suddenly increased in severity after a meal. Tests reveal she has a gallstone blocking her sphincter of Oddi. Which of the following substances would be found at reduced levels in her circulation?
  A. Unconjugated bile acids
  B. Conjugated bile acids
  C. Cholesterol
  D. Phosphatidylcholine
  E. Amylase

10. A newborn infant who was delivered vaginally is noted to be mildly jaundiced, but no bilirubin is found in the urine. The child's symptoms are most likely attributable to a developmental delay in the expression or establishment of which of the following:
  A. Colonic bacterial colonization
  B. MDR2
  C. UDP glucuronyl transferase
  D. Heme oxygenase
  E. Biliverdin reductase

ANSWERS

1. The correct answer is **E.** Urobilinogen is formed in the colon by the action of bacteria on released bilirubin; a portion is reabsorbed and enters the enterohepatic circulation from which some urobilinogen escapes to the systemic circulation and can be excreted by the kidneys because it is less firmly bound to plasma proteins than bilirubin. Bilirubin, on the other hand, is not absorbed intact from the colon (rules out option **D**). Colectomy will not affect the enterohepatic circulation of conjugated bile acids because they are absorbed in the terminal ileum; if anything, the production of bile acids from the liver may rise to compensate for the loss of absorption of unconjugated bile acids that would be formed by bacteria in the colon (rules out option **C**). Lipid absorption should be unaffected because it takes place in the small intestine and bile acid secretion should be maintained or even increased (rules out option **A**). In the presumed absence of any co-occuring liver disease, the synthesis of clotting factors should occur normally (rules out option **B**).

2. The correct answer is **E.** The liver is responsible for metabolizing steroid hormones, so estrogen levels will rise. On the other hand, with loss of the glucose buffer function as well as the capacity to synthesize plasma proteins, hypoglycemia and a fall in fibrinogen would be expected with an acute reduction in liver function (rules out options **A** and **B**). 25-Hydroxycholecalciferol is also produced in the liver from cholecalciferol produced in the skin (rules out option **C**). Finally, bilirubin is conjugated in hepatocytes, so this reaction will not occur (rules out option **D**).

3. The correct answer is **C.** Kupffer cells are phagocytes that are strategically located in the sinusoids to cleanse portal blood of low levels of particulate matter, such as bacteria that may escape intestinal barrier function. Hepatic stellate cells lie between the endothelium and hepatocytes and serve to store lipids; they also produce extracellular matrix proteins if the liver is injured (rules out option **A**). Cholangiocytes and gallbladder epithelial cells are concerned with the formation of bile and do not protect against bacterial dissemination (rules

out options **B** and **E**). Finally, hepatocytes perform the metabolic functions of the liver but do not actively phagocytose or defend against bacteria (rules out option **D**).

4. The correct answer is **D**. Encephalopathic symptoms imply that the animal's capacity for the detoxification of ammonia has been hampered, which is a function of hepatocytes. None of the other cell types listed participates in the conversion of ammonia to urea, the form in which it can be excreted in the urine (rules out options **A, B, C,** and **E**).

5. The correct answer is **E**. The pancreatic duct joins the bile duct just proximal to the sphincter of Oddi, so a stone lodged in the sphincter would impair the outflow of both bile and pancreatic juice and/or reflux of bile into the pancreas. Retention of pancreatic secretions can result in the premature activation of pancreatic enzymes and tissue injury. Gallstones in the right and left hepatic ducts would impair bile flow from the portions of the liver that they drain, but should not impair the flow of pancreatic juice (rules out options **A** and **B**). A stone in the cystic duct would prevent flow of bile into the gallbladder. It might cause cholecystitis if it happened acutely, but in general it would not impact pancreatic or biliary secretion (rules out option **C**). Finally, a stone in the common bile duct would be consistent with the patient's symptoms, including dilation of the gallbladder, but should not impair pancreatic secretion (rules out option **D**).

6. The correct answer is **B**. In the gallbladder, bile is concentrated via a process that removes NaCl via coupled sodium/proton and chloride/bicarbonate exchangers (rules out option **C**). The protons and bicarbonate in the lumen combine to form water and CO_2, which are then absorbed. However, bile acid anions are excluded by the gallbladder epithelial cells, meaning that chloride ions are absorbed while sodium (and calcium) ions are retained for electrical neutrality, such that sodium and calcium ion concentrations rise as the bile volume decreases (rules out option **E**). The concentration of bile acid anions rises markedly, although bile remains isotonic because most of these are in the form of micelles (rules out option **A**). There is little glucose in either hepatic or gallbladder bile in health, because it is reabsorbed by cholangiocytes (rules out option **D**).

7. The correct answer is **C**. Because the assimilation of fat-soluble vitamins, which depends completely on mixed micelles, is normal, bile must be flowing to the small intestine. This rules out locations that cause obstructive jaundice (options **B** and **E**). A stone in the cystic duct would still allow bile to flow to the intestine, and would not affect one side of the liver more than the other (rules out option **A**). Because bile is flowing to the intestine, the enterohepatic circulation is intact, and the bile acid pool must recycle through the side of the liver from which bile drainage is not obstructed. Thus, since flux is increased through the left side of the liver, the left hepatic duct cannot be blocked (rules out option **D**).

8. The correct answer is **C**. The patient's presentation is consistent with liver cirrhosis, which involves excessive deposition of extracellular matrix components in the liver secondary to the activation of hepatic stellate cells (rules out options **B** and **D**). The resulting hardening of the liver, combined with injury to sinusoids, increases portal pressures and causes fluid to weep from the surface of the liver into the abdominal cavity (rules out options **A** and **E**). On the other hand, the reduction in both numbers of viable hepatocytes as well as their function reduces the production of albumin, leading to hypoalbuminemia.

9. The correct answer is **A**. The patient has symptoms consistent with acute obstructive jaundice. Thus, substances that are normally eliminated in the bile, including conjugated bile acids, cholesterol, and phosphatidylcholine, will reflux into the systemic circulation and accumulate there (rules out options **B, C,** and **D**). The location of her gallstone will also prevent the release of pancreatic secretions, and amylase (and other pancreatic products) will rise in the circulation—some of her pain may also be attributable to pancreatitis. On the other hand, since bile cannot reach the small intestine, conjugated bile acids cannot be deconjugated by intestinal bacteria, and the level of unconjugated bile acids in the circulation should fall.

10. The correct answer is **C**. Because no bilirubin is found in the urine, the bilirubin in the circulation is unconjugated (unconjugated bilirubin is bound too tightly to albumin for any of it to be excreted via the kidneys). The causes of unconjugated bilirubinemia include overproduction, impaired conjugation or impaired hepatic uptake. Colonic bacteria deconjugate bilirubin glucuronides, but the released bilirubin is converted into urobilinogen, which is the form that can be reabsorbed. In addition, the child was delivered vaginally so is unlikely to have a delay in bacterial colonization (rules out option **A**). MDR2 transports bilirubin glucuronides into the bile, so decreased expression of this transporter would cause conjugated bilirubinemia (rules out option **B**). Heme oxygenase and biliverdin reductase are involved sequentially in the conversion of heme to bilirubin, so if they are reduced, less rather than more bilirubin would be produced (rules out options **D** and **E**). In fact, a developmental delay in the expression of UDP glucuronyl transferase is quite common in neonates.

SECTION V CARDIOVASCULAR PHYSIOLOGY

Cells exist within a body fluid compartment known as the interstitial fluid, and the cardiovascular system has evolved to ensure that the composition of the interstitial fluid is maintained within a narrow range. Homeostasis is accomplished by pumping a separate fluid compartment—plasma—around the body, where it can be "conditioned" as it passes through specific organs that add nutrients, oxygen, hormones and needed metabolites, and/or remove waste products. The plasma then delivers needed substances to other organs and tissues. Efficient transfer of substances between the cells and the plasma is accomplished by dense networks of capillaries, which offer little resistance to the transfer of substances across their walls, and provide for short diffusion distances between the capillaries and the sites at which products will be utilized. The pumping function in this system is provided by the heart, a four-chambered organ that drives blood around two circuits in series, one that perfuses the lungs and one that serves the remainder of the body.

In this section, the components of the cardiovascular system that permit it to serve the body's needs for substance transfer will be considered. First, the electrical activity that allows the chambers of the heart to contract in an ordered fashion, to move the circulation unidirectionally, will be discussed. Then, the properties of blood and its components that suit them to transport dissolved solutes to and from the interstitial fluid will be considered. The properties of the circulatory "plumbing," or blood vessels, will be addressed, along with the mechanisms that regulate them. Finally, the specialized properties of the circulation in areas of the body with unique needs will be discussed.

Origin of the Heartbeat & the Electrical Activity of the Heart

OBJECTIVES

After studying this chapter, you should be able to:

- Describe the structure and function of the conduction system of the heart and compare the action potentials in each part.
- Describe the way the electrocardiogram (ECG) is recorded, the waves of the ECG, and the relationship of the ECG to the electrical axis of the heart.

INTRODUCTION

The parts of the heart normally beat in orderly sequence: Contraction of the atria (**atrial systole**) is followed by contraction of the ventricles (**ventricular systole**), and during **diastole** all four chambers are relaxed. The heartbeat originates in a specialized **cardiac conduction system** and spreads via this system to all parts of the myocardium. The structures that make up the conduction system are the **sinoatrial node (SA node)**, the **internodal atrial pathways**, the **atrioventricular node (AV node)**, the **bundle of His** and its branches, and the **Purkinje system.** The SA node normally discharges most rapidly, with

depolarization spreading from it to the other regions before they discharge spontaneously. The SA node is therefore the normal **cardiac pacemaker,** with its rate of discharge determining the rate at which the heart beats. Impulses generated in the SA node pass through the atrial pathways to the AV node, through this node to the bundle of His, and through the branches of the bundle of His via the Purkinje system to the ventricular muscle. Each of the cell types in the heart contains a unique electrical discharge pattern; the sum of these electrical discharges can be recorded as the electrocardiogram (ECG).

■ ORIGIN & SPREAD OF CARDIAC EXCITATION

ANATOMIC CONSIDERATIONS

In the human heart, the SA node is located at the junction of the superior vena cava with the right atrium. The AV node is located in the right posterior portion of the interatrial septum (**Figure 29–1**). There are three bundles of atrial fibers that contain Purkinje-type fibers and connect the SA node to the AV node: the anterior, middle (tract of Wenckebach), and posterior (tract of Thorel) tracts. Bachmann bundle is sometimes used to identify a branch of the anterior internodal tract that connects the right and left atria. Conduction also occurs through atrial myocytes, but it is more rapid in these bundles. The AV node is continuous with the bundle of His, which gives off a left bundle branch at the top of the interventricular

septum and continues as the right bundle branch. The left bundle branch divides into an anterior fascicle and a posterior fascicle. The branches and fascicles run subendocardially down either side of the septum and come into contact with the Purkinje system, whose fibers spread to all parts of the ventricular myocardium.

Individual cells within regions of the heart have unique histologic features. Purkinje fibers, specialized conducting cells, are large with fewer mitochondria and striations and distinctly different from a myocyte specialized for contraction. Compared with Purkinje fibers, cells within the SA node and, to a lesser extent, the AV node are smaller and sparsely striated and are less conductive due to their higher internal resistance. The atrial muscle fibers are separated from those of the ventricles by a fibrous tissue ring, and normally the only conducting tissue between the atria and ventricles is the bundle of His.

The SA node develops from structures on the right side of the embryo and the AV node from structures on the left. This is why in

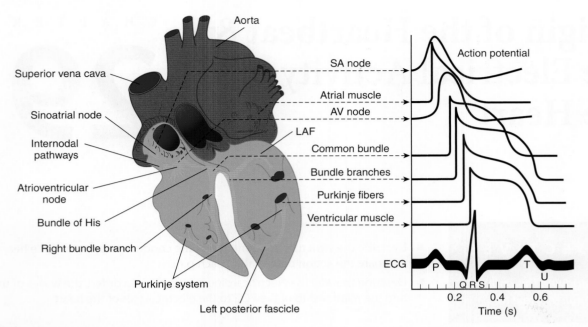

FIGURE 29–1   Conducting system of the heart. Left: Anatomic depiction of the human heart with additional focus on areas of the conduction system. **Right:** Typical transmembrane action potentials for the SA and AV nodes, other parts of the conduction system, and the atrial and ventricular muscles are shown along with the correlation to the extracellularly recorded electrical activity, that is, the electrocardiogram (ECG). The action potentials and ECG are plotted on the same time axis but with different zero points on the vertical scale for comparison. AV, atrioventricular; LAF, left anterior fascicle; SA, sinoatrial. (Data from Donahue JG, Choo PW, Manson JE, et al. The incidence of herpes zoster. *Arch Intern Med.* 155:1605–1609, 1995; Choo PW, Galil K, Donahue JG, et al. Risk factors for postherpetic neuralgia. *Arch Intern Med.* 1997;157:1217–1224.)

the adult the right vagus is distributed mainly to the SA node and the left vagus mainly to the AV node. Similarly, the sympathetic innervation on the right side is distributed primarily to the SA node and the sympathetic innervation on the left side primarily to the AV node. On each side, most sympathetic fibers come from the stellate ganglion. Noradrenergic fibers are epicardial, whereas the vagal fibers are endocardial. However, connections exist for reciprocal inhibitory effects of the sympathetic and parasympathetic innervation of the heart on each other. Thus, acetylcholine acts

presynaptically to reduce norepinephrine release from the sympathetic nerves, and conversely, neuropeptide Y released from noradrenergic endings may inhibit the release of acetylcholine.

PROPERTIES OF CARDIAC MUSCLE

Myocardial fibers have a resting membrane potential of approximately –90 mV **(Figure 29–2)**. The individual fibers are separated by membranes but depolarization spreads rapidly through

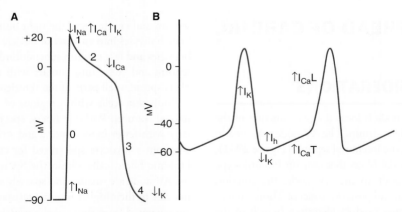

FIGURE 29–2   Comparison of action potentials in ventricular muscle and diagram of the membrane potential of pacemaker tissue. (A) Phases of action potential in ventricular myocyte (0–4, see text for details) are superimposed with principal changes in current that contribute to changes in membrane potential. **(B)** The principal current responsible for each part of the potential of pacemaker tissue is shown under or beside the component. L, long-lasting; T, transient. Other ion channels contribute to the electrical response. Note that the resting membrane potential of pacemaker tissue is somewhat lower than that of atrial and ventricular muscle.

them as if they were a syncytium because of the presence of gap junctions. The transmembrane action potential of single cardiac muscle cells is characterized by rapid depolarization (phase 0), an initial rapid repolarization (phase 1), a plateau (phase 2), and a slow repolarization process (phase 3) that allows return to the resting membrane potential (phase 4). The initial depolarization is due to Na^+ influx through rapidly opening Na^+ channels (the Na^+ current, I_{Na}). The inactivation of Na^+ channels contributes to the rapid repolarization phase. Ca^{2+} influx through more slowly opening Ca^{2+} channels (the Ca^{2+} current, I_{Ca}) produces the plateau phase, and repolarization is due to net K^+ efflux through multiple types of K^+ channels. Recorded extracellularly, the summed electrical activity of all the cardiac muscle fibers is the ECG. The timing of the discharge of the individual units relative to the ECG is shown in Figure 29–1. Note that the ECG is a combined electrical record and thus the overall shape reflects electrical activity from cells from different regions of the heart.

PACEMAKER POTENTIALS

Rhythmically discharging cells have a membrane potential that, after each impulse, declines to the firing level. Thus, this **prepotential** or **pacemaker potential** (Figure 29–2) triggers the next impulse. At the peak of each impulse, I_K begins and brings about repolarization. I_K then declines, and a channel permeable to both Na^+ and K^+ is activated. Because this channel is activated following hyperpolarization, it is referred to as an "h" channel. As I_h increases, the membrane begins to depolarize, forming the first part of the prepotential. Ca^{2+} channels then open. These are of two types in the heart, the **T** (for transient) **channels** and the **L** (for long-lasting) **channels.** The calcium current (I_{Ca}) due to opening of T channels completes the prepotential, and I_{Ca} due to opening of L channels produces the impulse. While these are the prominent changes, it should be noted that other ion channels and local Ca^{2+} release from the sarcoplasmic reticulum help shape potential changes. As can be seen in Figure 29–2, prepotentials are normally prominent in the SA and AV node cells and, action potentials in these cells are largely due to Ca^{2+} and not Na^+ influx. Consequently, there is no sharp, rapid depolarizing spike before the plateau. "Latent pacemakers" are present in other portions of the conduction system that can take over when the SA and AV nodes are depressed or conduction from them is blocked. Atrial and ventricular muscle fibers do not have prepotentials, and they discharge spontaneously only when injured or abnormal.

When the cholinergic vagal fibers to nodal tissue are stimulated, the membrane becomes hyperpolarized and the slope of the prepotentials is decreased because the acetylcholine released at the nerve endings increases the K^+ conductance of nodal tissue via M_2 muscarinic receptors. The resulting I_{KAch} slows the depolarizing effect of I_h. In addition, activation of the M_2 receptors decreases cyclic adenosine 3',5'-monophosphate (cAMP) in the cells, and this slows the opening of Ca^{2+} channels. The result is a decrease in firing rate. Strong vagal stimulation may abolish spontaneous discharge for some time. Conversely, stimulation of the sympathetic cardiac nerves speeds the depolarizing effect of I_h,

CLINICAL BOX 29-1

Use of Digitalis

Digitalis, or its clinically useful preparations (digoxin and digitoxin) has been described in medical literature for over 200 years. It was originally derived from the foxglove plant. (*Digitalis purpurea* is the name of the common foxglove.) Correct administration can strengthen contractions through digitalis inhibitory effects on the Na, K ATPase, resulting in greater amounts of Ca^{2+} release and subsequent changes in contraction forces. Digitalis can also have an electrical effect in decreasing AV nodal conduction velocity and thus altering AV transmission to the ventricles.

THERAPEUTIC HIGHLIGHTS

Digitalis has been used for treatment of systolic heart failure. It augments contractility, thereby improving cardiac output, improving left ventricle emptying, and decreasing ventricular filling pressures. Digitalis has also been used to treat atrial fibrillation and atrial flutter. In this scenario, digitalis reduces the number of impulses transmitted through the AV node and thus, provides effective rate control.

In both these instances alternative treatments developed over the past 20 years and the need to tightly regulate dose due to significant potential for side effects have reduced the use of digitalis. However, with better understanding of mechanism and toxicity, digitalis and its clinically prepared derivatives remain important drugs in modern medicine.

and the rate of spontaneous discharge increases. Norepinephrine secreted by the sympathetic endings binds to β_1 receptors, and the resulting increase in intracellular cAMP facilitates the opening of L channels, increasing I_{Ca} and the rapidity of the depolarization phase of the impulse.

The rate of discharge of the SA node and other nodal tissue is increased when the temperature rises, and this may contribute to the tachycardia associated with fever. Digitalis depresses nodal tissue and exerts an effect like that of vagal stimulation, particularly on the AV node (**Clinical Box 29–1**).

SPREAD OF CARDIAC EXCITATION

Depolarization initiated in the SA node spreads radially through the atria and converges on the AV node. Atrial depolarization is complete in about 0.1 s. Because conduction in the AV node is slow, a delay of about 0.1 s (**AV nodal delay**) occurs before excitation spreads to the ventricles. It is interesting to note here that when there is a lack of contribution of I_{Na} in the depolarization (phase 0) of the action potential, a marked loss of conduction is observed. This delay is shortened by stimulation of the sympathetic nerves to the heart and lengthened by stimulation of the vagi. From the top of the septum, the wave of depolarization spreads in the rapidly conducting Purkinje fibers to all parts of the ventricles in 0.08–0.1 s. In humans, depolarization of the ventricular muscle starts at the left side of the interventricular

septum and moves to the right across the mid portion of the septum. The wave of depolarization then spreads down the septum to the apex of the heart. It returns along the ventricular walls to the AV groove, proceeding from the endocardial to the epicardial surface (Figure 29–3). The last parts of the heart to be depolarized

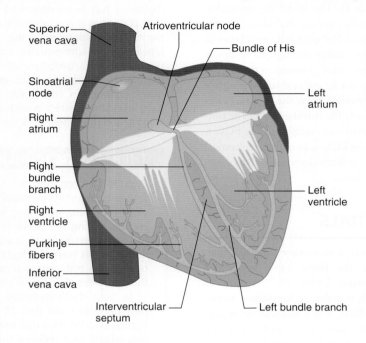

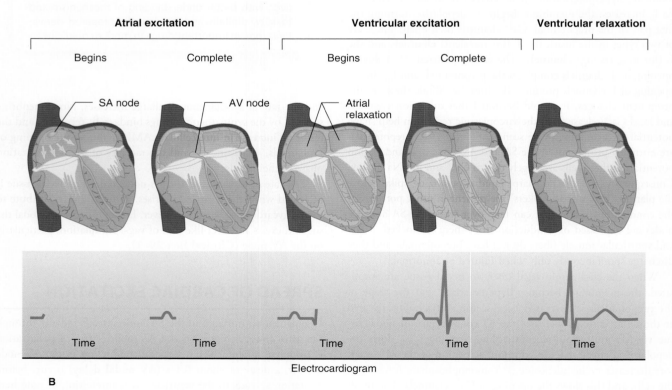

FIGURE 29–3 Normal spread of electrical activity in the heart. Conducting system of the heart paired with the sequence of cardiac excitation. **(A)** Anatomic position of electrical activity. **(B)** Corresponding electrocardiogram. The yellow color denotes areas that are depolarized. (Adapted with permission from Widmaier EP, Raff H, Strang KT: *Vander's human physiology,* 11th ed. New York: McGraw-Hill; 2008.)

are the posterobasal portion of the left ventricle, the pulmonary conus, and the uppermost portion of the septum.

■ THE ELECTROCARDIOGRAM

The electrocardiogram (**ECG**) may be recorded by using an **active** or **exploring electrode** connected to an indifferent electrode at zero potential (**unipolar recording**) or by using two active electrodes (**bipolar recording**). In a volume conductor, the sum of the potentials at the points of an equilateral triangle with a current source in the center is zero at all times. A triangle with the heart at its center (**Einthoven triangle,** see below) can be approximated by placing electrodes on both wrists (or shoulders) and on the left ankle (or left lower abdomen). These are the three **standard limb leads** used in electrocardiography. A fourth neutral lead is commonly connected to the right ankle. Alternatively, if the three standard limb electrodes are connected to a common terminal, an indifferent electrode ("V" electrode) that stays near zero potential is obtained. Depolarization moving toward an active electrode in a volume conductor produces a positive deflection, whereas depolarization moving in the opposite direction produces a negative deflection.

The names of the various waves and segments of the ECG in humans are shown in **Figure 29–4.** By convention, an upward deflection is written when the active electrode becomes positive relative to the indifferent electrode, and a downward deflection is written when the active electrode becomes negative. As can be seen in Figure 29–1, the P wave is primarily produced by atrial depolarization, the QRS complex is dominated by ventricular depolarization, and the T wave by ventricular repolarization. The U wave is an inconstant finding that may be due to Purkinje fiber repolarization, ventricular myocytes with long action potentials, or electrolyte imbalances. The intervals between the various waves of the ECG and the events in the heart that occur during these intervals are shown in **Table 29–1.**

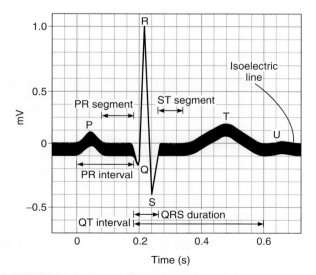

FIGURE 29–4 Waves of the ECG. Standard names for individual waves and segments that make up the ECG are shown. Electrical activity that contributes the observed deflections is discussed in the text and in Table 29–2.

TABLE 29–1 ECG intervals.

Intervals	Normal Durations		Events in the Heart during Interval
	Average	Range	
PR interval[a]	0.18[b]	0.12–0.20	Atrioventricular conduction
QRS duration	0.08	to 0.10	Ventricular depolarization
QT interval	0.40[c]	to 0.43	Ventricular action potential
ST interval (QT minus QRS)	0.32	…	Plateau portion of the ventricular action potential

[a]Measured from the beginning of the P wave to the beginning of the QRS complex.

[b]Shortens as heart rate increases from average of 0.18 s at a rate of 70 beats/min to 0.14 s at a rate of 130 beats/min.

[c]Can be lower (0.35) depending on the heart rate.

UNIPOLAR & BIPOLAR LEADS

Nine unipolar leads, that is, leads that record the potential difference between an **exploring electrode** and an **indifferent electrode,** are commonly used in clinical electrocardiography. There are six unipolar chest leads (precordial leads) designated V_1–V_6 (**Figure 29–5**) and three unipolar limb leads: VR (right arm), VL (left arm), and VF (left foot). The neutral lead or an indifferent electrode (the V lead that effectively records a "zero" potential because they are situated such that the electrical activity should be cancelled out) are used as reference electrodes. **Augmented limb leads,** designated by the letter a (aVR for augmented vector right—placed at the right wrist; aVL for augmented vector left—left wrist; and aVF for augmented vector foot—left foot), are generally used. The augmented limb leads do not use the neutral or V electrode as the zero, rather, they are recordings between the one, augmented limb and the other two limbs. This increases the size of the potentials by 50% without any change in configuration from the nonaugmented record.

With bipolar leads (discussed further), the **standard limb leads** each record the differences in potential between two limbs. Because current flows only in the body fluids, the records obtained are those that would be obtained if the electrodes were at the points of attachment of the limbs, no matter where on the limbs the electrodes are placed. In lead I, the electrodes are connected so that an upward deflection is inscribed when the left arm becomes positive relative to the right (left arm positive). In lead II, the electrodes are on the right arm and left leg, with the leg positive; and in lead III, the electrodes are on the left arm and left leg, with the leg positive.

NORMAL ECG

The sequence in which the parts of the heart are depolarized and the position of the heart relative to the electrodes are the important in interpreting the configurations of the waves in each lead (Figure 29–5). The atria are located posteriorly in the chest. The ventricles form the base and anterior surface of the heart with the right ventricle anterolateral to the left. Thus, aVR "looks at"

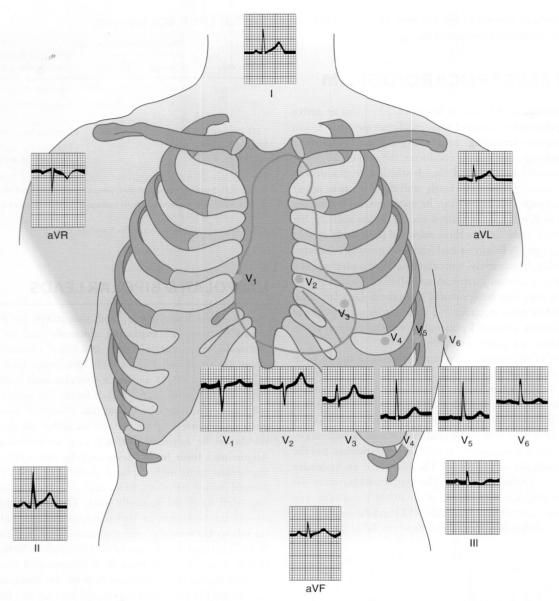

FIGURE 29–5 Normal ECG. Positional for standard unipolar leads are shown. The augmented extremity leads (aVR, aVL, and aVF) are shown on the right shoulder, left shoulder, and lower left abdomen, respectively (Note that these are usually placed on the arms and legs). The six chest leads (V_1–V_6) are shown in their proper placement. Tracings from individual electrodes (positions marked in figure) are shown for a normal ECG. See text for additional details. (Reproduced with permission from Goldman MJ: *Principles of Clinical Electrocardiography,* 12th ed. New York: McGraw-Hill; 1986.)

the cavities of the ventricles. Atrial depolarization, ventricular depolarization, and ventricular repolarization move away from the exploring electrode, and the P wave, QRS complex, and T wave are therefore all negative (downward) deflections; aVL and aVF look at the ventricles, and the deflections are therefore predominantly positive or biphasic. There is no Q wave in V_1 and V_2, and the initial portion of the QRS complex is a small upward deflection because ventricular depolarization first moves across the midportion of the septum from left to right toward the exploring electrode. The wave of excitation then moves down the septum

and into the left ventricle away from the electrode, producing a large S wave. Finally, it moves back along the ventricular wall toward the electrode, producing the return to the isoelectric line. Conversely, in the left ventricular leads (V_4–V_6) there may be an initial small Q wave (left to right septal depolarization), and there is a large R wave (septal and left ventricular depolarization) followed in V_4 and V_5 by a moderate S wave (late depolarization of the ventricular walls moving back toward the AV junction). It should be noted that there is considerable variation in the position of the normal heart, and the position affects the configuration of the electrocardiographic complexes in the various leads.

BIPOLAR LIMB LEADS & THE CARDIAC VECTOR

Because the standard limb leads are records of the potential differences between two points, the deflection in each lead at any instant indicates the magnitude and direction of the electromotive force generated in the heart in the axis of the lead **(cardiac vector or axis).** The vector at any given moment in the two dimensions of the frontal plane can be calculated from any two standard limb leads if it is assumed that the three electrode locations form the points of an equilateral triangle (Einthoven triangle) and that the heart lies in the center of the triangle **(Figure 29–6).** These assumptions are not completely warranted, but calculated vectors are useful approximations. An approximate **mean QRS vector** ("electrical axis of the heart") is often plotted by using the average QRS deflection in each lead (Figure 29–6). This is a **mean** vector as opposed to an **instantaneous** vector, and the average QRS deflections should be measured by integrating the QRS complexes. However, they can be approximated by measuring the net differences between the positive and negative peaks of the QRS. The normal direction of the mean QRS vector is generally said to be –30° to +110° on the coordinate system shown in Figure 29–6. **Left** or **right axis deviation** is said to be present if the calculated axis falls to the left of –30° or to the right of +110°, respectively. Right or left axis deviation is suggestive of right ventricular hypertrophy or left ventricular hypertrophy, but there are better and more reliable electrocardiographic criteria for these conditions.

HIS BUNDLE ELECTROGRAM

In patients with heart block, the electrical events in the AV node, bundle of His, and Purkinje system are frequently studied with a catheter containing an electrode at its tip that is passed through a vein to the right side of the heart and manipulated into a position close to the tricuspid valve. Three or more standard electrocardiographic leads are recorded simultaneously. The record of the electrical activity obtained with the catheter **(Figure 29–7)** is the **His bundle electrogram (HBE).** It normally shows an A deflection when the AV node is activated, an H spike during transmission through the His bundle, and a V deflection during ventricular depolarization. With the HBE and the standard electrocardiographic leads, it is possible to time three intervals accurately: (1) the PA interval, the time from the first appearance of atrial depolarization to the A wave in the HBE, which represents conduction time from the SA node to the AV node; (2) the AH interval, from the A wave to the start of the H spike, which represents the AV nodal conduction time; and (3) the HV interval, the time from the start of the H spike to the start of the QRS deflection in the ECG, which represents conduction in the bundle of His and the bundle branches. The approximate normal values for these intervals in adults are PA, 27 ms; AH, 92 ms; and HV, 43 ms. These values illustrate the relative slowness of conduction in the AV node.

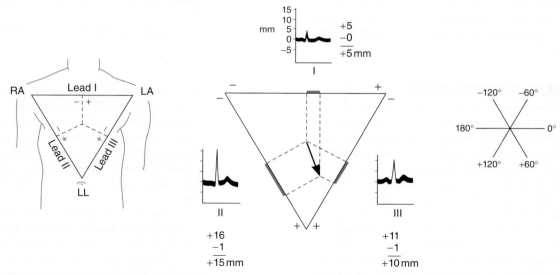

FIGURE 29–6 Cardiac vector. Left: Einthoven triangle. Perpendiculars dropped from the midpoints of the sides of the equilateral triangle intersect at the center of electrical activity. RA, right arm; LA, left arm; LL, left leg. **Center:** Calculation of mean QRS vector. In each lead, distances equal to the height of the R wave minus the height of the largest negative deflection in the QRS complex are measured off from the midpoint of the side of the triangle representing that lead. An arrow drawn from the center of electrical activity to the point of intersection of perpendiculars extended from the distances measured off on the sides represents the magnitude and direction of the mean QRS vector. **Right:** Reference axes for determining the direction of the vector.

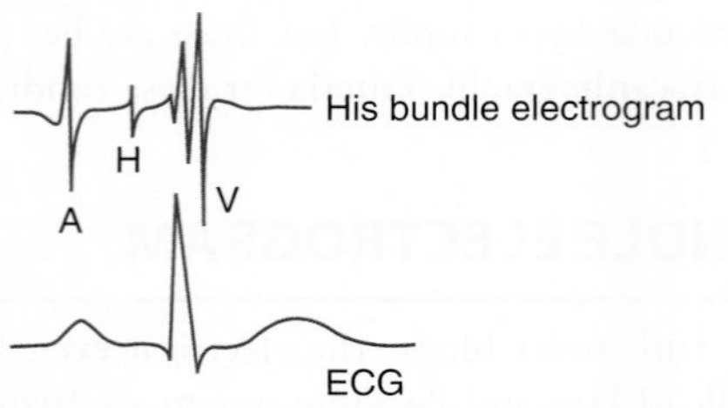

FIGURE 29–7 Normal His bundle electrogram (HBE) with simultaneously recorded ECG. An HBE recorded with an invasive electrode is superimposed on a standard ECG reading. Timing of depolarizations of the HBE is described in the text.

■ CLINICAL APPLICATIONS: CARDIAC ARRHYTHMIAS

NORMAL CARDIAC RATE

In the normal human heart, each beat originates in the SA node (**normal sinus rhythm**). The heart beats about 70 times per minute at rest. The rate is slowed (**bradycardia**) during sleep and accelerated (**tachycardia**) by emotion, exercise, fever, and many other stimuli. In healthy young individuals breathing at a normal rate, the heart rate varies with the phases of respiration: It accelerates during inspiration and decelerates during expiration, especially if the depth of breathing is increased. This **sinus arrhythmia** is a normal phenomenon and is primarily due to fluctuations in parasympathetic output to the heart. During inspiration, impulses in the vagi from the stretch receptors in the lungs inhibit the cardioinhibitory area in the medulla oblongata. The tonic vagal discharge that keeps the heart rate slow decreases, and the heart rate rises. Disease processes affecting the sinus node lead to marked bradycardia accompanied by dizziness and syncope (**Clinical Box 29–2**).

ABNORMAL PACEMAKERS

The AV node and other portions of the conduction system can, in abnormal situations, become the cardiac pacemaker. In addition, diseased atrial and ventricular muscle fibers can have their membrane potentials reduced and discharge repetitively.

Because the discharge rate of the SA node is more rapid than that of the other parts of the conduction system, the SA node normally controls the heart rate. Slowed conduction between the atria and ventricles is known as **incomplete heart block.** Examples of first-degree and second-degree incomplete heart block are described in **Figure 29–8.** When conduction from the atria to the ventricles is completely interrupted, **complete (third-degree) heart block** results, and the ventricles beat at a low rate (**idioventricular rhythm**) independently of the atria (Figure 29–8). The block may be due to disease in the AV node (**AV nodal block**) or in the conducting system below the node (**infranodal block**). In patients with AV nodal block, the remaining nodal tissue becomes the pacemaker and the rate of the idioventricular rhythm

CLINICAL BOX 29–2

Sick Sinus Syndrome

Sick sinus syndrome (bradycardia-tachycardia syndrome; sinus node dysfunction) is a collection of heart rhythm disorders that include **sinus bradycardia** (slow heart rates from the natural pacemaker of the heart), **tachycardias** (fast heart rates), and **bradycardia-tachycardia** (alternating slow and fast heart rhythms). Sick sinus syndrome is relatively uncommon and is usually found in people older than 50, in whom the cause is often a nonspecific, scarlike degeneration of the heart's conduction system. When found in younger people, especially in children, a common cause of sick sinus syndrome is heart surgery, especially on the upper chambers. Holter monitoring is an effective tool for diagnosing sick sinus syndrome because of the episodic nature of the disorder. Extremely slow heart rate and prolonged pauses may be seen during Holter monitoring, along with episodes of atrial tachycardias.

THERAPEUTIC HIGHLIGHTS

Treatment depends on the severity and type of disease. Tachycardias are frequently treated with medication. When there is marked bradycardia in patients with sick sinus syndrome or third-degree heart block, an electronic pacemaker is frequently implanted. These devices, which have become sophisticated and reliable, are useful in patients with sinus node dysfunction, AV block, and bifascicular or trifascicular block. They are useful also in patients with severe neurogenic syncope, in whom carotid sinus stimulation produces pauses of more than 3 s between heartbeats.

is approximately 45 beats/min. In patients with infranodal block due to disease in the bundle of His, the ventricular pacemaker is located more peripherally in the conduction system and the ventricular rate is lower; it averages 35 beats/min, but in individual cases it can be as low as 15 beats/min. In such individuals, there may also be periods of asystole lasting a minute or more. The resultant cerebral ischemia causes dizziness and fainting (**Stokes–Adams syndrome**).

Sometimes one branch of the bundle of His is interrupted, causing **right** or **left bundle branch block.** In bundle branch block, excitation passes normally down the bundle on the intact side and then sweeps back through the muscle to activate the ventricle on the blocked side. The ventricular rate is therefore normal, but the QRS complexes are prolonged and deformed (Figure 29–8). Block can also occur in the anterior or posterior fascicle of the left bundle branch, producing the condition called **hemiblock** or **fascicular block.** Left anterior hemiblock produces abnormal left axis deviation in the ECG, whereas left posterior hemiblock produces abnormal right axis deviation. It is not

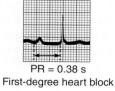
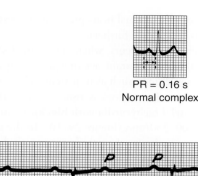

PR = 0.16 s
Normal complex

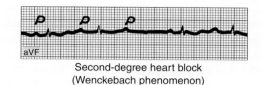

PR = 0.38 s
First-degree heart block

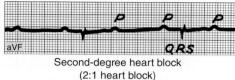
aVF   QRS

Second-degree heart block
(2:1 heart block)

aVF

Second-degree heart block
(Wenckebach phenomenon)

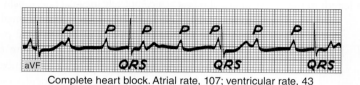
aVF   QRS   QRS   QRS

Complete heart block. Atrial rate, 107; ventricular rate, 43

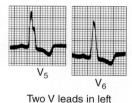
V_5 V_6

Two V leads in left
bundle branch block

FIGURE 29–8 **ECG with heart block.** Individual traces that depict normal ECG and various forms of heart block are shown. When conduction between the atria and ventricles is slowed but not completely interrupted, **incomplete heart block** is present. In first-degree heart block (upper right) atrial impulses reach the ventricles but the PR interval is abnormally long. In second-degree heart block (middle left) not all atrial impulses are conducted to the ventricles, eg, 2:1 block where a ventricular beat that follows every second atrial beat. Alternatively, there can be repeated sequences of beats in which the PR interval lengthens progressively until a ventricular beat is dropped (Wenckebach phenomenon, middle right). The PR interval of the cardiac cycle that follows each dropped beat is usually normal or only slightly prolonged. Complete heart block and left bundle block are discussed in the text. When appropriate, unipolar leads are noted.

uncommon to find combinations of fascicular and branch blocks (**bifascicular** or **trifascicular block**). The HBE permits detailed analysis of the site of block when there is a defect in the conduction system.

ECTOPIC FOCI OF EXCITATION & REENTRY

Normally, myocardial cells do not discharge spontaneously, and the possibility of spontaneous discharge of the His bundle and Purkinje system is low because the normal pacemaker discharge of the SA node is more rapid than their rate of spontaneous discharge. In abnormal conditions when the His–Purkinje fibers or the myocardial fibers discharge spontaneously, **increased automaticity** of the heart is said to be present. If an irritable **ectopic focus** discharges once, the result is a beat that occurs before the expected next normal beat and transiently interrupts the cardiac rhythm (atrial, nodal, or ventricular **extrasystole** or **premature beat**). If the focus discharges repetitively at a rate higher than that of the SA node, it produces rapid, regular tachycardia (atrial, ventricular, or nodal **paroxysmal tachycardia** or **atrial flutter**).

A more common cause of paroxysmal arrhythmias is a defect in conduction that permits a wave of excitation to propagate continuously within a closed circuit (**circus movement**). For example, if a transient block is present on one side of a portion of the conducting system, the impulse can go down the other side. If the block then wears off, the impulse may conduct in a retrograde direction in the previously blocked side back to the origin and then descend again, establishing a circus movement (**Figure 29–9**). If the reentry is in the AV node, the reentrant

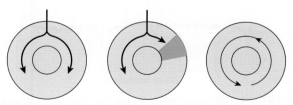

FIGURE 29–9 **Depolarization of a ring of cardiac tissue.** Normally, the impulse spreads in both directions in the ring (**left**) and the tissue immediately behind each branch of the impulse is refractory. When a transient block occurs on one side (**center**), the impulse on the other side goes around the ring, and if the transient block has now worn off (**right**), the impulse passes this area and continues to circle indefinitely (circus movement).

activity depolarizes the atrium, and the resulting atrial beat is called an echo beat. In addition, the reentrant activity in the node propagates back down to the ventricle, producing paroxysmal nodal tachycardia. Circus movements can also become established in the atrial or ventricular muscle fibers.

ATRIAL ARRHYTHMIAS

Excitation spreading from an independently discharging focus in the atria stimulates the AV node prematurely and is conducted to the ventricles. The P waves of atrial extrasystoles are abnormal, but the QRST configurations are usually normal (**Figure 29–10**). The excitation may depolarize the SA node, which must repolarize and then depolarize to the firing level before it can initiate the next normal beat. Consequently, a pause occurs between the extrasystole and the next normal beat that is usually equal in length to the interval between the normal beats preceding the extrasystole, and the rhythm is "reset" (see further).

Atrial tachycardia occurs when an atrial focus discharges regularly or there is reentrant activity producing atrial rates up to 220/min. Sometimes, such as in patients taking digitalis, some degree of atrioventricular block is associated with the tachycardia (**paroxysmal atrial tachycardia with block**). In atrial flutter, the atrial rate is 200–350/min (Figure 29–10). In the most common form of this arrhythmia, there is large counterclockwise circus movement in the right atrium. This produces a characteristic sawtooth pattern of flutter waves due to atrial contractions. It is almost always associated with 2:1 or greater AV block, because in adults the AV node cannot conduct more than about 230 impulses per minute. In **atrial fibrillation,** the atria beat very rapidly (300–500/min) in a completely irregular and disorganized fashion. Because the AV node discharges at irregular intervals, the ventricles also beat at a completely irregular rate, usually 80–160/min (Figure 29–10). The condition can be paroxysmal or chronic, and in some cases there appears to be a genetic predisposition. Occasional atrial extrasystoles occur from time to time in most normal humans and have no pathologic significance. In paroxysmal atrial tachycardia and flutter, the ventricular rate may be so high that diastole is too short for adequate filling of the ventricles with blood between contractions. Consequently, cardiac output is reduced and symptoms of heart failure appear.

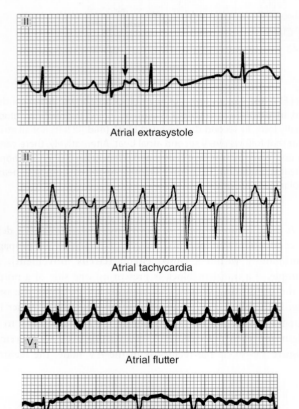

FIGURE 29–10 Atrial arrhythmias. The illustration shows an atrial premature beat with its P wave superimposed on the T wave of the preceding beat (*arrow*); atrial tachycardia; atrial flutter with 4:1 AV block; and atrial fibrillation with a totally irregular ventricular rate. Leads used to capture electrical activity are marked in each trace. (Reproduced with permission from Goldschlager N, Goldman MJ: *Principles of Clinical Electrocardiography,* 13th ed. New York: McGraw-Hill; 1989.)

VENTRICULAR ARRHYTHMIAS

Premature beats that originate in an ectopic ventricular focus usually have bizarrely shaped prolonged QRS complexes because of the slow spread of the impulse from the focus through the ventricular muscle to the rest of the ventricle. They are usually incapable of exciting the bundle of His, and retrograde conduction to the atria therefore does not occur. In the meantime, the next succeeding normal SA nodal impulse depolarizes the atria. The P wave is usually buried in the QRS of the extrasystole. If the normal impulse reaches the ventricles, they are still in the refractory period following depolarization from the ectopic focus.

However, the second succeeding impulse from the SA node produces a normal beat. Thus, ventricular premature beats are followed by a **compensatory pause** that is often longer than the pause after an atrial extrasystole. Furthermore, ventricular premature beats do not interrupt the regular discharge of the SA node, whereas atrial premature beats often interrupt and "reset" the normal rhythm.

Atrial and ventricular premature beats are not strong enough to produce a pulse at the wrist if they occur early in diastole, when the ventricles have not had time to fill with blood and the ventricular musculature is still in its relatively refractory period. They may not even open the aortic and pulmonary valves, in which case there is, in addition, no second heart sound.

Paroxysmal ventricular tachycardia is in effect a series of rapid, regular ventricular depolarizations usually due to a circus movement involving the ventricles. **Torsades de pointes** is a form of ventricular tachycardia in which the QRS morphology varies

(Figure 29–11). Tachycardias originating above the ventricles (supraventricular tachycardias such as paroxysmal nodal tachycardia) can be distinguished from paroxysmal ventricular tachycardia by use of the HBE; in supraventricular tachycardias, a His bundle H deflection is present, whereas in ventricular tachycardias, there is none. Ventricular premature beats are not uncommon and, in the absence of ischemic heart disease, usually benign. Ventricular tachycardia is more serious because cardiac output is decreased, and ventricular fibrillation is an occasional complication of ventricular tachycardia.

In **ventricular fibrillation** (Figure 29–11), the ventricular muscle fibers contract in a totally irregular and ineffective way because of the very rapid discharge of multiple ventricular ectopic foci or a circus movement. The fibrillating ventricles, like the fibrillating atria, look like a quivering "bag of worms." Ventricular fibrillation can be produced by an electric shock or an extrasystole during a critical interval, the **vulnerable period.** The vulnerable period coincides in time with the midportion of the T wave; that is, it occurs at a time when some of the ventricular myocardium is depolarized, some is incompletely repolarized, and some is completely repolarized. These are excellent conditions in which to establish reentry and a circus movement. The fibrillating ventricles cannot pump blood effectively, and circulation of the blood stops. Therefore, in the absence of emergency treatment, ventricular fibrillation that lasts more than a few minutes is fatal. The most frequent cause of sudden death in patients with myocardial infarcts is ventricular fibrillation.

LONG QT SYNDROME

An indication of vulnerability of the heart during repolarization is the fact that in patients in whom the QT interval is prolonged, cardiac repolarization is irregular and the incidence of ventricular arrhythmias and sudden death increases. The syndrome can be caused by a number of different drugs, by electrolyte abnormalities, by myocardial ischemia, or can be congenital. Mutations of eight different genes have been reported to cause the syndrome. Six cause reduced function of various K^+ channels by alterations in their structure; one inhibits a K^+ channel by reducing the amount of the ankyrin isoform that links it to the cytoskeleton; and one increases the function of the cardiac Na^+ channel.

ACCELERATED AV CONDUCTION

An interesting condition seen in some otherwise normal individuals who are prone to attacks of paroxysmal atrial arrhythmias is **accelerated AV conduction (Wolff–Parkinson–White syndrome).** Normally, the only conducting pathway between the atria and the ventricles is the AV node. Individuals with Wolff–Parkinson–White syndrome have an additional aberrant muscular or nodal tissue connection (**bundle of Kent**) between the atria and ventricles. This conducts more rapidly than the slowly conducting AV node, and one ventricle is excited early. The manifestations of its activation merge with the normal QRS pattern, producing a short PR interval and a prolonged QRS deflection slurred on the upstroke

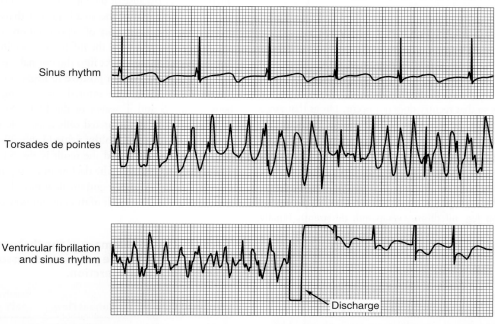

Sinus rhythm

Torsades de pointes

Ventricular fibrillation and sinus rhythm

Discharge

FIGURE 29–11 **Record obtained from an implanted cardioverter–defibrillator in a 12-year-old boy with congenital long QT syndrome who collapsed while answering a question in school. Top:** Normal sinus rhythm with long QT interval. **Middle:** Torsades de pointes. **Bottom:** Ventricular fibrillation with discharge of defibrillator, as programmed 7.5 s after the start of ventricular tachycardia, converting the heart to normal sinus rhythm. The boy recovered consciousness in 2 min and had no neurologic sequelae. (Reproduced with permission from Moss AJ, Daubert JP: Images in clinical medicine. Internal ventricular fibrillation, *N Engl J Med.* 2000 Feb 10;342(6):398.)

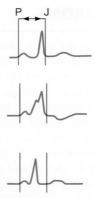

FIGURE 29–12 Accelerated AV conduction. Top: Normal sinus beat. **Middle:** Short PR interval; wide, slurred QRS complex; normal PJ interval (Wolff–Parkinson–White syndrome). **Bottom:** Short PR interval, normal QRS complex (Lown–Ganong–Levine syndrome). (Reproduced with permission from Goldschlager N, Goldman MJ: *Principles of Clinical Electrocardiography*, 13th ed. New York: McGraw-Hill; 1989.)

(Figure 29–12), with a normal interval between the start of the P wave and the end of the QRS complex ("PJ interval"). The paroxysmal atrial tachycardias seen in this syndrome often follow an atrial premature beat. This beat conducts normally down the AV node but spreads to the ventricular end of the aberrant bundle, and the impulse is transmitted retrograde to the atrium. A circus movement is thus established. Less commonly, an atrial premature beat finds the AV node refractory but reaches the ventricles via the bundle of Kent, setting up a circus movement in which the impulse passes from the ventricles to the atria via the AV node.

TREATMENTS FOR ARRHYTHMIAS

Many different drugs used in the treatment of arrhythmias slow conduction in the conduction system and the myocardium. This depresses ectopic activity and reduces the discrepancy between normal and reentrant paths so that reentry does not occur. Drugs that target Na^+ channels (eg, quinidine) can slow I_{Na} and prolong refractoriness (eg, quinidine, disopyramide), inhibit I_{Na} with minimal prolongation of refractoriness (eg, flecainide, propafenone) or shorten refractoriness in depolarized cells (eg, lidocaine, mexiletine). Drugs that target K^+ channels can prolong refractoriness (eg, amiodarone, sotalol, dofetilide). Drugs that block L-type Ca^{2+} channels can slow SA pacemaker and AV conduction (eg, nifedipine, verapamil, diltiazem). Finally, drugs that block β-adrenergic receptors reduce the activation of I_{CaL} (eg, propranolol, metoprolol). Interestingly, it has become clear that in some patients any of these drugs can be **proarrhythmic** rather than antiarrhythmic—that is, they can also cause various arrhythmias. Therefore, careful monitoring and alternative procedures are extremely important when using antiarrhythmic drugs.

An alternative treatment is radiofrequency catheter ablation of reentrant pathways. Catheters with electrodes at the tip can be inserted into the chambers of the heart and its environs and used to map the exact location of an ectopic focus or accessory bundle responsible for the production of reentry and supraventricular tachycardia. The pathway can then be ablated by passing radiofrequency current with the catheter tip placed close to the bundle or focus. In skilled hands, this form of treatment can be very effective and is associated with few complications.

■ ELECTROCARDIOGRAPHIC FINDINGS IN OTHER CARDIAC & SYSTEMIC DISEASES

MYOCARDIAL INFARCTION

When the blood supply to part of the myocardium is interrupted, profound changes take place in the myocardium that lead to irreversible changes and death of muscle cells. The ECG is very useful for diagnosing ischemia and locating areas of infarction. The underlying electrical events and the resulting electrocardiographic changes are complex, and only a brief review can be presented here.

The three major abnormalities that cause electrocardiographic changes in acute myocardial infarction are summarized in Table 29–2. The first change—abnormally rapid repolarization after discharge of the infarcted muscle fibers as a result of accelerated opening of K^+ channels—develops seconds after occlusion of a coronary artery in experimental animals. It lasts only a few minutes, but before it is over the resting membrane potential of the infarcted fibers declines because of the loss of intracellular K^+. Starting about 30 min later, the infarcted fibers also begin to depolarize more slowly than the surrounding normal fibers. All three of these changes cause current flow that produces elevation of the ST segment in electrocardiographic leads recorded with electrodes over the infarcted area. Because of the rapid repolarization in the infarct, the membrane potential of the area is greater than it is in the normal area during the latter part of repolarization, making the normal region negative relative to the infarct. Extracellularly, current therefore flows out of the infarct into the normal area (since, by convention, current flow is from positive to negative). This current flows toward electrodes over the injured area, causing increased positivity between the S and T waves of the ECG. Similarly, the delayed depolarization of the infarcted cells causes the infarcted area to be positive relative to the healthy tissue (Table 29–2) during the early part of repolarization, and the result is also ST segment elevation. The remaining change—the decline in resting membrane potential during diastole—causes a current flow into the infarct during ventricular diastole. The result of this current flow is a depression of the

TABLE 29–2 Summary of the three major abnormalities of membrane polarization associated with acute myocardial infarction.

Defect in Infarcted Cells	Current Flow	Resultant ECG Change in Leads Over Infarct
Rapid repolarization	Out of infarct	ST segment elevation
Decreased resting membrane potential	Into infarct	TQ segment depression (manifested as ST segment elevation)
Delayed depolarization	Out of infarct	ST segment elevation

TQ segment of the ECG. However, the electronic arrangement in electrocardiographic recorders is such that a TQ segment depression is recorded as an ST segment elevation. Thus, the hallmark of acute myocardial infarction is elevation of the ST segments in the leads overlying the area of infarction. Leads on the opposite side of the heart show ST segment depression.

After some days or weeks, the ST segment abnormalities subside. The dead muscle and scar tissue become electrically silent. The infarcted area is therefore negative relative to the normal myocardium during systole, and it fails to contribute its share of positivity to the electrocardiographic complexes. The manifestations of this negativity are multiple and subtle. Common changes include the appearance of a Q wave in some of the leads in which it was not previously present and an increase in the size of the normal Q wave in some of the other leads, although so-called non-Q-wave infarcts are also seen. These latter infarcts tend to be less severe, but there is a high incidence of subsequent reinfarction. Another finding in infarction of the anterior left ventricle is "failure of progression of the R wave"; that is, the R wave fails to become successively larger in the precordial leads as the electrode is moved from right to left over the left ventricle. If the septum is infarcted, the conduction system may be damaged, causing bundle branch block or other forms of heart block.

Myocardial infarctions are often complicated by serious ventricular arrhythmias, with the threat of ventricular fibrillation and death. In experimental animals, and presumably in humans, ventricular arrhythmias occur during three periods. During the first 30 min of an infarction, arrhythmias due to reentry are common. There follows a period relatively free from arrhythmias but, starting 12 h after infarction, arrhythmias occur as a result of increased automaticity. Arrhythmias occurring 3 days to several weeks after infarction are once again usually due to reentry.

EFFECTS OF CHANGES IN THE IONIC COMPOSITION OF THE BLOOD

Changes in the Na^+ and K^+ concentrations of the extracellular fluids would be expected to affect the potentials of the myocardial fibers because the electrical activity of the heart depends on the distribution of these ions across the muscle cell membranes. Clinically, a fall in the plasma level of Na^+ may be associated with low-voltage electrocardiographic complexes, but changes in the plasma K^+ level produce severe cardiac abnormalities. Hyperkalemia is a very dangerous and potentially lethal condition because of its effects on the heart. As the plasma K^+ level rises, the first change in the ECG is the appearance of tall peaked T waves, a manifestation of altered repolarization (**Figure 29–13**). At higher K^+ levels, paralysis of the atria and prolongation of the

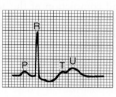

Normal tracing (plasma K⁺ 4–5.5 mEq/L). PR interval = 0.16 s; QRS interval = 0.06 s; QT interval = 0.4 s (normal for an assumed heart rate of 60).

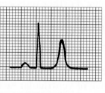

Hyperkalemia (plasma K⁺ ±7.0 mEq/L). The PR and QRS intervals are within normal limits. Very tall, slender peaked T waves are now present.

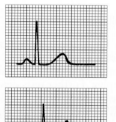

Hyperkalemia (plasma K⁺ ±8.5 mEq/L). There is no evidence of atrial activity; the QRS complex is broad and slurred and the QRS interval has widened to 0.2 s. The T waves remain tall and slender. Further elevation of the plasma K⁺ level may result in ventricular tachycardia and ventricular fibrillation.

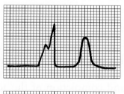

Hypokalemia (plasma K⁺ ±3.5 mEq/L). PR interval = 0.2 s; QRS interval = 0.06 s; ST segment depression. A prominent U wave is now present immediately following the T. The actual QT interval remains 0.4 s. If the U wave is erroneously considered a part of the T, a falsely prolonged QT interval of 0.6 s will be measured.

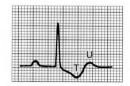

Hypokalemia (plasma K⁺ ±2.5 mEq/L). The PR interval is lengthened to 0.32 s; the ST segment is depressed; the T wave is inverted; a prominent U wave is seen. The true QT interval remains normal.

FIGURE 29–13 Correlation of plasma K⁺ level and the ECG, assuming that the plasma Ca²⁺ level is normal. The diagrammed complexes are left ventricular epicardial leads. (Reproduced with permission from Goldman MJ: *Principles of Clinical Electrocardiography*, 12th ed. New York: McGraw-Hill; 1986.)

QRS complexes occur. Ventricular arrhythmias may develop. The resting membrane potential of the muscle fibers decreases as the extracellular K^+ concentration increases. The fibers eventually become unexcitable, and the heart stops in diastole. Conversely, a decrease in the plasma K^+ level causes prolongation of the PR interval, prominent U waves, and, occasionally, late T wave inversion in the precordial leads. If the T and U waves merge, the apparent QT interval is often prolonged; if the T and U waves are separated, the true QT interval is seen to be of normal duration. Hypokalemia is a serious condition, but it is not as rapidly fatal as hyperkalemia.

Increases in extracellular Ca^{2+} concentration enhance myocardial contractility. When large amounts of Ca^{2+} are infused into experimental animals, the heart relaxes less during diastole and eventually stops in systole (**calcium rigor**). However, in clinical conditions associated with hypercalcemia, the plasma calcium level is rarely if ever high enough to affect the heart. Hypocalcemia causes prolongation of the ST segment and consequently of the QT interval, a change that is also produced by phenothiazines and tricyclic antidepressant drugs and by various diseases of the central nervous system.

CHAPTER SUMMARY

- Contractions in the heart are controlled via a well-regulated electrical signaling cascade that originates in pacemaker cells in the sinoatrial (SA) node and is passed via internodal atrial pathways to the atrioventricular (AV) node, the bundle of His, the Purkinje system, and to all parts of the ventricle.

- Most cardiac cells have an action potential that includes a rapid depolarization, an initial rapid repolarization, a plateau, and a slow repolarization process to return to resting potential. These changes are defined by sequential activation and inactivation of Na^+, Ca^{2+}, and K^+ channels.

- Compared to typical myocytes, pacemaker cells have a slightly different sequence of events. After repolarization to the resting potential, there is a slow depolarization that occurs due to a channel that can pass both Na^+ and K^+. As this "funny" current continues to depolarize the cell, Ca^{2+} channels are activated to rapidly depolarize the cell. The hyperpolarization phase is again dominated by K^+ current.

- Spread of the electrical signal from cell to cell is via gap junctions. The rate of spread is dependent on anatomic features, but also can be altered (to a certain extent) via neural input.

- The electrocardiogram (ECG) is an algebraic sum of the electrical activity in the heart. The normal ECG includes well-defined waves and segments, including the P wave (atrial depolarization), the QRS complex (ventricular depolarization), and the T wave (ventricular repolarization). Various arrhythmias can be detected in irregular ECG recordings.

- Because of the contribution of ionic movement to cardiac muscle contraction, heart tissue is sensitive to ionic composition of the blood. Most serious are increases in $[K^+]$ that can produce severe cardiac abnormalities, including paralysis of the atria and ventricular arrhythmias.

MULTIPLE-CHOICE QUESTIONS

For all questions, select the single best answer unless otherwise directed.

1. An older patient who had previously recovered from a heart attack was experiencing slight chest discomfort, dizziness, palpitations and shortness of breath. He was taken to the emergency room via ambulance where an electrocardiogram (ECG) showed increased heart rate (> 100 beats/min) and a long QRS (> 0.12 s). He was diagnosed with wide complex tachycardia with a ventricular origin and properly treated. Which part of his ECG corresponds to ventricular repolarization?
    A. The P wave
    B. The QRS duration
    C. The T wave
    D. The U wave
    E. The PR interval

2. A 50-year-old woman was recently prescribed disopyramide for cardiac arrhythmia. In a follow-up examination, the woman complained of faintness and confusion. A brief examination showed a low heart rate with sick sinus syndrome. Her disopyramide dosage was adjusted and a subsequent follow-up examination showed a normal ECG. In which of the following regions in the heart would you normally find a slowly depolarizing "prepotential"?
    A. Sinoatrial node
    B. Atrial muscle cells
    C. Bundle of His
    D. Purkinje fibers
    E. Ventricular muscle cells

3. An elite athlete came in for a routine physical examination. It was noticed on his ECG that there were progressive increases in the PR interval which were eventually followed by a skip of the QRS complex. Further tests determined the observed second-degree heart block to be consistent with a Wenckebach AV block. Which of the following would be associated with this second-degree heart block?
    A. The ventricular rate is lower than the atrial rate.
    B. The ventricular ECG complexes are distorted.
    C. There is a high incidence of ventricular tachycardia.
    D. Stroke volume is decreased.
    E. Cardiac output is increased.

4. A PhD student is able to measure ionic conductance in isolated muscle cells in his biophysical laboratory. A goal of the laboratory's work is to measure specific effects of cardiac drugs on the initiation and completion of the action potential. The student is able to evaluate several drugs acting on Na^+ current (I_{Na}), I_K, and I_{Ca}, and eventually determine the concentrations of drugs necessary to block individual channels contributing to the cardiomyocyte action potential. Currents caused by opening of which of the following channels contribute to the rapid depolarization phase of the action potential of ventricular muscle cells?
    A. Na^+ channels
    B. Cl^- channels
    C. Ca^{2+} channels
    D. K^+ channels
    E. HCO_3^- channels

5. A 45-year-old man from Connecticut experiences chest pain, dyspnea, confusion, and syncope shortly after one of

his lunch-time gardening sessions. He fears a heart attack and immediately is taken to the emergency room. His ECG shows third-degree atrioventricular (AV) block (ie, complete heart block), however, his blood work does not show evidence of ischemia, myocardial infarction or ionic imbalances. Further workup is negative for Lyme disease, however, traces of digoxin are in his blood. The man reveals he does have foxglove in his garden and frequently eats while he tends to the plants. He is instructed to stop eating while working in the garden, especially around the foxglove that may have provided the cardiac glycoside. Which of the following are consistent with complete heart block?

A. Fainting may occur because the atria are unable to pump blood into the ventricles.

B. Ventricular fibrillation is common.

C. The atrial rate is lower than the ventricular rate.

D. Fainting may occur because of prolonged periods during which the ventricles fail to contract.

6. An MD/PhD student is part of a heart laboratory where they can directly measure conduction in different regions of the heart. They are testing drugs that interrupt conduction from the atrioventricular (AV) node through the bundle of His and into the Purkinje fibers. They find novel drugs that can both slow and increase conduction, and begin to apply these to tachycardia and bradycardia animal models for pre-clinical development. They find that propagation of the action potential through the heart is fastest in which of the following cardiac structures?

A. Sinoatrial (SA) node

B. Atrial muscle

C. AV node

D. Purkinje fibers

E. Ventricular muscle

7. In a muscle physiology laboratory with a focus on regenerative medicine, a main project is centered on developing heart tissue from stem cells. A variety of growth factors and matrix proteins are evaluated for their ability to transform stem cells into the various cell types in the heart. A particular combination results in muscle cells that are unusually "stringy" and detailed microscopy shows that these cells, while consistently staining for cardiac muscle protein makers, contain fewer striations and mitochondria than the usual cardiomyocyte. Biophysical examination shows that these cells have a low internal resistance. Such findings are most consistent with cardiac muscle cells from which region of the heart?

A. Sinoatrial (SA) node

B. Atrial muscle

C. AV node

D. Purkinje fibers

E. Ventricular muscle

8. A patient with an inferior myocardial infarction develops a stable bradycardia of 50 beats/min. Her cardiologist orders an ECG to evaluate whether there is sinus node dysfunction or an atrioventricular conduction disturbance. Which of the following findings would lead to a diagnosis of a first-degree heart block?

A. Asynchrony of P waves and QRS complexes

B. Fixed, prolonged PR interval followed by a nonconducted QRS complex at a regular interval

C. Normal PR interval, normal QRS complex, increase R–R interval

D. Prolonged PR interval with every P wave followed by a QRS complex

E. The PR interval is progressively prolonged until a QRS complex is dropped

9. An otherwise healthy 35-year-old adult has recently moved and, for the first time in his life, experienced allergies. He obtains over-the-counter antihistamines at the pharmacy. While the antihistamines are successful in relieving his allergy symptoms, he discovers that he can no longer perform his typical light exercise without feeling faint. When he subsequently fainted after being scared in a friendly prank, his partner took him to the doctor. An ECG showed indications of Long QT syndrome (LQTS). Genetic tests showed that he had a mutation in a cardiomyocyte-expressed K^+ channel known to be associated with a mild form of LQTS. He was immediately taken off the antihistamines, prescribed β-blockers and informed of a list of medications to avoid. He was also recommended for follow-up treatment to control LQTS. His symptoms reflect the fact that cardiac K^+ channels dominate which part of the cardiomyocyte action potential?

A. Phase 0

B. Phase 1

C. Phase 2

D. Phase 3

E. Phase 4

10. A 55-year-old man recently contracted an infection and was prescribed antibiotics at a local clinic. Near the end of the antibiotic cycle, and as the infection subsided, the patient noticed symptoms of weakness and visited his family physician. Upon examination, the patient reported that he had recently taken an antibiotic (penicillin G) but had also been taking antihypertensive drugs (ACE inhibitors), which he had not disclosed at the clinic for fear of delaying receipt of his antibiotic prescription. Noting the drug combination, the physician suspected moderate hyperkalemia and ordered blood work and an ECG. Both were consistent with moderately high K^+. The patient was instructed to stop any penicillin treatments, put on a low K^+ diet for cautionary purposes and instructed on why it is important to disclose drug history during exams. How would the ECG for this patient with moderate hyperkalemia (plasma K^+ ~7.0 mEq/L) compare to a normal ECG?

A. The PR (~0.16 s), QRS (~0.06 s) and QT (~0.4 s) intervals would be normal. The T wave would be normal.

B. The PR and QRS intervals would be within normal limits. An exaggerated T wave (tall) would be prominent.

C. The QRS interval would be broadened and no PR interval would be visible. The T wave would be exaggerated.

D. A slightly larger PR interval (~0.2 s) with a normal QRS interval (~0.06 s) would exist. There would be a depression in the ST region and a limited T wave. The QT interval would be normal, but could be misread as extended if the U wave was prominent and the QU interval used instead.

ANSWERS

1. The correct answer is **C**. The deflection that characterizes the T wave is dominated by a collection of ventricular myocyte repolarizations. In a typical ECG, the deflections observed in the P wave **(A)** and the QRS duration **(B)** are primarily produced by atrial depolarization and ventricular depolarization, respectively. Thus,

these two answers are ruled out. Although understanding of the inconsistent U wave (**D**) is incomplete, it has been attributed to Purkinje fiber repolarization, ventricular myocytes with long action potentials, or electrolyte imbalances and can be excluded. The PR interval (**E**) represents the time between atrial and ventricular depolarization, and can be ruled out.

2. The correct answer is **A.** Cells in the sinoatrial node or atrioventricular node have pacemaker potential that is associated with a slowly depolarizing prepotential. Atrial muscle cells (**B**), cells in the His Bundle (**C**), Purkinje fiber cells (**D**) and ventricular muscle cells (**E**) all maintain a stable depolarization that is quickly polarized following activation of voltage-gated Na^+ channels.

3. The correct answer is **A.** In second-degree heart block, a subset of AV impulses fail to translate into a ventricular response, resulting in a lower ventricular contraction rate when compared to atrial contractions. The QRS readings, or the part of the ECG dominated by ventricular depolarization, are typically normal when they occur, ruling out **B**. Because these readings do not appear more frequently, ventricular tachycardia (**C**) is ruled out. The stroke volume (**D**) refers to the amount of blood pumped by the left ventricle during a single contraction. Since second-degree block alters the amount of contractions rather than the contraction itself, stroke volume is unchanged. Second-degree heart block would reduce the amount of blood pumped in one minute, or the cardiac output (**E**), ruling out this answer.

4. The correct answer is **A.** The action potential in ventricular muscle cells is initiated by activation of voltage-gated Na^+ channels, where the cell rapidly depolarizes from a resting potential near –90 mV to a value of +20 mV. At that time both Ca^{2+} (**C**) and K^+ channels (**D**) open, allowing for a slight repolarizations during a plateau phase. It is when the Ca^{2+} channels close and the K^+ channels are still opens that the large repolarization occurs, ruling out **C** and **D**. Cl^- channels (**B**) do not significantly contribute to the ventricular muscle cell action potential and HCO_3^- (**E**) is not carried by channels in the ventricular muscle fiber. Both of these can therefore be ruled out as answers.

5. The correct answer is **D.** The lack of signal from the AV node through to the ventricles limits contractions and subsequently, blood flow that can lead to fainting. The atria are properly excited and the passive flow of blood from the atria to the ventricle should be in order, thus option **A** could be ruled out. Ventricular fibrillation (**B**) refers to increased contractions of the ventricles while a reduced amount of contractions is the hallmark of complete heart block. The atrial rate is normal in complete heart block, but the transfer of this signal to the ventricles is blocked, thus, the atrial rate would be higher than the ventricular rate and (**C**) can be eliminated.

6. The correct answer is **D.** The most rapid conduction of the action potential (~4 m/s) occurs through the Purkinje fibers.

Depolarization is initiated in the SA node (**A**) with a conduction rate of ~0.05 m/s and then spreads radially through the atrial muscle cells (**B**) at ~1 m/s until it converges on the AV node. Conduction through the AV node (**C**) is slow (0.05 m/s), allowing for a delay of ~0.1 s before excitation is transferred to the His/Purkinje system and onto the ventricles. Conductance in ventricular cells (**E**) is similar to that in the atrial cells, ~1 m/s.

7. The correct answer is **D.** Purkinje fibers are specialized conducting cells that tend to be large and with fewer mitochondria and striations when compared to other cardiomyocytes. Compared with Purkinje fibers, cells within the SA node (**A**) and, to a lesser extent, the AV node (**C**), would also expect to show less striation, but be smaller in size and less conductive due to their higher internal resistance. Because they are primarily contracting cells, atrial muscle cells (**B**) and ventricular muscle cells (**E**) would be more compact and very highly striated with many mitochondria, and can be ruled out as answers.

8. The correct answer is **D.** First-degree heart block is characterized by prolonged PR intervals, which effectively slow the heart rate. P waves and QRS complex remain synchronized in first degree heart block, ruling out **A**. A fixed, prolonged PR interval (**B**) or an increasingly prolonged PR interval (**E**) followed by a drop of the QRS complex are indicative of a second-degree heart block and can be ruled out. An increase in an R - R interval with normal P wave and QRS complex (**C**) is indicative of a slower heart rate and can be ruled out.

9. The correct answer is **D.** It is in phase 3 where the K^+ channels dominate and allow for rapid repolarization to the resting potential, ~90 mv. Phase 0 (**A**) of the action potential refers to the rapid depolarization following the initiation of the action potential and can be ruled out. Phase 1 (**B**) refers to the initial repolarization following closure of Na^+ channels, and opening of both Ca^{2+} and K^+ channels. Phase 2 (**C**) refers to the plateau where repolarization is slowed due to the participation of both Ca^{2+} and K^+ conductances. Because activity of Ca^{2+} channels are equally as important as K^+ channels in phases 2 and 3, and **C** can be ruled out. In phase 4 (**E**), K^+ channels are closed and a resting potential is reached until the next action potential.

10. The correct answer is **B.** In moderate hyperkalemia, the exaggerated T wave, representing ventricular repolarization, is the prominent feature that differs from a normal ECG. Since there is a difference from normal, option **A** can be ruled out. The features described in option **C** are indicative of extreme hyperkalemia with very high plasma K^+ (8.5 mEq/L as opposed to 4–5.5 mEq/L). The changes noted in option **D** are indicative of hypokalemia (plasma K^+ ~2.5 mEq/L) and can be ruled out.

The Heart as a Pump

- Describe how the sequential pattern of contraction and relaxation in the heart results in a normal pattern of blood flow.
- Understand the pressure, volume, and flow changes that occur during the cardiac cycle.
- Explain the basis of the arterial pulse, heart sounds, and murmurs.
- Delineate the ways by which cardiac output can be upregulated in the setting of specific physiologic demands for increased oxygen supply to the tissues, such as exercise.
- Describe how the pumping action of the heart can be compromised in the setting of specific disease states.

■ MECHANICAL EVENTS OF THE CARDIAC CYCLE

Atrial systole starts after the p wave of the EKG; ventricular systole starts near the end of the R wave and ends just after the T wave. **SYSTOLIC PRESSURE** in the vascular system refers to the peak pressure reached during systole, not the mean pressure; similarly, the **DIASTOLIC PRESSURE** refers to the lowest pressure during diastole.

LATE DIASTOLE

Late in diastole, the mitral (bicuspid) and tricuspid valves between the atria and ventricles (atrioventricular [AV] valves) are open and the aortic and pulmonary valves are closed. Blood flows into the heart throughout diastole, filling the atria and ventricles. The rate of filling declines as the ventricles become distended and, especially when the heart rate is low, the cusps of the AV valves drift toward the closed position (**Figure 30–1**). The pressure in the ventricles remains low. About 70% of the ventricular filling occurs passively during diastole.

ATRIAL SYSTOLE

Contraction of the atria propels some additional blood into the ventricles. Contraction of the atrial muscle narrows the orifices of the superior and inferior vena cava and pulmonary veins, and the inertia of the blood moving toward the heart tends to keep blood in it. However, despite these inhibitory influences, there is some regurgitation of blood into the veins.

VENTRICULAR SYSTOLE

At the start of ventricular systole, the AV valves close. Ventricular muscle initially shortens relatively little, but intraventricular pressure rises sharply as the myocardium presses on the blood in the ventricle (**Figure 30–2**). This period of **isovolumetric (isovolumic, isometric) ventricular contraction** lasts about 0.05 s, until the pressures in the left and right ventricles exceed the pressures in the aorta (80 mm Hg; 10.6 kPa) and pulmonary artery (10 mm Hg), and the aortic and pulmonary valves open. During isovolumetric contraction, the AV valves bulge into the atria, causing a small but sharp rise in atrial pressure.

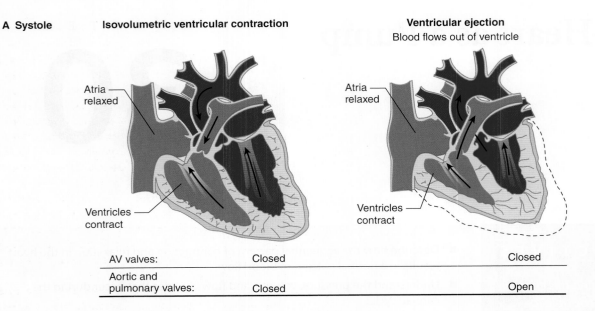

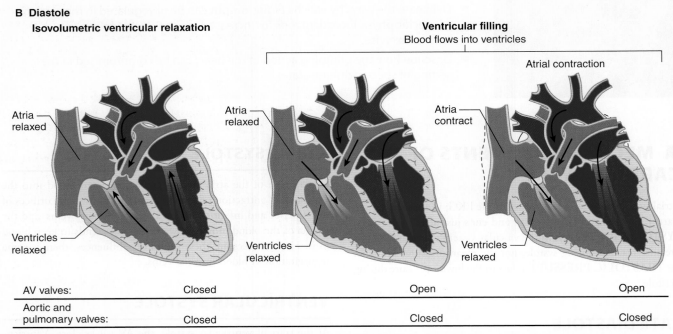

FIGURE 30–1 **Divisions of the cardiac cycle: (A) systole and (B) diastole.** The phases of the cycle are identical in both halves of the heart. The direction in which the pressure difference favors flow is denoted by an arrow; note, however, that flow will not actually occur if a valve prevents it. AV, atrioventricular.

When the aortic and pulmonary valves open, the phase of **ventricular ejection** begins. Ejection is rapid at first, slowing down as systole progresses. The intraventricular pressure rises to a maximum and then declines somewhat before ventricular systole ends. Peak pressures in the left and right ventricles are about 120 and 25 mm Hg, respectively. Late in systole, pressure in the aorta actually exceeds that in the left ventricle, but for a short period momentum keeps the blood moving forward. The

AV valves are pulled down by the contractions of the ventricular muscle, and atrial pressure drops. The amount of blood ejected by each ventricle per stroke at rest is 70–90 mL. The **end-diastolic ventricular volume** is about 130 mL. Thus, about 50 mL of blood remains in each ventricle at the end of systole **(end-systolic ventricular volume),** and the **ejection fraction,** the percentage of the end-diastolic ventricular volume that is ejected with each stroke, is about 65%. The ejection fraction is

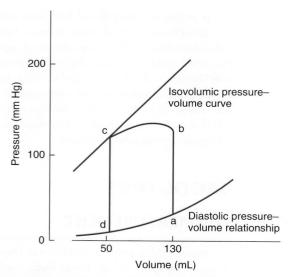

FIGURE 30–2 Normal pressure–volume loop of the left ventricle. During diastole, the ventricle fills and pressure increases from d to a. Pressure then rises sharply from a to b during isovolumetric contraction and from b to c during ventricular ejection. At c, the aortic valves close and pressure falls during isovolumetric relaxation from c back to d. (Reproduced with permission from McPhee SJ, Lingappa VR, Ganong WF [editors]: *Pathophysiology of Disease*, 6th ed. New York, NY: McGraw-Hill; 2010.)

a valuable index of ventricular function. It can be measured by injecting radionuclide-labeled red blood cells and imaging the cardiac blood pool at the end of diastole and the end of systole (equilibrium radionuclide angiocardiography), or by computed tomography.

EARLY DIASTOLE

Once the ventricular muscle is fully contracted, the already falling ventricular pressures drop more rapidly. This is the period of **protodiastole,** which lasts about 0.04 s. It ends when the momentum of the ejected blood is overcome and the aortic and pulmonary valves close, setting up transient vibrations in the blood and blood vessel walls. After the valves are closed, pressure continues to drop rapidly during the period of **isovolumetric ventricular relaxation.** Isovolumetric relaxation ends when the ventricular pressure falls below the atrial pressure and the AV valves open, permitting the ventricles to fill. Filling is rapid at first, then slows as the next cardiac contraction approaches. Atrial pressure continues to rise after the end of ventricular systole until the AV valves open, then drops and slowly rises again until the next atrial systole.

LENGTH OF SYSTOLE & DIASTOLE

Cardiac muscle has the unique property of contracting and repolarizing faster when the heart rate is high, and the duration

of systole decreases from 0.27 s at a heart rate of 65 beats/min to 0.16 s at a rate of 200 beats/min. The reduced time interval is mainly due to a decrease in the duration of systolic ejection. However, the duration of systole is more fixed than diastole, and when the heart rate is increased, diastole is shortened to a much greater degree. For example, at a heart rate of 65 beats/min, the duration of diastole is 0.62 s, whereas at a heart rate of 200 beats/min, it is only 0.14 s. This fact has important physiologic and clinical implications. It is during diastole that the heart muscle rests, and coronary blood flow to the subendocardial portions of the left ventricle occurs only during diastole. Furthermore, most of the ventricular filling occurs in diastole. At heart rates up to about 180 beats/min, filling is adequate as long as there is ample venous return, and cardiac output per minute is increased by an increase in rate. However, at very high heart rates, filling may be compromised to such a degree that cardiac output falls.

Because it has a prolonged action potential, cardiac muscle cannot contract in response to a second stimulus until near the end of the initial contraction. Therefore, cardiac muscle cannot be tetanized like skeletal muscle. The highest rate at which the ventricles can contract is theoretically about 400/min, but in adults the AV node will not conduct more than about 230 impulses/min because of its long refractory period. A ventricular contraction rate of more than 230/min is seen only in paroxysmal ventricular tachycardia.

Exact measurement of the duration of isovolumetric ventricular contraction is difficult in clinical situations, but it is relatively easy to measure the duration of **total electromechanical systole (QS₂),** the **preejection period (PEP),** and the **left ventricular ejection time (LVET)** by recording the ECG, phonocardiogram, and carotid pulse simultaneously. QS_2 is the period from the onset of the QRS complex to the closure of the aortic valves, as determined by the onset of the second heart sound. LVET is the period from the beginning of the carotid pressure rise to the dicrotic notch (see below). PEP is the difference between QS_2 and LVET and represents the time for the electrical as well as the mechanical events that precede systolic ejection. The ratio PEP/LVET is normally about 0.35, and it increases without a change in QS_2 when left ventricular performance is compromised in a variety of cardiac diseases.

ARTERIAL PULSE

The blood forced into the aorta during systole not only moves the blood in the vessels forward but also sets up a pressure wave that travels along the arteries. The pressure wave expands the arterial walls as it travels, and the expansion is palpable as the **pulse.** The rate at which the wave travels, which is independent of and much higher than the velocity of blood flow, is about 4 m/s in the aorta, 8 m/s in the large arteries, and 16 m/s in the small arteries of young adults. Consequently, the pulse is felt in the radial artery at the wrist about 0.1 s after the peak of systolic ejection into the aorta. With advancing age, the arteries become more or less distensible, and the pulse wave moves faster.

ATRIAL PRESSURE CHANGES & THE JUGULAR PULSE

Atrial pressure rises during atrial systole and continues to rise during isovolumetric ventricular contraction when the AV valves bulge into the atria. When the AV valves are pulled down by the contracting ventricular muscle, pressure falls rapidly and then rises as blood flows into the atria until the AV valves open early in diastole. The return of the AV valves to their relaxed position also contributes to this pressure rise by reducing atrial capacity. The atrial pressure changes are transmitted to the great veins, producing three characteristic waves in the record of jugular pressure. The **a wave** is due to atrial systole. The **c wave** is the transmitted manifestation of the rise in atrial pressure produced by the bulging of the tricuspid valve into the atria during isovolumetric ventricular contraction. The **v wave** mirrors the rise in atrial pressure before the tricuspid valve opens during diastole. The jugular pulse waves are superimposed on the respiratory fluctuations in venous pressure. Venous pressure falls during inspiration as a result of the increased negative intrathoracic pressure and rises again during expiration.

HEART SOUNDS

Two sounds are normally heard through a stethoscope during each cardiac cycle. The first is a low, slightly prolonged "lub" (**first sound**), caused by vibrations set up by the sudden closure of the AV valves at the start of ventricular systole (**Figure 30–3**). The second is a shorter, high-pitched "dup" (**second sound**), caused by vibrations associated with closure of the aortic and pulmonary valves just after the end of ventricular systole. A soft, low-pitched **third sound** is heard about one-third of the way through diastole in many normal young individuals. It coincides with the period of rapid ventricular filling and is probably due to vibrations set up by the inrush of blood. A **fourth sound** can sometimes be heard immediately before the first sound when atrial pressure is high or the ventricle is stiff in conditions such as ventricular hypertrophy. It is due to ventricular filling and is rarely heard in normal adults.

MURMURS

Murmurs, or **bruits**, are abnormal sounds heard in various parts of the vascular system caused by high blood flow that is turbulent and creates sounds. Examples include: when an artery or a heart valve is narrowed; over a large, highly vascular goiter; over the carotid artery when its lumen is narrowed and distorted by atherosclerosis, and the bruits heard over an aneurysmal dilation of one of the large arteries, an arteriovenous (A-V) fistula, or a patent ductus arteriosus.

ECHOCARDIOGRAPHY

Wall movement and other aspects of cardiac function can be evaluated by the noninvasive technique of **echocardiography.** Pulses of ultrasonic waves are emitted from a transducer that also functions as a receiver to detect waves reflected back from various parts of the heart. Reflections occur wherever acoustic impedance changes, and a recording of the echoes displayed against time on an oscilloscope provides a record of the movements of the ventricular wall, septum, and valves during the cardiac cycle. When combined with Doppler techniques, echocardiography can be used to measure velocity and volume of flow through valves. It has considerable clinical usefulness, particularly in evaluating and planning therapy in patients with valvular lesions.

■ CARDIAC OUTPUT

METHODS OF MEASUREMENT

Two methods of measuring cardiac output, in addition to Doppler combined with echocardiography, are the **direct Fick's method** and the **indicator dilution method.**

Fick's principle states that the amount of a substance taken up by an organ (or by the whole body) per unit of time is equal to the arterial level of the substance minus the venous level (**A-V difference**) times the blood flow. This principle can be applied, of course, only in situations in which the arterial blood is the sole source of the substance taken up. The principle can be used to determine cardiac output by measuring the amount of O_2 consumed by the body in a given period and dividing this value by the A-V difference across the lungs. Because systemic arterial blood has effectively the same O_2 content in all parts of the body, the arterial O_2 content can be measured in a sample obtained from any convenient artery. A sample of venous blood in the pulmonary artery is obtained by means of a cardiac catheter. It has now become commonplace to insert a catheter through a forearm vein and to guide its tip into the heart with the aid of a fluoroscope. The procedure is generally benign. Catheters can be inserted through the right atrium and ventricle into the small branches of the pulmonary artery. An example of the calculation of cardiac output using a typical set of values is as follows:

Output of le ventricle

$$= \frac{O_2 \text{ consumption (mL/min)}}{[A_{O_2}] - [V_{O_2}]}$$

$$= \frac{250 \text{ mL/min}}{190 \text{ mL/L arterial blood} - 140 \text{ mL/L venous blood in pulmonary artery}}$$

$$= \frac{250 \text{ mL/min}}{50 \text{ mL/L}}$$

$$= 5 \text{ L/min}$$

In the indicator dilution technique, a known amount of a substance, such as a dye or, more commonly, a radioactive isotope, is injected into an arm vein and the concentration of the indicator in serial samples of arterial blood is determined. The output of the heart is equal to the amount of indicator injected divided by its average concentration in arterial blood after a single circulation through the heart. In practice, the log of the indicator concentration in the serial arterial samples is plotted against time as the concentration rises, falls, and then rises again as the indicator recirculates. The initial decline in concentration, linear on a semilog plot, is extrapolated to the abscissa, giving the time for first passage of the indicator through the circulation. The cardiac output for that period is calculated and then converted to output per minute.

A popular indicator dilution technique is **thermodilution,** in which the indicator used is cold saline. The saline is injected into the right atrium through one channel of a double-lumen catheter, and the temperature change in the blood is recorded in the pulmonary artery, using a thermistor in the other, longer side of the catheter. The temperature change is inversely proportional to the amount of blood flowing through the pulmonary artery; that is, to the extent that the cold saline is diluted by blood. This technique has two important advantages: (1) the saline is completely innocuous; and (2) the cold is dissipated in the tissues so recirculation is not a problem, and it is easy to make repeated determinations.

FACTORS CONTROLLING CARDIAC OUTPUT

Changes in cardiac output can be produced by changes in cardiac rate, or stroke volume, or both. The cardiac rate is controlled primarily by autonomic nerves, with sympathetic stimulation increasing the rate and parasympathetic stimulation decreasing it. Stroke volume is also determined in part by neural input, with sympathetic stimuli making the myocardial muscle fibers contract with greater strength at any given length and parasympathetic stimuli having the opposite effect. When the strength of contraction increases without an increase in fiber length, more of the blood that normally remains in the ventricles is expelled; that is, the ejection fraction increases.

The force of contraction of cardiac muscle depends on its preloading and its afterloading. The **preload** is the degree to which the myocardium is stretched before it contracts and the **afterload** is the resistance against which blood is expelled.

RELATION OF TENSION TO LENGTH IN CARDIAC MUSCLE

The length–tension relationship in cardiac muscle is similar to that in skeletal muscle; when the muscle is stretched, the developed tension increases to a maximum and then declines as stretch becomes more extreme. Starling pointed this out when he stated that the "energy of contraction is proportional to the initial length of the cardiac muscle fiber" **(Starling's law of the heart** or the **Frank–Starling law).** For the heart, the length of the muscle fibers (ie, the extent of the preload) is proportional to the end-diastolic volume. The relation between ventricular stroke volume and end-diastolic volume is called the **Frank–Starling curve.**

When cardiac output is regulated by changes in cardiac muscle fiber length, this is referred to as **heterometric regulation.**

Conversely, regulation due to changes in contractility independent of length is sometimes called **homometric regulation.**

FACTORS AFFECTING END-DIASTOLIC VOLUME

The myocardium is covered by a fibrous layer known as the epicardium. This, in turn, is surrounded by the pericardium, which separates the heart from the rest of the thoracic viscera. The space between the epicardium and pericardium (the pericardial sac) normally contains 5–30 mL of clear fluid, which lubricates the heart and permits it to contract with minimal friction.

An increase in intrapericardial pressure (eg, as a result of infection or pressure from a tumor) limits the extent to which the ventricle can fill, as does a decrease in ventricular compliance (ie, an increase in ventricular stiffness produced by myocardial infarction, infiltrative disease, and other abnormalities). Atrial contractions aid ventricular filling. Factors affecting the amount of blood returning to the heart likewise influence the degree of cardiac filling during diastole. An increase in total blood volume increases **venous return.** Constriction of the veins reduces the size of the venous reservoirs, decreasing venous pooling and thus increasing venous return. An increase in the normal negative intrathoracic pressure increases the pressure gradient along which blood flows to the heart, whereas a decrease impedes venous return. Standing decreases venous return, and muscular activity increases it as a result of the pumping action of skeletal muscle.

The effects of systolic and diastolic dysfunction on the pressure–volume loop of the left ventricle are summarized in **Figure 30–3.**

MYOCARDIAL CONTRACTILITY

The contractility of the myocardium exerts a major influence on stroke volume. When the sympathetic nerves to the heart are stimulated, the whole length–tension curve shifts upward and to the left **(Figure 30–4).**

Changes in cardiac rate and rhythm also affect myocardial contractility (known as the force–frequency relation, Figure 30–8). Ventricular extrasystoles condition the myocardium in such a way that the next succeeding contraction is stronger than the preceding normal contraction. This **postextrasystolic potentiation** is independent of ventricular filling, since it occurs in isolated cardiac muscle and is due to increased availability of intracellular Ca^{2+}.

OXYGEN CONSUMPTION BY THE HEART

Basal O_2 consumption by the myocardium is about 2 mL/100 g/min, that is considerably higher than that of resting skeletal muscle. O_2 consumption by the beating heart is about 9 mL/100 g/min at rest. Increases occur during exercise and in a number of different states. Cardiac venous O_2 tension is low, and little additional O_2 can be extracted from the blood in the coronaries, so increases in O_2 consumption require increases in coronary blood flow.

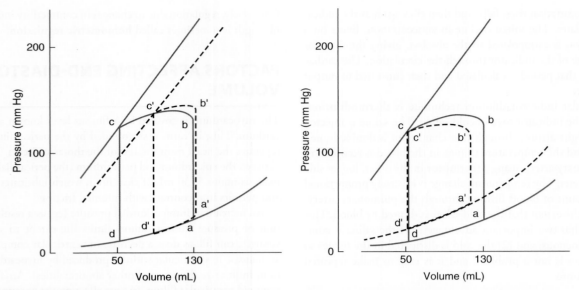

FIGURE 30–3 **Effect of systolic and diastolic dysfunction on the pressure–volume loop of the left ventricle.** In both panels, the solid lines represent the normal pressure–volume loop (equivalent to that shown in Figure 30–2) and the dashed lines show how the loop is shifted by the disease process represented. **Left:** Systolic dysfunction shifts the isovolumic pressure–volume curve to the right, decreasing the stroke volume from b–c to b′–c′. **Right:** Diastolic dysfunction increases end-diastolic volume and shifts the diastolic pressure–volume relationship upward and to the left. This reduces the stroke volume from b–c to b′–c′. (Reproduced with permission from McPhee SJ, Lingappa VR, Ganong WF [editors]: *Pathophysiology of Disease*, 6th ed. New York, NY: McGraw-Hill; 2010.)

O_2 consumption by the heart is determined primarily by intramyocardial tension, the contractile state of the myocardium, and the heart rate. Ventricular work per beat correlates with O_2 consumption. The work is the product of stroke volume and mean arterial pressure in the pulmonary artery or the aorta (for the right and left ventricle, respectively). Because aortic pressure is seven times greater than pulmonary artery pressure, the stroke work of the left ventricle is approximately seven times the stroke work of the right. In theory, a 25% increase in stroke volume without a change in arterial pressure should produce the same increase in O_2 consumption as a 25% increase in arterial pressure without a change in stroke volume. However, for reasons that

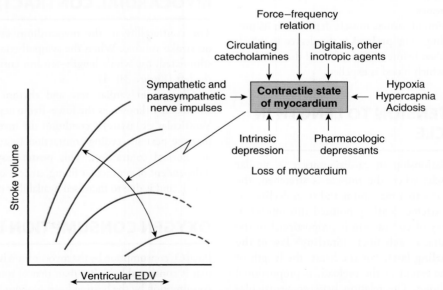

FIGURE 30–4 **Effect of changes in myocardial contractility on the Frank–Starling curve.** The curve shifts downward and to the right as contractility is decreased. The major factors influencing contractility are summarized on the right. The dashed lines indicate portions of the ventricular function curves where maximum contractility has been exceeded; that is, they identify points on the "descending limb" of the Frank–Starling curve. EDV, end-diastolic volume. (Reproduced with permission from Braunwald E, Ross J, Sonnenblick EH: Mechanisms of contraction of the normal and failing heart. N Engl J Med 1967; Oct 12; 277(15):794–800.)

are incompletely understood, pressure work produces a greater increase in O_2 consumption than volume work.

It is worth noting that the increase in O_2 consumption produced by increased stroke volume when the myocardial fibers are stretched is an example of the operation of Laplace's law which states that the tension developed in the wall of a hollow viscus is proportional to the radius of the viscus. When the heart is dilated, its radius is increased.

CHAPTER SUMMARY

■ Blood flows into the atria and then the ventricles of the heart during diastole and atrial systole, and is ejected during systole when the ventricles contract and pressure exceeds the pressures in the pulmonary artery and aorta.

■ Careful timing of the opening and closing of the AV, pulmonary, and aortic valves allows blood to move in an appropriate direction through the heart with minimal regurgitation.

■ The proportion of blood leaving the ventricles in each cardiac cycle is called the ejection fraction and is a sensitive indicator of cardiac health.

■ The arterial pulse represents a pressure wave set up when blood is forced into the aorta; it travels much faster than the blood itself.

■ Heart sounds reflect the normal vibrations set up by abrupt valve closures; heart murmurs can arise from abnormal flow often (although not exclusively) caused by diseased valves.

■ Changes in cardiac output reflect variations in heart rate, stroke volume, or both; these are controlled, in turn, by neural and hormonal input to cardiac myocytes.

■ Cardiac output is strikingly increased during exercise.

■ In heart failure, the ejection fraction of the heart is reduced due to impaired contractility in systole or reduced filling during diastole; this results in inadequate blood supplies to meet the body's needs. Initially, this is manifested only during exercise, but eventually the heart will not be able to supply sufficient blood flow even at rest.

MULTIPLE-CHOICE QUESTIONS

For all questions, select the single best answer unless otherwise directed.

1. The second heart sound is caused by
   A. closure of the aortic and pulmonary valves.
   B. vibrations in the ventricular wall during systole.
   C. ventricular filling.
   D. closure of the mitral and tricuspid valves.
   E. retrograde flow in the vena cava.

2. The fourth heart sound is caused by
   A. closure of the aortic and pulmonary valves.
   B. vibrations in the ventricular wall during systole.
   C. ventricular filling.
   D. closure of the mitral and tricuspid valves.
   E. retrograde flow in the vena cava.

3. The dicrotic notch on the aortic pressure curve is caused by
   A. closure of the mitral valve.
   B. closure of the tricuspid valve.
   C. closure of the aortic valve.
   D. closure of the pulmonary valve.
   E. rapid filling of the left ventricle.

4. During exercise, a man consumes 1.8 L of oxygen per minute. His arterial O_2 content is 190 mL/L, and the O_2 content of his mixed venous blood is 134 mL/L. His cardiac output is approximately
   A. 3.2 L/min.
   B. 16 L/min.
   C. 32 L/min.
   D. 54 L/min.
   E. 160 mL/min.

5. A 75 year old woman with a history of chronic congestive heart failure undergoes cardia catheterization t determine the extent of cardiac dysfunction. During estimation of systolic function, in what phase of the cardiac cycle should her peak left ventricular systolic pressure occur?
   A. Rapid filling
   B. Isovolumetric contraction
   C. Ventricular ejection
   D. Atrial systole
   E. Isovolumetric relaxation

6. A patient with congestive heart failure has an ejection fraction of 0.3 and an end-diastolic volume of 180 mL. In what phase of the cardiac cycle was the end-diastolic volume measured?
   A. Before filling phase
   B. At the end of ventricular ejection
   C. Before atrial systole
   D. After isovolumetric relaxation
   E. At the end of atrial systole

7. A 21-year-male athlete is running up and down the stairs of in a stadium. His baseline heart rate was 66 beats/min, but increased to 175 beats/min. How did the duration of systole and diastole change in this athlete from the start of the exercise to the end?
   A. No changes in systole or diastole
   B. Systole slightly increased; diastole significantly decreased
   C. Systole slightly decreased; diastole significantly increased
   D. Systole slightly decreased; diastole significantly decreased
   E. Systole slightly increased; diastole significantly increased

8. A 54-year-old man presents to the primary care physician with dyspnea upon exertion. He also notes palpitations some times when he works too hard in the garden. On cardiac examination, a systolic murmur is heard. What valvular abnormality is this man likely experiencing?
   A. Tricuspid valve stenosis.
   B. Mitral valve stenosis.
   C. Aortic valve stenosis.
   D. Pulmonary valve insufficiency.
   E. Aortic valve insufficiency.

9. A 60-year-old woman comes to her physician for routine checkup. She has a history of MI 7 years previously but currently has no complaints or symptoms. She undergoes an echocardiogram. Which measurement would be the best index of preload in this woman?
   A. End-systolic volume
   B. Mean aortic pressure
   C. End-diastolic volume
   D. Cardiac output
   E. Stroke volume

10. A 21-year man is getting a mandatory physical in order to participate in the football program at his college. The physician listens to heart and asks him to inspire. She hears a slitting of the second heart sound (S2). What sequence of valve closings would account for this sound heard during inspiration?
    A. The tricuspid closing before the mitral valve.
    B. Pulmonic valve closing before the aortic valve.
    C. Aortic valve closing before the pulmonic valve.
    D. Aortic valve closing before the tricuspid valve.
    E. Aortic valve closing before the mitral valve.

ANSWERS

1. Correct answer is **A.** Closure of the aortic and pulmonary valves causes the characteristic second heart sound.

2. Correct answer is **C.** Ventricular filling causes the fourth heart sound, which is due to either increased atrial pressure or stiffened ventricles.

3. Correct answer is **C.** The dicrotic notch is evident when vibrations occur due to closure of the aortic valve.

4. Correct answer is **C.** O_2 consumption/(Arterial-venous O_2 content) = 1.8 L/min = 1800 ml/min/(190 – 134 ml/L) = 32 L/min.

5. Correct answer is **C.** Peak left ventricular systolic pressure occurs during ejection with the aortic valve open. Ventricular pressures are low during diastolic filling, isovolumetric contraction and relaxation.

6. Correct answer is **E.** At the end of ventricular ejection, the ventricle has ejected the blood and is at the end systolic volume. Diastolic filling includes a rapid passive filling phase followed by atrial systole and the heart should be at the end-diastolic volume at the end of atrial systole.

7. Correct answer is **D.** Increased heart rate decreases diastolic filling times more that systolic ejection times within the heart.

8. Correct answer is **C.** Tricuspid valve stenosis murmur would occur during diastole, as would murmurs due to mitral valve stenosis, pulmonary valve insufficiency or aortic valve insufficiency.

9. Correct answer is **C.** Preload is the due to the amount of stretch on myocytes during filling, prior to contraction. End-diastolic volume is the measurement of preload.

10. Correct answer is **C.** Splitting of S2 sound on inspiration is due to aortic valve closing before the pulmonic valve.

Blood as a Circulatory Fluid & the Dynamics of Blood & Lymph Flow

CHAPTER

31

OBJECTIVES

After studying this chapter, you should be able to:

- Describe the components of blood and lymph and the role of hemoglobin in transporting oxygen.
- Understand blood groups and the reasons for transfusion reactions.
- Delineate the process of hemostasis and the adverse consequences of intravascular thrombosis.
- Identify the types of blood and lymphatic vessels that make up the circulatory system and the regulation of their constituent cell types.
- Describe how physical principles dictate the flow of blood and lymph.
- Understand the basis of methods used to measure blood flow and blood pressure.
- Understand the basis of disease states where components of the blood and vasculature are abnormal.

INTRODUCTION

The **circulatory system** supplies inspired O_2 as well as substances absorbed from the gastrointestinal tract to the tissues, returns CO_2 to the lungs and other products of metabolism to the kidneys, functions in the regulation of body temperature, and distributes hormones and other agents that regulate cell function, all via the blood. Blood is pumped through a closed system by the heart. From the left ventricle, blood is pumped through the arteries and arterioles to the capillaries, where it equilibrates with interstitial fluid. The capillaries drain through venules into the veins and back to the right atrium. Some tissue fluids enter another system of vessels, the lymphatics, which drain lymph via the thoracic duct and the right lymphatic duct into the venous system. The circulation is controlled by multiple regulatory systems to maintain adequate capillary blood flow when possible in all organs, but particularly in the heart and brain.

Blood flows through the circulation primarily because of the forward motion imparted to it by the heart, although diastolic recoil of the walls of the arteries, compression of the veins by skeletal muscles during exercise, and the negative pressure in the thorax during inspiration also move the blood forward. The resistance to flow depends mostly on the diameter of the vessels, and principally that of the arterioles. The blood flow to each tissue is regulated by mechanisms that dilate or constrict its vessels. All of the blood flows through the lungs, but the systemic circulation is made up of numerous different circuits in parallel (Figure 31–1). The arrangement permits wide variations in regional blood flow.

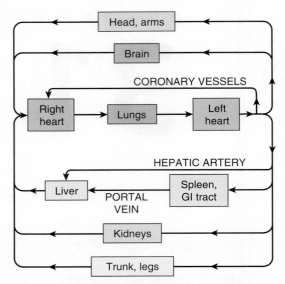

FIGURE 31–1   Diagram of the circulation in the adult.

TABLE 31–1   Normal values for the cellular elements in human blood.

Cell	Cells/µL (average)	Approximate Normal Range	Percentage of Total White Cells
Total white blood cells	9000	4000–11,000	100
Granulocytes			
Neutrophils	5400	3000–6000	50–70
Eosinophils	275	150–300	1–4
Basophils	35	0–100	0.4
Lymphocytes	2750	1500–4000	20–40
Monocytes	540	300–600	2–8
Erythrocytes			
Females	4.8×10^6	NA	NA
Males	5.4×10^6	NA	NA
Platelets	300,000	200,000–500,000	NA

NA, not applicable.

BLOOD AS A CIRCULATORY FLUID

Blood consists of a protein-rich fluid known as plasma, in which are suspended cellular elements: white blood cells, red blood cells, and platelets. The normal total circulating blood volume is about 8% of the body weight (5600 mL in a 70-kg man). About 55% of this volume is plasma.

BONE MARROW

In the adult, red blood cells, many white blood cells, and platelets are formed in the bone marrow. In the fetus, blood cells are also formed in the liver and spleen. In children, blood cells are actively produced in the marrow cavities of all the bones. By age 20, the marrow in the cavities of the long bones, except for the upper humerus and femur, has become inactive. The bone marrow is actually one of the largest organs in the body, approaching the size and weight of the liver. Seventy-five percent of the cells in the marrow belong to the white blood cell–producing myeloid series and only 25% are maturing red cells, even though there are over 500 times as many red cells in the circulation than white cells. This difference reflects the fact that the average lifespan of white cells is short, whereas that of red cells is long.

Hematopoietic stem cells (HSCs) are bone marrow cells capable of producing all types of blood cells. They differentiate into committed stem cells **(progenitor cells)** which in turn form the various types of blood cells. There are separate progenitor cells for megakaryocytes, lymphocytes, erythrocytes, eosinophils, and basophils; neutrophils and monocytes arise from a common precursor. The bone marrow stem cells are also the source of osteoclasts (see Chapter 21), Kupffer cells (see Chapter 28), mast cells, dendritic cells, and Langerhans cells. The HSCs are few in number but are capable of completely replacing the bone marrow when injected into a patient whose own bone marrow has been destroyed.

WHITE BLOOD CELLS

Normally, human blood contains 4000–11,000 white blood cells per microliter (Table 31–1). Of these, the **granulocytes (polymorphonuclear leukocytes, PMNs)** are the most numerous. Young granulocytes have horseshoe-shaped nuclei that become multilobed as the cells grow older (Figure 31–2). Most of them contain neutrophilic granules **(neutrophils),** but a few contain granules that stain with acidic dyes **(eosinophils),** and some have basophilic granules **(basophils).** The other two cell types found in peripheral blood are **lymphocytes,** which have large round nuclei and scanty cytoplasm, and **monocytes,** which have abundant agranular cytoplasm and kidney-shaped nuclei (Figure 31–2).

PLATELETS

Platelets are small, granulated bodies that aggregate at sites of vascular injury. They lack nuclei and are 2–4 µm in diameter (Figure 31–2). They normally have a half-life of about 4 days. The **megakaryocytes,** giant cells in the bone marrow, form platelets by pinching off bits of cytoplasm and extruding them into the circulation.

RED BLOOD CELLS

The red blood cells **(erythrocytes)** carry hemoglobin. They are biconcave disks that are manufactured in the bone marrow. They lose their nuclei before entering the circulation and survive for an average of 120 days in humans. The number of red cells is conveniently expressed as the **hematocrit,** or the percentage of the blood, by volume, that is occupied by erythrocytes. There are thus about 3×10^{13} red blood cells and about 900 g of hemoglobin in the circulating blood of an adult man.

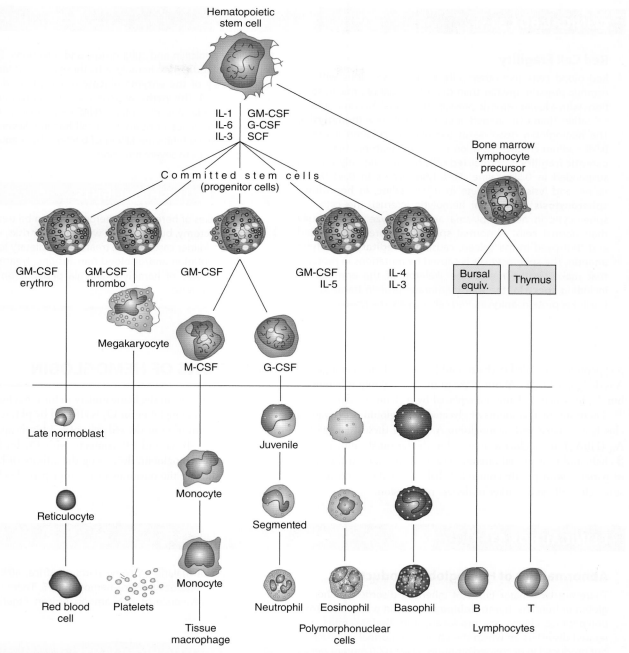

FIGURE 31–2 **Development of various formed elements of the blood from bone marrow cells.** Cells below the horizontal line are found in normal peripheral blood. The principal sites of action of erythropoietin (erythro) and the various colony-stimulating factors (CSF) that stimulate the differentiation of the components are indicated. Erythro, erythropoietin; G, granulocyte; IL, interleukin; M, macrophage; SCF, stem cell factor; thrombo, thrombopoietin.

ROLE OF THE SPLEEN

The spleen is an important blood filter that removes aged or abnormal red cells. It also contains many platelets and plays a significant role in the immune system. Abnormal red cells are removed if they are not as flexible as normal red cells and consequently are unable to squeeze through the slits between the endothelial cells that line the splenic sinuses (Clinical Box 31–1).

HEMOGLOBIN

The red, oxygen-carrying pigment in the red blood cells of vertebrates is **hemoglobin** (Clinical Box 31-2). It is a globular molecule made up of four subunits. Each subunit contains **heme,** an iron-containing porphyrin derivative, conjugated to a polypeptide. There are two pairs of polypeptides in each hemoglobin molecule. In normal adult hemoglobin (**hemoglobin A),** the two

CLINICAL BOX 31–1

Red Cell Fragility

Red blood cells, like other cells, shrink in solutions with an osmotic pressure greater than that of normal plasma. In solutions with a lower osmotic pressure they swell, become spherical rather than disk-shaped, and eventually lyse **(hemolysis).** The hemoglobin dissolves in the plasma, coloring it red. A 0.9% sodium chloride solution is isotonic with plasma. When **osmotic fragility** is normal, red cells begin to hemolyze when suspended in 0.5% saline; 50% lysis occurs in 0.40–0.42% saline, and lysis is complete in 0.35% saline. In **hereditary spherocytosis** (congenital hemolytic icterus), the cells are spherocytic in normal plasma and hemolyze more readily than normal cells. Abnormal spherocytes are also trapped and destroyed in the spleen, causing **hereditary hemolytic anemia.** The spherocytosis is caused by mutations in proteins that make up the membrane skeleton of the erythrocyte, including **spectrin,** the transmembrane protein **band 3,** and the linker protein, **ankyrin.** Red cells can also be lysed by drugs

(especially penicillin and sulfa drugs) and infections. The susceptibility of red cells to hemolysis by these agents is increased by deficiency of the enzyme glucose-6-phosphate dehydrogenase (G6PD). This pathway generates dihydronicotinamide adenine dinucleotide phosphate (NADPH), which is needed for the maintenance of normal red cell fragility. Severe G6PD deficiency also inhibits the killing of bacteria by granulocytes and predisposes to severe infections.

THERAPEUTIC HIGHLIGHTS

Severe cases of hereditary spherocytosis can be treated by splenectomy, but this is not without other risks, such as sepsis. Milder cases can be treated with dietary folate supplementation and/or blood transfusions. Treatment of other forms of hemolytic anemia depends on the underlying cause.

---

polypeptides are called α chains and β chains. Thus, hemoglobin A is designated $\alpha_2\beta_2$. About 2.5% of the hemoglobin is hemoglobin A_2, in which β chains are replaced by δ chains ($\alpha_2\delta_2$).

There are small amounts of glycated hemoglobin A derivatives closely associated with hemoglobin A. One of these, hemoglobin A_{1c} (HbA_{1c}), has a glucose attached to the terminal valine in each β chain and is of special interest because it increases in the blood of patients with poorly controlled diabetes mellitus and is measured clinically as a marker of disease progression.

REACTIONS OF HEMOGLOBIN

O_2 binds to the Fe^{2+} in the heme moiety to form **oxyhemoglobin.** The affinity of hemoglobin for O_2 is affected by pH, temperature, and the concentration in the red cells of 2,3-bisphosphoglycerate (2,3-BPG). 2,3-BPG and H^+ compete with O_2 for binding to deoxygenated hemoglobin, decreasing the affinity of hemoglobin for O_2 by shifting the positions of the four peptide chains (quaternary structure).

CLINICAL BOX 31–2

Abnormalities of Hemoglobin Production

There are two major types of inherited disorders of hemoglobin in humans: **hemoglobinopathies,** in which abnormal polypeptide chains are produced, and **thalassemias** and related disorders, in which the chains are normal in structure but produced in decreased amounts. Over 1000 mutant genes that cause the production of abnormal hemoglobins have been described. In one of the most common, hemoglobin S, the α chains are normal but the β chains have a single substitution of a valine residue for one glutamic acid, leading to **sickle cell anemia.** When an individual is heterozygous for the mutation, half the circulating hemoglobin is abnormal. Many of the abnormal hemoglobins are harmless; however, some have abnormal O_2 equilibria, while others cause anemia. For example, hemoglobin S polymerizes at low O_2 tensions, and causes red cells to become sickle-shaped, hemolyze, and form aggregates that block blood vessels. The sickle cell gene is an example of a gene that has persisted due to its beneficial effect when present in heterozygous form, conferring resistance

to one type of malaria. In some parts of Africa, 40% of the population is heterozygous for hemoglobin S. There is a corresponding prevalence of 10% among African Americans in the United States.

THERAPEUTIC HIGHLIGHTS

Hemoglobin F decreases the polymerization of deoxygenated hemoglobin S, and hydroxyurea stimulates production of hemoglobin F in children and adults. Hydroxyurea is therefore valuable for the treatment of sickle cell disease. In severe sickle cell disease, hematopoietic stem cell transplantation also has some benefit, and prophylactic treatment with antibiotics is helpful. The clinically important thalassemias result in severe anemia, often requiring repeated blood transfusions. Hematopoietic stem cell transplantation is also being explored.

When blood is exposed to various drugs and other oxidizing agents, the ferrous iron (Fe^{2+}) normally present in hemoglobin is converted to ferric iron (Fe^{3+}), forming **methemoglobin.** Methemoglobin is dark-colored, and when present in large quantities causes a dusky discoloration of the skin. Some oxidation of hemoglobin to methemoglobin occurs normally, but the dihydronicotinamide adenine dinucleotide (NADH)-methemoglobin reductase system converts methemoglobin back to hemoglobin. Congenital absence of this system is one cause of hereditary methemoglobinemia.

Carbon monoxide reacts with hemoglobin to form **carbon monoxyhemoglobin (carboxyhemoglobin).** The affinity of hemoglobin for O_2 is much lower than its affinity for carbon monoxide.

HEMOGLOBIN IN THE FETUS

The blood of the human fetus normally contains **fetal hemoglobin (hemoglobin F).** Its structure is similar to that of hemoglobin A except that the β chains are replaced by γ chains. The γ chains have 37 amino acid residues that differ from those in the β chain. Fetal hemoglobin is normally replaced by adult hemoglobin soon after birth. In the body, its O_2 content at a given Po_2 is greater than that of adult hemoglobin because it binds 2,3-BPG less avidly. Hemoglobin F is therefore critical to facilitate movement of O_2 from the maternal to the fetal circulation.

CATABOLISM OF HEMOGLOBIN

When old red blood cells are destroyed by tissue macrophages, the globin portion of the hemoglobin molecule is split off, and the heme is converted to **biliverdin.** In humans, most of the biliverdin is converted to **bilirubin** and excreted in the bile (see Chapter 28). The iron from the heme is reused for hemoglobin synthesis.

■ BLOOD TYPES

The membranes of human red cells contain a variety of **blood group antigens,** which are also called **agglutinogens.** The most important and best known of these are the A and B antigens.

The A and B antigens are inherited as mendelian dominants, and define four major **blood types.** Type A individuals have the A antigen, type B have the B, type AB have both, and type O have neither. The A and B antigens are complex oligosaccharides that differ in their terminal sugar. An *H* gene codes for a fucose transferase that adds a terminal fucose, forming the H antigen that is usually present in individuals of all blood types. Individuals who are type A also express a second transferase that catalyzes placement of a terminal N-acetylgalactosamine on the H antigen, whereas individuals who are type B express a transferase that places a terminal galactose. Individuals who are type AB have both transferases. Individuals who are type O have neither, so the H antigen persists.

Antibodies against red cell agglutinogens are called **agglutinins.** Antigens very similar to A and B are common in intestinal bacteria and possibly in foods. Therefore, infants rapidly develop antibodies against the antigens not present in their own cells. Thus, type A individuals develop anti-B antibodies, type B individuals develop anti-A antibodies, type O individuals develop both, and type AB individuals develop neither. When the plasma of a type A individual is mixed with type B red cells, the anti-B antibodies cause the type B red cells to clump (agglutinate). ABO **blood typing** is performed by mixing an individual's red blood cells with antisera containing the various agglutinins and checking for agglutination.

TRANSFUSION REACTIONS

Dangerous **hemolytic transfusion reactions** occur when blood is transfused into an individual who has agglutinins against the red cells in the transfusion. The plasma in the transfusion is usually so diluted in the recipient that it rarely causes agglutination. However, when the recipient's plasma has agglutinins against the donor's red cells, the cells agglutinate and hemolyze. The severity of the resulting transfusion reaction may vary from an asymptomatic minor rise in plasma bilirubin to severe jaundice and renal tubular damage leading to anuria and death.

Persons with type AB blood are "universal recipients" because they have no circulating agglutinins and can be given blood of any type. Type O individuals are "universal donors" because they lack A and B antigens, and type O blood can be given to anyone without producing a transfusion reaction due to ABO incompatibility. However, the possibility of reactions due to incompatibilities in systems other than ABO always exists. In cross-matching, donor red cells are mixed with recipient plasma on a slide and checked for agglutination.

THE RH GROUP

Aside from the antigens of the ABO system, those of the Rh system are of the greatest clinical importance. The Rh factor is composed primarily of the C, D, and E antigens, although it actually contains many more. D is by far the most antigenic component, and the term Rh-positive as it is generally used means that the individual has agglutinogen D. The Rh-negative individual has no D antigen and forms the anti-D agglutinin when injected with D-positive cells. Eighty-five percent of whites are D-positive and 15% are D-negative; over 99% of Asians are D-positive. Unlike the ABO system, anti-D antibodies do not develop without exposure of a D-negative individual to D-positive red cells.

HEMOLYTIC DISEASE OF THE NEWBORN

A complication due to Rh incompatibility arises when an Rh-negative mother carries an Rh-positive fetus. Small amounts of fetal blood leak into the maternal circulation at the time of delivery, and some mothers develop significant titers of anti-Rh agglutinins. During the next pregnancy, the mother's agglutinins cross the placenta to the fetus, and can cause hemolysis and various forms of **hemolytic disease of the newborn (erythroblastosis** fetalis) in an Rh-positive fetus. If hemolysis is severe, the infant may die in utero or may develop anemia, severe jaundice, and edema (**hydrops fetalis**). **Kernicterus,** a neurologic syndrome in which unconjugated bilirubin is deposited in the basal ganglia, may also develop. Bilirubin rarely penetrates the brain in adults, but it does in infants with erythroblastosis, possibly because the blood–brain barrier is more permeable. The concentration of unconjugated bilirubin is very high in this condition because production is increased and the bilirubin-conjugating system is not yet mature.

Fortunately, it is usually possible to prevent sensitization from occurring in Rh-negative mothers with a single dose of anti-Rh antibodies during the postpartum period. Such passive immunization does not harm the mother and prevents active antibody formation. The institution of such treatment on a routine basis to unsensitized Rh-negative women who have delivered an Rh-positive baby has reduced the incidence of hemolytic disease by more than 90%. In addition, fetal Rh typing is now possible, and treatment with a small dose of Rh immune serum will prevent sensitization during pregnancy.

■ PLASMA

The fluid portion of the blood, the **plasma,** is a remarkable solution containing ions, inorganic molecules, and organic molecules that are in transit to various parts of the body. Normal plasma volume is about 5% of body weight. Plasma clots on standing, remaining fluid only if an anticoagulant is added. If whole blood is allowed to clot and the clot is removed, the remaining fluid is called **serum.** Serum has essentially the same composition as plasma, except that its fibrinogen and clotting factors II, V, and VIII (Table 31–2) have been removed and it has a higher serotonin content because of the breakdown of platelets during clotting.

PLASMA PROTEINS

The plasma proteins consist of **albumin, globulin,** and **fibrinogen** fractions. Most capillary walls are relatively impermeable to these, so they exert an osmotic force of about 25 mm Hg across the capillary wall (**oncotic pressure;** see Chapter 1) that pulls water into the blood. The plasma proteins are also responsible for 15% of the buffering capacity of proteins in the blood (including hemoglobin; see Chapter 39) because of the weak ionization of their substituent COOH and NH_2 groups. Plasma proteins may have specific functions (eg, antibodies and clotting factors), whereas others function as nonspecific carriers for various solutes.

ORIGIN OF PLASMA PROTEINS

Circulating antibodies are manufactured by lymphocytes. Most of the other plasma proteins are synthesized in the liver.

Synthesis plays an important role in the maintenance of albumin levels. In normal adult humans, the plasma albumin

TABLE 31–2 System for naming blood-clotting factors.

Factor[a]	Names
I	Fibrinogen
II	Prothrombin
III	Thromboplastin
IV	Calcium
V	Proaccelerin, labile factor, accelerator globulin
VII	Proconvertin, serum prothrombin conversion accelerator (SPCA), stable factor
VIII	Antihemophilic factor (AHF), antihemophilic factor A, antihemophilic globulin (AHG)
IX	Plasma thromboplastic component (PTC), Christmas factor, antihemophilic factor B
X	Stuart-Prower factor
XI	Plasma thromboplastin antecedent (PTA), antihemophilic factor C
XII	Hageman factor, glass factor
XIII	Fibrin-stabilizing factor, Laki-Lorand factor
HMW-K	High-molecular-weight kininogen, Fitzgerald factor
PreKa	Prekallikrein, Fletcher factor
Ka	Kallikrein
PL	Platelet phospholipid

[a]Factor VI is not a separate entity and has been dropped.

level is 3.5–5.0 g/dL, and the total exchangeable albumin pool is 4.0–5.0 g/kg body weight; 38–45% of this albumin is intravascular, and much of the rest of it is in the skin. Between 6% and 10% of the exchangeable pool is degraded per day, and the degraded albumin is replaced by hepatic synthesis. Albumin synthesis is carefully regulated. It is decreased during fasting and increased in conditions where there is excessive albumin loss.

HYPOPROTEINEMIA

Plasma protein levels are maintained during starvation until body protein stores are markedly depleted. However, in prolonged starvation and in malabsorption syndromes, plasma protein levels are low (**hypoproteinemia**). They are also low in liver disease, and in nephrosis, because large amounts of albumin are lost in the urine. Because of the decrease in the plasma oncotic pressure, edema tends to develop. Rarely, there is congenital absence of a specific plasma protein. An example is **afibrinogenemia**, characterized by defective blood clotting.

■ HEMOSTASIS

Hemostasis is the process of forming clots in the walls of damaged blood vessels and preventing blood loss while maintaining blood in a fluid state within the vascular system. A collection of complex mechanisms operates to balance coagulation and anticoagulation.

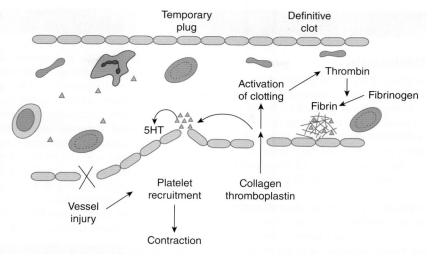

FIGURE 31–3 Summary of reactions involved in hemostasis. Injury to a blood vessel exposes collagen and thromboplastin, recruiting platelets to the site of injury to form a temporary plug. Platelets release 5-hydroxytryptamine, among other factors, resulting in smooth muscle contraction and vasoconstriction. Activation of the clotting cascade in response to collagen and thromboplastin activates thrombin, which converts circulating fibrinogen to fibrin monomers. Fibrin monomers polymerize and are cross-linked and accumulate with platelets at the site of injury to form the definitive clot.

RESPONSE TO INJURY

When a small blood vessel is damaged, the injury initiates a series of events (Figure 31–3) that lead to the formation of a clot. This seals off the damaged region and prevents further blood loss. The initial event is constriction of the vessel and formation of a temporary **hemostatic plug** of platelets that is triggered when platelets bind to collagen and aggregate. This is followed by conversion of the plug into the definitive clot. Vasoconstriction is due to serotonin and other vasoconstrictors liberated from platelets that adhere to the walls of the damaged vessels.

THE CLOTTING MECHANISM

The temporary plug is bound together and converted into the definitive clot by **fibrin.** Fibrin formation involves a cascade of enzymatic reactions and a series of numbered clotting factors (Table 31–2). The fundamental reaction is conversion of the soluble plasma protein fibrinogen to insoluble fibrin. The process involves the release of two pairs of polypeptides from each fibrinogen molecule. The remaining portion, **fibrin monomer,** then polymerizes with other monomers to form **fibrin.** The fibrin is initially a loose mesh of interlacing strands. It is converted by the formation of covalent cross linkages to a dense, tight aggregate (stabilization). This latter reaction is catalyzed by activated factor XIII and requires Ca^{2+}.

The conversion of fibrinogen to fibrin is catalyzed by thrombin. Thrombin is a serine protease that is formed from its circulating precursor, prothrombin, by the action of activated factor X. It has additional actions, including activation of platelets, endothelial cells, and leukocytes via the so-called proteinase-activated receptors, which are G-protein–coupled.

Factor X can be activated by either the intrinsic and extrinsic systems. The initial reaction in the **intrinsic system** is conversion of inactive factor XII to active factor XII (XIIa). This activation, which is catalyzed by high-molecular-weight kininogen and kallikrein (see Chapter 32), can be brought about by collagen fibers underlying the endothelium. Active factor XII then activates factor XI, and active factor XI activates factor IX. Activated factor IX forms a complex with active factor VIII, which is activated when it is separated from von Willebrand factor. The complex of IXa and VIIIa activate factor X. Phospholipids (PL) from aggregated platelets and Ca^{2+} are necessary for full activation of factor X. The **extrinsic system** is triggered by the release of tissue thromboplastin (TPL), a protein–phospholipid mixture that activates factor VII. TPL and factor VII activate factors IX and X. In the presence of PL, Ca^{2+}, and factor V, activated factor X catalyzes the conversion of prothrombin to thrombin. The extrinsic pathway is inhibited by a **tissue factor pathway inhibitor** that forms a quaternary structure with TPL, factor VIIa, and factor Xa.

ANTICLOTTING MECHANISMS

The tendency of blood to clot is balanced in vivo by reactions that prevent clotting, break down any clots that do form, or both. These reactions include the interaction between the platelet-aggregating effect of thromboxane A_2 and the antiaggregating effect of prostacyclin (**Clinical Box 31–3**).

Antithrombin III is a circulating protease inhibitor that binds to serine proteases in the coagulation system, blocking their activity as clotting factors. This binding is facilitated by **heparin,** a naturally occurring anticoagulant. The clotting factors that are inhibited are the active forms of factors IX, X, XI, and XII.

Abnormalities of Hemostasis

In addition to clotting abnormalities due to platelet disorders, hemorrhagic diseases can be produced by selective deficiencies of clotting factors. Hemophilia A, caused by factor VIII deficiency, is relatively common. von Willebrand factor deficiency likewise causes a bleeding disorder by reducing platelet adhesion and lowering plasma factor VIII. Finally, when absorption of fat-soluble vitamin K is depressed, the resulting clotting factor deficiencies may cause a significant bleeding tendency.

Formation of clots inside blood vessels is called **thrombosis** to distinguish it from the normal extravascular clotting of blood. Thromboses are a major medical problem. They occur particularly where blood flow is sluggish, or in vessels when the intima is damaged by atherosclerotic plaques, and over areas of damage to the endocardium. They frequently occlude the arterial supply to organs, and bits of thrombus **(emboli)** sometimes break off and travel in the bloodstream to damage other organs, for example, obstruction of the pulmonary artery or its branches by thrombi from the leg veins **(pulmonary embolism)**. Congenital absence of protein C leads to uncontrolled intravascular coagulation and, in general, death in

infancy. If this condition is diagnosed and treatment is instituted, the coagulation defect disappears. Resistance to APC is another cause of thrombosis, and this condition is common. It is due to a point mutation in the gene for factor V, which prevents APC from inactivating the factor.

Disseminated intravascular coagulation is another serious complication of septicemia, extensive tissue injury, and other diseases in which fibrin is deposited in the vascular system. The increased consumption of platelets and coagulation factors causes bleeding to occur at the same time. The cause of the condition appears to be increased generation of thrombin due to increased TPL activity without adequate tissue factor inhibitory pathway activity.

THERAPEUTIC HIGHLIGHTS

Hemophilia has been treated with factor VIII–rich preparations or, more recently, recombinant factor VIII. Some patients with von Willebrand disease are treated with desmopressin, which stimulates production of factor VIII. Thrombotic disorders, on the other hand, are treated with anticoagulants.

The endothelium of the blood vessels also plays an active role in preventing the extension of clots. All endothelial cells except those in the cerebral microcirculation produce **thrombomodulin**, a thrombin-binding protein, on their surfaces. In circulating blood, thrombin is a procoagulant that activates factors V and VIII, but when it binds to thrombomodulin, it becomes an anticoagulant that activates protein C. Activated protein C (APC), along with its cofactor protein S, inactivates factors V and VIII and inactivates an inhibitor of tissue plasminogen activator, increasing the formation of plasmin.

Plasmin (fibrinolysin) is the active component of the **plasminogen (fibrinolytic) system.** This enzyme lyses fibrin and fibrinogen, with the production of fibrinogen degradation products (FDPs) that inhibit thrombin. Plasmin is formed from its inactive precursor, plasminogen, by the action of thrombin and **tissue-type plasminogen activator (t-PA).** It is also activated by **urokinase-type plasminogen activator (u-PA).** If the t-PA gene or the u-PA gene is knocked out in mice, some fibrin deposition occurs and clot lysis is slowed. However, when both are knocked out, spontaneous fibrin deposition is extensive.

Plasminogen receptors are located on the surfaces of many different types of cells and are plentiful on endothelial cells. When plasminogen binds to its receptor, it is activated, so intact blood vessel walls are provided with a mechanism that discourages clot formation.

Human recombinant t-PA is used clinically in myocardial infarction and stroke.

ANTICOAGULANTS

Heparin is a naturally occurring anticoagulant that facilitates the action of antithrombin III. Low-molecular-weight fragments of heparin have a longer half-life and produce a more predictable anticoagulant response than unfractionated heparin. The highly basic protein protamine forms an irreversible complex with heparin and is used clinically to neutralize heparin.

In vivo, a plasma Ca^{2+} level low enough to interfere with blood clotting is incompatible with life, but clotting can be prevented in vitro if Ca^{2+} is removed from the blood. Coumarin derivatives such as **dicumarol** and **warfarin** are also effective anticoagulants. They inhibit vitamin K, a necessary cofactor for the enzyme that catalyzes the conversion of glutamic acid residues to γ-carboxyglutamic acid residues. Six of the proteins involved in clotting (factors II (prothrombin), VII, IX, and X, protein C, and protein S) require conversion of glutamic acid residues to γ-carboxyglutamic acid residues before being released into the circulation, and hence all six are vitamin K dependent.

■ LYMPH

Lymph is tissue fluid that enters the lymphatic vessels. It drains into the venous blood via the thoracic and right lymphatic ducts. It contains clotting factors and clots on standing. In most locations, it also contains proteins that have traversed capillary walls and can then return to the blood via the lymph. Nevertheless, its protein content is generally lower than that of plasma. Lipids are absorbed from the intestine into the lymphatics, and the lymph in the thoracic duct after a meal is milky because of its high fat content. Lymphocytes also enter the circulation principally through the lymphatics.

STRUCTURAL FEATURES OF THE CIRCULATION

Here, the two major cell types that make up the blood vessels and how they are arranged into the various vessel types will be described.

ENDOTHELIUM

Located between the circulating blood and the media and adventitia of the blood vessels, endothelial cells constitute a large and important organ. They respond to flow changes, stretch, a variety of circulating substances, and inflammatory mediators. They secrete growth regulators and vasoactive substances.

VASCULAR SMOOTH MUSCLE

The smooth muscle in blood vessel walls is important in the regulation of blood pressure and hypertension. The membranes of the muscle cells contain various types of K^+, Ca^{2+}, and Cl^- channels. Contraction is produced primarily by the myosin light chain mechanism described in Chapter 5. However, vascular smooth muscle also undergoes prolonged contractions that determine vascular tone. These may be due in part to the latch-bridge mechanism (see Chapter 5), but other factors also play a role.

Vascular smooth muscle cells provide an interesting example of the way high and low cytosolic Ca^{2+} can have different and even opposite effects (see Chapter 2). In these cells, influx of Ca^{2+} via voltage-gated Ca^{2+} channels produces a diffuse increase in cytosolic Ca^{2+} that initiates contraction. However, the Ca^{2+} influx also initiates Ca^{2+} release from the sarcoplasmic reticulum via ryanodine receptors (see Chapter 5), and the high local Ca^{2+} concentration produced by these Ca^{2+} sparks increases the activity of Ca^{2+}-activated K^+ channels in the cell membrane. K^+ efflux increases the membrane potential, shutting off voltage-gated Ca^{2+} channels and producing relaxation. Ca^{2+} sparks act on the β_1-subunit of the BK channel, and mice lacking this subunit show increased vascular tone and blood pressure.

ARTERIES & ARTERIOLES

The characteristics of the various types of blood vessels are listed in Table 31–3. Artery walls have an outer layer of connective tissue, the adventitia; a middle layer of smooth muscle, the media; and an inner layer, the intima, made up of the endothelium and underlying connective tissue. The aorta and other large diameter arteries contain a relatively large amount of elastic tissue, primarily located in the inner and external elastic laminas. They are stretched during systole and recoil on the blood during diastole. Arterioles contain less elastic tissue but much more smooth muscle. The muscle is innervated by noradrenergic nerve fibers, which function as constrictors, and in some instances by cholinergic fibers, which dilate the vessels. The arterioles are the major site of the resistance to blood flow, and small changes in their caliber cause large changes in the total peripheral resistance.

CAPILLARIES

The arterioles divide into smaller muscle-walled vessels, sometimes called **metarterioles,** and these in turn feed into capillaries. The upstream openings of capillaries are surrounded by smooth muscle **precapillary sphincters.** Precapillary sphincters are not innervated, but can respond to local or circulating vasoconstrictor substances. The capillaries are about 5 μm in diameter at the arterial end and 9 μm in diameter at the venous end. When the sphincters are dilated, the diameter of the capillaries is just sufficient to permit red blood cells to squeeze through in "single file."

The capillary walls, which are about 1 μm thick, are made up of a single layer of endothelial cells. In skeletal, cardiac, and smooth muscle, the junctions between the endothelial cells permit the passage of molecules up to 10 nm in diameter. It also appears that plasma and its dissolved proteins can be taken up by endocytosis, transported

TABLE 31–3 Characteristics of various types of blood vessels in humans.

Vessel	Lumen Diameter	Wall Thickness	All Vessels of Each Type	
			Approximate Total Cross-Sectional Area (cm²)	Percentage of Blood Volume Contained[a]
Aorta	2.5 cm	2 mm	4.5	2
Artery	0.4 cm	1 mm	20	8
Arteriole	30 μm	20 μm	400	1
Capillary	5 μm	1 μm	4500	5
Venule	20 μm	2 μm	4000	54
Vein	0.5 cm	0.5 mm	40	
Vena cava	3 cm	1.5 mm	18	

[a]In systemic vessels, there is an additional 12% in the heart and 18% in the pulmonary circulation.

across the endothelial cells, and discharged by exocytosis (**vesicular transport;** see Chapter 2). However, this process can account for only a small portion of the transport across the endothelium. In the brain, the junctions between endothelial cells are tighter, and transport across them is largely limited to small molecules (although pathological conditions may open these junctions). In most endocrine glands, the intestinal villi, and parts of the kidneys, on the other hand, the cytoplasm of the endothelial cells is attenuated to form gaps called **fenestrations.** These fenestrations are 20–100 nm in diameter and may be opened to permit the passage of larger molecules, although their permeability is likely significantly reduced by a thick layer of endothelial glycocalyx. An exception to this is found in the liver, where the sinusoidal capillaries are extremely porous, the endothelium is discontinuous, and gaps occur between endothelial cells that are not closed by membranes. Some of the gaps are 600 nm in diameter, and others may be as large as 3000 nm. They therefore permit the passage of large molecules, including plasma proteins, which is important for hepatic function (see Chapter 28).

Capillaries and postcapillary venules have **pericytes** around their endothelial cells. These cells have long processes that wrap around the vessels. They are contractile and release a wide variety of vasoactive agents. They also synthesize and release constituents of the basement membrane and extracellular matrix. One of their physiologic functions appears to be regulation of flow through the junctions between endothelial cells, particularly in the presence of inflammation.

LYMPHATICS

The lymphatics collect plasma and its constituents that have exuded from the capillaries into the interstitial space (ie, the lymph). They drain via a system of vessels that coalesce and eventually enter the right and left subclavian veins at their junctions with the respective internal jugular veins. The lymph vessels contain valves and regularly traverse lymph nodes. Small lymph vessels differ from capillaries in several details: No fenestrations are visible in the lymphatic endothelium; very little basal lamina is present under the endothelium; and the junctions between endothelial cells are open, with no tight intercellular connections.

ARTERIOVENOUS ANASTOMOSES

In the fingers, palms, and ear lobes, short channels connect arterioles to venules, bypassing the capillaries. These **arteriovenous (A-V) anastomoses,** or **shunts,** have thick, muscular walls and are abundantly innervated, presumably by vasoconstrictor nerve fibers.

VENULES & VEINS

The walls of venules are only slightly thicker than those of capillaries. The walls of the veins are also thin and easily distended. They contain relatively little smooth muscle, but considerable venoconstriction is produced by activity in the noradrenergic nerves to the veins and by circulating vasoconstrictors such as endothelins. Variations in venous tone are important in circulatory adjustments.

The intima of the limb veins is folded at intervals to form **venous valves** that prevent retrograde flow. No valves are present in the very small veins, the great veins, or the veins from the brain and viscera.

ANGIOGENESIS

When tissues grow, blood vessels must proliferate to maintain a normal blood supply. Therefore, angiogenesis, the formation of new blood vessels, is important during fetal life and growth to adulthood. It is also important for processes such as wound healing, formation of the corpus luteum after ovulation, and formation of new endometrium after menstruation. Abnormally, it is important in tumor growth; if tumors do not develop a blood supply, they do not grow.

During embryonic development, a network of leaky capillaries is formed in tissues from angioblasts. Vessels then branch off, hook up with the capillaries, and provide them with smooth muscle, which brings about their maturation. Angiogenesis in adults is presumably similar; new vessels are formed by branching from preexisting vessels rather than from angioblasts.

Many factors are involved in angiogenesis. A key compound is **vascular endothelial growth factor (VEGF).** This factor exists in multiple isoforms, and there are three VEGF receptors that are tyrosine kinases. VEGF appears to be primarily responsible for vasculogenesis, whereas the budding of vessels that connect to the immature capillary network is regulated by other as yet unidentified factors. Some VEGF isoforms and receptors may play a more prominent role in the formation of lymphatic vessels (**lymphangiogenesis**) than that of blood vessels.

The actions of VEGF and related factors have received considerable attention because of the requirement for angiogenesis in tumor development. VEGF antagonists and other angiogenesis inhibitors have now entered clinical practice as therapies for many malignancies.

■ BIOPHYSICAL CONSIDERATIONS FOR CIRCULATORY PHYSIOLOGY

FLOW, PRESSURE, & RESISTANCE

Blood flows from areas of high pressure to areas of low pressure, except when momentum transiently sustains flow. The relationship between mean flow, mean pressure, and resistance in the blood vessels can be stated as:

$$\text{Flow (F)} = \frac{\text{Pressure (P)}}{\text{Resistance (R)}}$$

Flow is therefore equal to the **effective perfusion pressure** divided by the **resistance.** The effective perfusion pressure is the intraluminal pressure at the arterial end minus the pressure at the venous end. The units of resistance (pressure divided by flow) are dyne·s/cm^5. To avoid dealing with such complex units, resistance in the cardiovascular system is sometimes expressed in **R units,** which are obtained by dividing pressure in mm Hg by flow in mL/s (see also Table 33–1). Thus, for example, when the mean aortic pressure is 90 mm Hg and the left ventricular output is 90 mL/s, the total peripheral resistance is

$$\frac{90\,\text{mm Hg}}{90\,\text{mL/s}} = 1\,\text{R unit}$$

METHODS FOR MEASURING BLOOD FLOW

Various noninvasive devices can measure flow. Most commonly, blood velocity can be measured with **Doppler flow meters.** Ultrasonic waves are sent into a vessel diagonally, and the waves reflected from the red and white blood cells are picked up by a downstream sensor. The frequency of the reflected waves is higher by an amount that is proportional to the rate of flow because of the Doppler effect.

Indirect methods for measuring the blood flow of various organs in humans include the Kety N_2O method for measuring cerebral blood flow. Another is determination of the renal blood flow by measuring the clearance of para-aminohippuric acid. A considerable amount of data on blood flow in the extremities has been obtained by **plethysmography.** The forearm, for example, is sealed in a watertight chamber. When venous drainage of the forearm is occluded, the rate of increase in the volume of the forearm is a function of arterial blood flow.

APPLICABILITY OF PHYSICAL PRINCIPLES TO FLOW IN BLOOD VESSELS

Physical principles and equations that describe the behavior of perfect fluids in rigid tubes have often been used indiscriminately to explain the behavior of blood in blood vessels. Blood vessels are not rigid tubes, and the blood is not a perfect fluid but a two-phase system of liquid and cells. Therefore, the behavior of the circulation deviates, sometimes markedly, from that predicted by these principles. However, the physical principles are of value when used as an aid to understanding what goes on in the body.

LAMINAR FLOW

The flow of blood in straight blood vessels is normally **laminar.** Within the vessels, an infinitely thin layer of blood in contact with the wall of the vessel does not move. The next layer within the vessel has a low velocity, the next a higher velocity, and so forth, velocity being greatest in the center of the stream. Laminar flow occurs up to a certain **critical velocity.** At or above this velocity, flow is turbulent. The probability of turbulence is also related to the diameter of the vessel and the viscosity of the blood. This probability can be expressed by the ratio of inertial to viscous forces as follows:

$$\text{Re} = \frac{\rho D \dot{V}}{\eta}$$

where Re is the Reynolds number, named for the man who described the relationship; ρ is the density of the fluid; D is the diameter of the tube under consideration; $\dot{V}$ is the velocity of the flow; and η is the viscosity of the fluid. The higher the value of Re, the greater the probability of turbulence. When D is in cm, $\dot{V}$ is in cm s^{-1}, and η is in poise; flow is usually not turbulent if Re is less than 2000. When Re is more than 3000, turbulence is almost always present. Laminar flow can be disturbed at the branching points of arteries, increasing the likelihood that atherosclerotic plaques will be deposited. Constriction of an artery likewise increases the velocity of blood flow through the constriction, producing turbulence and sound beyond the constriction. Examples are bruits heard over arteries constricted by atherosclerotic plaques and the sounds of Korotkoff heard when measuring blood pressure (see below). In healthy humans, the critical velocity is sometimes exceeded in the ascending aorta at the peak of systolic ejection, but it is usually exceeded only when an artery is constricted.

SHEAR STRESS & GENE ACTIVATION

Flowing blood creates a force on the endothelium that is parallel to the long axis of the vessel. This **shear stress** (γ) is proportional to viscosity (η) times the shear rate (dy/dr), which is the rate at which the axial velocity increases from the vessel wall toward the lumen.

$$\gamma = \eta(dy/dr)$$

Change in shear stress and other physical variables, such as cyclic strain and stretch, produces marked changes in the expression of genes by endothelial cells. The genes that are activated include those that produce growth factors, integrins, and related molecules. Recent evidence has implicated endothelial surface structures known as **primary cilia** as sensors of shear stress, which in turn activate signaling pathways to alter cell function.

AVERAGE VELOCITY

When considering flow in a system of tubes, it is important to distinguish between velocity, which is displacement per unit time (eg, cm/s), and flow, which is volume per unit time (eg, cm^3/s). Velocity ($\dot{V}$) is proportional to flow (Q) divided by the area of the conduit (A):

$$\dot{V} = \frac{Q}{A}$$

Therefore, $Q = A \times \dot{V}$, and if flow stays constant, velocity increases in direct proportion to any decrease in A.

The average velocity of fluid movement at any point in a system of tubes in parallel is inversely proportional to the *total* cross-sectional area at that point. Therefore, the average velocity of the blood is high in the aorta, declines steadily in the smaller vessels, and is lowest in the capillaries, which have 1000 times the *total* cross-sectional area of the aorta (Table 31–3). The average velocity of blood flow increases again as the blood enters the veins and is relatively high in the vena cava, although not so high as in the aorta.

POISEUILLE–HAGEN FORMULA

The relationship between the flow in a long narrow tube, the viscosity of the fluid, and the radius of the tube is expressed mathematically in the **Poiseuille–Hagen formula:**

$$F = (P_A - P_B) \times \left(\frac{\pi}{8}\right) \times \left(\frac{1}{\eta}\right) \times \left(\frac{r^4}{L}\right)$$

where

F = flow

$P_A - P_B$ = pressure difference between two ends of the tube

η = viscosity

r = radius of tube

L = length of tube

Because flow is equal to pressure difference divided by resistance (R),

$$R = \frac{8\eta L}{\pi r^4}$$

Because flow varies directly and resistance inversely with the fourth power of the radius, blood flow and resistance in vivo are markedly affected by small changes in the caliber of the vessels. Thus, for example, flow through a vessel is doubled by an increase of only 19% in its radius; and when the radius is doubled, resistance is reduced to 6% of its previous value. This is why organ blood flow and systemic arterial pressure are so effectively regulated by small changes in the caliber of the arterioles.

VISCOSITY & RESISTANCE

The resistance to blood flow is determined not only by the radius of the blood vessels (**vascular hindrance**) but also by the viscosity of the blood. Plasma is about 1.8 times as viscous as water, whereas whole blood is 3–4 times as viscous as water. Thus, viscosity depends on the **hematocrit.** The effect of viscosity in vivo deviates from that predicted by the Poiseuille–Hagen formula. In large vessels, increases in hematocrit cause appreciable increases in viscosity. However, in vessels smaller than 100 μm in diameter—that is, in arterioles, capillaries, and venules—the viscosity change per unit change in hematocrit is much less than it is in large-bore vessels. This is due to a difference in the nature of flow through the small vessels, known as the Fahraeus-Lindqvist effect. This holds that in small vessels, erythrocytes move to the center of the vessel, leaving cell-free plasma at the vessel wall. Therefore, the net change in viscosity per unit change in hematocrit is considerably smaller in the body than it is in vitro. Hematocrit changes thus have relatively little effect on the peripheral resistance except when the changes are large. In severe polycythemia (excessive production of red blood cells), the increase in resistance does increase the work of the heart. Conversely, in marked anemia, peripheral resistance is decreased, in part because of the decline in viscosity. Of course, the decrease in hemoglobin decreases the O_2-carrying ability of the blood, but the improved blood flow due to the decrease in viscosity partially compensates for this.

Viscosity is also affected by the composition of the plasma and the resistance of the cells to deformation. Clinically significant increases in viscosity are seen in diseases in which plasma proteins such as immunoglobulins are markedly elevated as well as when red blood cells are abnormally rigid (hereditary spherocytosis).

CRITICAL CLOSING PRESSURE

In rigid tubes, the relationship between pressure and flow of homogeneous fluids is linear, but in thin-walled blood vessels it is not. When the pressure in a small blood vessel is reduced, a point is reached at which no blood flows, even though the pressure is not zero. This is because the vessels are surrounded by tissues that exert a small but definite pressure on them, and when the intraluminal pressure falls below the tissue pressure, they collapse. The pressure at which flow ceases is called the **critical closing pressure.**

LAW OF LAPLACE

It is perhaps surprising that structures as delicate as capillaries are not more prone to rupture. The principal reason is their small diameter. The protective effect of small size is reflective of the **law of Laplace.** This states that tension in the wall of a cylinder (T) is equal to the product of the transmural pressure (P) and the radius (r) divided by the wall thickness (w):

$$T = Pr/w$$

The **transmural pressure** is the pressure inside the cylinder minus the pressure outside the cylinder, but because tissue pressure in the body is low, it can generally be ignored. In a thin-walled vessel, w is very small and it too can be ignored, but it becomes a significant factor in vessels such as arteries. Therefore, in a thin-walled vessel, P = T divided by the two principal radii of curvature:

$$P = T\left(\frac{1}{r_1} + \frac{1}{r_2}\right)$$

In a cylinder such as a blood vessel, one radius is infinite, so

$$P = \frac{T}{r}$$

Consequently, the smaller the radius of a blood vessel, the lower the tension in the wall necessary to balance the distending pressure. In the human aorta, for example, the tension at normal pressures is about 170,000 dynes/cm, and in the vena cava it is about 21,000 dynes/cm; but in the capillaries, it is approximately 16 dynes/cm.

The law of Laplace also makes clear a disadvantage faced by dilated hearts. When the radius of a cardiac chamber is increased, a greater tension must be developed in the myocardium to produce any given pressure; consequently, a dilated heart must do more work.

RESISTANCE & CAPACITANCE VESSELS

In vivo, the veins are an important blood reservoir. Normally, they are partially collapsed and oval in cross section. A large amount of blood can be added to the venous system before the veins become distended to the point where further increments in volume produce a large rise in venous pressure. The veins are therefore called **capacitance vessels.** The small arteries and arterioles are referred to as **resistance vessels** because they are the principal site of the peripheral resistance (see below).

At rest, at least 50% of the circulating blood volume is in the systemic veins, 12% is in the heart cavities, and 18% is in the low-pressure pulmonary circulation. Only 2% is in the aorta, 8% in the arteries, 1% in the arterioles, and 5% in the capillaries (Table 31–3).

VELOCITY & FLOW OF BLOOD

Although the mean velocity of the blood in the proximal portion of the aorta is 40 cm/s, the flow is phasic, and velocity ranges from 120 cm/s during systole to a negative value at the time of the transient backflow before the aortic valve closes in diastole. In the distal portions of the aorta and in the large arteries, velocity is also much greater in systole than it is in diastole. However, the vessels are elastic, and forward flow is continuous because of the recoil during diastole of the vessel walls that have been stretched during systole. Pulsatile flow appears to maintain optimal function of the tissues, apparently via distinct effects on gene transcription.

ARTERIAL PRESSURE

The pressure in the aorta and in the brachial and other large arteries in a young adult human rises to a peak value (**systolic pressure**) of about 120 mm Hg during each heart cycle and falls to a minimum (**diastolic pressure**) of about 70 mm Hg. The arterial pressure is conventionally written as systolic pressure over diastolic pressure, for example, 120/70 mm Hg. The **pulse pressure,** the difference between the systolic and diastolic pressures, is normally about 50 mm Hg. The **mean pressure** is the average pressure throughout the cardiac cycle. Because systole is shorter than diastole, the mean pressure is slightly less than the value halfway between systolic and diastolic pressure. As an approximation, mean pressure equals the diastolic pressure plus one-third of the pulse pressure.

The pressure falls very slightly in the large- and medium-sized arteries because their resistance to flow is small, but it falls rapidly in the small arteries and arterioles, which are the main sites of the peripheral resistance against which the heart pumps. The mean pressure at the end of the arterioles is 30–38 mm Hg. Pulse pressure also declines rapidly to about 5 mm Hg at the ends of the arterioles. The magnitude of the pressure drop along the arterioles depends on whether they are constricted or dilated.

EFFECT OF GRAVITY

The pressure in any vessel below the heart is increased and that in any vessel above heart level is decreased by the effect of gravity. The magnitude of the gravitational effect is 0.77 mm Hg/cm of vertical distance above or below the heart. Thus, in an adult human in the upright position, when the mean arterial pressure at heart level is 100 mm Hg, the mean pressure in a large artery in the head (50 cm above the heart) is 62 mm Hg ($100 - [0.77 \times 50]$) and the pressure in a large artery in the foot (105 cm below the heart) is 180 mm Hg ($100 + [0.77 \times 105]$). The effect of gravity on venous pressure is similar.

METHODS OF MEASURING BLOOD PRESSURE

If a cannula is inserted into an artery, the arterial pressure can be measured directly. When an artery is tied off beyond the point at which the cannula is inserted, an **end pressure** is recorded, flow in the artery is interrupted, and all the kinetic energy of flow is converted into pressure energy. If, alternatively, a T tube is inserted into a vessel and the pressure is measured in the side arm of the tube, the recorded **side pressure**, under conditions where pressure drop due to resistance is negligible, is lower than the end pressure by the kinetic energy of flow. This is because in a tube or a blood vessel the total energy—the sum of the kinetic energy of flow and the potential energy—is constant (**Bernoulli's principle).**

It is worth noting that the pressure drop in any segment of the arterial system is due both to resistance and to conversion of potential into kinetic energy. The pressure drop due to energy lost in overcoming resistance is irreversible, since the energy is dissipated as heat; but the pressure drop due to conversion of potential to kinetic energy as a vessel narrows is reversed when the vessel widens out again.

The Bernoulli principle also has a significant application in pathophysiology. According to the principle, the greater the velocity of flow in a vessel, the lower the lateral pressure distending its walls. When a vessel is narrowed, the velocity of flow in the narrowed portion increases and the distending pressure decreases. Therefore, when a vessel is narrowed by a pathologic process such as an atherosclerotic plaque, the lateral pressure at the constriction is decreased and the narrowing tends to maintain itself.

AUSCULTATORY METHOD

The arterial blood pressure in humans is routinely measured by the **auscultatory method.** An inflatable cuff attached to a mercury manometer (**sphygmomanometer**) is wrapped around the arm and a stethoscope is placed over the brachial artery at the elbow. The cuff is rapidly inflated until the pressure is well above the expected systolic pressure in the brachial artery. The artery is occluded by the cuff, and no sound is heard with the stethoscope. The pressure in the cuff is then lowered slowly. At the point at which systolic pressure in the artery just exceeds the cuff pressure, a spurt of blood passes through with each heartbeat and a tapping sound is heard below the cuff. The cuff pressure at which the sounds are first heard is the systolic pressure. As the cuff pressure is lowered further, the sounds become louder, then dull and muffled. These are the **sounds of Korotkoff.** Finally, in most individuals, they disappear. The diastolic pressure in resting adults correlates best with the pressure at which the sound disappears. However, in adults after exercise and in children, the diastolic pressure correlates best with the pressure at which the sounds become muffled. This is also true in diseases such as hyperthyroidism and aortic regurgitation.

The sounds of Korotkoff are produced by turbulent flow in the brachial artery. When the artery is narrowed by the cuff, the velocity of flow through the constriction exceeds the **critical velocity** and turbulent flow results. At cuff pressures just below the systolic pressure, flow through the artery occurs only at the peak of systole, and the intermittent turbulence produces a tapping sound. As long as the pressure in the cuff is above the diastolic pressure in the artery, flow is interrupted at least during part of diastole,

and the intermittent sounds have a staccato quality. When the cuff pressure is near the arterial diastolic pressure, the vessel is still constricted, but the turbulent flow is continuous.

NORMAL ARTERIAL BLOOD PRESSURE

Because the arterial pressure is the product of the cardiac output and the peripheral resistance, it is affected by conditions that affect either or both of these factors. Emotion increases the cardiac output and peripheral resistance, and about 20% of hypertensive patients have blood pressures that are higher in the doctor's office than at home. Blood pressure normally falls up to 20 mm Hg during sleep. This fall is reduced or absent in hypertension.

There is general agreement that blood pressure rises with advancing age, but the magnitude of this rise is uncertain because hypertension is a common disease and its incidence increases with advancing age (Clinical Box 31–4). Individuals who have

---

CLINICAL BOX 31–4

Hypertension

Hypertension is a sustained elevation of the systemic arterial pressure. It is most commonly due to increased peripheral resistance and is a very common abnormality in humans. It can be produced by many diseases and causes a number of serious disorders. When the resistance against which the left ventricle must pump (afterload) is elevated for a long period, the cardiac muscle hypertrophies. Left ventricular hypertrophy is associated with a poor prognosis. The total O_2 consumption of the heart, already increased by the work of expelling blood against a raised pressure, is increased further because there is more muscle. Therefore, any decrease in coronary blood flow has more serious consequences in hypertensive patients than it does in normal individuals.

The incidence of atherosclerosis increases in hypertension, and myocardial infarcts are common even when the heart is not enlarged. Eventually, the ability to compensate for the high peripheral resistance is exceeded, and the heart fails. Hypertensive individuals are also predisposed to thromboses of cerebral vessels and cerebral hemorrhage. An additional complication is chronic kidney disease. However, disease incidence can be markedly reduced by active treatment of hypertension. In most patients with elevated blood pressure, the cause of the hypertension is unknown, and they are said to have **essential hypertension.** At present, essential hypertension is treatable but not curable.

In other, less common forms of hypertension, the cause is known. A review of these is helpful because it emphasizes ways disordered physiology can lead to disease. Pathology that compromises the renal blood supply leads to renal hypertension, as does narrowing (coarctation) of the thoracic aorta, which both increases renin secretion and increases peripheral resistance. Pheochromocytomas, adrenal medullary tumors

that secrete norepinephrine and epinephrine, can cause sporadic or sustained hypertension. Increased secretion of aldosterone or other mineralocorticoids causes renal Na^+ retention, which leads to hypertension. A primary increase in plasma mineralocorticoids inhibits renin secretion. For unknown reasons, plasma renin is also low in 10–15% of patients with essential hypertension and normal circulating mineralocortical levels (low renin hypertension). Mutations in a number of single genes are also known to cause hypertension. These cases of monogenic hypertension are rare but informative. One of these is glucocorticoid-remediable aldosteronism (GRA), in which a hybrid gene encodes an adrenocorticotropic hormone (ACTH)-sensitive aldosterone synthase, with resulting hyperaldosteronism. 11-β hydroxylase deficiency also causes hypertension by increasing the secretion of deoxycorticosterone. Normal blood pressure is restored when ACTH secretion is inhibited by administering a glucocorticoid. Mutations that decrease 11-β hydroxysteroid dehydrogenase cause loss of specificity of the mineralocorticoid receptors with stimulation of them by cortisol and, in pregnancy, by the elevated circulating levels of progesterone. Finally, mutations of the genes for ENaCs that reduce degradation of the β- or γ-subunits increase ENaC activity and lead to excess renal Na^+ retention and hypertension (Liddle syndrome).

THERAPEUTIC HIGHLIGHTS

Effective lowering of the blood pressure can be produced by drugs that block α- or β-adrenergic receptors; drugs that inhibit the activity of angiotensin-converting enzyme; and calcium channel blockers that relax vascular smooth muscle.

systolic blood pressures less than 120 mm Hg at age 50–60 and never develop clinical hypertension still have systolic pressures that rise throughout life. This rise may be the closest approximation to the rise in normal individuals. Diastolic pressure also rises, but then starts to fall in middle age as the stiffness of arteries increases. Consequently, pulse pressure rises with advancing age.

Systolic and diastolic blood pressures are lower in young women than in young men until age 55–65, after which they become comparable. Because there is a positive correlation between blood pressure and the incidence of heart attacks and strokes, the lower blood pressure before menopause in women may be one reason that, on average, they live longer than men.

■ CAPILLARY CIRCULATION

The 5% of the circulating blood that is in the capillaries is in a sense the most important part of the blood volume because it is the only pool from which O_2 and nutrients can enter the interstitial fluid and into which CO_2 and waste products can enter the bloodstream.

METHODS OF STUDY

It is difficult to obtain accurate measurements of capillary pressures and flows. Capillary pressure has been estimated by determining the amount of external pressure necessary to occlude the capillaries or the amount of pressure necessary to make saline start to flow through a micropipette inserted so that its tip faces the arteriolar end of the capillary.

CAPILLARY PRESSURE & FLOW

Capillary pressures vary considerably, but typical values in human nail bed capillaries are 32 mm Hg at the arteriolar end and 15 mm Hg at the venous end. The pulse pressure is approximately 5 mm Hg at the arteriolar end and zero at the venous end. The capillaries are short, but blood moves slowly (about 0.07 cm/s) because the total cross-sectional area of the capillary bed is large. Transit time from the arteriolar to the venular end of an average-sized capillary is 1–2 s.

EQUILIBRATION WITH INTERSTITIAL FLUID

The factors other than vesicular transport responsible for transport across the capillary wall are diffusion and filtration. Diffusion is quantitatively much more important. O_2 and glucose are in higher concentration in the bloodstream than in the interstitial fluid and diffuse into the interstitial fluid, whereas CO_2 diffuses in the opposite direction.

The rate of filtration at any point along a capillary depends on a balance of forces sometimes called the **Starling forces.** One of these forces is the **hydrostatic pressure gradient** (the hydrostatic pressure in the capillary minus the hydrostatic pressure of the interstitial fluid). The interstitial fluid pressure varies from one organ to another, and there is considerable evidence that it is subatmospheric (about −2 mm Hg) in subcutaneous tissue. It is, however, positive in the liver and kidneys and as high as 6 mm Hg in the brain. The other force is the **osmotic pressure gradient** across the capillary wall (colloid osmotic pressure of plasma minus colloid osmotic pressure of interstitial fluid). This component is directed inward.

Thus:

$$\text{Fluid movement} = k[(P_c - P_i) - (\pi_c - \pi_i)]$$

where k = capillary filtration coefficient
P_c = capillary hydrostatic pressure
P_i = interstitial hydrostatic pressure
π_c = capillary colloid osmotic pressure
π_i = interstitial colloid osmotic pressure

π_i is usually negligible, so the osmotic pressure gradient $(\pi_c - \pi_i)$ usually equals the oncotic pressure. The capillary filtration coefficient takes into account, and is proportional to, the permeability of the capillary wall and the area available for filtration. Fluid moves into the interstitial space at the arteriolar end of the capillary and into the capillary at the venular end. In other capillaries, the balance of Starling forces may be different. For example, fluid moves out of almost the entire length of the capillaries in the renal glomeruli, and into the capillaries through almost their entire length in the intestines. About 24 L of fluid is filtered through the capillaries per day. This is about 0.3% of the cardiac output. About 85% of the filtered fluid is reabsorbed into the capillaries, and the remainder returns to the circulation via the lymphatics.

Small molecules often equilibrate with the tissues near the arteriolar end of each capillary. In this situation, total diffusion can be increased by increasing blood flow; that is, exchange is **flow-limited.** Conversely, transfer of substances that do not reach equilibrium with the tissues during their passage through the capillaries is said to be **diffusion-limited.**

■ VENOUS CIRCULATION

Blood flows through the blood vessels, including the veins, primarily because of the pumping action of the heart. However, venous flow is aided by the heartbeat, the increase in the negative intrathoracic pressure during each inspiration, and contractions of skeletal muscles that compress the veins (**muscle pump**).

VENOUS PRESSURE & FLOW

The pressure in the venules is 12–18 mm Hg. It falls steadily in the larger veins to about 5.5 mm Hg in the great veins outside the thorax. The pressure in the great veins at their entrance into the right atrium (**central venous pressure**) averages 4.6 mm Hg, but fluctuates with respiration and heart action. Peripheral venous pressure, like arterial pressure, is affected by gravity. On a proportional basis, gravity has a greater effect on venous than on arterial pressures.

When blood flows from the venules to the large veins, its average velocity increases as the total cross-sectional area of the vessels decreases. In the great veins, the velocity of blood is about one-fourth that in the aorta, averaging about 10 cm/s.

Central venous pressure is decreased during negative pressure breathing and shock. It is increased by positive pressure breathing, straining, expansion of the blood volume, and heart failure. In advanced heart failure or obstruction of the superior vena cava, the pressure in the antecubital vein may reach values of 20 mm Hg or more.

THORACIC PUMP

During inspiration, the intrapleural pressure falls from −2.5 to −6 mm Hg. This negative pressure is transmitted to the great veins and, to a lesser extent, the atria, so that central venous pressure fluctuates from about 6 mm Hg during expiration to approximately 2 mm Hg during quiet inspiration. The drop in venous pressure during inspiration aids venous return. When the diaphragm descends during inspiration, intra-abdominal pressure rises, and this also squeezes blood toward the heart because backflow into the leg veins is prevented by the venous valves.

EFFECTS OF HEARTBEAT

The variations in atrial pressure are transmitted to the great veins, producing the **a, c,** and **v waves** of the venous pressure–pulse curve (see Chapter 30). Atrial pressure drops sharply during the ejection phase of ventricular systole because the atrioventricular valves are pulled downward, increasing the capacity of the atria. This action sucks blood into the atria from the great veins. The sucking of the blood into the atria during systole contributes appreciably to venous return.

Close to the heart, venous flow becomes pulsatile. When the heart rate is slow, two periods of peak flow are detectable, one during ventricular systole, due to pulling down of the atrioventricular valves, and one in early diastole, during the period of rapid ventricular filling.

MUSCLE PUMP

In the limbs, the veins are surrounded by skeletal muscles, and contraction of these muscles during activity compresses the veins. Pulsations of nearby arteries may also compress veins. Because the venous valves prevent reverse flow, blood moves toward the heart. During quiet standing, when the full effect of gravity is manifest, venous pressure at the ankle is 85–90 mm Hg. Rhythmic contractions of the leg muscles while the person is standing serve to lower the venous pressure in the legs to less than 30 mm Hg by propelling blood toward the heart. This heartward movement of the blood is decreased in patients with **varicose veins** because their valves are incompetent. These patients may develop stasis and ankle edema. However, even when the valves are incompetent, muscle contractions continue to produce a basic heartward movement of the blood because the resistance of the larger veins in the direction of the heart is less than the resistance of the small vessels away from the heart.

VENOUS PRESSURE IN THE HEAD

In the upright position, venous pressure above the heart is decreased by the force of gravity. The neck veins collapse above the point where the venous pressure is close to zero. However, the dural sinuses have rigid walls and cannot collapse. The pressure in them in the standing or sitting position is therefore subatmospheric. The magnitude of the negative pressure is proportional to the vertical distance above the top of the collapsed neck veins, and in the superior sagittal sinus may be as much as −10 mm Hg. This fact must be kept in mind by neurosurgeons. Neurosurgical procedures are sometimes performed with the patient seated. If one of the sinuses is opened during such a procedure it sucks air, causing **air embolism.**

AIR EMBOLISM

Because air, unlike fluid, is compressible, its presence in the circulation has serious consequences. The forward movement of the blood depends on the fact that blood is incompressible. Large amounts of air fill the heart and effectively stop the circulation, causing sudden death because most of the air is compressed by the contracting ventricles rather than propelled into the arteries. Small amounts of air are swept through the heart with the blood, but bubbles lodge in small blood vessels. The surface capillarity of the bubbles markedly increases the resistance to blood flow, and flow is reduced or abolished. Blockage of small vessels in the brain leads to serious and even fatal neurologic abnormalities. Treatment with hyperbaric oxygen is of value because the pressure reduces the size of the gas emboli.

■ LYMPHATIC CIRCULATION & INTERSTITIAL FLUID VOLUME

LYMPHATIC CIRCULATION

Fluid efflux normally exceeds influx across the capillary walls, but the extra fluid enters the lymphatics and drains through them back into the blood. This keeps the interstitial fluid pressure from rising and promotes the turnover of tissue fluid. The normal 24-h lymph flow is 2–4 L.

Lymphatic vessels can be divided into two types: initial lymphatics and collecting lymphatics. The former lack valves and smooth muscle in their walls, and they are found in regions such as the intestine or skeletal muscle. Tissue fluid appears to enter them through loose junctions between the endothelial cells that form their walls. The fluid in them apparently is massaged by muscle contractions of the organs and contraction of arterioles and venules, with which they are often associated. They drain into the collecting lymphatics, which have valves and smooth muscle in their walls and contract in a peristaltic fashion, propelling the lymph. Flow in the collecting lymphatics is further aided by movements of skeletal muscle, the negative intrathoracic pressure during inspiration, and the suction effect of high velocity flow of blood in the veins in which the lymphatics terminate. However, the contractions are the principal factor propelling the lymph.

OTHER FUNCTIONS OF THE LYMPHATIC SYSTEM

Appreciable quantities of protein enter the interstitial fluid in the liver and intestine, and smaller quantities enter from the blood in other tissues. The macromolecules enter the lymphatics, presumably at the junctions between the endothelial cells, and the proteins are returned to the bloodstream via the lymphatics. The amount of protein returned in this fashion in 1 day is equal to 25–50% of the total circulating plasma protein. Absorbed long-chain fatty acids and cholesterol from the intestine are also transported to the blood via the lymphatics.

INTERSTITIAL FLUID VOLUME

The amount of fluid in the interstitial spaces depends on the capillary pressure, the interstitial fluid pressure, the oncotic pressure, the capillary filtration coefficient, the number of active capillaries, lymph flow, and the total extracellular fluid (ECF) volume. The ratio of precapillary to postcapillary venular resistance is also important. Precapillary constriction lowers filtration pressure, whereas postcapillary constriction raises it. Changes in any of these variables lead to changes in the volume of interstitial fluid. Factors promoting an increase in this volume are summarized in Table 31–4. **Edema** is the accumulation of interstitial fluid in abnormally large amounts.

TABLE 31–4 Causes of increased interstitial fluid volume and edema.

Increased filtration pressure
Venular constriction
Increased venous pressure (heart failure, incompetent valves, venous obstruction, increased total ECF volume, effect of gravity, etc.)
Decreased osmotic pressure gradient across capillary
Decreased plasma protein level
Accumulation of osmotically active substances in interstitial space
Increased capillary permeability
Substance P
Histamine and related substances
Kinins, etc.
Inadequate lymph flow

In active tissues, capillary pressure rises, often to the point where it exceeds the oncotic pressure throughout the length of the capillary. In addition, osmotically active metabolites may temporarily accumulate in the interstitial fluid because they cannot be washed away as rapidly as they are formed. To the extent that they accumulate, they decrease the magnitude of the osmotic gradient due to the oncotic pressure. The amount of fluid leaving the capillaries is therefore markedly increased. Lymph flow is increased, decreasing the degree to which the fluid would otherwise accumulate, but exercising muscle, for example, still increases in volume by as much as 25%.

Interstitial fluid tends to accumulate in dependent parts because of the effect of gravity. In the upright position, the capillaries in the legs are protected from the high arterial pressure by the arterioles, but the high venous pressure is transmitted to them through the venules. Skeletal muscle contractions keep the venous pressure low by pumping blood toward the heart (see above) when the individual moves about; however, if one stands still for long periods, fluid accumulates and edema eventually develops. The ankles also swell when travelers sit for prolonged periods with their feet in a dependent position. Venous obstruction may contribute to the edema in these situations.

Whenever there is abnormal retention of salt in the body, water is also retained. The salt and water are distributed throughout the ECF, and since the interstitial fluid volume is increased, there is a predisposition to edema. Salt and water retention is a factor in the edema seen in heart failure, nephrosis, and cirrhosis, but there are also variations in fluid movement across the capillary walls in these diseases. In heart failure, for example, venous pressure is usually elevated, with a consequent elevation in capillary pressure. In cirrhosis of the liver, oncotic pressure is low because hepatic synthesis of plasma proteins is depressed; and in nephrosis, oncotic pressure is low because large amounts of protein are lost in the urine.

Another cause of edema is inadequate lymphatic drainage. Edema caused by lymphatic obstruction is called **lymphedema,** and the edema fluid has a high-protein content. If it persists, it causes a chronic inflammatory condition that leads to fibrosis of the interstitial tissue.

CHAPTER SUMMARY

- Blood is a suspension of red blood cells (erythrocytes), white blood cells, and platelets in a protein-rich fluid known as plasma.
- Blood cells arise in the bone marrow and are subject to regular renewal; the majority of plasma proteins are synthesized by the liver.
- Hemoglobin in red blood cells transports oxygen to peripheral tissues. Fetal hemoglobin is specialized to facilitate diffusion of oxygen from mother to fetus. Mutated forms of hemoglobin lead to red cell abnormalities and anemia.
- Complex oligosaccharide structures form the basis of the ABO blood group system. AB blood group oligosaccharides, as well as other blood group molecules, can trigger the production of antibodies in naïve individuals following inappropriate transfusions.
- Blood flows from the heart to arteries and arterioles, thence to capillaries, and eventually to venules and veins and back to the heart. Each segment of the vasculature has specific contractile

properties and regulatory mechanisms. Physical principles govern the flow of blood through each segment of the circulation.

■ Transfer of oxygen and nutrients from the blood to tissues, as well as collection of metabolic wastes, occurs exclusively in the capillary beds.

■ Fluid also leaves the circulation across the walls of capillaries. Some is reabsorbed; the remainder enters the lymphatic system, which eventually returns fluid to the bloodstream.

■ Hypertension is an increase in mean blood pressure that is usually chronic and is common in humans. Hypertension can result in serious health consequences if left untreated, which control the dynamics of the circulatory system and its integration with other organs.

MULTIPLE-CHOICE QUESTIONS

For all questions, select the single best answer unless otherwise directed.

1. A student uses a variety of experimental approaches in a research project designed to analyze blood flow rates in healthy subjects. In which of the following types of blood vessel will flow be the slowest?
   A. Arteries
   B. Arterioles
   C. Capillaries
   D. Venules
   E. Veins

2. In the experiment described in Question 1, which of the following statements will be true about the measured velocity of blood flow?
   A. It is higher in the capillaries than the arterioles.
   B. It is higher in the veins than in the venules.
   C. It is higher in the veins than the arteries.
   D. It falls to zero in the descending aorta during diastole.
   E. It is reduced in a constricted area of a blood vessel.

3. A 50-year-old woman comes to her physician complaining of swelling of her feet and ankles. After ruling out heart and kidney problems, he tells her that lymph flow from the foot can be increased by which of the following?
   A. Rising from the supine to the standing position.
   B. Massaging the foot.
   C. Administration of a drug that decreases capillary permeability.
   D. Surgery to ablate varicose veins.
   E. Abstaining from exercise.

4. The pressure in a capillary in skeletal muscle is 35 mm Hg at the arteriolar end and 14 mm Hg at the venular end. The interstitial pressure is 0 mm Hg. The colloid osmotic pressure is 25 mm Hg in the capillary and 1 mm Hg in the interstitium. The net force producing fluid movement across the capillary wall at its arteriolar end is
   A. 3 mm Hg out of the capillary.
   B. 3 mm Hg into the capillary.
   C. 10 mm Hg out of the capillary.
   D. 11 mm Hg out of the capillary.
   E. 11 mm Hg into the capillary.

5. When the radius of the resistance vessels is increased, which of the following is increased?
   A. Systolic blood pressure
   B. Diastolic blood pressure
   C. Viscosity of the blood
   D. Hematocrit
   E. Capillary blood flow

6. A 30-year-old patient comes to her primary care clinician complaining of headaches and vertigo. A blood test reveals a hematocrit of 65%, and a diagnosis of polycythemia is made. Which of the following would also be increased?
   A. Mean blood pressure
   B. Radius of the resistance vessels
   C. Radius of the capacitance vessels
   D. Central venous pressure
   E. Capillary blood flow

7. A pharmacologist discovers a drug that stimulates the production of VEGF receptors. He is excited because the drug might be of value in the treatment of
   A. coronary artery disease.
   B. cancer.
   C. diabetic retinopathy.
   D. macular degeneration.
   E. dysmenorrhea.

8. In an experiment, a scientist measured the diameter of the femoral artery in an anesthetized dog both prior to and after the arterial endothelium was damaged by mechanically rubbing the arterial lumen. The dilator response to injected acetylcholine changed to a constrictor response when the endothelium was damaged. What is the basis for this effect?
   A. More Na^+ is generated.
   B. More bradykinin is generated.
   C. The damage elevates cyclic guanosine monophosphate (cGMP) in the remaining vascular smooth muscle.
   D. The damage augments the production of endothelin by the endothelium.
   E. The damage interferes with the production of NO by the endothelium.

9. A 40-year-old man with long-standing diabetes comes to his primary care physician complaining of swelling in his feet and ankles that makes it hard for him to wear shoes. He notes that his urine has developed a foamy appearance, and a blood test reveals that his blood urea nitrogen is increased. The primary cause of edema in this patient is most likely a reduction in which of the following:
   A. Lymph flow
   B. Barrier function of the capillaries
   C. Venous hydrostatic pressure
   D. Capillary oncotic pressure
   E. Interstitial oncotic pressure

10. A 2-year-old African American boy is brought to his pediatrician because of acute fever, apparent bone pain, and painful swelling of his hands and feet. A physical examination reveals splenomegaly and a blood test shows the presence of hemoglobin S. After the acute symptoms subside with rest, hydration, and the use of analgesics, hydroxyurea is prescribed. This drug would be expected to reduce the risk of further acute episodes of disease via which mechanism?
    A. Increasing the synthesis of hemoglobin S
    B. Increasing the oxygen-carrying capacity of hemoglobin
    C. Reducing the oxygen-carrying capacity of hemoglobin
    D. Increasing the levels of hypoxia-inducible factor
    E. Increasing the synthesis of hemoglobin F.

ANSWERS

1. The correct answer is **C**. The velocity of blood flow depends on the pressure in a particular segment, which is highest in the arteries and next highest in the arterioles (rules out options **A** and **B**). Pressure in the venules and veins is even lower than in the capillaries, and these "capacitance vessels" serve as a reservoir for the majority of blood in the systemic circulation. However, flow is also determined by the cross-sectional area of the vessel bed in question. Although each capillary is small, in aggregate their cross-sectional area exceeds that of all other vessel types listed, in some cases, by a considerable margin (rules out options **D** and **E**).

2. The correct answer is **B**. The rate of blood flow depends on the pressure in a given vessel and inversely upon the total cross-sectional area. The pressure in the veins and venules is relatively comparable, but the latter have a larger cross-sectional area. The capillaries have the largest cross-sectional area and pressure is also lower here than in the arterioles, and so flow will be slowest through the capillaries (rules out option **A**). The cross-sectional area of the veins and arteries is comparable, but the arteries reflect the pressure imparted by the heart (rules out option **C**). In the descending aorta, the elasticity of the walls provides recoil during diastole, meaning that flow continues despite the cessation of outflow from the heart (rules out option **D**). Finally, when a blood vessel is constricted, the reduction in cross-sectional area will speed blood flow for a given pressure (rules out option **E**).

3. The correct answer is **B**. The lymphatic system collects fluid that has escaped from the capillaries and returns it to the vascular system. Edema, or an abnormal accumulation of interstitial fluid, occurs when fluid volume increases faster than lymphatic function can remove it, or if there is inadequate lymphatic flow. Flow can be increased by massage because the lymphatics lie close to the surface. Edema is particularly common in the extremities, particularly after prolonged standing, because of the effect of gravity. The lymphatic system also needs to fight against gravity to return fluid to the circulation via the subclavian veins (rules out option **A**). Exercise and varicose vein surgery increases venous return, maintaining a lower pressure in the venous system and reducing the formation of lymph (rules out options **D** and **E**). Lymph formation also depends on capillary permeability; if this is reduced, less lymph will be formed (rules out option **C**).

4. The correct answer is **D**. Fluid movement into or out of the capillary is proportional to the difference between the capillary and interstitial hydrostatic pressure at any given point, minus the difference between the capillary and interstitial oncotic pressure. In the example given, the respective pressures are $(35 - 0) - (25 - 1) = 11$ mm Hg (rules out options **A**, **B**, and **C**). A positive value means that fluid will be forced out of the capillary (rules out option **E**). Note that the difference in pressure from the arteriolar to the venular end of the capillary is irrelevant, and that in health, fluid is usually forced from the capillary at its arteriolar end and reclaimed to some extent at the venular end as the capillary hydrostatic pressure falls and the capillary oncotic pressure is either constant, or even increased, as fluid is lost.

5. The correct answer is **E**. The principal site of peripheral resistance is the arterioles and small arteries. An increase in the radius of these resistance vessels will reduce resistance, decreasing both the systolic and diastolic pressures (rules out options **A** and **B**). The viscosity of the blood and its hematocrit should be unaffected by the caliber of the resistance vessels (rules out options **C** and **D**). However, as resistance in the arterial system decreases, more blood will be delivered to the capillaries.

6. The correct answer is **A**. In polycythemia, there is excessive production of red blood cells resulting in a meaningful increase in blood viscosity. Although the effects of hematocrit on viscosity are blunted by the Fahraeus–Lindqvist effect in small vessels, eventually this is overcome when changes in hematocrit are large, leading to an increase in peripheral resistance and the mean blood pressure. The excess red cells may also lead to thrombosis in some capillary beds, particularly in the kidneys leading to the release of vasoconstrictors (rules out option **B**). Similarly, the capacitance vessels will not be dilated (rules out option **C**). The increased viscosity of the blood will also slow blood flow through the capillaries and reduce venous return, and thus would not increase central venous pressure (rules out options **D** and **E**).

7. The correct answer is **A**. VEGF is a key factor involved in angiogenesis, or the development of new blood vessels. It also enhances vascular permeability. Its synthesis is promoted by hypoxia. In that coronary artery disease results from blockage of some of the vessels that supply oxygen to the heart, triggering angiogenesis to bypass blocked vessels could at least theoretically be of therapeutic benefit, particularly if the effect could be targeted specifically to the heart. In cancer, tumor growth depends on the formation of new blood vessels to support the growing tumor mass, which has effectively been targeted with VEGF antagonists. So the drug described could actually worsen disease in cancer by enhancing tumor oxygenation (rules out option **B**). A similar scenario relates to macular degeneration and diabetic retinopathy, where retinal injury has been attributed to excessive production of VEGF, growth of leaky vessels, and scarring (rules out options **C** and **D**). Dysmenorrhea, or excessive menstrual bleeding, has also been correlated with microvascular density in the uterine endometrium (rules out option **E**).

8. The correct answer is **E**. Acetylcholine acts on vascular smooth muscle to induce its contraction, but in intact vessels, its more prominent effect is to induce the release of NO from the endothelium, resulting in vasodilatation. Sodium influx can induce endothelial stiffness and reduce NO generation, but this effect depends on the endothelium (rules out option **A**). Bradykinin induces vasodilatation in an endothelium-dependent manner, but acts in parallel to the effect of acetylcholine (rules out option **B**). Endothelial damage should not increase cGMP *per se*; even if it did, cGMP results in smooth muscle relaxation and vasodilatation (indeed, it mediates the effects of NO) (rules out option **C**). Finally, endothelin is predominantly a vasoconstrictor, but it does not participate in the response to acetylcholine. In fact, endothelin reduces the vasodilatory response to exogenous acetylcholine in intact vessels (rules out option **D**).

9. The correct answer is **D**. The patient is displaying signs of kidney damage, a serious complication of diabetes that can develop over time. Elevated glucose in the kidneys and accompanying inflammation damages the glomeruli, rendering them incapable of excluding albumin from the urine. Eventually, the liver cannot keep pace with this protein loss, and the hypoalbuminemia means that fluid cannot be retained in the capillaries. Edema can also result from lymphatic

obstruction, but this should not be accompanied by evidence of kidney injury (rules out option **A**). Similarly, an increase in capillary permeability can result in tissue edema, but this is typically the result of allergic and/or inflammatory reactions that release histamine in the tissues, and is not accompanied by loss of protein in the urine (rules out option **B**). Finally, a decrease in venous pressure or the interstitial oncotic pressure would oppose, rather than promote, edema formation (rules out options **C** and **E**).

10. The correct answer is **E**. The presentation of the patient is consistent with a diagnosis of sickle cell anemia. In this genetic disorder, the β chains of hemoglobin carry a mutation that causes the resulting hemoglobin, hemoglobin S, to polymerize at low oxygen levels and deform red blood cells into a sickle shape. These cells may hemolyze, leading to anemia, and form aggregates that block blood vessels. Hydroxyurea induces the synthesis of the fetal form of hemoglobin, hemoglobin F, which decreases the polymerization of deoxygenated hemoglobin S. Increasing hemoglobin S synthesis is not an effect of hydroxyurea and in any case would be expected to worsen, rather than benefit, disease (rules out option **A**). Hydroxyurea has no direct effect on the affinity of hemoglobin for oxygen (rules out options **B** and **C**). Further, to the extent that hydroxyurea improves tissue oxygenation by reducing sickling and red cell destruction, it would be expected to suppress rather than increase levels of hypoxia-inducible factor (rules out option **D**).

Cardiovascular Regulatory Mechanisms

OBJECTIVES

After studying this chapter, you should be able to:

- Describe the neural mechanisms that control arterial blood pressure and heart rate, including the receptors, afferent and efferent pathways, central integrating pathways, and effector mechanisms involved.
- Describe the direct effects of CO_2 and hypoxia on the rostral ventrolateral medulla.
- Define how the process of autoregulation contributes to control of vascular caliber.
- Identify the paracrine factors and hormones that regulate vascular tone, their sources, and their mechanisms of action.

INTRODUCTION

Multiple cardiovascular regulatory mechanisms are able to increase the blood supply to active tissues and increase or decrease heat loss from the body by redistributing the blood. In the face of challenges such as hemorrhage, they maintain the blood flow to the heart and brain. When the challenge faced is severe, flow to these vital organs is maintained at the expense of the circulation to the rest of the body. Circulatory adjustments are effected by altering the output of the pump (the heart), changing the diameter of the resistance vessels (primarily the arterioles), or altering the amount of blood pooled in the capacitance vessels (the veins). Regulation of cardiac output is discussed in Chapter 30. This chapter reviews the systemic regulatory mechanisms that synergize with the local mechanisms to adjust vascular responses throughout the body.

■ NEURAL CONTROL OF THE CARDIOVASCULAR SYSTEM

The cardiovascular system is under neural influences coming from several parts of the brainstem, forebrain, and insular cortex. The brainstem receives feedback from sensory receptors in the vasculature (eg, baroreceptors and chemoreceptors). A simplified model of the feedback control circuit is shown in Figure 32–1.

INNERVATION OF THE BLOOD VESSELS & THE HEART

Most vascular beds receive input only from the sympathetic division of the autonomic nervous system, and the activation of these sympathetic nerves release norepinephrine that acts on α_1-adrenoceptors to mediate vasoconstriction. The nerves to the resistance vessels regulate tissue blood flow and arterial pressure and those to the venous capacitance vessels vary the volume of blood "stored" in the veins. A change in the level of activity (increase or decrease) in sympathetic nerves is one of the many factors that mediate vasoconstriction or vasodilation (Table 32–1).

The heart receives opposing influences from the two divisions of the autonomic nervous system. Release of norepinephrine from postganglionic sympathetic nerves activates β_1-adrenoceptors in the heart, notably on the sinoatrial (SA) node, atrioventricular (AV) node, His-Purkinje conductive tissue, and atrial and ventricular contractile tissue. In response to stimulation of sympathetic nerves, the heart rate (chronotropy), rate of transmission in the cardiac conductive tissue (dromotropy), and the force of ventricular contraction (inotropy) are increased. Release of acetylcholine from postganglionic parasympathetic (vagus) nerves activates

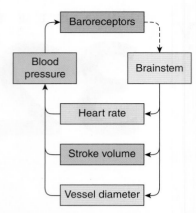

FIGURE 32–1 Feedback control of blood pressure. Brainstem excitatory input to sympathetic nerves to the heart and vasculature increases heart rate and stroke volume and reduces vessel diameter. Together these increase blood pressure, which activates the baroreceptor reflex to reduce the activity in the brainstem.

muscarinic receptors in the heart to reduce heart rate, the rate of transmission through the AV node, and atrial contractility.

NEURAL CONTROL OF THE CARDIOVASCULAR SYSTEM

Neurons in the rostral ventrolateral medulla (RVLM) release glutamate on preganglionic sympathetic neurons that control the vasculature (Figure 32–2). RVLM neurons are a major source

TABLE 32–1 Summary of factors affecting the caliber of the arterioles.

Vasoconstriction	Vasodilation
Local factors	
Decreased local temperature	Increased CO_2 and decreased O_2
Autoregulation	Increased K^+, adenosine, lactate
	Decreased local pH
	Increased local temperature
Endothelial products	
Endothelin-1	Nitric oxide
Locally released platelet serotonin	Kinins
Thromboxane A_2	Prostacyclin
Circulating neurohumoral agents	
Epinephrine (except in skeletal muscle and liver)	Epinephrine in skeletal muscle and liver
Norepinephrine	Calcitonin G-related protein
Arginine vasopressin	Substance P
Angiotensin II	Histamine
Endogenous digitalis-like substance	Atrial natriuretic peptide
Neuropeptide Y	Vasoactive intestinal polypeptide
Neural factors	
Increased sympathetic nerve activity	Decreased sympathetic nerve activity

of excitatory input to sympathetic nerves. Neurovascular compression of the RVLM has been linked to some cases of essential hypertension in humans (Clinical Box 32–1). The activity of RVLM neurons is determined by many factors (see Table 32–2). The pathway from the limbic cortex via the hypothalamus mediates the blood pressure (BP) rise and tachycardia produced by emotions such as stress, sexual excitement, and anger. Pain usually causes a rise in BP via afferent impulses converging in the RVLM, but prolonged severe pain may cause vasodilation and fainting. Activation of afferents from exercising muscles also increases RVLM neuronal activity and BP (somatosympathetic reflex).

Table 32–3 summarizes factors that affect the heart rate. In general, stimuli that increase the heart rate also increase BP, whereas those that decrease the heart rate lower BP. However, there are exceptions, such as the production of hypotension and tachycardia by stimulation of atrial stretch receptors and the production of hypertension and bradycardia by increased intracranial pressure.

BARORECEPTORS

The baroreceptors are stretch receptors in the walls of the heart and blood vessels. The carotid sinus and aortic arch receptors monitor the arterial circulation. Receptors in the low-pressure part of the circulation (eg, walls of the atria and the pulmonary circulation) are called cardiopulmonary receptors. The baroreceptors are activated when the pressure in the carotid sinus and aortic arch rises. The afferent fibers in the glossopharyngeal and vagus nerves release glutamate to excite neurons in the nucleus of the tractus solitarius (NTS; Figure 32–2). Excitatory (glutamate) projections extend from the NTS to the caudal ventrolateral medulla (CVLM), where they stimulate γ-aminobutyric acid (GABA)-secreting inhibitory neurons that project to the RVLM. Excitatory projections also extend from the NTS to the cardiac vagal motor neurons in the nucleus ambiguus. Thus, increased baroreceptor discharge *inhibits* sympathetic nerve activity and *excites* vagal nerve activity to produce vasodilation, hypotension, bradycardia, and a decrease in cardiac output.

ROLE OF BARORECEPTORS IN SHORT-TERM CONTROL OF BLOOD PRESSURE

The changes in heart rate and BP that occur in humans on standing up or lying down are due in part to baroreceptor reflexes. The function of the receptors can be tested by monitoring changes in heart rate as a function of increasing arterial pressure during infusion of the α-adrenoceptor agonist phenylephrine. A normal response is shown in Figure 32–3; between a systolic pressure of 120 and 150 mm Hg, there is a linear relation between pressure and lowering of the heart rate (longer R-R interval). Baroreceptors are very important in short-term control of arterial pressure. Activation of the reflex allows for rapid adjustments in BP in response to abrupt changes in posture, blood volume, cardiac output, or peripheral resistance during exercise.

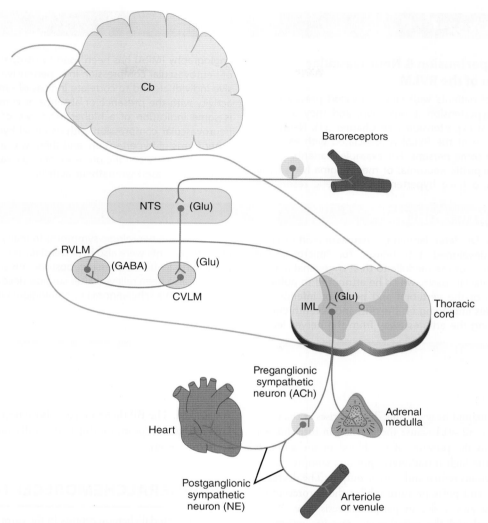

FIGURE 32-2 Basic neural pathways involved in the control of blood pressure. The drawing shows a parasagittal section of the brainstem and its connections to the thoracic spinal cord. The rostral ventrolateral medulla (RVLM) is one of the major sources of excitatory input to sympathetic nerves controlling the vasculature. These neurons receive inhibitory input from the baroreceptors via an inhibitory (GABAergic) neuron in the caudal ventrolateral medulla (CVLM). The nucleus of the tractus solitarius (NTS) is the site of termination of baroreceptor afferent fibers that release glutamate. ACh, acetylcholine; GABA, γ-aminobutyric acid; Glu, glutamate; IML, intermediolateral cell column; NE, norepinephrine.

Removal of the baroreceptor reflex prevents an individual from adjusting their BP in response to stimuli that cause abrupt changes in blood volume, cardiac output, or peripheral resistance, including exercise and postural changes. A long-term change in BP resulting from loss of baroreceptor reflex control is called neurogenic hypertension.

ATRIAL STRETCH & CARDIOPULMONARY RECEPTORS

Atrial stretch receptors respond primarily to distension of the atrial walls. The reflex circulatory adjustments initiated by increased discharge from these receptors include vasodilation, a fall in BP, and an increase in heart rate. Receptors in the endocardial surfaces

of the ventricles are activated during ventricular distension. The response is a vagal bradycardia and hypotension, comparable to a baroreceptor reflex. Left ventricular stretch receptors may play a role in the maintenance of vagal tone that keeps the heart rate low at rest. Various chemicals are known to elicit reflexes due to activation of cardiopulmonary chemoreceptors and may play a role in various cardiovascular disorders (Clinical Box 32–2).

VALSALVA MANEUVER

The function of the receptors can be tested by monitoring the changes in heart rate and BP that occur in response to brief periods of straining (forced expiration against a closed glottis: the Valsalva maneuver). Valsalva maneuvers occur regularly during

CLINICAL BOX 32–1

Essential Hypertension & Neurovascular Compression of the RVLM

In about 88% of patients with elevated blood pressure, the cause of the hypertension is unknown, and they are said to have essential hypertension (see Chapter 31). Neurovascular compression of the RVLM is associated with essential hypertension in some persons. For example, patients with a schwannoma (acoustic neuroma) or meningioma lying close to the RVLM also have hypertension. Magnetic resonance angiography (MRA) has been used to compare the incidence of neurovascular compression in hypertensive and normotensive individuals and to correlate indices of sympathetic nerve activity with the presence or absence of compression. There is some indication of a higher incidence of coexistence of neurovascular compression with essential hypertension than other forms of hypertension, and there was a strong positive relationship between the presence of neurovascular compression and increased sympathetic activity.

THERAPEUTIC HIGHLIGHTS

In the 1970s, Dr. Peter Jannetta, a neurosurgeon in Pittsburgh, PA developed a technique for "microvascular decompression" of the medulla to treat trigeminal neuralgia and hemifacial spasm, which he attributed to pulsatile compression of the vertebral and posterior inferior cerebellar arteries impinging on the fifth and seventh cranial nerves. Moving the arteries away from the nerves led to reversal of the neurologic symptoms in many cases. Some of these patients were also hypertensive, and they showed reductions in blood pressure postoperatively. Hypertension has also been relieved after surgical decompression in patients with a schwannoma or meningioma in the vicinity of the RVLM.

---

coughing, defecation, and heavy lifting. The BP rises at the onset of straining (Figure 32–4) because the increase in intrathoracic pressure is added to the pressure of the blood in the aorta. It then falls because the high intrathoracic pressure compresses the veins, decreasing venous return and cardiac output. The decreases in arterial pressure and pulse pressure inhibit the baroreceptors, causing tachycardia and a rise in peripheral resistance. When the glottis is opened and the intrathoracic pressure returns to normal, cardiac output is restored but the peripheral vessels are constricted. The BP therefore rises above normal, and this stimulates the baroreceptors, causing bradycardia and a drop in pressure to normal levels.

PERIPHERALCHEMORECEPTOR REFLEX

Peripheral arterial chemoreceptors in the carotid and aortic bodies have very high rates of blood flow. These receptors are primarily activated by a reduction in partial pressure of oxygen (PaO_2), but they also respond to an increase in the partial pressure of carbon dioxide ($PaCO_2$) and pH. Chemoreceptors exert their main effects on respiration; however, their activation also leads to

TABLE 32–2 Factors affecting the activity of RVLM neurons.

Direct stimulation
CO_2
Hypoxia
Excitatory inputs
Cortex via hypothalamus
Mesencephalic periaqueductal gray
Brainstem reticular formation
Pain pathways
Somatic afferents (somatosympathetic reflex)
Carotid and aortic chemoreceptors
Inhibitory inputs
Cortex via hypothalamus
Caudal ventrolateral medulla
Caudal medullary raphe nuclei
Lung inflation afferents
Carotid, aortic, and cardiopulmonary baroreceptors

TABLE 32–3 Factors affecting heart rate.

Heart rate accelerated by:	Heart rate slowed by:
Decreased activity of arterial baroreceptors	Increased activity of arterial baroreceptors
Increased activity of atrial stretch receptors	Expiration
Inspiration	Fear
Excitement	Grief
Anger	Stimulation of pain fibers in trigeminal nerve
Most painful stimuli	Increased intracranial pressure
Hypoxia	
Exercise	
Thyroid hormones	
Fever	

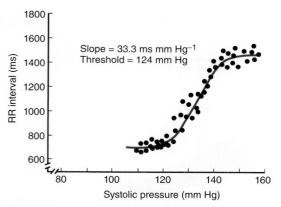

FIGURE 32–3 Baroreflex-mediated lowering of the heart rate during infusion of phenylephrine in a human subject. Note that the values for the R-R interval of the electrocardiogram, which are plotted on the vertical axis, are inversely proportional to the heart rate. (Adapted with permission from Kotrly KJ, Ebert TJ, Vucins EJ, et al: Effects of fentanyl-diazepam-nitrous oxide anesthesia on arterial baroreflex control of heart rate in man, *Br J Anaesth.* 1986 Apr;58(4):406-414.)

vasoconstriction. Heart rate changes are variable and depend on various factors, including changes in respiration. A direct effect of chemoreceptor activation is to increase vagal nerve activity. However, hypoxia also produces hyperpnea and increased catecholamine secretion from the adrenal medulla, both of which produce tachycardia and an increase in cardiac output. Hemorrhage that produces hypotension leads to chemoreceptor stimulation due to decreased blood flow to the chemoreceptors and consequent stagnant anoxia of these organs.

CENTRAL CHEMORECEPTORS

When intracranial pressure is increased, the blood supply to RVLM neurons is compromised, and the local hypoxia and hypercapnia increase their activity. The resultant rise in systemic arterial pressure (Cushing reflex) tends to restore the blood flow to the medulla. Over a considerable range, the BP rise is proportional to the increase in intracranial pressure. The rise in BP causes a reflex decrease in heart rate via the arterial baroreceptors. This is why bradycardia rather than tachycardia is characteristically seen in patients with increased intracranial pressure.

A rise in arterial PCO_2 stimulates the RVLM, but the direct peripheral effect of hypercapnia is vasodilation. Therefore, the peripheral and central actions tend to cancel each other out. Moderate hyperventilation, which significantly lowers the CO_2 tension of the blood, causes cutaneous and cerebral vasoconstriction in humans, but there is little change in BP. Exposure to high concentrations of CO_2 is associated with marked cutaneous and cerebral vasodilation, but vasoconstriction occurs elsewhere and usually there is a slow rise in BP.

CLINICAL BOX 32–2

Cardiopulmonary Chemosensitive Receptors

Activation of chemosensitive vagal C fibers in the cardiopulmonary region (eg, juxtacapillary region of alveoli, ventricles, atria, great veins, and pulmonary artery) causes profound bradycardia, hypotension, and a brief period of apnea followed by rapid shallow breathing (Bezold-Jarisch reflex). This reflex can be elicited by a variety of substances including capsaicin, serotonin, phenylbiguanide, and veratridine. This reflex may be activated during myocardial ischemia and reperfusion as a result of increased production of oxygen radicals and by agents used as radiocontrast for coronary angiography. This can contribute to the hypotension that is frequently a stubborn complication of heart disease. Activation of cardiopulmonary chemosensitive receptors may also be part of a defense mechanism protecting individuals from toxic chemical hazards. Activation of cardiopulmonary reflexes may help reduce the amount of inspired pollutants that gets absorbed into the blood, protecting vital organs from potential toxicity of these pollutants, and facilitating their elimination. Finally, the syndrome of cardiac slowing with hypotension (vasovagal syncope) has also been attributed to activation of the Bezold-Jarisch reflex. Vasovagal syncope can occur after prolonged upright posture that results in pooling of blood in the lower extremities and diminished intracardiac blood volume (also

called postural syncope). This phenomenon is exaggerated if combined with dehydration. The resultant arterial hypotension is sensed in the carotid sinus baroreceptors, and afferent fibers from these receptors trigger autonomic signals that increase heart rate and contractility. However, pressure receptors in the wall of the left ventricle respond by sending signals that trigger paradoxical bradycardia and decreased contractility, resulting in sudden marked hypotension. The individual also feels lightheaded and may experience a brief episode of loss of consciousness.

THERAPEUTIC HIGHLIGHTS

The most critical intervention for individuals who experience episodes of neurogenic syncope is to avoid dehydration and to avoid situations that trigger the adverse event. Episodes of syncope may be reduced or prevented by an increased dietary salt intake or administration of mineralocorticoids. Vasovagal syncope has been treated with the use of β-adrenoceptor antagonists and disopyramide, an antiarrhythmic agent that blocks Na^+ channels. Cardiac pacemakers have also been used to stabilize the heart rate during episodes that normally trigger bradycardia.

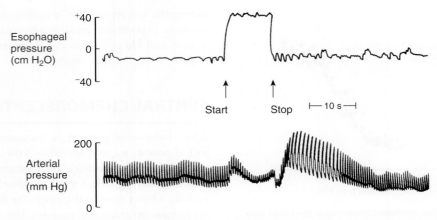

FIGURE 32-4 **Diagram of the response to straining (the Valsalva maneuver) in a healthy man, recorded with a needle in the brachial artery.** Blood pressure rises at the onset of straining because increased intrathoracic pressure is added to the pressure of the blood in the aorta. It then falls because the high intrathoracic pressure compresses veins, decreasing venous return, and cardiac output. (Used with permission from M McIlroy.)

■ LOCAL REGULATION

AUTOREGULATION

The capacity of tissues to regulate their own blood flow is referred to as autoregulation. Most vascular beds have an intrinsic capacity to compensate for moderate changes in perfusion pressure by changes in vascular resistance, so that blood flow remains relatively constant. This capacity is well developed in the kidneys (see Chapter 37), but it has also been observed in the mesentery, skeletal muscle, brain, liver, and myocardium. It is probably due in part to the intrinsic contractile response of smooth muscle to stretch (myogenic theory of autoregulation). As the pressure rises, the blood vessels are distended and the vascular smooth muscle fibers that surround the vessels contract. If it is postulated that the muscle responds to the tension in the vessel wall, this theory could explain the greater degree of contraction at higher pressures; the wall tension is proportional to the distending pressure times the radius of the vessel (law of Laplace; see Chapter 31), and the maintenance of a given wall tension as the pressure rises would require a decrease in radius. Vasodilator substances tend to accumulate in active tissues, and these "metabolites" also contribute to autoregulation (metabolic theory of autoregulation). When blood flow decreases, they accumulate and the vessels dilate; when blood flow increases, they tend to be washed away.

VASODILATOR METABOLITES

The metabolic changes that produce vasodilation include, in most tissues, decreases in O_2 tension and pH. These changes cause relaxation of the arterioles and precapillary sphincters. A local fall in O_2 tension, in particular, can initiate a program of vasodilatory gene expression secondary to production of hypoxia-inducible factor-1α (HIF-1α), a transcription factor with multiple targets. Increases in CO_2 tension and osmolality also dilate the vessels.

The direct dilator action of CO_2 is most pronounced in the skin and brain. The neurally mediated vasoconstrictor effects of systemic as opposed to local hypoxia and hypercapnia have been discussed above. A rise in temperature exerts a direct vasodilator effect, and the temperature rise in active tissues (due to the heat of metabolism) may contribute to the vasodilation. K^+ is another substance that accumulates locally, and has demonstrated dilator activity secondary to the hyperpolarization of vascular smooth muscle cells. Lactate may also contribute to the dilation. In injured tissues, histamine released from damaged cells increases capillary permeability. Thus, it is probably responsible for some of the swelling in areas of inflammation. Adenosine may play a vasodilator role in cardiac muscle but not in skeletal muscle. It also inhibits the release of norepinephrine.

LOCALIZED VASOCONSTRICTION

Injured arteries and arterioles constrict strongly. The constriction appears to be due in part to the local liberation of serotonin from platelets that stick to the vessel wall in the injured area. Injured veins also constrict.

A drop in tissue temperature causes vasoconstriction, and this local response to cold plays a part in temperature regulation (see Chapter 17).

■ SUBSTANCES SECRETED BY THE ENDOTHELIUM

ENDOTHELIAL CELLS

As noted in Chapter 31, the endothelial cells constitute a large and important tissue. They secrete many growth factors and vasoactive substances. The vasoactive substances include prostaglandins and thromboxane, nitric oxide (NO), and endothelin (ET).

PROSTACYCLIN & THROMBOXANE A$_2$

Prostacyclin is produced by endothelial cells and thromboxane A$_2$ by platelets from their common precursor arachidonic acid via the cyclooxygenase pathway. Thromboxane A$_2$ promotes platelet aggregation and vasoconstriction, whereas prostacyclin inhibits platelet aggregation and promotes vasodilation. The balance between platelet thromboxane A$_2$ and prostacyclin fosters localized platelet aggregation and consequent clot formation (see Chapter 31) while preventing excessive extension of the clot and maintaining blood flow around it.

The thromboxane A$_2$–prostacyclin balance can be shifted toward prostacyclin by administration of low doses of aspirin. Aspirin produces irreversible inhibition of cyclooxygenase by acetylating a serine residue in its active site. Obviously, this reduces production of both thromboxane A$_2$ and prostacyclin. However, endothelial cells produce new cyclooxygenase in a matter of hours, whereas platelets cannot manufacture the enzyme, and the level rises only as new platelets enter the circulation. This is a slow process because platelets have a half-life of about 4 days. Therefore, administration of small amounts of aspirin for prolonged periods reduces clot formation and has been shown to be of value in preventing myocardial infarctions, unstable angina, transient ischemic attacks, and stroke.

NITRIC OXIDE

A chance observation led to the discovery that the endothelium plays a key role in vasodilation. Many different stimuli act on endothelial cells to produce endothelium-derived relaxing factor (EDRF), a substance that is now known to be nitric oxide (NO). NO is synthesized from arginine (Figure 32–5) in a reaction catalyzed by nitric oxide synthase (NO synthase, NOS). Three isoforms of NOS have been identified: NOS 1, or neuronal NOS, found in the nervous system; NOS 2, inducible NOS, found in macrophages and other immune cells; and NOS 3, endothelial NOS, found in endothelial cells. NOS 1 and NOS 3 are activated by agents that increase intracellular Ca^{2+}, including the vasodilators acetylcholine and bradykinin. NOS 2 in immune cells is not activated by Ca^{2+} but is induced by cytokines. The NO that is formed in the endothelium diffuses to smooth muscle cells, where it activates soluble guanylyl cyclase, producing cyclic 3,5-guanosine monophosphate (cGMP; see Figure 32–5), which in turn mediates the relaxation of vascular smooth muscle. NO is short-lived and is inactivated by hemoglobin and superoxide.

Adenosine, atrial natriuretic peptide (ANP), and histamine via H$_2$ receptors produce relaxation of vascular smooth muscle that is independent of the endothelium. However, acetylcholine, histamine via H$_1$ receptors, bradykinin, vasoactive intestinal peptide (VIP), substance P, and some other polypeptides act via the endothelium, and various vasoconstrictors that act directly on vascular smooth muscle would produce much greater constriction if their effects were not limited by their ability simultaneously to cause release of NO. When flow to a tissue

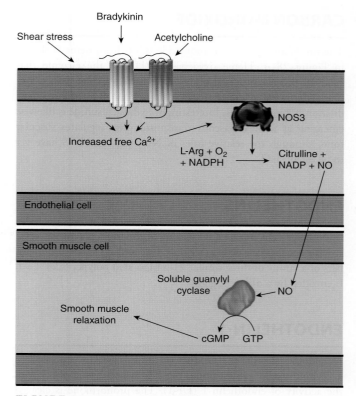

FIGURE 32–5 Endothelial-derived NO leads to smooth muscle relaxation. The endothelial form of nitric oxide synthase (NOS3) is activated by increased free Ca^{2+} and can be induced by a variety of extracellular signals. NOS3 acts on L-arginine, NADPH, and O$_2$ to yield citrulline, NADP, and NO. A variety of cofactors are required for this reaction (not shown). NO can diffuse to adjacent smooth muscle cells where it activates soluble guanylyl cyclase. This leads to the production of cGMP and subsequent smooth muscle relaxation.

is suddenly increased by arteriolar dilation, the large arteries to the tissue also dilate. This flow-induced dilation is due to local release of NO. Products of platelet aggregation also cause release of NO, and the resulting vasodilation helps keep blood vessels with an intact endothelium patent. This is in contrast to injured blood vessels, where the endothelium is damaged at the site of injury and platelets aggregate and produce vasoconstriction (see Chapter 31). Nitroglycerin and other nitrovasodilators that are of great value in the treatment of angina act by stimulating guanylyl cyclase in the same manner as NO. NO is also involved in vascular remodeling and angiogenesis, and may be involved in the pathogenesis of atherosclerosis.

Further evidence for a physiologic role of NO is the observation that mice lacking NOS 3 are hypertensive. This suggests that tonic release of NO is necessary to maintain normal BP.

Penile erection is also produced by release of NO, with consequent vasodilation and engorgement of the corpora cavernosa (see Chapter 23). This accounts for the efficacy of drugs such as phosphodiesterase 5 inhibitors, which slow the breakdown of cGMP.

CARBON MONOXIDE

The production of carbon monoxide (CO) from heme is shown in Figure 28–4. Heme oxygenase-2 (HO-2) the enzyme that catalyzes this reaction is also present in cardiovascular tissues, and there is growing evidence that CO as well as NO produces local dilation of blood vessels. Interestingly, hydrogen sulfide is likewise emerging as a third gaseous transmitter that regulates vascular tone, although the relative roles of NO, CO, and H_2S have yet to be established.

ENDOTHELINS

Endothelial cells produce ET-1, one of the most potent vasoconstrictor agents yet isolated. ET-1, ET-2, and ET-3 are the members of a family of three similar 21-amino-acid polypeptides. Each is encoded by a different gene.

ENDOTHELIN-1

In endothelial cells, the product of the ET gene is processed to a 39-amino-acid prohormone, big ET, which has about 1% of the activity of endothelin-1 (ET-1). The prohormone is cleaved by endothelin-converting enzyme (ECE) to form ET-1. Small amounts of big ET and ET-1 are secreted into the blood, but for the most part, they are secreted locally and act in a paracrine fashion.

Two different ET receptors have been cloned, both of which are coupled via G-proteins to phospholipase C (see Chapter 2). The ET_A receptor, which is specific for ET-1, is found in many tissues and mediates the vasoconstriction produced by ET-1. The ET_B receptor responds to all three ETs, and is coupled to G_i. It may mediate vasodilation, and may mediate the developmental effects of the ETs (see below).

REGULATION OF SECRETION

ET-1 is not stored in secretory granules, and most regulatory factors alter the transcription of its gene, with changes in secretion occurring promptly thereafter. Factors activating and inhibiting the gene are summarized in Table 32–4.

CARDIOVASCULAR FUNCTIONS

As noted above, ET-1 appears primarily to be a paracrine regulator of vascular tone. However, ET-1 is not increased in hypertension, and in mice in which one allele of the ET-1 gene is knocked out, BP is actually elevated rather than reduced. The concentration of circulating ET-1 is elevated in heart failure and after myocardial infarction, so it may play a role in the pathophysiology of these diseases.

TABLE 32–4 Regulation of endothelin-1 secretion via transcription of its gene.

Stimulators	Inhibitors
Angiotensin II	NO
Catecholamines	ANP
Growth factors	PGE_2
Hypoxia	Prostacyclin
Insulin	
Oxidized LDL	
HDL	
Shear stress	
Thrombin	

ANP, atrial natriuretic peptide; HDL, high-density lipoprotein; LDL, low-density lipoprotein; NO, nitric oxide; PGE_2, prostaglandin E_2; VIP, vasoactive intestinal polypeptide.

OTHER FUNCTIONS OF ENDOTHELINS

ET-1 is found in brain, kidneys, and endothelial cells. ET-2 is produced primarily in the kidneys and intestine. ET-3 is present in the blood, the brain, kidneys, and gastrointestinal tract. In the brain, ETs are abundant and, in early life, are produced by both astrocytes and neurons. They are found in the dorsal root ganglia, ventral horn cells, the cortex, the hypothalamus, and cerebellar Purkinje cells. They also play a role in regulating transport across the blood–brain barrier. There are ET receptors on mesangial cells (see Chapter 37), and the polypeptide participates in tubuloglomerular feedback.

Mice that have both alleles of the ET-1 gene deleted have severe craniofacial abnormalities and die of respiratory failure at birth. They also have megacolon (Hirschsprung disease), apparently because the cells that normally form the myenteric plexus fail to migrate to the distal colon (see Chapter 27). In addition, ETs play a role in closing the ductus arteriosus at birth.

■ SYSTEMIC REGULATION BY NEUROHUMORAL AGENTS

Many circulating substances affect the vascular system. The vasodilator regulators include kinins, VIP, and ANP. Circulating vasoconstrictor hormones include vasopressin, norepinephrine, epinephrine, and angiotensin II (Ang II).

KININS

Two related vasodilator peptides called kinins are found in the body, bradykinin and kallidin. Kallidin can be converted to bradykinin by aminopeptidase. Both peptides are metabolized to forms that are active at the type 1 bradykinin receptor by kininase I, a carboxypeptidase that removes the carboxyl terminal arginine (Arg). In addition, the dipeptidylcarboxypeptidase kininase II (also known as angiotensin-converting enzyme (ACE) that converts Ang I to Ang II) inactivates bradykinin and kallidin.

Bradykinin and kallidin are formed from two precursor proteins: high-molecular-weight kininogen and low-molecular-weight kininogen, which are hydrolyzed by proteases called kallikreins to produce the active peptides. There are two types of kallikreins: plasma kallikrein, which circulates in an inactive form, and tissue kallikrein, which appears to be located primarily on the apical membranes of cells concerned with transcellular electrolyte transport. Tissue kallikrein is found in many tissues, including sweat and salivary glands, the pancreas, the prostate, the intestine, and the kidneys. Tissue kallikrein acts on high-molecular-weight kininogen to form bradykinin and low-molecular-weight kininogen to form kallidin. When activated, plasma kallikrein acts on high-molecular-weight kininogen to form bradykinin.

Inactive plasma kallikrein (prekallikrein) is converted to the active form, kallikrein, by active factor XII, the factor that initiates the intrinsic blood clotting cascade. Kallikrein also activates factor XII in a positive feedback loop, and high-molecular-weight kininogen has a factor XII–activating action. This system is normally kept in check by the C1-esterase inhibitor (C1INH), which is a member of the serpin protease family that inhibits several enzymes in the clotting cascade by binding irreversibly to their active sites. The enzyme responsible for converting tissue prekallikrein into tissue kallikrein is not known.

The actions of both kinins resemble those of histamine. They are primarily paracrines, although small amounts are also found in the circulating blood. They cause contraction of visceral smooth muscle, but they relax vascular smooth muscle via NO, lowering BP. They also significantly increase vascular permeability resulting in edema, attract leukocytes, and cause pain upon injection under the skin. They are formed during active secretion in sweat glands, salivary glands, and the exocrine portion of the pancreas, and they are probably responsible for the increase in blood flow when these tissues are actively secreting their products.

Two bradykinin receptors, B1R and B2R, have been identified. Their amino acid residues are 36% identical, and both are coupled to G-proteins. B1 receptor may mediate the pain-producing effects of the kinins, and antagonists have entered clinical trials for the treatment of pain and inflammation. The B2 receptor has strong homology to the H_2 receptor and is found in many different tissues.

NATRIURETIC HORMONES

There is a family of natriuretic peptides involved in vascular regulation, including ANP secreted by the heart, B-type natriuretic peptide (BNP), and C-type natriuretic peptide (CNP). They are released in response to hypervolemia or increase in local pressure. ANP and BNP circulate, whereas CNP acts predominantly in a paracrine fashion. In general, these peptides antagonize the action of various vasoconstrictor agents and lower BP. ANP and BNP also serve to coordinate the control of vascular tone with fluid and electrolyte homeostasis via actions on the distal nephron of the kidney.

CIRCULATING VASOCONSTRICTORS

Vasopressin is a potent vasoconstrictor, but when injected into healthy individuals, there is a compensating decrease in cardiac output, so that there is little change in BP. Its role in BP regulation is discussed in Chapter 17.

Norepinephrine has a generalized vasoconstrictor action, whereas epinephrine dilates the vessels in skeletal muscle and the liver. The relative unimportance of circulating norepinephrine, as opposed to norepinephrine released from vasomotor nerves, is pointed out in Chapter 20, where the cardiovascular actions of catecholamines are discussed in detail.

Ang II is the most important vasoconstrictor in the body. It is formed by the action of ACE on Ang I, which is produced by hydrolysis of angiotensinogen by renin (see Chapter 38). The action of renin is the rate-limiting step in production of Ang II. Renin secretion and Ang II synthesis are increased when BP falls or extracellular fluid (ECF) volume is reduced, and is reduced with high salt diet or hypervolemia. Ang II also increases water intake and stimulates aldosterone secretion (see Chapter 20).

Urotensin-II, a polypeptide first isolated from the spinal cord of fish, is present in human cardiac and vascular tissue. It is one of the most potent mammalian vasoconstrictors known, and is being explored for its role in a large range of different human disease states. For example, levels of both urotensin-II and its receptor have been shown to be elevated in hypertension and heart failure, and may be markers of disease in these and other conditions.

MULTIPLE-CHOICE QUESTIONS

For all questions, select the single best answer unless otherwise directed.

1. A 49-year-old woman was admitted to the hospital after experiencing recurrent episodes of shortness of breath, severe headache, sweating, and abdominal pain. These episodes occurred primarily during physical exertion. Vitals were taken and included a BP recording of 160/95 mm Hg. She underwent a series of exams including imaging studies that showed a tumor on her adrenal medulla (pheochromocytoma). When this tumor suddenly releases a large amount of epinephrine into the circulation, the patient's heart rate would be expected to
   A. increase because the increase in BP stimulates the carotid and aortic baroreceptors.
   B. increase because epinephrine has a direct chronotropic effect on the heart.
   C. increase because of increased tonic vagal nerve activity to the heart.
   D. decrease because the increase in BP reduces activity in the carotid and aortic chemoreceptors.
   E. decrease because of increased vagal activity to the AV node.

2. A 69-year-old man made an appointment with his primary care physician after he began to experience syncope when he got out of bed in the mornings. Vitals at rest were normal for a man at this age and included a BP reading of 135/85 mm Hg. The physician asked him to lie down for a few minutes and then to stand up quickly. Upon standing, his BP was

80/50 mm Hg. The physician said he likely was experiencing episodes of orthostatic hypotension which is not uncommon in individuals over the age of 65 due to dysfunction of the baroreceptor reflex. Where are the arterial baroreceptors located, what are the afferent fibers, and where do the afferent fibers terminate?

A. Atria and pulmonary veins, vagus nerve, and nucleus ambiguus

B. Carotid body and aortic body, glossopharyngeal nerve and vagus nerve, and NTS

C. Carotid sinus and aortic arch, carotid sinus nerve and aortic depressor nerve, and NTS

D. Carotid sinus and atria, glossopharyngeal and vagus nerves, and nucleus ambiguus

E. Carotid body and ventricle, dorsal root fibers, and RVLM

3. A 45-year-old woman had a BP of 155/95 mm Hg when she was sitting in a chair at her clinician's office for a physical. It was her first time to see this clinician and her first physical in over 10 years. She was advised to begin monitoring her BP at home. While at home her systolic BP while seated was usually between 110 and 130 mm Hg and her diastolic pressure was between 75 and 85 mm Hg. Stress-induced activation of which neurons might contribute to the higher BP while in her physician's office?

A. Limbic cortex and NTS

B. Hypothalamus and CVLM

C. NTS and CVLM

D. Hypothalamus and RVLM

E. Limbic cortex and nucleus ambiguus

4. An MD/PhD candidate was studying neurotransmission with central pathways that control sympathetic nerve activity. She was particularly interested in studying the neurotransmitters within this pathway. Which group of neurons within central autonomic pathways release glutamate and which release GABA on their postsynaptic targets?

A. GABA is released by NTS neurons projecting to the RVLM; RVLM neurons release glutamate in the intermediolateral cell column (IML).

B. Glutamate is released by CVLM neurons projecting to the RVLM; RVLM neurons release GABA in the IML.

C. GABA is released by NTS neurons projecting to the nucleus ambiguus; nucleus ambiguus neurons release glutamate in the IML.

D. GABA is released by CVLM neurons projecting to the RVLM; RVLM neurons release glutamate in the IML.

E. Glutamate is released by CVLM neurons projecting to the NTS; NTS neurons release GABA in the RVLM.

5. A 53-year-old woman with chronic lung disease was experiencing difficulty breathing. Her partial pressure of oxygen and carbon dioxide in her arterial blood (PaO_2, $PaCO_2$) were 50 mm Hg and 60 mm Hg, respectively. What is the most potent stimulus of peripheral and central chemoreceptors?

A. Peripheral chemoreceptors are very sensitive to small increases in $PaCO_2$; central chemoreceptors are very sensitive to small decreases in PaO_2.

B. Peripheral chemoreceptors are very sensitive to small decreases in $PaCO_2$; central chemoreceptors are very sensitive to small increases in PaO_2.

C. Peripheral chemoreceptors are very sensitive to small decreases in PaO_2; central chemoreceptors are very sensitive to small increases in $PaCO_2$.

D. Peripheral chemoreceptors are very sensitive to small increases in PaO_2; central chemoreceptors are very sensitive to small decreases in $PaCO_2$.

E. Peripheral chemoreceptors are very sensitive to small decreases in arterial pH; central chemoreceptors are very sensitive to small increases in arterial pH.

6. A 57-year-old man had an acoustic neuroma that initially was associated with the loss of hearing and tinnitus. As the tumor grew larger it compressed the ventrolateral brainstem and he experienced severe hypertension, headaches, facial weakness, vertigo, and unsteady gait due to raised intracranial pressure. Why might an increase in intracranial pressure cause an increase in BP?

A. When intracranial pressure is increased, the blood supply to RVLM neurons is compromised, and the local hypoxia and hypercapnia increase their activity.

B. When intracranial pressure is increased, cortical neurons that project to the RVLM are activated.

C. When intracranial pressure is increased, the blood supply to NTS neurons is compromised, and the local hypoxia and hypercapnia decrease their activity.

D. When intracranial pressure is increased, the blood supply to CVLM neurons is compromised, and the local hypoxia and hypercapnia increase their activity.

7. A neurophysiology professor was demonstrating the role of the baroreceptors in the control of heart rate (measured from an electrocardiogram; R-R interval) to a group of medical students in a human physiology laboratory. BP was measured using a noninvasive approach, and the level of BP was changed by administering varying doses of phenylephrine, an α_1-adrenocepotor agonist to increase BP and varying doses of nitroprusside, a vasodilator, to reduce BP. A graph was drawn depicting the changes in heart rate as a function of systolic BP. What is the likely result when studying systolic BP in the range of 80–160 mm Hg?

A. R-R interval will be highest at 80 mm Hg; it will decrease linearly up to about 150 mm Hg and no further change in R-R interval as pressure increases to 160 mm Hg.

B. R-R interval will be lowest at 80 mm Hg; it will increase linearly between about 120 and 150 mm Hg; and R-R interval will be similar at BP levels of 150 and 160 mm Hg.

C. R-R interval will be lowest at 80 mm Hg and the highest R-R interval will be reached near a systolic pressure of 130 mm Hg because all baroreceptors would be maximally activated by this pressure level.

D. R-R interval will be highest at 80 mm Hg and the lowest R-R interval will be reached near a systolic pressure of 130 mm Hg because all baroreceptors would be maximally activated by this pressure level.

E. R-R interval will similar between a systolic BP of 80 and 100 mm Hg because the threshold for activating baroreceptors is about 100 mm Hg; R-R interval will increase linearly as systolic pressure increases from 100 to 160 mm Hg.

8. A 55-year-old man comes to his primary care clinician complaining of erectile dysfunction. He is given a prescription for a phosphodiesterase 5 inhibitor, and on follow-up, reports that his ability to sustain an erection has been improved markedly by this treatment. The action of which of the following vasoactive mediators would primarily be increased in this patient?

A. Histamine

B. Endothelin-1

C. Prostacyclin
D. cGMP
E. Atrial natriuretic peptide

9. A 60-year-old woman with hypertension is prescribed an angiotensin II (Ang II) receptor blocker or antagonist (ARB), losartan. What changes in BP, renin, and circulating aldosterone would you expect?
   A. Increased BP, reduced renin, increased aldosterone
   B. Decreased BP, reduced renin, increased aldosterone
   C. Increased BP, increased renin, decreased aldosterone
   D. Decreased BP, increased renin, decreased aldosterone

10. A 67-year-old man presents to the ED with severe shortness of breath. Past medical history is significant for heart failure. Physical examination shows bilateral peripheral edema, and crackles on lung auscultation. Laboratory data are significant for elevated ANP. What is the likely cause of the elevated ANP in this patient?
    A. Increased blood volume
    B. Constricted airways
    C. Increased renin levels
    D. Decreased BP
    E. Decreased venous blood volume

11. A 45-year-old woman comes to her family physician for a yearly checkup. Her BP is noted to be the same while lying or while standing. What changes in heart rate, preload, and pulse pressure most likely occur in going from lying to standing positions?
    A. Heart rate decreased; preload decreased; pulse pressure increased
    B. Heart rate increased; preload decreased; pulse pressure decreased
    C. Heart rate increased; preload increased; pulse pressure increased
    D. No change in any variable
    E. Heart rate decreased; preload increased; pulse pressure increased

ANSWERS

1. The best answer is **B.** The binding of epinephrine to the β_1-adrenoceptors in the SA node will increase heart rate. The increase in BP would lead to an increase in baroreceptor nerve activity that would activate vagal nerve activity to the heart and potentially decrease heart rate, but the direct action of epinephrine on the heart would likely overcome the reflex-induced change (rules out options A and C). The increase in BP would not activate the carotid and aortic chemoreceptors; they are activated by reduction in the partial pressure of oxygen in the arterial circulation (rules out option D). An increase in vagal nerve activity to the AV node would reduce conduction velocity through the AV node but would not reduce heart rate (rules out option E).

2. The best answer is **C.** The carotid sinus and aortic arch baroreceptors monitor the arterial circulation. The carotid sinus is a small dilation of the internal carotid artery just above the bifurcation of the common carotid into external and internal carotid branches; baroreceptors are located in this dilation as well as in the wall of the arch of the aorta. The afferent nerve fibers from the carotid sinus form a distinct branch of the glossopharyngeal nerve (carotid sinus nerve). The fibers from the aortic arch form a branch of the vagus nerve (aortic depressor nerve). These afferent fibers terminate in the NTS. Cardiopulmonary receptors are located in the low-pressure part of the circulation within the walls of the right and left atria at the entrance of the superior and inferior venae cavae. They respond primarily to changes in blood volume rather than BP (rules out option A and D). The carotid body and aortic body contain chemoreceptors rather than baroreceptors (rules out options B and E). Baroreceptors, chemoreceptors, or cardiopulmonary receptors terminate in the NTS not the nucleus ambiguus which is the location of cardiac vagal motor neurons (rules out option A and D).

3. The best answer is **D.** A pathway from the cerebral cortex (particularly the limbic cortex) to the RVLM with a relay in the hypothalamus is responsible for the rise in BP rise and tachycardia produced by emotions such as stress, sexual excitement, and anger. Activation of the NTS and CVLM would decrease BP (rules out options A, B, and C). Activation of the nucleus ambiguus decreases heart rate and does not directly affect BP (rules out option E).

4. The best answer is **D.** Neurons in the NTS project to and excite (via release of glutamate) neurons in the CVLM. CVLM neurons are GABA-secreting neurons that project to and inhibit RVLM neurons. The axons of RVLM neurons course dorsally and medially and then descend in the lateral column of the spinal cord to the thoracolumbar IML. They contain phenylethanolamine-N-methyltransferase, but glutamate is the excitatory transmitter they secrete to activate preganglionic sympathetic neurons. NTS neurons also release glutamate in the nucleus ambiguus to excite cardiac vagal preganglionic neurons that release acetylcholine on postganglionic parasympathetic neurons in the heart. This description rules out options A, B, C, and E.

5. The best answer is **C.** Peripheral arterial chemoreceptors in the carotid and aortic bodies have very high rates of blood flow. These receptors are primarily activated by a reduction in PaO_2, but they also respond to an increase in the $PaCO_2$ and pH of the arterial blood. Central chemoreceptors along the surface of the ventrolateral medullary are primarily activated by an increase in the $PaCO_2$ and pH of the arterial blood. This description rules out options A, B, D, and E.

6. The best answer is **A.** Patients with a schwannoma (acoustic neuroma) or meningioma lying close to the RVLM also can have hypertension. As the tumor enlarges it can cause an increase in intracranial pressure that causes compression of the RVLM and a reduced blood supply to RVLM neurons. RVLM neurons are directly activated by hypoxia and hypercapnia. The increase in RVLM neuronal activity increases sympathetic nerve activity and thus BP. Cortical neurons do not directly connect with the RVLM; the pathway from the limbic cortex to the RVLM includes a synapse in the hypothalamus (rules out option B). The NTS is in the dorsomedial not ventrolateral medulla so it would not be directly impacted by the acoustic neuroma (rules out option C). If the blood supply to CVLM neurons were compromised and their activity increased, RVLM neuronal activity would be reduced not increased and hypotension would result (rules out option D).

7. The best answer is **B.** The threshold for activating baroreceptors is about 50 mm Hg (rules out option E), and baroreceptors are maximally activated at a pressure of about

150 mm Hg (rules out option C). Between a systolic pressure of 120 and 150 mm Hg, there is a linear relation between pressure and lowering of the heart rate (longer R-R interval). The heart rate will be highest (R-R interval will be lowest) at 80 mm Hg (rules out options A and D).

8. The best answer is **D**. PDE5 inhibitors reduce hydrolysis of cGMP that leads to sustained effects of its mediators like NO causing sustained engorgement of the corpus cavernous in the penis.

9. The best answer is **D**. ARBs reduce BP but cause an increase in renin. The Ang II produced by the increase in renin is inactive because of the ARB. Because aldosterone is synthesized via Ang II mediated by AT1 receptor, circulating aldosterone would be decreased.

10. The best answer is **A**. Increased blood volume causes an increase in intra-atrial pressure, leading to release of ANP.

11. The best answer is **B**. Initially upon standing preload is reduced, and therefore stroke volume and BP are decreased. Baroreceptor firing increases sympathetic outflow to increase heart rate and vascular tone. Pulse pressure decreases both because systolic pressure is lower when stroke volume is decreased and because baroreceptor response increases diastolic pressure when arterioles are constricted.

Circulation Through Special Regions

- Define the special features of the circulation in the brain, coronary vessels, skin, and fetus.
- Describe how cerebrospinal fluid (CSF) is formed and reabsorbed, and its role in protecting the brain from injury.
- Understand the function of the blood–brain barrier.
- Delineate how the oxygen needs of the contracting myocardium are met by the coronary arteries, and consequences of their occlusion.
- List the vascular reactions of the skin and the reflexes that mediate them.
- Understand how the fetus is supplied with oxygen and nutrients in utero, and the circulatory events required at birth.

INTRODUCTION

The vascular supplies of many organs have special features that are important to their physiology. The portal circulation of the anterior pituitary is discussed in Chapter 18; the pulmonary circulation in Chapter 34; the renal circulation in Chapter 37; and the circulation of the splanchnic area, particularly the intestines and liver, in Chapters 25 and 28. This chapter is concerned with the special circulations of the brain, the heart, and the skin, as well as the placenta and fetus.

■ CEREBRAL CIRCULATION: ANATOMIC CONSIDERATIONS

VESSELS

The principal arterial inflow to the brain in humans is via two internal carotid arteries and two vertebral arteries, with the carotid arteries quantitatively the most significant. The vertebral arteries unite to form the basilar artery, and the basilar artery and the carotids form the **circle of Willis** below the hypothalamus. The circle of Willis is the origin of the six large vessels supplying the cerebral cortex. Substances injected into one carotid artery are distributed almost exclusively to the cerebral hemisphere on that side. Occlusion of one carotid artery, particularly in older patients, often causes serious symptoms of cerebral ischemia. Venous drainage from the brain by way of the deep veins and dural sinuses empties principally into the internal jugular veins.

The cerebral vessels have a number of unique anatomic features. In the choroid plexuses, there are gaps between the capillary endothelial cells, but the choroid epithelial cells that separate them from the cerebrospinal fluid (CSF) are connected to one another by tight junctions. The capillaries in the brain substance resemble nonfenestrated capillaries in muscle, but tight junctions between the endothelial cells limit the passage of substances via the paracellular route. In addition, there is little vesicular transport. However, multiple transport systems are present. The brain capillaries are also surrounded by the endfeet of astrocytes that are closely applied to the basal lamina of the capillaries, but with gaps of about 20 nm between endfeet.

INNERVATION

Three systems of nerves innervate the cerebral blood vessels. Postganglionic sympathetic neurons have their cell bodies in the superior cervical ganglia, and their endings contain norepinephrine. Many also contain neuropeptide Y. Cholinergic neurons also innervate the cerebral vessels. Many also contain vasoactive intestinal peptide (VIP) and peptide histidyl methionine (PHM-27). These nerves end primarily on large arteries. Sensory nerves are found on more distal arteries. They have their cell bodies in the trigeminal ganglia and contain substance P, neurokinin A, and calcitonin gene-related peptide (CGRP). Substance P, CGRP, VIP, and PHM-27 cause vasodilation, whereas neuropeptide Y is a vasoconstrictor.

■ CEREBROSPINAL FLUID

FORMATION & ABSORPTION

CSF fills the ventricles and subarachnoid space. In humans, the volume of CSF is about 150 mL and the rate of CSF production is about 550 mL/day. It has been estimated that 50–70% of the CSF is formed in the choroid plexuses and the remainder is formed around blood vessels and along ventricular walls. The CSF in the ventricles flows through the foramens of Magendie and Luschka to the subarachnoid space and is absorbed through the **arachnoid villi** into veins. Another important route for CSF reabsorption into the bloodstream is via the cribriform plate above the nose and thence into the cervical lymphatics. However, reabsorption via the arachnoid villi may assume a greater role if CSF pressure is elevated. Likewise, when CSF builds up abnormally, aquaporin water channels may be expressed in the choroid plexus and brain microvessels to compensate.

CSF is formed continuously in two stages. First, plasma is passively filtered across the choroidal capillary endothelium. Next, secretion of water and ions across the choroidal epithelium provides for active control of CSF composition and quantity. Bicarbonate, chloride, and potassium ions enter the CSF via channels in the epithelial cell apical membranes. Aquaporins provide for water movement to balance osmotic gradients. The composition of CSF is essentially the same as that of brain extracellular fluid (ECF), which makes up 15% of the brain volume. In adults, free communication appears to take place between the brain interstitial fluid and CSF.

Lumbar CSF pressure is normally 70–180 mm H_2O. Up to pressures well above this range, the rate of CSF formation is independent of intraventricular pressure. However, absorption is proportional to the pressure. At a pressure of 112 mm H_2O, which is the average normal CSF pressure, filtration and absorption are equal. Below a pressure of approximately 68 mm H_2O, absorption stops. Large amounts of fluid accumulate when the capacity for CSF reabsorption is decreased (**external hydrocephalus**). Fluid also accumulates proximal to the block and distends the ventricles when the foramens of Luschka and Magendie are blocked or there is obstruction within the ventricular system (**internal hydrocephalus**).

PROTECTIVE FUNCTION

The most critical role for CSF (and the meninges) is to protect the brain. The dura is attached firmly to bone. Normally, there is no "subdural space," with the arachnoid being held to the dura by the surface tension of the thin layer of fluid between the two membranes. The brain itself is supported within the arachnoid by the blood vessels and nerve roots and by the multiple fine fibrous **arachnoid trabeculae.** The buoyancy of the brain in the CSF permits its relatively flimsy attachments to suspend it very effectively. When the head receives a blow, the arachnoid slides on the dura and the brain moves, but its motion is gently checked by the CSF cushion and by the arachnoid trabeculae.

The pain produced by spinal fluid deficiency illustrates the importance of CSF in supporting the brain. Removal of CSF during lumbar puncture can cause a severe headache. The pain can be relieved by intrathecal injection of sterile isotonic saline.

HEAD INJURIES

Without the protection of the spinal fluid and the meninges, the brain would probably be unable to withstand even minor traumas; but with this protection, it takes a fairly severe blow to produce cerebral damage. The brain is damaged most commonly when the skull is fractured and bone is driven into neural tissue (depressed skull fracture), when the brain moves far enough to tear the delicate bridging veins from the cortex to the bone, or when the brain is accelerated by a blow on the head and is driven against the skull opposite where the blow was struck (**contrecoup injury**).

■ THE BLOOD–BRAIN BARRIER

The tight junctions between capillary endothelial cells in the brain and between the epithelial cells in the choroid plexus prevent proteins from entering the brain in adults and slow the penetration of some smaller molecules. This uniquely limited exchange of substances into the brain is referred to as the **blood–brain barrier.**

PENETRATION OF SUBSTANCES INTO THE BRAIN

Water, CO_2, and O_2 penetrate the brain with ease, as do the lipid-soluble free forms of steroid hormones, whereas proteins and polypeptides do not. The passive penetration of CO_2 contrasts with the regulated transcellular penetration of H^+ and HCO_3^- and has physiologic significance in the regulation of respiration.

Glucose is the major source of energy for nerve cells. Its transport into the CSF is markedly enhanced by the presence of specific transporters, including the glucose transporter 1 (GLUT1). Infants with congenital GLUT1 deficiency have low CSF glucose concentrations in the presence of normal plasma glucose, and they have seizures and delayed development. Transporters for thyroid hormones; several organic acids; choline; nucleic acid precursors;

and neutral, basic, and acidic amino acids are present at the blood–brain barrier.

Some drugs and peptides cross the cerebral capillaries but are promptly transported back into the blood by a multidrug nonspecific **P-glycoprotein** transporter in the apical membranes of the endothelial cells. In the absence of this transporter in mice, larger proportions of systemically administered doses of various drugs are found in the brain than in controls. Pharmacologic agents inhibiting this transporter could be of value in the treatment of central nervous system (CNS) diseases by ensuring adequate accumulation of therapeutic agents in the brain.

CIRCUMVENTRICULAR ORGANS

Four small areas in or near the brainstem are permeable to polypeptides: (1) the **posterior pituitary** (neurohypophysis) and the adjacent ventral part of the **median eminence** of the hypothalamus, (2) the **area postrema**, (3) the **organum vasculosum of the lamina terminalis (OVLT,** supraoptic crest), and (4) the **subfornical organ (SFO).**

These areas are referred to as the **circumventricular organs**. All have fenestrated capillaries, and are said to be "outside the blood–brain barrier." Some of them function as **neurohemal organs;** where polypeptides secreted by neurons enter the circulation. Others function as chemoreceptor zones such that circulating substances can trigger changes in brain function without penetrating the blood–brain barrier. For example, the area postrema initiates vomiting in response to chemical changes in the plasma. It is also concerned with cardiovascular control—circulating angiotensin II acts here to produce a neurally mediated increase in blood pressure. Angiotensin II also acts on the SFO and possibly on the OVLT to increase water intake. The OVLT is the site of the osmoreceptor controlling vasopressin secretion, and interleukin-1 (IL-1) produces fever by acting here too.

FUNCTION OF THE BLOOD–BRAIN BARRIER

The blood–brain barrier strives to maintain the constancy of the environment of the neurons in the CNS (Clinical Box 33–1). The constancy of the composition of the ECF in all parts of the body is maintained by multiple homeostatic mechanisms, but because of the sensitivity of the cortical neurons to ionic change, it is not surprising that an additional defense has evolved to protect them. Other functions of the blood–brain barrier include protection of the brain from toxins in the blood and prevention of the escape of neurotransmitters into the general circulation.

DEVELOPMENT OF THE BLOOD–BRAIN BARRIER

The blood–brain barrier is immature at birth. For example, in severely jaundiced infants with high plasma levels of free bilirubin, this substance enters the brain and can damage the basal ganglia (**kernicterus).**

■ CEREBRAL BLOOD FLOW & ITS REGULATION

KETY METHOD

According to **Fick's principle** (see Chapter 30), the blood flow of any organ can be measured by determining the amount of a given substance (Q_x) removed from the bloodstream by the organ per unit of time and dividing that value by the difference between the concentration of the substance in arterial blood and the concentration in the venous blood from the organ ($[A_x] - [V_x]$). Thus:

$$\text{Cerebral blood flow (CBF)} = \frac{Q_x}{[A_x] - [V_x]}$$

This can be applied clinically using inhaled nitrous oxide (N_2O) (**Kety's method**). The average cerebral blood flow in young adults is 54 mL/100 g/min. Note that the Kety method gives no information about regional differences in blood flow. It also can only measure flow to perfused parts of the brain. In spite of the marked local fluctuations in brain blood flow with neural activity, the cerebral circulation is regulated in such a way that total blood flow remains relatively constant. The factors involved in regulating the flow are summarized in Figure 33–1.

ROLE OF INTRACRANIAL PRESSURE

In adults, the brain is encased in a rigid enclosure. The cranial cavity normally contains a brain weighing approximately 1400 g, 75 mL of blood, and 75 mL of spinal fluid. Because brain tissue and spinal fluid are essentially incompressible, the volume of blood, spinal fluid, and brain in the cranium at any time must be relatively constant. The cerebral vessels are compressed whenever

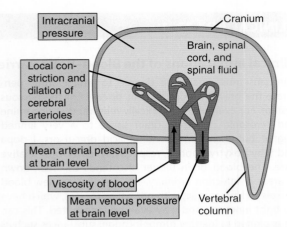

FIGURE 33–1 Diagrammatic summary of the factors affecting overall cerebral blood flow.

the intracranial pressure rises. Any change in venous pressure causes a similar change in intracranial pressure. Thus, a rise in venous pressure decreases cerebral blood flow both by decreasing the effective perfusion pressure and by compressing the cerebral vessels. This relationship helps compensate for changes in arterial blood pressure at the level of the head. For example, if the body is accelerated upward (positive *g*), blood moves toward the feet and arterial pressure at the level of the head decreases. However, venous pressure also falls and intracranial pressure falls, so that the pressure on the vessels decreases and blood flow is less severely compromised. Conversely, during acceleration downward, force acting toward the head (negative *g*) increases arterial pressure at head level, but intracranial pressure also rises, so that the vessels are supported and do not rupture.

ROLE OF VASOMOTOR & SENSORY NERVES

In addition to direct effects, nerves may modulate the tone of cerebral vessels indirectly, via release of paracrine substances from astrocytes. The precise role of these nerves, however, remains a matter of debate. Noradrenergic discharge occurs when the blood pressure is markedly elevated, reducing the passive increase in blood flow and helping to protect the blood–brain barrier from disruption. With sympathetic stimulation, greater increases in pressure can occur without an increase in flow. Finally, neurovascular coupling may adjust local perfusion in response to changes in brain activity (see below).

BLOOD FLOW IN VARIOUS PARTS OF THE BRAIN

Positron emission tomography (PET) can be used to determine regional blood flow in conscious humans. Because blood flow is tightly coupled to brain metabolism, local uptake of 2-deoxyglucose is also a good index of blood flow. Another valuable technique involves magnetic resonance imaging (MRI). **Functional magnetic resonance imaging (fMRI)** measures the amount of oxygenated

CLINICAL BOX 33-2

Changes in Cerebral Blood Flow in Disease

Several disease states are known to be associated with localized or general changes in cerebral blood flow. For example, epileptic foci are hyperemic during seizures, whereas flow is reduced in other parts of the brain. Parietooccipital flow is decreased in patients with symptoms of agnosia. In Alzheimer disease, the earliest change is decreased metabolism and blood flow in the superior parietal cortex, with later spread to the temporal lobe and finally the frontal cortex. In Huntington disease, blood flow is reduced bilaterally in the caudate nucleus early in the disease. In manic depressives there is a general decrease in cortical blood flow when the patients are depressed. In schizophrenia, some evidence suggests decreased blood flow in the frontal lobes, temporal lobes, and basal ganglia. Finally, during the aura in patients with migraine, a bilateral decrease in blood flow starts in the occipital cortex and spreads anteriorly to the temporal and parietal lobes.

blood in a tissue area. When neurons become active, their increased discharge triggers an increase in local blood flow and oxygen. PET scanning can be used to measure not only blood flow but the concentration of molecules, such as dopamine, in various regions of the living brain. On the other hand, fMRI does not involve the use of radioactivity. Consequently, it can be used at frequent intervals to measure changes in regional blood flow in a single individual.

In resting humans, the average blood flow in gray matter is 69 mL/100 g/min compared with 28 mL/100 g/min in white matter. At rest, blood flow is greatest in the premotor and frontal regions. During voluntary clenching of the right hand, flow is increased in the hand area of the left motor cortex and the corresponding sensory areas in the postcentral gyrus. When persons talk, there is a bilateral increase in blood flow in the face, tongue, and mouth-sensory and motor areas and the upper premotor cortex in the categorical (usually the left) hemisphere. Reading produces widespread increases in blood flow. Problem solving, reasoning, and motor ideation without movement produce increases in selected areas of the premotor and frontal cortex. In anticipation of a cognitive task, many of the brain areas that will be activated during the task are activated beforehand, as if the brain produces an internal model of the expected task. Blood flow also changes during diseases (**Clinical Box 33–2**).

■ BRAIN METABOLISM & OXYGEN REQUIREMENTS

OXYGEN CONSUMPTION

O_2 consumption by the human brain (cerebral metabolic rate for O_2, CMRO$_2$) averages approximately 20% of the total body resting O_2 consumption. The brain is extremely sensitive to hypoxia, and occlusion of its blood supply produces unconsciousness in a

CLINICAL BOX 33-3

Stroke

When the blood supply to a part of the brain is interrupted, ischemia damages or kills the cells in the area, producing the signs and symptoms of a stroke. There are two general types of strokes: hemorrhagic and ischemic. Hemorrhagic stroke occurs when a cerebral artery or arteriole ruptures, sometimes but not always at the site of a small aneurysm. Ischemic stroke occurs when flow in a vessel is compromised. Thrombi may pass to the brain as emboli where they then lodge and interrupt flow. In the past, little could be done to modify the course of a stroke and its consequences. However, it has become clear that in the penumbra, the area surrounding the most severe brain damage, ischemia reduces glutamate uptake by astrocytes, and the increase in local glutamate causes excitotoxic damage to neurons (see Chapter 7).

THERAPEUTIC HIGHLIGHTS

The clot-lysing drug, tissue-type plasminogen activator (t-PA) (see Chapter 31) is of great benefit in ischemic strokes. In animals, drugs that prevent excitotoxic damage can reduce the effects of strokes. t-PA and presumably antiexcitotoxic treatment must be given early in the course of a stroke to be of maximum benefit. This is why stroke has become a condition in which rapid diagnosis and treatment are extremely important. In addition, of course, it is important to determine if a stroke is thrombotic or hemorrhagic.

period as short as 10 s. The vegetative structures in the brainstem are more resistant to hypoxia than the cerebral cortex, and patients may recover from accidents causing fairly prolonged hypoxia with normal vegetative functions but permanent intellectual deficiencies. The basal ganglia use O_2 at a very high rate, and symptoms of Parkinson disease as well as intellectual deficits can be produced by chronic hypoxia. The thalamus and the inferior colliculus are also very susceptible to hypoxic damage (Clinical Box 33–3).

ENERGY SOURCES

Glucose is the major source of energy for the brain; under normal conditions, 90% of the energy needed to maintain ion gradients across cell membranes and transmit electrical impulses comes from this source. Glucose enters the brain via GLUT1 in cerebral capillaries (see above). Other transporters then distribute it to neurons and glial cells.

Glucose is taken up from the blood in large amounts, and the RQ (respiratory quotient; see Chapter 26) of cerebral tissue is 0.95–0.99. Importantly, insulin is not required for most cerebral cells to utilize glucose. In general, glucose utilization at rest parallels blood

flow and O_2 consumption. This does not mean that the source of energy is always glucose. During prolonged starvation, appreciable utilization of other substances occurs. The consequences of hypoglycemia in terms of neural function are discussed in Chapter 24.

GLUTAMATE & AMMONIA REMOVAL

The brain's uptake of glutamate is approximately balanced by its output of glutamine. Glutamate entering the brain associates with ammonia and leaves as glutamine. The glutamate–glutamine conversion in the brain—the opposite of the reaction in the kidney that produces some of the ammonia entering the tubules—serves as a detoxifying mechanism to keep the brain free of ammonia, which is very toxic to nerve cells.

■ CORONARY CIRCULATION

ANATOMIC CONSIDERATIONS

The two coronary arteries that supply the myocardium arise from the sinuses behind two of the cusps of the aortic valve at the root of the aorta. The valves are patent throughout the cardiac cycle. Most of the venous blood returns to the heart through the coronary sinus and anterior cardiac veins (**Figure 33–2**), which drain into the right atrium. In addition, there are **arteriosinusoidal vessels,** sinusoidal capillary-like vessels that connect arterioles to the chambers; **thebesian veins** that connect capillaries to the chambers; and a few **arterioluminal vessels** that are small arteries draining directly into the chambers. A few anastomoses occur between coronary arterioles and extracardiac arterioles. These channels enlarge and increase in number in patients with coronary artery disease.

PRESSURE GRADIENTS & FLOW IN THE CORONARY VESSELS

The heart compresses its blood vessels when it contracts. The pressure inside the left ventricle is slightly higher than in the aorta during systole. Consequently, flow occurs in the arteries

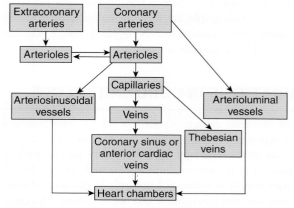

FIGURE 33–2 **Diagram of the coronary circulation.**

supplying the subendocardial portion of the left ventricle only during diastole, although the force is sufficiently dissipated in the more superficial portions to permit some flow throughout the cardiac cycle. Because diastole is shorter when the heart rate is high, left ventricular coronary flow is reduced during tachycardia. On the other hand, the pressure differential between the aorta and the right ventricle, and the differential between the aorta and the atria, are somewhat greater during systole than during diastole. Consequently, coronary flow in those parts of the heart is not appreciably reduced during systole. Because no blood flow occurs during systole in the subendocardial portion of the left ventricle, this region is prone to ischemic damage and is the most common site of myocardial infarction. Blood flow to the left ventricle is decreased in patients with stenotic aortic valves. These patients are particularly prone to develop symptoms of myocardial ischemia, in part because of compression and in part because the myocardium requires more O_2 to expel blood through the stenotic aortic valve. Coronary flow is also decreased when the aortic diastolic pressure is low. The rise in venous pressure in conditions such as heart failure reduces coronary flow because it decreases effective coronary perfusion pressure (Clinical Box 33–4).

Coronary blood flow has been measured by inserting a catheter into the coronary sinus and applying the Kety method to the heart on the assumption that the N_2O content of coronary venous blood is typical of the entire myocardial effluent. Coronary flow at rest in humans is about 250 mL/min (5% of the cardiac output). Techniques utilizing **radionuclides** have been used to study regional blood flow in the heart and to detect areas of ischemia and infarct. Radionuclides such as thallium-201 (^{201}Tl) are pumped into cardiac muscle cells by Na, K ATPase and equilibrate with the intracellular K^+ pool. For the first 10–15 min after intravenous injection, ^{201}Tl distribution is directly proportional to myocardial blood flow, and areas of ischemia can be detected by their low uptake. The uptake of this isotope is often determined soon after exercise and again several hours later to bring out areas in which exertion leads to compromised flow. Conversely, radiopharmaceuticals such as technetium-99m stannous pyrophosphate (^{99m}Tc-PYP) are selectively taken up by infarcted tissue and make infarcts stand out as "hot spots" on scintigrams of the chest. Coronary angiography can be combined with measurement of ^{133}Xe washout to provide detailed analysis of coronary blood flow. Radiopaque contrast medium is first injected into the coronary arteries, and radiographs are used to outline their distribution. The angiographic camera is then replaced with a scintillation camera, and ^{133}Xe washout is measured.

VARIATIONS IN CORONARY FLOW

At rest, the heart extracts 70–80% of the O_2 from each unit of blood delivered to it. O_2 delivery can only be increased significantly by increasing blood flow. Blood flow increases when the metabolism of the myocardium is increased. The caliber of the coronary vessels is influenced not only by pressure changes in the aorta but also by chemical and neural factors. The coronary circulation also shows considerable autoregulation.

CHEMICAL FACTORS

The close relationship between coronary blood flow and myocardial O_2 consumption indicates that one or more of the products of metabolism cause coronary vasodilation. Factors suspected of playing this role include a lack of O_2 and increased local concentrations of CO_2, H^+, K^+, lactate, prostaglandins, adenine nucleotides, and adenosine. Likely several or all of these act in an integrated fashion, redundant fashion, or both. Asphyxia, hypoxia, and intracoronary injections of cyanide increase coronary blood flow 200–300% in denervated as well as intact hearts. A similar increase in flow is produced in the area supplied by a coronary artery if the artery is occluded and then released. This **reactive hyperemia** is likely due to release of adenosine.

NEURAL FACTORS

The coronary arterioles contain α-adrenergic receptors, which mediate vasoconstriction, and β-adrenergic receptors, which mediate vasodilation. Noradrenergic nerve activity and injections of norepinephrine cause coronary vasodilation. However, norepinephrine increases the heart rate and the force of cardiac contraction, and the vasodilation is due to production of vasodilator metabolites in the myocardium. When the inotropic and chronotropic effects of noradrenergic discharge are blocked by a β-adrenergic blocking drug, norepinephrine elicits coronary vasoconstriction. Thus, the direct effect of noradrenergic stimulation is constriction of the coronary vessels. On the other hand, stimulation of vagal fibers dilates the coronaries.

When the systemic blood pressure falls, the reflex increase in noradrenergic discharge increases coronary blood flow secondary to the metabolic changes in the myocardium at a time when the cutaneous, renal, and splanchnic vessels are constricted. In this way the circulation of the heart, like that of the brain, is preserved when flow to other organs is compromised.

■ CUTANEOUS CIRCULATION

The amount of heat lost from the body is regulated to a large extent by varying the amount of blood flowing through the skin. The fingers, toes, palms, and earlobes contain well-innervated arteriovenous anastomoses. Thermoregulatory stimuli can vary blood flow from 1 to as much as 150 mL/100 g of skin/min.

WHITE REACTION

When a pointed object is drawn lightly over the skin, the stroke lines become pale (**white reaction**). The mechanical stimulus apparently initiates contraction of the precapillary sphincters, and blood drains out of the capillaries and small veins. The response appears in about 15 s.

TRIPLE RESPONSE

When the skin is stroked more firmly with a pointed instrument, instead of the white reaction there is reddening that appears in about 10 s (**red reaction**). This is followed in a few minutes by local swelling and diffuse, mottled reddening around the injury. The initial redness is due to capillary dilation, a direct response of the capillaries to pressure. The swelling (**wheal**) is local edema due to increased permeability of the capillaries and venules. The redness spreading out from the injury (**flare**) is due to arteriolar dilation. This three-part response—red reaction, wheal, and flare—is called the **triple response** and is part of the normal reaction to injury that persists after total sympathectomy. The flare is due to an **axon reflex,** a response in which impulses initiated in sensory nerves by the injury are relayed antidromically down other branches of the sensory nerve fibers. The transmitter released at the central termination of the sensory C fiber neurons is substance P, and substance P and CGRP are present in all parts of the neurons. Both dilate arterioles and, in addition, substance P causes extravasation of fluid.

REACTIVE HYPEREMIA

Reactive hyperemia is the increase in the amount of blood in a region when its circulation is reestablished after a period of occlusion, which occurs in many organs. When the blood supply to a limb is occluded, the cutaneous arterioles below the occlusion dilate. When the circulation is reestablished, blood flowing into the dilated vessels makes the skin become fiery red. The arteriolar dilation is apparently due to a local effect of hypoxia.

GENERALIZED RESPONSES

Noradrenergic nerve stimulation and circulating epinephrine and norepinephrine constrict cutaneous blood vessels. No known vasodilator nerve fibers extend to the cutaneous vessels, and thus vasodilation is brought about by a decrease in constrictor tone as well as the local production of vasodilator metabolites. Skin color and temperature also depend on the state of the capillaries and venules. A cold blue or gray skin is one in which the arterioles are constricted and the capillaries dilated; a warm red skin is one in which both are dilated.

Because painful stimuli cause diffuse noradrenergic discharge, a painful injury causes generalized cutaneous vasoconstriction in addition to the local triple response. When the body temperature rises during exercise, the cutaneous blood vessels dilate in spite of continuing noradrenergic discharge in other parts of the body. Dilation of cutaneous vessels in response to a rise in hypothalamic temperature overcomes other reflex activity. Cold causes cutaneous vasoconstriction; however, with severe cold, superficial vasodilation may supervene. Shock is more profound in patients with elevated temperatures because of cutaneous vasodilation, and patients in shock should not be warmed to the point that their body temperature rises.

■ PLACENTAL & FETAL CIRCULATION

UTERINE CIRCULATION

The blood flow of the uterus parallels its metabolic activity and undergoes cyclic fluctuations that correlate with the menstrual cycle. The function of the spiral and basilar arteries of the endometrium in menstruation is discussed in Chapter 22. During pregnancy, blood flow increases rapidly as the uterus increases in size. Vasodilator metabolites are undoubtedly produced in the uterus, as they are in other active tissues. In early pregnancy, estrogens act on the blood vessels to increase uterine blood flow in excess of tissue O_2 needs. However, even though uterine blood flow increases 20-fold during pregnancy, the size of the conceptus increases much more. Consequently, more O_2 is extracted from the uterine blood during the latter part of pregnancy, and the O_2 saturation of uterine blood falls. Corticotrophin-releasing hormone appears to play an important role in upregulating uterine blood flow.

PLACENTA

The placenta is the "fetal lung" **(Figures 33–3** and **33–4)**. Its maternal portion is in effect a large blood sinus. Into this "lake" project the villi of the fetal portion containing the small branches

of the fetal umbilical arteries and vein (Figure 33–3). O_2 is taken up by the fetal blood and CO_2 is discharged into the maternal circulation across the walls of the villi. The placenta is also the route by which all nutritive materials enter the fetus and by which fetal wastes are discharged to the maternal blood.

FETAL CIRCULATION

The arrangement of the circulation in the fetus is shown diagrammatically in Figure 33–4. Fifty-five percent of the fetal cardiac output goes through the placenta. The blood in the

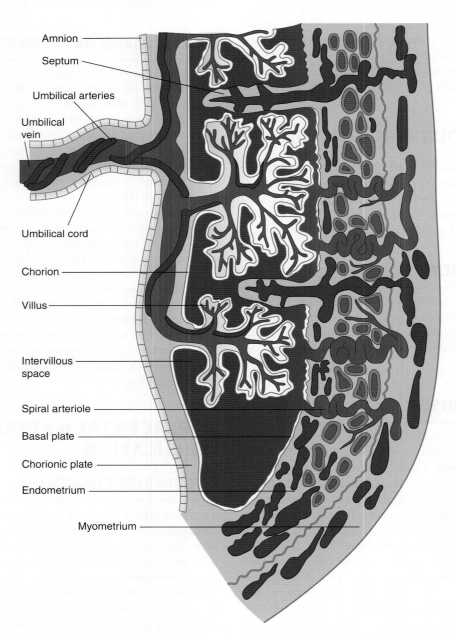

Amnion

Septum

Umbilical arteries

Umbilical vein

Umbilical cord

Chorion

Villus

Intervillous space

Spiral arteriole

Basal plate

Chorionic plate

Endometrium

Myometrium

FIGURE 33–3 Diagram of a section through the human placenta, showing the way the fetal villi project into the maternal sinuses.

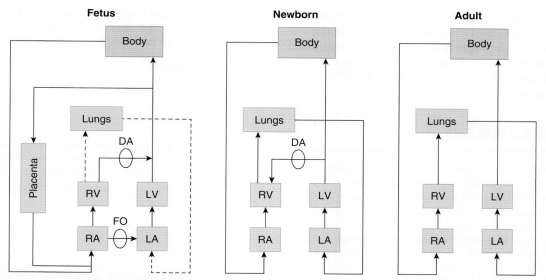

FIGURE 33–4 Diagram of the circulation in the fetus, the newborn infant, and the adult. DA, ductus arteriosus; FO, foramen ovale; LA, left atrium; LV, left ventricle; RA, right atrium; RV, right ventricle. Note that circulation to the fetal liver is not shown for simplicity.

umbilical vein in humans is believed to be about 80% saturated with O_2, compared with 98% saturation in the arterial circulation of the adult. The ductus venosus diverts some of this blood directly to the inferior vena cava, and the remainder mixes with the portal blood of the fetus. The portal and systemic venous blood of the fetus is only 26% saturated, and the saturation of the mixed blood in the inferior vena cava is approximately 67%. Most of the blood entering the heart through the inferior vena cava is diverted directly to the left atrium via the patent foramen ovale. Most of the blood from the superior vena cava enters the right ventricle and is expelled into the pulmonary artery. The resistance of the collapsed lungs is high, and the pressure in the pulmonary artery is several mm Hg higher than it is in the aorta, so that most of the blood in the pulmonary artery passes through the **ductus arteriosus** to the aorta. In this fashion, the relatively unsaturated blood from the right ventricle is diverted to the trunk and lower body of the fetus, while the head of the fetus receives the better-oxygenated blood from the left ventricle. From the aorta, some of the blood is pumped into the umbilical arteries and back to the placenta. The O_2 saturation of the blood in the lower aorta and umbilical arteries of the fetus is approximately 60%.

FETAL RESPIRATION

The tissues of fetal and newborn mammals have a remarkable resistance to hypoxia. However, the O_2 saturation of the maternal blood in the placenta is so low that the fetus might suffer hypoxic damage if fetal red cells did not have a greater O_2 affinity than adult red cells. The fetal red cells contain fetal hemoglobin (hemoglobin F), whereas the adult cells contain adult hemoglobin (hemoglobin A).

CHANGES IN FETAL CIRCULATION & RESPIRATION AT BIRTH

Because of the patent ductus arteriosus and foramen ovale (Figure 33–4), the left heart and right heart pump in parallel in the fetus. At birth, the circulation has to change rapidly from a parallel to a serial system and from placental to pulmonary gas exchange. The essential element initiating the changes is the fall in the pulmonary vascular resistance when the lungs are first filled with a gas. The pulmonary vascular resistance falls to less than 20% of the value in utero after the lungs are expanded by the first few breaths.

The stimulus for the baby to initiate breathing after birth is not fully understood. It is likely that the sudden exposure to light, sound, cold air, and other tactile stimuli are the most important triggers. Oxygen is a strong vasodilator of the pulmonary vascular tree, operating through the production of nitric oxide (NO). The high arterial oxygen tension and bradykinin, which is released from the lungs during their initial inflation, are vasoconstrictors for the umbilical arteries and ductus arteriosus.

Blood returning from the lungs raises the pressure in the left atrium, closing the foramen ovale. The ductus arteriosus constricts and this, together with the fall in pulmonary vascular resistance, directs most of the output of the right ventricle through the lungs. The ductus arteriosus is functionally closed within a few hours of birth and permanent anatomic closure follows in the next 24–48 h. In addition, relatively high concentrations of vasodilators are present in the ductus in utero—especially prostaglandin $F_{2\alpha}$—and synthesis of this prostaglandin is blocked at birth.

After established pulmonary respiration, highly oxygenated blood containing pulmonary bradykinin reaches the umbilical arteries, initiating constriction. Further constriction is also stimulated by cold and handling of the cord and the arteries are completely constricted within 3–5 min. Venous flow continues as a result of the increased placental pressure within the contracted uterus and the negative intrathoracic pressure of the baby's respiratory efforts. Within 5 min, flow ceases within the umbilical cord and there is little residual blood remaining within the placenta.

CHAPTER SUMMARY

- CSF is produced predominantly in the choroid plexus of the brain. Fluid is reabsorbed into the bloodstream to maintain appropriate pressure in the setting of continuous production.

- The permeation of circulating substances into the brain is tightly controlled. Water, CO_2, and O_2 permeate freely. Other substances (such as glucose) require specific transport mechanisms, whereas entry of macromolecules is negligible. The effectiveness of the blood–brain barrier in preventing entry of xenobiotics is bolstered by active efflux.

- The coronary circulation supplies oxygen to the contracting myocardium. Metabolic products and neural input induce vasodilation as needed. Blockage of coronary arteries may lead to irreversible injury to heart tissue.

- Control of cutaneous blood flow is a key facet of temperature regulation, and is underpinned by shunting through arteriovenous anastomoses. Hypoxia, axon reflexes, and sympathetic input are all important determinants of flow through the cutaneous vasculature.

- The fetal circulation cooperates with that of the placenta and uterus to deliver oxygen and nutrients to the growing fetus, as well as carrying away waste products. Unique anatomic features of the fetal circulation as well as biochemical properties of fetal hemoglobin serve to ensure adequate O_2 supply. At birth, the foramen ovale and the ductus arteriosus close such that the neonatal lungs now serve as the site for oxygen exchange.

MULTIPLE-CHOICE QUESTIONS

For all questions, select the single best answer unless otherwise directed.

1. A scientist uses the model of a pregnant sheep to understand how oxygen is delivered from the mother to the developing fetus. She measures Po_2 in various vessels of the maternal–fetal circulation. Which of the following blood vessels would be expected to have the lowest Po_2 value?
   A. Maternal artery
   B. Maternal uterine vein
   C. Maternal femoral vein
   D. Umbilical artery
   E. Umbilical vein

2. The pressure differential between the heart and the aorta is least in the
   A. left ventricle during systole.
   B. left ventricle during diastole.
   C. right ventricle during systole.
   D. right ventricle during diastole.
   E. left atrium during systole.

3. A scientist injects a rat intravenously with Evans blue, a dye that binds to serum albumin, then euthanizes the animal 1 h later. When she examines sections of the brain, where would blue staining be expected?
   A. Medulla
   B. Area postrema
   C. Motor area
   D. Parietal lobe
   E. Thalamus

4. Using Fick's principle, a physiology student measures blood flow to various tissues and organs at rest. Which of the following would be expected to have the greatest blood flow per 100 g of tissue?
   A. Brain
   B. Heart muscle
   C. Skin
   D. Liver
   E. Kidneys

5. Following a motor vehicle accident and severe hemorrhage, a 20-year-old male victim is found to have a rapid, weak pulse, cold, clammy skin, and low blood pressure. He is judged to be suffering from hypovolemic shock. Which of the following might be expected to worsen the consequences of this shock?
   A. Increasing his core body temperature
   B. Laying the patient down and elevating his feet by 12 in
   C. Preventing further blood loss
   D. Giving a sports drink containing glucose and electrolytes by mouth
   E. Administering a blood transfusion

6. A baby boy is brought to the hospital because of convulsions. In the course of a workup, his body temperature and plasma glucose are found to be normal, but his CSF glucose is 12 mg/dL (normal, 65 mg/dL). A possible explanation of his condition is
   A. constitutive activation of GLUT3 in neurons.
   B. SGLT-1 deficiency in astrocytes.
   C. GLUT5 deficiency in cerebral capillaries.
   D. GLUT1 deficiency in cerebral capillaries.
   E. GLUT1 deficiency in microglia.

7. A 50-year-old man is brought to the emergency room complaining of severe chest pain, shortness of breath, nausea, and anxiety. He is obese and his skin is clammy. In a clear voice, he tells the physician that his symptoms began shortly after he tried to run after a man who had stolen a woman's purse, and admits that he has not been taking the statin drug that his primary care physician prescribed because he believed it was causing muscle weakness. Blood tests reveal elevated levels of troponins and creatine kinase. What is the most likely diagnosis?
   A. Exercise-induced asthma
   B. Stroke
   C. Acute myocardial infarction
   D. Food poisoning
   E. Acute kidney failure

8. The patient in Question 7 is found to have a clot occluding the coronary vessel that supplies the subendocardial portion of the left ventricle. This is a particularly vulnerable site for a myocardial infarct because of which of the following factors?
   A. Because the patient is bradycardic
   B. Because flow in the right coronary artery is reduced to zero at the start of systole

C. Because pressure in the left ventricle is slightly higher than in the aorta during systole
D. Because the aortic diastolic pressure is high
E. Because venous pressure is reduced

9. For the patient in question 7, injection of t-PA would probably be most beneficial
    A. after at least 1 year of uncomplicated recovery.
    B. after at least 2 months of rest and recuperation.
    C. during the second week after occlusion of his coronary artery.
    D. during the second day after occlusion of his coronary artery.
    E. during the second hour after occlusion of his coronary artery.

10. A female infant is delivered at a gestational age of 32 weeks, weighing 1 kg. Forty-eight hours after birth, the baby is noted to have a heart murmur and a bounding pulse, and is feeding poorly. Indomethacin is administered and the symptoms resolve. What is the most likely diagnosis?
    A. Necrotizing enterocolitis
    B. Bronchopulmonary dysplasia
    C. Apnea
    D. Patent ductus arteriosus
    E. Respiratory distress syndrome

ANSWERS

1. The correct answer is **D.** Oxygenated blood flows from the maternal arteries and its oxygen tension will be progressively reduced as it traverses various vascular beds (rules out option **A**). Maternal arteries supply oxygenated blood to the placenta, where it equilibrates with the fetal blood in the fetal villi and drains into the umbilical veins (rules out option **E**). Blood draining from the uterus via the uterine veins will have a lower oxygen tension than that in the femoral veins, due to delivery of oxygen to the fetus (rules out option **C**). However, the specific properties of fetal hemoglobin compared to that in the maternal circulation allow for oxygen delivery to the fetal tissues and will significantly deplete oxygen in the blood returning to the placenta via the umbilical artery (rules out option **B**). It is important to recall that the designation of vein and artery in the fetal circulation refers to their anatomical relationship to the fetal heart, and unlike adult arteries, the umbilical artery in the fetus carries deoxygenated blood.

2. The correct answer is **A.** Blood flows to the coronary circulation from the aorta, and aortic pressure declines from a high of around 120 mm Hg during systole to a low of around 80 mm Hg during diastole. Left ventricular pressure is minimal during diastole, when the ventricle relaxes to allow for filling (rules out option **B**). It then rises during systole until it exceeds the pressure in the aorta, when the aortic valve opens. The pressure continues to increase to allow for ventricular ejection. On the other hand, the right ventricle needs to pump only against the low pressure pulmonary circulation during systole, and is relaxed during diastole (rules out options **C** and **D**). The atria are also relaxed during systole, allowing for a larger pressure gradient between them and the aorta (rules out option **E**).

3. The correct answer is **B.** The area postrema is one of the so-called circumventricular organs, parts of the brain that contain fenestrated capillaries and thus are accessible to plasma proteins. The area postrema is a chemoreceptor trigger zone that senses toxins in the plasma to trigger vomiting, among other regulatory functions. Thus, its access to blood components is important to its physiological function, and it is said to lie "outside the blood–brain barrier." All of the other brain regions listed are higher areas that have essentially no passive permeability to proteins, protein-bound lipids or small, water-soluble solutes. Specific active transport mechanisms transfer needed solutes, such as glucose, while excluding those that might be harmful to the brain (rules out options **A, C, D,** and **E**).

4. The correct answer is **E.** The kidneys act to filter the blood of harmful water-soluble metabolites, as well as maintaining water and electrolyte homeostasis. These functions require a very high rate of blood flow to allow precise, minute-to-minute control of plasma composition. However, the kidney extracts relatively little oxygen from the blood that passes through it. This can be compared to the brain and liver, which have a blood flow per unit mass that is only around 10–12% of that flowing to the kidneys, but consume almost 20% of total oxygen (rules out options **A** and **D**). Heart muscle has a blood flow that is approximately 20% of that flowing to the kidneys (rules out option **B**). The skin is the least well-perfused, with a blood flow that is less than 5% of that flowing to the kidneys per unit mass (rules out option **C**).

5. The correct answer is **A.** Blood flow to the skin is controlled primarily as an adaptive response to thermoregulatory stimuli. When the core temperature rises, skin vessels dilate and blood flow increases markedly to increase the rate of heat loss. This would increase the blood volume that is distributed to the skin, further depriving vital organs of adequate perfusion. On the other hand, raising the feet will increase venous return to the heart, as will preventing further blood loss (rules out options **B** and **C**). Blood transfusions (or IV fluids for less severe cases) can also be used to sustain an adequate circulatory volume (rules out option **E**). Finally, giving a sports drink would likely not worsen shock, although it is not advised because of the risk of aspiration if the victim loses consciousness or requires subsequent surgery (rules out option **D**).

6. The correct answer is **D.** The blood–brain barrier ensures that there is limited passive permeability for water-soluble solutes to enter the brain. Needed solutes, such as glucose, are actively transported across the capillary endothelial cells and into the CSF via GLUT1 transport molecules. GLUT3 is present in neurons, but even if constitutively active, uptake of glucose from the CSF into neurons would simply increase the gradient driving additional glucose transport across the capillaries assuming they were otherwise normal (rules out option **A**). SGLT1 is a sodium-coupled glucose transporter than can be induced in astrocytes by hypoxia, but its deficiency would initially increase rather than decrease CSF glucose concentrations before re-equilibration occurred (rules out option **B**). The same can be said for the expected effects of GLUT1 deficiency in microglia (rules out option **E**). Finally, while GLUT5 participates in glucose uptake by microglia, it is not normally expressed by cerebral capillaries (rules out option **C**).

7. The correct answer is **C.** Myocardial infarction is common in men above the age of 45, and particularly those who are

overweight and hypercholesterolemic. Stress and exercise are often precipitating factors. The patient's symptoms might be consistent with exercise-induced asthma, but chest pain would not be severe and cardiac enzymes would not be elevated (rules out option **A**). It is unlikely that he is suffering from a stroke in the absence of signs of one-sided weakness or slurred speech (rules out option **B**) although strokes can be a later complication of a myocardial infarction. Food poisoning could be accompanied by nausea and fever, but not the other symptoms listed (rules out option **D**). Acute kidney failure can cause shortness of breath and disturb heart rhythms, but would not be expected to elevate cardiac enzymes (rules out option **E**).

8. The correct answer is **C**. During systole, the pressure inside the left ventricle is slightly higher than that in the aorta, and the contracting heart muscle compresses the coronary vessels, temporarily preventing flow to the subendocardial region of the left ventricle. In more superficial regions of the left ventricle, the forces are dissipated and some flow occurs throughout the cardiac cycle. The right coronary artery also remains patent throughout the cardiac cycle because of the low pressure in the right ventricle (rules out option **B**). Diastole is shortened when the heart rate is high, meaning that bradycardia would reduce, rather than increase, the length of time when flow to the left ventricle is restricted (rules out option **A**). Aortic pressures are highest during systole rather than diastole (rules out option **D**). Finally, if venous pressure was reduced, this would be expected to increase the effective coronary perfusion pressure, thereby decreasing the risk of infarction (rules out option **E**).

9. The correct answer is **E**. Treatment of myocardial infarction aims to restore flow to the affected area of heart muscle as soon as possible while avoiding reperfusion injury, because prolonged hypoxia results in myocyte death and irreversible changes in cardiac function in the affected region. t-PA acts by binding with plasminogen to the fibrin surface of a clot, facilitating the conversion of plasminogen to plasmin and dissolving the clot. It has a short plasma half-life but does increase the risk of bleeding, especially if cardiac surgery is subsequently needed. Nevertheless, it is frequently administered in the emergency room setting and would not be expected to have any therapeutic effect if administration was delayed, even if only by days (rules out options **A, B, C,** and **D**).

10. The correct answer is **D**. The failure of the ductus arteriosus to close spontaneously after birth is a relatively common complication in premature infants, and particularly in girls and/or those that have very low birth weights. In utero, high concentrations of vasodilatory prostaglandins are present in the ductus and may contribute to its patency. At birth, cyclooxygenase that produces these prostaglandins is normally inhibited but this mechanism may fail with prematurity; therapy with indomethacin, a cyclooxygenase inhibitor, can replace this step. Indomethacin may be injurious to the bowel, and would not therefore be indicated in the setting of necrotizing enterocolitis (rules out option **A**). Further, the symptoms as well as the efficacy of indomethacin are not consistent with the respiratory complications of prematurity (rules out options **B, C,** and **E**).

SECTION VI RESPIRATORY PHYSIOLOGY

The uptake of O_2 and removal of CO_2 from the body is the primary goal of the lung. At rest, a normal human breathes 12–15 times a minute. With each breath containing ~500 mL of air, this translates to 6–8 L of air that is inspired and expired every minute. On average, 250 mL of O_2 enters the body per minute and 200 mL of CO_2 is excreted. In addition to the O_2 that enters the respiratory system, inspired air also contains a variety of particulates that must be properly filtered and/or removed to maintain lung health. Although humans have a certain amount of control over breathing, most functions, including the fine adjustments necessary for proper lung function, are accomplished independent of voluntary control. The goal of this section is to review basic concepts that underlie important aspects of the control and outcome of breathing and introduce other important functions of the lung.

The respiratory system is connected to the outside world by the upper airway that leads down a set of conduits before reaching the gas-exchanging areas (the alveoli). The function of the lungs is supported by a variety of anatomic features that serve to inflate/deflate the lung, thereby allowing the movement of gases to and from the rest of the body. Supporting features include the chest wall, the respiratory muscles, the areas in the brain that control the muscles, and the tracts and nerves that connect the brain to the muscles. The lung also supports the pulmonary circulation, which allows for movement of gases to other organs and tissues of the body. In the first chapter of this section, the unique anatomic and cellular makeup of the respiratory system and how the intricate structure of the lung contributes to respiratory physiology will be explored.

The discussion will continue with an overview of the primary function of the respiratory system—the capture of O_2 from the outside environment and its delivery to tissues, as well as the simultaneous removal of CO_2 from the tissues to the outside environment. During this discussion, the critical role of pH in gas exchange as well as the ability of the lung to contribute to pH regulation of the blood is examined.

The final chapter in this section begins with an overview of some of the key factors that aid in the control of breathing. This will include the repetitive neuronal firing that controls muscle movements that inflate/deflate the lung and the series of feedback loops that increase/decrease deflation depending on the gas content of the blood. Specific examples of common respiratory abnormalities and how they relate to altered regulation of breathing are also discussed to better understand the intricate feedback loops that help regulate breathing.

Due to the complexity of the lung there is a wide-ranging list of diseases that impact its function. Such diseases include common (and uncommon) respiratory infections, asthma, chronic obstructive pulmonary disease, acute respiratory distress syndrome, pulmonary hypertension, and lung cancer. The health burden from such a diverse collection of disorders cannot be overstated. The continued and improved understanding of respiratory physiology and lung function will provide opportunities to develop new strategies for treatment of the myriad of lung diseases.

Introduction to Pulmonary Structure & Mechanics

C H A P T E R

34

OBJECTIVES

After studying this chapter, you should be able to:

- List the passages through which air passes from the exterior to the alveoli, and describe the cells that line each of them.
- List the major muscles involved in respiration, and state the role of each.
- Define the basic measures of lung volume and give approximate values for each in a normal adult.
- Define lung compliance and airway resistance.
- Compare the pulmonary and systemic circulations, and list some major differences between them.
- Describe basic lung defense and metabolic functions.
- Define partial pressure and calculate the partial pressure of each of the important gases in the atmosphere at sea level.

INTRODUCTION

The structure of the respiratory system is uniquely suited to its primary function, the transport of gases in and out of the body. The respiratory system provides a large volume of tissue that is constantly exposed to the outside environment, and thus, to potential infection and injury. The pulmonary system includes a unique circulation that must handle the blood flow.

This chapter begins with the basic anatomy and cellular physiology that contribute to the respiratory system and some of their unique features. The chapter also includes discussion of how the anatomic features contribute to the basic mechanics of breathing, as well as some highlights of nonrespiratory physiology in the pulmonary system.

■ ANATOMY OF THE LUNGS

REGIONS OF THE RESPIRATORY TRACT

Airflow through the respiratory system can be broken down into three interconnected regions: the **upper airway,** the **conducting airway,** and the **alveolar airway.** The upper airway consists of the entry systems, the nose/nasal cavity and mouth that lead into the pharynx. The larynx extends from the lower part of the pharynx to complete the upper airway. The nose is the primary point of entry for inhaled air; therefore, the mucosal epithelium lining the nasopharyngeal airways is exposed to the highest concentration of inhaled allergens, toxicants, and particulate matter. With this in

mind, it is easy to understand that in addition to olfaction, the nose and upper airway provides two additional crucial functions in airflow—(1) filtering out large particulates to prevent them from reaching the conducting and alveolar airways and (2) serving to warm and humidify air as it enters the body. Particulates larger than 30–50 μm in size tend to not to be inhaled through the nose whereas particulates on the order of 5–10 μm impact on the nasopharynx and do enter the conducting airway. Most of these latter particles settle on mucous membranes in the nose and pharynx. Because of their momentum, they do not follow the airstream as it curves downward into the lungs, and they impact on or near the **tonsils** and **adenoids,** large collections of immunologically active lymphoid tissue in the back of the pharynx.

CONDUCTING AIRWAY

The conducting airway begins at the trachea and branches dichotomously to greatly expand the surface area of the tissue in the lung. The first 16 generations of passages form the conducting zone of the airways that transports gas from and to the upper airway described above (**Figure 34–1**). These branches are made up of bronchi, bronchioles, and terminal bronchioles. The conducting airway is made up of a variety of specialized cells that provide more than simply a conduit for air to reach the lung (**Figure 34–2**). The mucosal epithelium is attached to a thin basement membrane, and beneath this, the lamina propria. Collectively these are referred to as the "airway mucosa." Smooth muscle cells are found beneath the epithelium and an enveloping connective tissue is likewise interspersed with cartilage that is more predominant in the portions of the conducting airway of greater caliber. The epithelium is organized as a pseudostratified epithelium and contains several cell types, including ciliated and secretory cells (eg, goblet cells and glandular acini) that provide key components for airway innate immunity, and basal cells that can serve as progenitor cells during injury. As the conducting airway transitions to terminal and transitional bronchioles, the histologic appearance of the conducting tubes change. Secretory glands are absent from the epithelium of the bronchioles and terminal bronchioles, smooth muscle plays a more prominent role and cartilage is largely absent from the underlying tissue. Club cells (formerly termed "Clara cells"), nonciliated cuboidal epithelial cells that secrete important defense markers and serve as progenitor cells after injury, make up a large portion of the epithelial lining in the latter portions of the conducting airway.

Epithelial cells in the conducting airway can secrete a variety of molecules that aid in lung defense. These secretions can act directly as antimicrobials to help keep the airway free of infection. Airway epithelial cells also secrete a variety of chemokines and cytokines that recruit traditional immune cells and other immune effector cells to site of infections. The smaller particles that make it through the upper airway, ~2–5 μm in diameter, generally fall on the walls of the bronchi as the airflow slows in the smaller passages. There they can initiate reflex bronchial constriction and coughing. Alternatively, they can be moved away from the lungs by the "mucociliary escalator." The epithelium of the respiratory passages from the anterior third of the nose to the beginning of the respiratory bronchioles is ciliated (Figure 34–2). The cilia are bathed in a periciliary fluid where they typically beat at rates of 10–15 Hz. On top of the periciliary layer and the beating cilia rests a mucus layer, a complex mixture of proteins and polysaccharides secreted from specialized cells, glands, or both in the conducting airway. This combination allows for the trapping of foreign particles (in the mucus) and their transport out of the airway (powered by ciliary beat). The ciliary mechanism is capable of moving particles away from the lungs at a rate of at least 16 mm/min. When ciliary motility is defective mucus transport is virtually absent (**Clinical Box 34–1**).

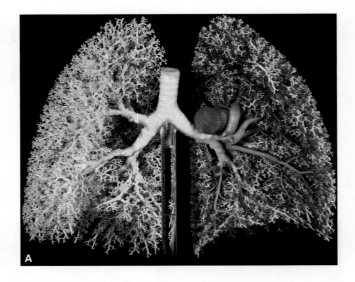

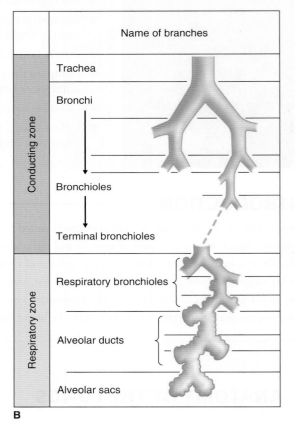

FIGURE 34–1 Conducting and respiratory zones in the airway. (A) Resin cast of the human airway tree shows dichotomous branching beginning at the trachea. Note the added pulmonary arteries (red) and veins (blue) displayed in the left lung. **(B)** The branching pattern of the airway is sketched with individual regions of the conducting and respiratory airways identified. (A, Reproduced with permission from Fishman AP: Fishman's Pulmonary Disease and Disorders, 4th ed. New York, NY: McGraw-Hill Medical; 2008; B, Reproduced with permission from Crystal RG, West JB: The Lung: scientific foundations. New York: Raven Press; 1991.)

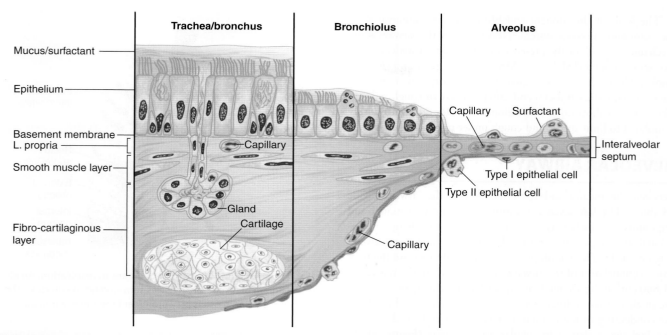

FIGURE 34–2 **Cellular transition from conducting airway to the alveolus.** The epithelial layer transitions from pseudostratified layer with submucosal glands to a cuboidal epithelium and then to a squamous epithelium. The underlying mesenchymal tissue and capillary structure also changes with the airway transition. (Adapted with permission from Fishman AP: *Fishman's Pulmonary Diseases and Disorders*, 4th ed. New York, NY: McGraw-Hill Medical; 2008.)

CLINICAL BOX 34–1

Cystic Fibrosis

Among whites, cystic fibrosis is one of the most common genetic disorders; greater than 3% of the United States population are carriers for this autosomal recessive disease.

The gene that is abnormal in cystic fibrosis is located on the long arm of chromosome 7 and encodes the **cystic fibrosis transmembrane conductance regulator (CFTR),** a regulated Cl⁻ channel located on the apical membrane of various secretory and absorptive epithelia. The number of reported mutations in the *CFTR* gene that cause cystic fibrosis is large (>1000) and the mutations are now grouped into five classes (I–V) based on their cellular function. Class I mutations do not allow for synthesis of the protein. Class II mutations have protein processing defects. Class III mutations have a block in their channel regulation. Class IV mutations display altered conductance of the ion channel. Class V mutations display reduced synthesis of the protein. The severity of the defect varies with the class and the individual mutation. The most common mutation causing cystic fibrosis is loss of the phenylalanine residue at amino acid position 508 of the protein (ΔF508), a Class II mutation that limits the amount of protein that gets to the plasma membrane.

One outcome of cystic fibrosis is repeated pulmonary infections, particularly with *Pseudomonas aeruginosa*, and progressive, eventually fatal destruction of the lungs. There is also suppressed chloride secretion across the wall of the airways.

One would expect Na⁺ reabsorption to be depressed as well, and indeed in sweat glands it is. However, in the lungs, it is enhanced, so that the Na⁺ and water move out of airways, leaving their other secretions inspissated and sticky. This results in a reduced periciliary layer that inhibits function of the mucociliary escalator, and alters the local environment to reduce the effectiveness of antimicrobial secretions.

THERAPEUTIC HIGHLIGHTS

Traditional treatments of cystic fibrosis address the various symptoms. Chest physiotherapy and mucolytics are used to loosen thick mucus and aid lung clearance. Antibiotics are used to prevent new infections and keep chronic infections in check. Bronchodilators and anti-inflammatory medications are used to help expand and clear air passages. Pancreatic enzymes and nutritive supplements are used to increase nutrient absorption and promote weight gain. Because of the "single gene" mutation of this disease, gene therapy has been closely examined; however, results have not been successful. More recently, drugs that target the molecular defects have been advancing in clinical trials and are showing great promise for better treatments.

The walls of the bronchi and bronchioles are innervated by the autonomic nervous system. Nerve cells in the airways sense mechanical stimuli or the presence of unwanted substances in the airways such as inhaled dusts, cold air, noxious gases, and cigarette smoke. These neurons can signal the respiratory centers to contract the respiratory muscles and initiate sneeze or cough reflexes. The receptors show rapid adaptation when they are continuously stimulated to limit sneeze and cough under normal conditions.

ALVEOLAR AIRWAY

Between the trachea and the alveolar sacs, the airways divide 23 times. The last seven generations form the transitional and respiratory zones where gas exchange occurs are made up of transitional and respiratory bronchioles, alveolar ducts, and alveoli (Figure 34–1). These multiple divisions greatly increase the total cross-sectional area of the airways, from 2.5 cm^2 in the trachea to 11,800 cm^2 in the alveoli. Consequently, the velocity of airflow in the small airways declines to very low values. The transition from the conducting to the respiratory region that ends in the alveoli also includes a change in cellular arrangements (Figure 34–2). Humans have 300 million alveoli, and the total area of the alveolar walls in contact with capillaries in both lungs is about 70 m^2.

The alveoli are lined by two types of epithelial cells. **Alveolar type I (ATI) cells** are flat cells with large cytoplasmic extensions and are the primary lining cells of the alveoli, covering approximately 95% of the alveolar epithelial surface area. **Alveolar type II (ATII) cells** are thicker and contain numerous lamellar inclusion bodies. Although these cells make up only 5% of the surface area, they represent approximately 60% of the epithelial cells in the alveoli. ATII cells are important in alveolar repair as well as other cellular physiology. One prime function of the ATII cell is the production of **surfactant.** This surfactant layer plays an important role in maintaining alveolar structure by reducing surface tension (see below).

The alveoli are surrounded by pulmonary capillaries. In most areas, air and blood are separated only by the alveolar epithelium and the capillary endothelium about 0.5 μm apart. The alveoli also contain other specialized cells, including pulmonary alveolar macrophages (PAMs), lymphocytes, plasma cells, neuroendocrine cells, and mast cells. PAMs are an important component of the pulmonary defense system. Like other macrophages, these cells come originally from the bone marrow. PAMs are actively phagocytic and ingest small particles that evade the mucociliary escalator and reach the alveoli. They also help process inhaled antigens for immunologic attack, and they secrete substances that attract granulocytes to the lungs as well as substances that stimulate granulocyte and monocyte formation in the bone marrow. Over-recruitment or dysregulation of PAMs may result in improper release lysosomal products into the extracellular space to cause alveolar damage and inflammation.

RESPIRATORY MUSCLES

The lungs are positioned within the thoracic cavity. The lungs are surrounded by a variety of muscles that contribute to breathing (**Figure 34–3**). The diaphragm is the major respiratory

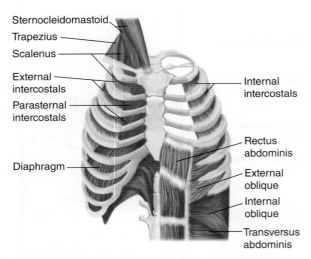

FIGURE 34–3 Muscles and movement in respiration. An idealized diagram of respiratory muscles surrounding the rib cage. The diaphragm and intercostals play prominent roles in respiration.

muscle and is situated at the base of the lungs. The diaphragm has three parts: the costal portion, made up of muscle fibers that are attached to the ribs around the bottom of the thoracic cage; the crural portion, made up of fibers that are attached to the ligaments along the vertebrae; and the central tendon, into which the costal and the crural fibers insert. The central tendon is also the inferior part of the pericardium. The crural fibers pass on either side of the esophagus and can compress it when they contract. The costal and crural portions are innervated by different parts of the phrenic nerve and can contract separately. For example, during vomiting and eructation, intra-abdominal pressure is increased by contraction of the costal fibers but the crural fibers remain relaxed, allowing material to pass from the stomach into the esophagus. Movement of the diaphragm accounts for 75% of the change in intrathoracic volume during quiet inspiration. The diaphragm is innervated by the phrenic nerves, arising from cervical segments 3–5. Thus, transection of the spinal cord above the third cervical segment is fatal without artificial respiration, however, transection below the fifth cervical segment still allows for respiratory drive to the diaphragm.

Other important **inspiratory muscles** include the **external intercostal muscles,** which run obliquely downward and forward from rib to rib. The ribs pivot as if hinged at the back, so that when the external intercostals contract they elevate the lower ribs. This pushes the sternum outward and increases the anteroposterior diameter of the chest. In patients with bilateral phrenic nerve palsy but intact innervation of their intercostal muscles, respiration is somewhat labored but adequate to maintain life.

Contraction of the **expiratory muscles** results in a decrease in intrathoracic volume and forced expiration. The internal intercostals have this action because they pass obliquely downward and posteriorly from rib to rib and therefore pull the rib cage downward when they contract. Contractions of the muscles of the anterior abdominal wall also aid expiration by pulling the rib cage downward and inward and by increasing the intra-abdominal pressure, which pushes the relaxing diaphragm upward.

In order for air to get into the conducting airway it must pass through the **glottis,** defined as the area including and between the vocal folds within the larynx. The abductor muscles in the larynx contract early in inspiration, pulling the vocal cords apart and opening the glottis. During swallowing or gagging, a reflex contraction of the adductor muscles closes the glottis and prevents aspiration of food, fluid, or vomitus into the lungs. In unconscious or anesthetized patients, glottic closure may be incomplete and vomitus may enter the trachea, causing an inflammatory reaction in the lung (**aspiration pneumonia**).

LUNG PLEURA

The **pleural cavity** serves as a lubricating fluid/area that allows for lung movement within the thoracic cavity (**Figure 34–4**). There are two layers that contribute to the pleural cavity: the **parietal pleura** and the **visceral pleura.** The parietal pleura lines the chest cavity containing the lungs and the visceral pleura lines the lung surface. The pleural fluid (~15–20 mL) forms a thin layer between the pleural membranes and prevents friction between surfaces during inspiration and expiration.

The lung itself contains a vast amount of free space—it is ~80% air. Although this maximizes surface area for gas exchange, it also requires an extensive support network to maintain lung shape and function. The **connective tissue** within the visceral pleura contains three layers that help support the lung. Elastic fibers follow the mesothelium effectively wrap the three lobes of the right lung and the two lobes of the left lung. A deep sheet of fine fibers that follow the outline of the alveoli provides support

to individual air sacks. Between these two separate sheets lies connective tissue that is interspersed with individual cells for support and lung maintenance/function.

Blood & Lymph in the Lung

Both the **pulmonary circulation** and the **bronchial circulation** contribute to blood flow in the lung. In the pulmonary circulation, almost all the blood in the body passes via the pulmonary artery to the pulmonary capillary bed, where it is oxygenated and returned to the left atrium via the pulmonary veins. The pulmonary arteries follow the branching of the bronchi down to the respiratory bronchioles. The pulmonary veins, however, are spaced between the bronchi on their return to the heart. The separate and much smaller bronchial circulation includes the bronchial arteries that come from systemic arteries. They form capillaries, which drain into bronchial veins or anastomose with pulmonary capillaries or veins. The bronchial veins drain into the azygos vein. The bronchial circulation nourishes the trachea down to the terminal bronchioles and also supplies the pleura and hilar lymph nodes. Lymphatic channels are more abundant in the lungs than in any other organ. Lymph nodes are arranged along the bronchial tree and extend down until the bronchi; node sizes can range from 1 mm in diameter at the bronchial periphery to 10 mm along the trachea. The nodes are connected by lymph vessels and allow for unidirectional flow of lymph to the subclavian veins.

■ MECHANICS OF RESPIRATION

INSPIRATION & EXPIRATION

The lungs and the chest wall are elastic structures. Because of the thin layer of fluid in the intrapleural space, the lungs slide easily on the chest wall, but resist being pulled away from it in the same way that two moist pieces of glass slide on each other but resist separation. The pressure in the "space" between the lungs and chest wall (intrapleural pressure) is subatmospheric (**Figure 34–5**). At the end of quiet expiration, the tendency of the lungs to recoil from the chest wall is just balanced by the tendency of the chest wall to recoil in the opposite direction.

Inspiration is an active process. The intrapleural pressure at the base of the lungs, which is normally about –2.5 mm Hg (relative to atmospheric) at the start of inspiration, decreases to about –6 mm Hg. The pressure in the airway becomes slightly negative, and air flows into the lungs. At the end of inspiration, the lung recoil begins to pull the chest back to the expiratory position, where the recoil pressures of the lungs and chest wall balance (see below). The pressure in the airway becomes slightly positive, and air flows out of the lungs. Expiration during quiet breathing is passive in the sense that no muscles that decrease intrathoracic volume contract. However, some contraction of the inspiratory muscles that occurs in the early part of expiration exerts a braking action on the recoil forces and slows expiration. Strong inspiratory efforts reduce intrapleural pressure to values as low as –30 mm Hg, producing correspondingly greater degrees of lung

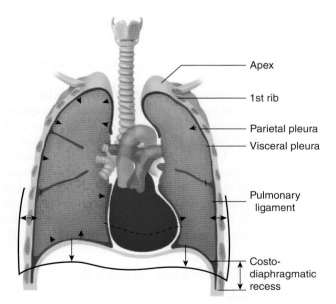

FIGURE 34–4 Pleural space and connective fibers. Front sectional drawing of lung within the rib cage. Note the parietal and visceral pleura and the infoldings around the lung lobes that include pleural space.

Labels: Apex; 1st rib; Parietal pleura; Visceral pleura; Pulmonary ligament; Costo-diaphragmatic recess

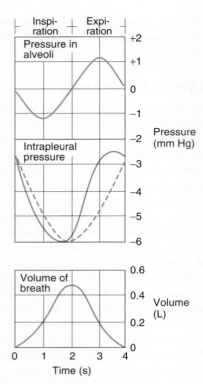

FIGURE 34–5 **Pressure in the alveoli and the pleural space relative to atmospheric pressure during inspiration and expiration.** The dashed line indicates what the intrapleural pressure would be in the absence of airway and tissue resistance; the actual curve (solid line) is skewed to the left by the resistance. Volume of breath during inspiration/expiration is graphed for comparison.

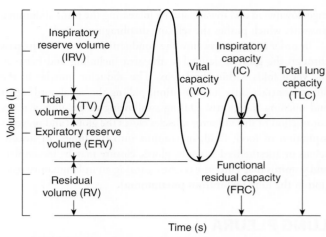

FIGURE 34–6 **Lung volumes and capacity measurements.** Lung volumes recorded by a spirometer. Lung capacities are determined from volume recordings. The amount of air that moves into the lungs with each inspiration (or out with each expiration) during quiet breathing is called the **tidal volume** (TV). Typical values for TV are on the order of 500–750 mL. The air inspired with a maximal inspiratory effort in excess of the TV is the **inspiratory reserve volume** (IRV; typically ~2 L). The volume expelled by an active expiratory effort after passive expiration is the **expiratory reserve volume** (ERV; ~1 L), and the air left in the lungs after a maximal expiratory effort is the **residual volume** (RV; ~1.3 L). When all four of the above components are taken together, they make up the **total lung capacity** (~5 L). The **vital lung capacity** (~3.5 L) refers to the maximum amount of air expired from the fully inflated lung, or maximum inspiratory level (this represents TV + IRV + ERV). The **inspiratory capacity** (~2.5 L) is the maximum amount of air inspired from the end-expiratory level (IRV + TV). The **functional residual capacity** (FRC; ~2.5 L) represents the volume of the air remaining in the lungs after expiration of a normal breath (RV + ERV). (Reproduced with permission from Fishman AP: *Fishman's Pulmonary Diseases and Disorders*, 4th ed. New York, NY: McGraw-Hill Medical; 2008.)

inflation. When ventilation is increased, the extent of lung deflation is also increased by active contraction of expiratory muscles that decrease intrathoracic volume.

QUANTITATING RESPIRATORY PHENOMENA

Modern spirometers permit direct measurement of gas intake and output. Modern techniques for gas analysis make possible rapid, reliable measurements of the composition of gas mixtures and the gas content of body fluids. For example, O_2 and CO_2 electrodes can be inserted into the airway or into blood vessels or tissues allowing for continual recording of P_{O_2} and P_{CO_2}. Assessment of blood oxygenation can be carried out noninvasively with a **pulse oximeter,** which can be easily placed on a fingertip.

Lung Volumes & Capacities

Important quantitation of lung function can be gleaned from the displacement of air volume during inspiration and/or expiration. Lung capacities refer to subdivisions that contain two or more volumes. Volumes and capacities recorded on a spirometer from a healthy individual are shown in **Figure 34–6**. Diagnostic spirometry is used to assess a patient's lung function for purposes of

comparison with a normal population, or with previous measures from the same patient.

Dynamic measurements of lung volumes and capacities have been used to help determine lung dysfunction. The **forced vital capacity (FVC),** the largest amount of air that can be expired after a maximal inspiratory effort, is frequently measured clinically as an index of pulmonary function. It gives useful information about the strength of the respiratory muscles and other aspects of pulmonary function. The fraction of the vital capacity expired during the first second of a forced expiration is referred to as **FEV$_1$** (forced expiratory volume in the first second). The FEV$_1$-to-FVC ratio (FEV$_1$/FVC) is a useful tool in the recognizing classes of airway disease (Clinical Box 34–2).

COMPLIANCE OF THE LUNGS & CHEST WALL

Compliance is developed due to the tendency for tissue to resume its original position after an applied force has been removed. After an expiration during quiet breathing, the lungs

CLINICAL BOX 34-2

Altered Airflow in Disease:

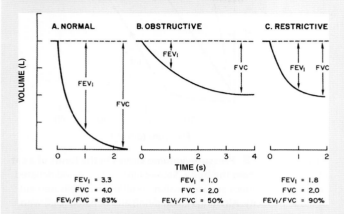

FEV₁ = 3.3
FVC = 4.0
FEV₁/FVC = 83%

FEV₁ = 1.0
FVC = 2.0
FEV₁/FVC = 50%

FEV₁ = 1.8
FVC = 2.0
FEV₁/FVC = 90%

Representative lung volume expired over time in normal and diseased lungs during respiratory testing. (A) Healthy patient. **(B)** Obstructive disease patient. **(C)** Restrictive disease patient. Note the differences in FEV_1, FVC, and FEV_1/FVC at the bottom of the figure. FEV_1, forced expiratory volume in the first second; FVC, forced vital capacity. (Reproduced with permission from Fishman AP: *Fishman's Pulmonary Disease and Disorders*, 4th ed. New York, NY: McGraw-Hill Medical, 2008.)

Airflow Measurements of Obstructive & Restrictive Disease

In the example above, a healthy FVC is ~4.0 L and a healthy FEV_1 is ~3.3 L. The calculated FEV_1/FVC is ~80%. Patients with obstructive or restrictive diseases can display reduced FVC, on the order of 2.0 L in the example above. Measurement of FEV_1, however, tends to vary significantly between the two diseases. In obstructive disorders, patients tend to show a slow, steady slope to the FVC, resulting in a small FEV_1, on the order of 1.0 L in the example. However, in the restrictive disorder, patient's airflow tends to be fast at first, and then quickly level out to approach FVC.

The resultant FEV_1 is much greater, on the order of 1.8 L in the example, even though FVC is equivalent (compare **B** and **C**). A quick calculation of FEV_1/FVC for patients with obstructive (50%) versus restrictive (90%) patterns defines the hallmark measurements in evaluating these two diseases. Obstructive disorders result in a marked decrease in both FVC and FEV_1/FVC, whereas restrictive disorders result in a loss of FVC without loss in FEV_1/FVC. It should be noted that these examples are idealized and several disorders can show mixed readings.

Obstructive Disease—Asthma

Asthma is characterized by episodic or chronic wheezing, cough, and a feeling of tightness in the chest as a result of bronchoconstriction. Although the disease is not fully understood, three airway abnormalities are present: **airway obstruction** that is at least partially reversible, **airway inflammation,** and **airway hyperresponsiveness** to a variety of stimuli. A link to allergy has long been recognized, and plasma IgE levels are often elevated. Proteins released from eosinophils in the inflammatory reaction may damage the airway epithelium and contribute to the hyperresponsiveness. Leukotrienes are released from eosinophils and mast cells, and can enhance bronchoconstriction. Numerous other amines, neuropeptides, chemokines, and interleukins have effects on bronchial smooth muscle or produce inflammation, and they may be involved in asthma.

THERAPEUTIC HIGHLIGHTS

Because β_2-adrenergic receptors mediate bronchodilation, β_2-adrenergic agonists have long been the mainstay of "rescue" treatment for mild to moderate asthma attacks. Inhaled steroids are used even in mild to moderate cases to reduce inflammation; they are very effective, but their side effects can be a problem. Agents that block synthesis of leukotrienes or their $CysLT_1$ receptor have also proved useful in some cases.

---

have a tendency to collapse and the chest wall has a tendency to expand. The interaction between the recoil of the lungs and recoil of the chest can be determined by measuring the pressure in the airway at various lung volumes, and a **pressure–volume (PV) curve** of the total respiratory system can be determined (P_{TR} in **Figure 34–7**). The pressure is zero at a lung volume that corresponds to the volume of gas in the lungs at **FRC (relaxation volume).** As can be noted from Figure 34–7, this relaxation pressure is the sum of slightly negative pressure component from the chest wall (P_w) and a slightly positive pressure from the lungs (P_L). P_{TR} is positive at greater volumes and negative at smaller volumes. **Compliance** of the lung and chest wall is measured as the slope of the P_{TR} curve, or, as a change in lung volume per unit change in airway pressure ($\Delta V/\Delta P$). It is normally measured in the pressure range where the relaxation

pressure curve is steepest, and normal values are ~0.2 L/cm H_2O in a healthy adult man. However, compliance depends on lung volume and thus can vary. In an extreme example, an individual with only one lung has approximately half the ΔV for a given ΔP. Compliance is also slightly greater when measured during deflation than when measured during inflation. Consequently, it is more informative to examine the whole PV curve. The curve is shifted downward and to the right (compliance is decreased) by pulmonary edema and interstitial pulmonary fibrosis. Pulmonary fibrosis is a progressive restrictive airway disease in which there is stiffening and scarring of the lung. The curve is shifted upward and to the left (compliance is increased) in emphysema. Emphysema is an obstructive lung disease in which the lung loses stiffness and takes on a more "floppy" character when compared with a healthy lung.

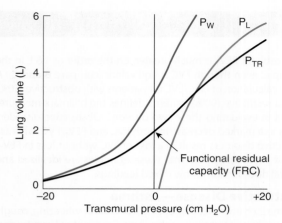

FIGURE 34–7 Pressure–volume curves in the lung. The pressure–volume curves of the total respiratory system (P_{TR}, black line), the lungs (P_L, blue line), and the chest (P_W, green line) are plotted together with standard volumes for functional residual capacity and tidal volume. The transmural pressure is intrapulmonary pressure minus intrapleural pressure in the case of the lungs, intrapleural pressure minus outside (barometric) pressure in the case of the chest wall, and intrapulmonary pressure minus barometric pressure in the case of the total respiratory system. From these curves, the total and actual elastic work associated with breathing can be derived. (Modified with permission from Mines AH: *Respiratory Physiology*, 3rd ed. New York, NY: Raven Press; 1993.)

Airway Resistance

Airway resistance is defined as the change of pressure (ΔP) from the alveoli to the mouth divided by the change in flow rate ($\dot{V}$). Measurements where alveolar and intrapleural pressure can be compared to actual pressure (eg, Figure 34–5 middle panel) illustrate the contribution of airway resistance. Airway resistance is increased as lung volume is reduced. The extensive bronchiole network that relies on smooth muscle as a primary support mechanism significantly contributes to airway resistance. Note that contraction of the smooth muscle that lines the bronchial airways will reduce the airway diameter, increase airway resistance, and make breathing more difficult.

Role of Surfactant in Alveolar Surface Tension

An important factor affecting the compliance of the lungs is the surface tension of the film of fluid that lines the alveoli. The magnitude of this component at various lung volumes can be measured by removing the lungs from the body of an experimental animal and distending them alternately with saline and with air while measuring the intrapulmonary pressure. Because saline reduces the surface tension to nearly zero, the PV curve obtained with saline measures only the tissue elasticity (**Figure 34–8**), whereas the curve obtained with air measures both tissue elasticity and surface tension. The difference between the saline and air curves is much smaller when lung volumes are small. Differences are also obvious in the curves generated during inflation and deflation. This difference is termed **hysteresis,** and notably is not

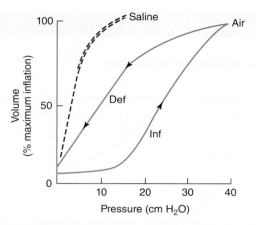

FIGURE 34–8 Pressure–volume curves in the lungs of a cat after removal from the body. Saline: lungs inflated and deflated with saline to reduce surface tension, resulting in a measurement of tissue elasticity. **Air:** lungs inflated (Inf) and deflated (Def) with air results in a measure of both tissue elasticity and surface tension. (Reproduced with permission from Morgan TE: Pulmonary surfactant. *N Engl J Med.* 1971; May 27; 284(21):1185–1193.)

present in the saline generated curves. The alveolar environment, and specifically the secreted factors that help reduce surface tension and keep alveoli from collapsing, contribute to hysteresis.

The low surface tension when the alveoli are small is due to the presence of **surfactant** in the fluid lining the alveoli. Surfactant is a mixture of dipalmitoylphosphatidylcholine (DPPC), other lipids, and proteins. If the surface tension is not kept low when the alveoli become smaller during expiration, they collapse in accordance with the law of Laplace. In spherical structures like an alveolus, the distending pressure (P) equals two times the tension (T) divided by the radius (r; $P = 2T/r$); if T is not reduced as r is reduced, the tension overcomes the distending pressure. Some clinical aspects of surfactant are discussed in **Clinical Box 34–3**.

DEAD SPACE & UNEVEN VENTILATION

Because gaseous exchange in the respiratory system occurs only in the terminal portions of the airways, the gas that occupies the rest of the respiratory system after inhalation is not available for gas exchange with pulmonary capillary blood. This **anatomic dead space** measured in mL is approximately equal to the body weight in pounds in a healthy individual. Thus, a normal sized man of 150 lb (68 kg) would have an anatomic dead space of 150 mL. Consequently, the **alveolar ventilation,** ie, the amount of air reaching the alveoli per minute, is less than the respiratory minute volume (RMV). Note that because of the dead space, rapid shallow breathing produces much less alveolar ventilation than slow deep breathing at the same RMV (**Table 34–1**).

It is important to distinguish between the **anatomic dead space** and the **total (physiologic) dead space** (volume of gas not equilibrating with blood, ie, wasted ventilation). In healthy individuals, the two dead spaces are identical and can be estimated by body weight. However, in disease states, no exchange may take place between the gas in some of the alveoli and the blood. The volume

Surfactant

Surfactant is important at birth. The fetus makes respiratory movements in utero, but the lungs remain collapsed until birth. After birth, the infant makes several strong inspiratory movements and the lungs expand. Surfactant keeps them from collapsing again. Surfactant deficiency is an important cause of **infant respiratory distress syndrome** (IRDS, also known as **hyaline membrane disease**), the serious pulmonary disease that develops in infants born before their surfactant system is functional. Surface tension in the lungs of these infants is high, and the alveoli are collapsed in many areas **(atelectasis).** An additional factor in IRDS is retention of fluid in the lungs. During fetal life, Cl^- is secreted with fluid by the pulmonary epithelial cells. At birth, there is a shift to Na^+ absorption by these cells via the epithelial Na^+ channels (ENaCs), and fluid is absorbed with the Na^+. Prolonged immaturity of the ENaCs contributes to the pulmonary abnormalities in IRDS.

Overproduction/dysregulation of surfactant proteins can also lead to respiratory distress and is the cause of pulmonary alveolar proteinosis (PAP).

THERAPEUTIC HIGHLIGHTS

Treatment of IRDS is commonly done with surfactant replacement therapy. Interestingly, such surfactant replacement therapy has not been as successful in clinical trials for adults experiencing respiratory distress due to surfactant dysfunction.

of gas in nonperfused alveoli and any volume of air in the alveoli in excess of that necessary to arterialize the blood in the alveolar capillaries is part of the dead-space gas volume. The total dead space can be calculated from the P_{CO_2} of expired air, the P_{CO_2} of arterial blood, and the tidal volume (V_T). The V_T times the P_{CO_2} of the expired gas (P_{ECO_2}) equals the arterial P_{CO_2} (Pa_{CO_2}) times the difference between the V_T and the dead space (V_D) plus the P_{CO_2} of inspired air (P_{ICO_2}) times V_D **(Bohr equation):**

$$P_{ECO_2} \times V_T = Pa_{CO_2} \times (V_T - V_D) + P_{ICO_2} \times V_D$$

The term $P_{ICO_2} \times V_D$ is so small that it can be ignored and the equation solved for V_D, where $V_D = V_T - (P_{ECO_2} \times V_T)/(Pa_{CO_2})$.

TABLE 34–1 Effect of variations in respiratory rate and depth on alveolar ventilation.

Respiratory rate	30/min	10/min
Tidal volume	200 mL	600 mL
Minute volume	6 L	6 L
Alveolar ventilation	(200 − 150) × 30 = 1500 mL	(600 − 150) × 10 = 4500 mL

If, for example: $P_{ECO_2} = 28$ mm Hg; $Pa_{CO_2} = 40$ mm Hg and $V_T = 500$ mL, then $V_D = 150$ mL.

The equation can also be used to measure the anatomic dead space if one replaces Pa_{CO_2} with alveolar P_{CO_2} (PA_{CO_2}; the P_{CO_2} of the last 10 mL of expired gas). P_{CO_2} is an average of gas from different alveoli in proportion to their ventilation regardless of whether they are perfused. This is in contrast to Pa_{CO_2}, which is gas equilibrated only with perfused alveoli, and consequently, in individuals with underperfused alveoli, is greater than P_{CO_2}.

■ GAS EXCHANGE IN THE LUNGS

PARTIAL PRESSURES

Unlike liquids, gases expand to fill the volume available to them, and the volume occupied by a given number of gas molecules at a given temperature (T, absolute temperature) and pressure (P) is (ideally) the same regardless of the composition of the gas. **Partial pressures** are frequently used to describe gases in respiration. The pressure of a gas is proportional to its temperature and number of moles (n) occupying a certain volume (V). From the equation state of ideal gas then: $P = \dfrac{nRT}{V}$. The pressure exerted by any one gas in a mixture of gases (its partial pressure) is equal to the total pressure times the fraction of the total amount of gas it represents. The partial pressure of a gas in a liquid is the pressure that, in the gaseous phase in equilibrium with the liquid, would produce the concentration of gas molecules found in the liquid.

The composition of dry air is 20.98% O_2, 0.04% CO_2, 78.06% N_2, and 0.92% other inert constituents. The barometric pressure (P_B) at sea level is 760 mm Hg (1 atm). The partial pressure (indicated by the symbol P) of O_2 (ie, P_{O_2}) in dry air at sea level is therefore (0.21 × 760), or 160 mm Hg. The P_{N_2} and the other inert gases are (0.79 × 760), or 600 mm Hg; and the P_{CO_2} is (0.0004 × 760), or 0.3 mm Hg. The water vapor in the air in most climates reduces these percentages, and therefore the partial pressures, to a slight degree. Air equilibrated with water is saturated with water vapor, and inspired air is saturated by the time it reaches the lungs. The P_{H_2O} at body temperature (37°C) is 47 mm Hg. Therefore, the partial pressures at sea level of the other gases in the air reaching the lungs are P_{O_2}, 150 mm Hg; P_{CO_2}, 0.3 mm Hg; and P_{N_2} (including the other inert gases), 563 mm Hg.

SAMPLING AND COMPOSITION OF ALVEOLAR AIR

Theoretically, all but the first 150 mL expired from a normal sized man (ie, the dead space) with each expiration is the gas that was in the alveoli **(alveolar air),** but some mixing always occurs at the interface between the dead-space gas and the alveolar air. A later portion of expired air is therefore the portion taken for analysis. Using modern apparatus with a suitable automatic valve, it is possible to collect the last 10 mL expired during quiet breathing.

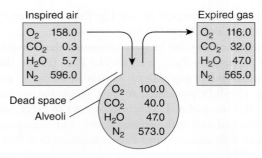

FIGURE 34–9 Partial pressures of gases (mm Hg) in various parts of the respiratory system. Typical partial pressures for inspired air, alveolar air, and expired air are given. See the text for additional details.

The composition of alveolar gas is compared with that of inspired and expired air in **Figure 34–9**.

P_{AO_2} can also be calculated from the **alveolar gas equation:**

$$P_{AO_2} = P_{IO_2} - P_{ACO_2}\left(F_{IO_2} + \frac{1 - F_{IO_2}}{R}\right)$$

where F_{IO_2} is the fraction of O_2 molecules in the dry gas, P_{IO_2} is the inspired P_{O_2}, and R is the respiratory exchange ratio; that is, the flow of CO_2 molecules across the alveolar membrane per minute divided by the flow of O_2 molecules across the membrane per minute.

Oxygen continuously diffuses out of the gas in the alveoli into the bloodstream, and CO_2 continuously diffuses into the alveoli from the blood. In the steady state, inspired air mixes with the alveolar gas, replacing the O_2 that has entered the blood and diluting the CO_2 that has entered the alveoli. Part of this mixture is expired. The O_2 content of the alveolar gas then falls and its CO_2 content rises until the next inspiration. Because the volume of gas in the alveoli is about 2 L at the end of expiration (FRC), each 350 mL increment of inspired and expired air has relatively little effect on P_{O_2} and P_{CO_2}.

DIFFUSION ACROSS THE ALVEOLOCAPILLARY MEMBRANE

Gases diffuse from the alveoli to the blood in the pulmonary capillaries or vice versa across the thin alveolocapillary membrane made up of the pulmonary epithelium, the capillary endothelium, and their fused basement membranes. Whether or not substances passing from the alveoli to the capillary blood reach equilibrium in the 0.75 s that blood takes to traverse the pulmonary capillaries at rest depends on their reaction with substances in the blood. Thus, for example, the anesthetic gas nitrous oxide (N_2O) does not react and reaches equilibrium in about 0.1 s (**Figure 34–10**). In this situation, the amount of N_2O taken up is not limited by diffusion but by the amount of blood flowing through the pulmonary capillaries; that is, it is **flow-limited.** On the other hand, carbon monoxide (CO) is taken up by hemoglobin in the red blood cells at such a high rate that the partial pressure of CO in the capillaries stays very low and equilibrium is not reached in the 0.75 s

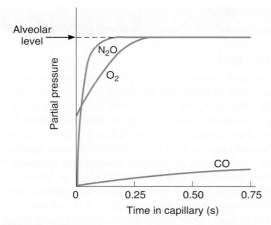

FIGURE 34–10 Uptake of various substances during the 0.75 s they are in transit through a pulmonary capillary. N_2O is not bound in blood, so its partial pressure in blood rises rapidly to its partial pressure in the alveoli. Conversely, CO is avidly taken up by red blood cells, so its partial pressure reaches only a fraction of its partial pressure in the alveoli. O_2 is intermediate between the two.

the blood is in the pulmonary capillaries. Therefore, the transfer of CO is not limited by perfusion at rest and instead is **diffusion-limited.** O_2 is intermediate between N_2O and CO; it is taken up by hemoglobin, but much less avidly than CO, and it reaches equilibrium with capillary blood in about 0.3 s. Thus, its uptake is **perfusion-limited.**

The **diffusing capacity** of the lung for a given gas is directly proportional to the surface area of the alveolocapillary membrane and inversely proportional to its thickness. The diffusing capacity for CO (D_{LCO}) is measured as an index of diffusing capacity because its uptake is diffusion-limited. D_{LCO} is proportional to the amount of CO entering the blood ($\dot{V}_{CO}$) divided by the partial pressure of CO in the alveoli minus the partial pressure of CO in the blood entering the pulmonary capillaries. Except in habitual cigarette smokers, this latter term is close to zero, so it can be ignored and the equation becomes:

$$D_{LCO} = \frac{\dot{V}_{CO}}{P_{ACO}}$$

The normal value of D_{LCO} at rest is about 25 mL/min/mm Hg. It increases up to threefold during exercise because of capillary dilation and recruitment. The P_{O_2} of alveolar air is normally 100 mm Hg, and the P_{O_2} of the blood entering the pulmonary capillaries is 40 mm Hg. The diffusing capacity for O_2, like that for CO at rest, is about 25 mL/min/mm Hg, and the P_{O_2} of blood is raised to 97 mm Hg, a value just under the alveolar P_{O_2}.

The P_{CO_2} of venous blood is 46 mm Hg, whereas that of alveolar air is 40 mm Hg, and CO_2 diffuses from the blood into the alveoli along this gradient. The P_{CO_2} of blood leaving the lungs is 40 mm Hg. CO_2 passes through all biologic membranes with ease, and the diffusing capacity of the lung for CO_2 is much greater than the capacity for O_2. It is for this reason that CO_2 retention is rarely a problem in patients with alveolar fibrosis even when the reduction in diffusing capacity for O_2 is severe.

PULMONARY CIRCULATION

PULMONARY BLOOD VESSELS

The pulmonary vascular bed resembles the systemic one, except that the walls of the pulmonary artery and its large branches are about 30% as thick as the wall of the aorta, and the small arterial vessels, unlike the systemic arterioles, are endothelial tubes with relatively little muscle in their walls. The walls of the postcapillary vessels also contain some smooth muscle. The pulmonary capillaries are large, and there are multiple anastomoses, so that each alveolus sits in a capillary basket.

PRESSURE, VOLUME, & FLOW

With two quantitatively minor exceptions, the blood put out by the left ventricle returns to the right atrium and is ejected by the right ventricle, making the pulmonary vasculature unique in that it accommodates a blood flow that is almost equal to that of all the other organs in the body. One of the exceptions is part of the bronchial blood flow. There are anastomoses between the bronchial capillaries and the pulmonary capillaries and veins, and although some of the bronchial blood enters the bronchial veins, some enters the pulmonary capillaries and veins, bypassing the right ventricle. The other exception is blood that flows from the coronary arteries into the chambers of the left side of the heart. Because of the small **physiologic shunt** created by those two exceptions, the blood in systemic arteries has a Po_2 about 2 mm Hg lower than that of blood that has equilibrated with alveolar air, and the saturation of hemoglobin is 0.5% less.

The pressure gradient in the pulmonary system is about 7 mm Hg, compared with a gradient of about 90 mm Hg in the systemic circulation. Pulmonary capillary pressure is about 10 mm Hg, whereas the oncotic pressure is 25 mm Hg, so that an inward-directed pressure gradient of about 15 mm Hg keeps the alveoli free of all but a thin film of fluid. When the pulmonary capillary pressure is more than 25 mm Hg, pulmonary congestion and edema result. The volume of blood in the pulmonary vessels at any one time is about 1 L, of which less than 100 mL is in the capillaries. The mean velocity of the blood in the root of the pulmonary artery is the same as that in the aorta (about 40 cm/s). It falls off rapidly, then rises slightly again in the larger pulmonary veins. It takes a red cell about 0.75 s to traverse the pulmonary capillaries at rest and 0.3 s or less during exercise.

EFFECT OF GRAVITY

Gravity has a relatively marked effect on the pulmonary circulation. In the upright position, the upper portions of the lungs are well above the level of the heart, and the bases are at or below it. Consequently, in the upper part of the lungs, the blood flow is less, the alveoli are larger, and ventilation is less than at the base. The pressure in the capillaries at the top of the lungs is close to the atmospheric pressure in the alveoli. Pulmonary arterial pressure is

normally just sufficient to maintain perfusion, but if it is reduced or if alveolar pressure is increased, some of the capillaries collapse. Under these circumstances, no gas exchange takes place in the affected alveoli and they become part of the physiologic dead space.

In the middle portions of the lungs, the pulmonary arterial and capillary pressure exceeds alveolar pressure, but the pressure in the pulmonary venules may be lower than alveolar pressure during normal expiration, so they are collapsed. Under these circumstances, blood flow is determined by the pulmonary artery–alveolar pressure difference rather than the pulmonary artery–pulmonary vein difference. Beyond the constriction, blood "falls" into the pulmonary veins, which are compliant and take whatever amount of blood the constriction lets flow into them. This has been called the **waterfall effect.** Obviously, the compression of vessels produced by alveolar pressure decreases and pulmonary blood flow increases as the arterial pressure increases toward the base of the lung. In the lower portions of the lungs, alveolar pressure is lower than the pressure in all parts of the pulmonary circulation and blood flow is determined by the arterial–venous pressure difference. Examples of diseases affecting the pulmonary circulation are given in Clinical Box 34–4.

VENTILATION/PERFUSION RATIOS

The ratio of pulmonary ventilation to pulmonary blood flow for the whole lung at rest is about 0.8 (4.2 L/min ventilation divided by 5.5 L/min blood flow). However, relatively marked differences occur in this **ventilation/perfusion ratio** in various parts of the

---

CLINICAL BOX 34–4

Diseases Affecting the Pulmonary Circulation

Pulmonary Hypertension

Sustained idiopathic pulmonary hypertension can occur at any age. Like systemic arterial hypertension, it is a syndrome with multiple causes. However, the causes are different from those causing systemic hypertension. They include hypoxia, inhalation of cocaine, treatment with dexfenfluramine and related appetite-suppressing drugs that increase extracellular serotonin, and systemic lupus erythematosus. Some cases are familial and appear to be related to mutations that increase the sensitivity of pulmonary vessels to growth factors or cause deformations in the pulmonary vascular system.

All these conditions lead to increased pulmonary vascular resistance. If appropriate therapy is not initiated, the increased right ventricular afterload can lead eventually to right heart failure and death. Treatment with vasodilators such as prostacyclin and prostacyclin analogs is effective. Until recently, these had to be administered by continuous intravenous infusion, but aerosolized preparations that appear to be effective are now available.

normal lung as a result of the effect of gravity, and/or disease. If the ventilation to an alveolus is reduced relative to its perfusion, the P_{O_2} in the alveolus falls because less O_2 is delivered to it and the P_{CO_2} rises because less CO_2 is expired. Conversely, if perfusion is reduced relative to ventilation, the P_{CO_2} falls because less CO_2 is delivered and the P_{O_2} rises because less O_2 enters the blood. When widespread, nonuniformity of ventilation and perfusion in the lungs can cause CO_2 retention and lowers systemic arterial P_{O_2}.

REGULATION OF PULMONARY BLOOD FLOW

Pulmonary blood flow is affected by both active and passive factors. There is an extensive autonomic innervation of the pulmonary vessels, and stimulation of the cervical sympathetic ganglia reduces pulmonary blood flow by as much as 30%. The vessels also respond to a wide variety of circulating humoral agents. Many of the dilator responses are endothelium-dependent and presumably operate via release of nitric oxide (NO).

Passive factors such as cardiac output and gravitational forces also have significant effects on pulmonary blood flow. Local adjustments of perfusion to ventilation occur with local changes in O_2. With exercise, cardiac output increases and pulmonary arterial pressure rises. More red cells move through the lungs without any reduction in the O_2 saturation of the hemoglobin in them, and consequently, the total amount of O_2 delivered to the systemic circulation is increased. Capillaries dilate, and previously underperfused capillaries are "recruited" to carry blood. The net effect is a marked increase in pulmonary blood flow with few, if any, alterations in autonomic outflow to the pulmonary vessels.

When a bronchus or a bronchiole is obstructed, hypoxia develops in the underventilated alveoli beyond the obstruction. The O_2 deficiency apparently acts directly on vascular smooth muscle in the area to produce constriction, shunting blood away from the hypoxic area. Accumulation of CO_2 leads to a drop in pH in the area, and a decline in pH also produces vasoconstriction in the lungs, as opposed to the vasodilation it produces in other tissues. Conversely, reduction of the blood flow to a portion of the lung lowers the alveolar P_{CO_2} in that area, and this leads to constriction of the bronchi supplying it, shifting ventilation away from the poorly perfused area. Systemic hypoxia also causes the pulmonary arterioles to constrict, with a resultant increase in pulmonary arterial pressure.

METABOLIC & ENDOCRINE FUNCTIONS OF THE LUNGS

In addition to their functions in gas exchange, the lungs have a number of metabolic functions. They manufacture surfactant for local use, as noted above. They also contain a fibrinolytic system that lyses clots in the pulmonary vessels. They release a variety of substances that enter the systemic arterial blood (Table 34–2), and they remove other substances from the systemic venous blood that reach them via the pulmonary artery. Prostaglandins are

TABLE 34–2 Biologically active substances metabolized by the lungs.

| **Synthesized and used in the lungs** |
| Surfactant |
| **Synthesized or stored and released into the blood** |
| Prostaglandins |
| Histamine |
| Kallikrein |
| **Partially removed from the blood** |
| Prostaglandins |
| Bradykinin |
| Adenine nucleotides |
| Serotonin |
| Norepinephrine |
| Acetylcholine |
| **Activated in the lungs** |
| Angiotensin I → angiotensin II |

removed from the circulation, but they are also synthesized in the lungs and released into the blood when lung tissue is stretched.

The lungs play an important role in activating angiotensin. The physiologically inactive decapeptide angiotensin I is converted to the pressor, aldosterone-stimulating octapeptide angiotensin II in the pulmonary circulation. The reaction occurs in other tissues as well, but it is particularly prominent in the lungs. Large amounts of the angiotensin-converting enzyme responsible for this activation are located on the surface of the endothelial cells of the pulmonary capillaries. The converting enzyme also inactivates bradykinin. Circulation time through the pulmonary capillaries is less than 1 s, yet 70% of the angiotensin I reaching the lungs is converted to angiotensin II in a single trip through the capillaries. Four other peptidases have been identified on the surface of the pulmonary endothelial cells, but their full physiologic role is unsettled.

Removal of serotonin and norepinephrine reduces the amounts of these vasoactive substances reaching the systemic circulation. However, many other vasoactive hormones pass through the lungs without being metabolized. These include epinephrine, dopamine, oxytocin, vasopressin, and angiotensin II. In addition, various amines and polypeptides are secreted by neuroendocrine cells in the lungs.

CHAPTER SUMMARY

- Air enters the respiratory system in the upper airway, proceeds to the conducting airway and then on to the respiratory airway that ends in the alveoli. The cross-sectional area of the airway gradually increases through the conducting zone, and then rapidly increases during the transition from conducting to respiratory zones.
- The mucociliary escalator in the conducting airway helps keep particulates out of the respiratory zone.
- There are several important measures of lung volume, including tidal volume, inspiratory volume, expiratory reserve

volume, FVC, the forced expiratory volume in the first second (FEV_1), RMV, and maximal voluntary ventilation.

- Net "driving pressure" for air movement into the lung includes the force of muscle contraction, lung compliance ($\Delta P/\Delta V$), and airway resistance ($\Delta P/\Delta V$).

- Surfactant decreases surface tension in the alveoli and helps keep them from deflating.

- Not all air that enters the airway is available for gas exchange. The regions where gas is not exchanged in the airway are termed "dead space." The conducting airway represents anatomic dead space. Increased dead space can occur in response to disease that affects air exchange in the respiratory zone (physiologic dead space).

- The pressure gradient in the pulmonary circulation system is much less than that in the systemic circulation.

- There are a variety of biologically activated substances that are metabolized in the lung. These include substances that are made and function in the lung (eg, surfactant), substances that are released or removed from the blood (eg, prostaglandins), and substances that are activated as they pass through the lung (eg, angiotensin II).

MULTIPLE-CHOICE QUESTIONS

For all questions, select the single best answer unless otherwise directed.

1. A group of friends from San Francisco, California, where the sea level barometric pressure is 760 mm Hg traveled to the summit of Mt. Everest, where the barometric pressure is about 250 mm Hg. Before leaving the Bay Area, the travelers measure the partial pressure of O_2 (Po_2) and they again measure Po_2 at the top of Mt. Everest. Assuming they are measuring "dry air," what is the difference in Po_2 at the two sites?
   A. 21%
   B. 52.5 mm Hg
   C. 107.5 mm Hg
   D. 160 mm Hg
   E. 510 mm Hg

2. A nurse in the pulmonology clinic administered respiratory tests on a subject. After speaking with the subject, he reported to the patient that the FVC measured at 4 L. Which statement below best describes what the nurse measured?
   A. The amount of air that normally moves into (or out of) the lung with each respiration.
   B. The amount of air that enters the lung but does not participate in gas exchange.
   C. The amount of air expired after maximal expiratory effort.
   D. The largest amount of gas that can be moved into and out of the lungs in 1 min.

3. You visit a grade school classroom with a homemade spirometer consisting of a tub of water, tube, and jug filled with water. You fill the jug with water and invert it into the tub and connect the tube. You ask each child to breath normally for five breaths, then, after a normal inhalation, have them exhale normally into the tube to displace water from the jug. You have the child repeat this five times. Upon completion of this exercise, you recover the jug and measure how much water has been displaced and divide by 5. You report to the

student their number. At the end of the class you ask all the students of their number and present a class average. What is it that you measured?
   A. Minute ventilatory volume
   B. Tidal volume
   C. Forced vital capacity (FVC)
   D. Dead space

4. In the laboratory, two students were able to model the movement of O_2 from the alveoli into the blood in the pulmonary capillaries by setting up a simple system. Their system contained two O_2 "tight" containers on either side of an O_2 permeable membrane such that O_2 could only pass between the two containers, but could not leave the containers. When they injected O_2 into one container, they noted a very fast equilibration of O_2 between the two sides. Which of the following explains the movement of O_2 across the membrane in their model and across the aveolocapillary membrane?
   A. Active transport
   B. Filtration
   C. Secondary active transport
   D. Facilitated diffusion
   E. Passive diffusion

5. In a classical physiology experiment the lungs were removed from a cadaver and PV curves were constructed (eg, Figure 34-8). When the lungs were filled with saline, PV curves for inflation and deflation were well-aligned and required minimal pressure. However, when lungs underwent PV testing with air, the curves were shifted to the right (more pressure required for similar volume change) and a clear hysteresis was observed (ie, inflation curves were shifted right of the deflation curves). Which of the following characteristics of the lung contributes to the saline shift and hysteresis?
   A. Collagen lining the trachea and primary/secondary bronchi is stiffened by saline.
   B. Lung inflation of collapsed alveoli requires more pressure to change initial volume, this is not observed during deflation.
   C. Dilution of mucus in the airways by saline allows for more laminar flow of liquid in the lung and reduces pressure differences between inflation and deflation.
   D. Airway resistance in the conducting airway is much higher for air compared to saline.

6. A baby born prematurely is taken to the intensive care unit and diagnosed with respiratory distress syndrome. The baby is quickly intubated through the nose to the airways, is given surfactant and is treated with noninvasive positive pressure ventilation to aid in breathing. Surfactant replacement and aided breathing continue until the baby can breathe on its own. The purpose of the surfactant treatment is to:
   A. help prevent alveolar collapse during breathing.
   B. stimulate ATI cells to secrete natural surfactant into the alveolus.
   C. increase mucus lining to allow for laminar airflow into the airway.
   D. stimulate innate immunity in the lung to prevent infections during treatment.

7. A patient enters the clinic complaining of dyspnea and persistent, nonproductive cough. After discussion, the patient reveals that the dyspnea has gotten progressively worse over the past year and he has additionally experienced weight loss,

fatigue, joint, and muscular pain. Which of the following spirometry and lung compliance measurements consistent with idiopathic pulmonary fibrosis were obtained from this patient?

A. A high FEV_1 and high lung compliance
B. A high FEV_1 and a low lung compliance
C. A normal FEV_1 and a high compliance
D. A low FEV_1 and a low lung compliance
E. A low FEV_1 and a high lung compliance

8. A 180-lb male patient comes in for surgical correction of a traumatic hernia sustained from a mountain biking accident. His chest X-ray is normal and has the following results from room air pulmonary function testing: tidal volume, 600 mL; respiratory rate, 12 breaths/min; vital capacity, 5L; Pao_2, 90 mm Hg; $Paco_2$, 40 mm Hg; $PEco_2$, 28 mm Hg. As a measure of lung health, you calculate his physiologic dead space and compare this to an estimate for his anatomical dead space. What do you find as his physiological dead space and anatomical dead space estimate, respectively?

A. 150 mL, 450 mL
B. 150 mL, 180 mL
C. 180 mL, 150 mL
D. 450 mL, 180 mL
E. 180 mL, 180 mL

9. A young adult male takes advantage of the free clinic to discuss recurring symptoms with a doctor. He explains that although he feels well at the moment, he sometimes hears some sound upon exhalation, and also can experience slight chest tightness and shortness of breath on occasion. The patient states that breathing symptoms come and go but tend to worsen seasonally. Standard spirometry tests are taken before and after inhalation of an β-adrenergic receptor agonist. Which of the following would be consistent with the diagnosis of asthma?

A. Initial tests: normal FEV_1, normal FVC, normal FEV_1/FVC; after inhalation treatment: no change.
B. Initial tests: normal FEV_1, normal FVC, normal FEV_1/FVC; after inhalation treatment: increased FEV_1, increased FVC, normal FEV_1/FVC.
C. Initial tests: low FEV_1, low FVC, normal FEV_1/FVC; after inhalation treatment: low FEV_1, low FVC, normal FEV_1/FVC.
D. Initial tests: low FEV_1, low FVC, low FEV_1/FVC; after inhalation treatment: improved FEV_1, slightly improved FVC, near normal FEV_1/FVC.

10. A scientist has isolated bronchial airway epithelial cells from a patient with cystic fibrosis (CF) and his parent who has shown no symptoms into her 50s. The scientist is able to form fully differentiated cells representing the airway in the laboratory using advanced tissue culture techniques. She sets out to make some comparative measurements between tissue cultures derived from the CF patient and those derived from the parent. Assuming the cultures faithfully reproduce what was observed in vivo, which of the following might the scientist expect to see in the epithelium derived from the CF patient when compared to that derived from the parent?

A. Higher mucus secretion
B. Altered potassium ion movement
C. Reduced chloride ion movement
D. Increased development of mucus secreting cells
E. Increased calcium ion movement

ANSWERS

1. The correct answer is **C**. The O_2 composition in dry air is the same at sea level or on top of Mt. Everest, 21%. The Po_2 is calculated by the multiplying the O_2 composition by the barometric pressure. Thus, at sea level, $Po_2 = 0.21 \times 760$ mm Hg, or 160 mm Hg (ruling out **D**); and on top of Mt. Everest, $Po_2 = 0.21 \times 250$ mm Hg, or 52.5 mm Hg (ruling out **B**). The difference, then, between sea level and Mt. Everest is $160 - 52.5 = 107.5$ mm Hg. The barometric pressure difference shown in (**E**) does not take into account the 21% oxygen in the air (**B**), both of which can be used to arrive at the correct answer (0.21×510 mm Hg = 107.1 mm Hg).

2. The correct answer is **C**. The maneuver is described is generally used to measure both the maximal respiratory effort, or FVC, and the forced expiratory volume during the first second (FEV_1). Both measurements, and more specifically, the ratio, FEV_1/FVC are important indicators of lung health. Answer **A** refers to the tidal volume, and is a measure of quiet respiration. Answer **B** refers to the dead space, and in healthy patients is a measure of the conducting airways. Answer **D** is referred to as the maximal minute volume.

3. The correct answer is **B**. You have asked the students to participate in quiet breathing and have measured the exhaled volume during this maneuver, also known as tidal volume. The minute ventilatory volume is the tidal volume collected over a minute of quiet breathing. Since you are averaging single breaths during quiet breathing, **A** can be ruled out. The FVC (**B**) refers to the maximum amount of air that can be exhaled after a full inhalation, and can be ruled out by the stated protocol of quiet breathing. Dead space (**D**) refers to the amount of air that enters the lung but does not participate in gas exchange, this cannot be inferred from the above maneuver and can be ruled out.

4. The correct answer is **E**. When O_2 reaches the alveoli it can freely move down its concentration gradient and across the alveolocapillary membrane via passive diffusion. As long as the membrane in the experimental box is permeable to oxygen, it will act similarly to the alveolocapillary membrane. Primary or secondary active transport as well as facilitated diffusion require proteins that specifically bind molecules for transport across membranes, none of these were provided, nor needed, in the experiment and thus, **A**, **C**, and **D** could be eliminated. Filtration refers to active removal of particles from a solution, in contrast, O_2 is able to freely move down its concentration gradient from one box to the other, ruling out **B**.

5. The correct answer is **B**. Collapsed alveoli, as might be encountered with a fully deflated lung, will have to overcome surface tension when inflated with air, but not with saline. As more pressure is exerted, more alveoli are recruited until the lung is fully inflated. This explains the shift to the right in the saline vs air experiments. Surface tension and the surfactant that naturally reduces surface tension in the lung also contribute to hysteresis, as compression of an expanded alveolus requires less pressure change than expansion and recruitment of alveoli during lung inflation. **A** is ruled out because the trachea and primary/secondary bronchi are stiff structures that are not collapsible with pressures used for inflation/deflation of the lung, and saline does not alter this stiffness. The presence or absence of normal amounts of mucus would not significantly alter air flow between inflation and deflation, ruling out **C**. Airway

resistance would be higher in a fluid-filled conduit compared to an air-filled conduit, ruling out **D**.

6. The correct answer is **A**. Surfactant is a lipid/protein mixture that is naturally secreted by ATII cells (ruling out **B**) in the epithelial lining of the lung to reduce surface tensions and keep alveoli from collapsing. Maturation of ATII cells occurs later in gestation and lack of surfactant secretion is common in premature births. Although some surfactant proteins can be found in the mucus lining of the conducting airway and can contribute to innate immunity via opsonization properties, they are a minimal component of mucus that does not affect airflow (ruling out **C**) nor stimulate other cells in the airway for innate immune purposes (eliminating **D**).

7. The correct answer is **D**. Idiopathic pulmonary fibrosis is associated with scarring of the alveoli that results in lung stiffness and limited lung expansion. A stiff lung would show lower changes in lung volume in response to increased pressure (ie, low compliance eliminating **A, C,** and **D**). Although the spirometry test might show a normal, or even high FEV_1/FVC ratio, the absolute measurements of FEV_1 and FVC would be reduced due to the limited ability to fully expand the lung (eliminating **A** and **B**).

8. The correct answer is **E**. Physiological dead space (V_D) can be calculated using the modified Bohr equation and measurements for expired P_{CO_2} (P_{ECO_2}), tidal volume (V_T), and arterial P_{CO_2} (P_{aCO_2}) as follows: $P_{ECO_2} \times V_T = P_{aCO_2} \times (V_T - V_D)$.

Rearranging this equation and solving for V_D yields: $V_D = V_T - (P_{ECO_2} \times V_T / P_{aCO_2})$. Putting in values from the tests above yields: $VD = 600$ mL $- (28$ mm Hg $\times 600$ mL$)/40$ mm Hg; $VD = 180$. This value is consistent with estimating anatomic dead space estimated by body weight (eg, 1 mL VD/1 lb body weight), and representative of a healthy individual.

9. The correct answer is **D**. Asthma is characterized by an obstructive airflow pattern (low FEV_1, low FVC and low FEV_1/FVC) when left untreated. Inhalation of β-adrenergic receptor agonists allows for bronchial smooth muscle relaxation and increased airflow, and can reverse obstructive airflow readings in asthmatics. Because airflow patterns in **A** and **B** are both normal before treatment, they are not indicative of asthma, and thus, can be ruled out. Although **C** does show reduced FEV_1 and FVC measurements at rest, the normal (or even a high) reading of FEV_1/FVC is more indicative of a restrictive airway disease and would not be expected for an asthmatic, and thus can be ruled out.

10. The correct answer is **C**. While it is true that CF patients suffer from increased mucus in the airway, this increase is not due to overproduction of mucus from airway epithelial cells, ruling out **A** and **D**. The primary defect in CF is lack of Cl^- movement due to a mutation in a Cl^- channel, the cystic fibrosis transmembrane conductance regulator (CFTR). It is the loss of Cl^- movement that limits water movement into the airway that subsequently traps mucus, ruling out **B** and **E**.

Gas Transport & pH

- Describe the manner in which O_2 flows "downhill" from the lungs to the tissues and CO_2 flows "downhill" from the tissues to the lungs.
- Explain the role for hemoglobin in O_2 transport.
- List the reactions that increase the amount of CO_2 in the blood, and draw the CO_2 dissociation curve for arterial and venous blood.
- Define alkalosis and acidosis; list typical causes and compensatory responses to each.
- Describe the effects of hypercapnia and hypocapnia, and give examples of conditions that can cause them.

INTRODUCTION

The concentrations for O_2 and CO_2 (measured as partial pressures, or Po_2 and Pco_2) change within each region of the lung, allowing for these gases to flow "downhill" or from higher partial pressures to lower partial pressures. For example, Po_2 is highest in the alveoli upon inspiration and lowest in the deoxygenated blood, whereas Pco_2 is exactly opposite. This allows for O_2 to cross the alveoli and re-oxygenate the blood in the pulmonary vasculature, while CO_2 leaves the bloodstream and enters the alveoli where it is expired. However, the amount of both these gases transported to and from the tissues would

be grossly inadequate if it were not for the fact that about 99% of the O_2 that dissolves in the blood combines with the O_2-carrying protein hemoglobin and that about 94.5% of the CO_2 that dissolves enters into a series of reversible chemical reactions that convert it into other compounds. Thus, the presence of hemoglobin increases the O_2-carrying capacity of the blood 70-fold, and the reactions of CO_2 increase the blood CO_2 content 17-fold. In this chapter, physiologic details that underlie O_2 and CO_2 movement under various conditions are discussed.

■ OXYGEN TRANSPORT

OXYGEN DELIVERY TO THE TISSUES

Oxygen delivery—the volume of oxygen delivered to the systemic vascular bed per minute—is the product of cardiac output and arterial oxygen concentration. The ability to deliver O_2 in the body depends on both the respiratory and the cardiovascular system. O_2 delivery to a particular tissue depends on the amount of O_2 entering the lungs, the adequacy of pulmonary gas exchange, the blood flow to the tissue, and the capacity of the

blood to carry O_2. Blood flow to an individual tissue depends on cardiac output and the degree of constriction of the vascular bed in the tissue. The amount of O_2 in the blood is determined by the amount of dissolved O_2, the amount of hemoglobin in the blood, and the affinity of the hemoglobin for O_2.

REACTION OF HEMOGLOBIN & OXYGEN

The dynamics of the reaction of hemoglobin with O_2 make it a particularly suitable O_2 carrier. Hemoglobin is a protein made up of four subunits, each of which contains a **heme** moiety attached to a polypeptide chain. In normal adults, most of the hemoglobin molecules contain two α and two β chains. Heme is a porphyrin ring complex that includes one atom of ferrous iron. Each of the four iron atoms in hemoglobin can reversibly bind one O_2 molecule. Because the iron stays in the ferrous state the reaction is **oxygenation** and not oxidation. It has been customary to write the reaction of hemoglobin with O_2 as $Hb + O_2 \rightleftarrows HbO_2$. Because it contains four deoxyhemoglobin (Hb) units, the hemoglobin molecule can also be represented as Hb_4, and it actually reacts with four molecules of O_2 to form Hb_4O_8. The reaction is rapid, requiring less than 0.01 s. The deoxygenation of Hb_4O_8 is also very rapid.

The quaternary structure of hemoglobin determines its affinity for O_2. In deoxyhemoglobin, the globin units are tightly bound in a **tense (T) configuration,** which reduces the affinity of the molecule for O_2. When O_2 is first bound, the bonds holding the globin units are released, producing a **relaxed (R) configuration,** which exposes more O_2 binding sites. The net result is a 500-fold increase in O_2 affinity. In tissues, these reactions are reversed, resulting in O_2 release. The transition from one state to another has been calculated to occur about 10^8 times in the life of a red blood cell (RBC). The **oxygen–hemoglobin dissociation curve** relates percentage saturation of the O_2-carrying power of hemoglobin (abbreviated as SaO_2) to the PO_2 (**Figure 35–1**). This curve has a characteristic sigmoid shape due to the T–R configuration interconversion. Note that small changes at low PO_2 lead to large changes in SaO_2.

When blood is equilibrated with 100% O_2, the normal hemoglobin becomes 100% saturated. When fully saturated, each gram of normal hemoglobin contains 1.39 mL of O_2. However, blood normally contains small quantities of inactive hemoglobin derivatives, and the measured value in vivo is thus slightly lower. Using the traditional estimate of saturated hemoglobin in vivo, 1.34 mL of O_2, the hemoglobin concentration in normal blood is about 15 g/dL (14 g/dL in women and 16 g/dL in men). Therefore, 1 dL of blood contains 20.1 mL (1.34 mL × 15) of O_2 bound to hemoglobin when the hemoglobin is 100% saturated. The amount of dissolved O_2 is a linear function of the PO_2 (0.003 mL/dL blood/mm Hg PO_2).

In vivo, the hemoglobin in the blood at the ends of the pulmonary capillaries is about 97.5% saturated with O_2 (PO_2 = 100 mm Hg). Because of a slight admixture with venous blood that bypasses the pulmonary capillaries (ie, physiologic shunt), the hemoglobin in systemic arterial blood is only 97%

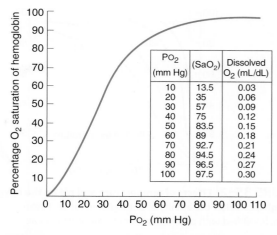

FIGURE 35–1 **Oxygen–hemoglobin dissociation curve.** pH 7.40, temperature 38°C. Inset table relates the percentage of saturated hemoglobin (SaO_2) to PO_2 and dissolved O_2. (Modified with permission from Comroe JH Jr, et al: *The Lung: Clinical Physiology and Pulmonary Function Tests*, 2nd ed. Year Book; 1962.)

saturated. The arterial blood therefore contains a total of about 19.8 mL of O_2 per dL: 0.29 mL in solution and 19.5 mL bound to hemoglobin. In venous blood at rest, the hemoglobin is 75% saturated and the total O_2 content is about 15.2 mL/dL: 0.12 mL in solution and 15.1 mL bound to hemoglobin. Thus, at rest the tissues remove about 4.6 mL of O_2 from each deciliter of blood passing through them (**Table 35–1**); 0.17 mL of this total represents O_2 that was in solution in the blood, and the remainder represents O_2 that was liberated from hemoglobin. In this way, 250 mL of O_2 per minute is transported from the blood to the tissues at rest.

FACTORS AFFECTING THE AFFINITY OF HEMOGLOBIN FOR OXYGEN

Three important conditions affect the oxygen–hemoglobin dissociation curve: the **pH,** the **temperature,** and the concentration of **2,3-diphosphoglycerate (2,3-DPG).** A rise in temperature or a fall in pH shifts the curve to the right (**Figure 35–2**). When the curve is shifted in this direction, a higher PO_2 is required for hemoglobin to bind a given amount of O_2. Conversely, a fall in

TABLE 35–1 **Gas content of blood.**

	mL/dL of Blood Containing 15 g of Hemoglobin			
	Arterial Blood (PO_2 95 mm Hg; PCO_2 40 mm Hg; Hb 97% Saturated)		Venous Blood (PO_2 40 mm Hg; PCO_2 46 mm Hg; Hb 75% Saturated)	
Gas	Dissolved	Combined	Dissolved	Combined
O_2	0.29	19.5	0.12	15.1
CO_2	2.62	46.4	2.98	49.7
N_2	0.98	0	0.98	0

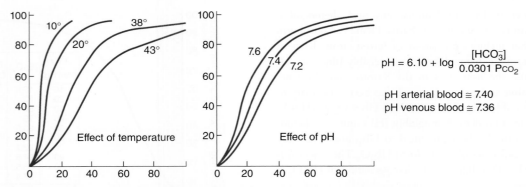

FIGURE 35–2 Effects of temperature and pH on the oxygen–hemoglobin dissociation curve. Both changes in temperature **(left)** and pH **(right)** can alter the affinity of hemoglobin for O_2. Plasma pH can be estimated using the modified Henderson–Hasselbalch equation, as shown. (Modified with permission from Comroe JH Jr, et al: *The Lung: Clinical Physiology and Pulmonary Function Tests*, 2nd ed. Year Book; 1962.)

temperature or a rise in pH shifts the curve to the left, and a lower P_{O_2} is required to bind a given amount of O_2. A convenient index for comparison of such shifts is the P_{50}, the P_{O_2} at which hemoglobin is half saturated with O_2. The higher the P_{50}, the lower the affinity of hemoglobin for O_2.

The decrease in O_2 affinity of hemoglobin when the pH of blood falls is called the **Bohr effect** and is closely related to the fact that deoxyhemoglobin binds H^+ more actively than does oxyhemoglobin. The pH of blood falls as its CO_2 content increases, so that when the P_{CO_2} rises, the curve shifts to the right and the P_{50} rises. Most of the unsaturation of hemoglobin that occurs in the tissues is secondary to the decline in the P_{O_2}, but an extra 1–2%

unsaturation is due to the rise in P_{CO_2} and consequent shift of the dissociation curve to the right.

2,3-DPG is plentiful in red cells. It is a highly charged anion that binds to the β chains of deoxyhemoglobin. One mole of deoxyhemoglobin binds 1 mol of 2,3-DPG. In effect,

$$HbO_2 + 2,3\text{-DPG} \rightleftarrows Hb - 2,3\text{-DPG} + O_2$$

In this equilibrium, an increase in the concentration of 2,3-DPG shifts the reaction to the right, causing more O_2 to be liberated. Some clinical features of hemoglobin are discussed in **Clinical Box 35–1**.

CLINICAL BOX 35–1

Hemoglobin & O_2 Binding In Vivo

Cyanosis
Reduced hemoglobin has a dark color, and a dusky bluish discoloration of the tissues (**cyanosis**), appears when the reduced hemoglobin concentration of the blood in the capillaries is more than 5 g/dL. Its occurrence depends on the total amount of hemoglobin in the blood, the degree of hemoglobin unsaturation, and the state of the capillary circulation. Cyanosis is most easily seen in the nail beds and mucous membranes and in the earlobes, lips, and fingers, where the skin is thin. Although visible observation is indicative of cyanosis, it is not fully reliable. Further tests of arterial oxygen tension and saturation, blood and hemoglobin counts can provide more reliable diagnoses.

Effects of 2,3-DPG on Fetal & Stored Blood
The affinity of fetal hemoglobin (hemoglobin F) for O_2 is greater than that for adult hemoglobin (hemoglobin A) and facilitates the movement of O_2 from the mother to the fetus. One cause of this greater affinity is the poor binding of 2,3-DPG by the γ polypeptide chains that replace β chains in fetal hemoglobin. Some abnormal hemoglobins in adults have low P_{50} values, and the resulting high O_2 affinity of the hemoglobin

causes enough tissue hypoxia to stimulate increased red cell formation, with resulting polycythemia.

Red cell 2,3-DPG concentration is increased in anemia and in a variety of diseases in which there is chronic hypoxia. This facilitates the delivery of O_2 to the tissues by raising the P_{O_2} at which O_2 is released in peripheral capillaries. In stored blood the 2,3-DPG level falls and the ability of this blood to release O_2 to the tissues is reduced. This decrease, which obviously limits the benefit of the blood if it is transfused into a hypoxic patient, is less if the blood is stored in citrate–phosphate–dextrose solution rather than the usual acid–citrate–dextrose solution.

THERAPEUTIC HIGHLIGHTS
Cyanosis is an indication of poorly oxygenated hemoglobin rather than a disease, and thus can have many causes, from cold exposure to drug overdose to chronic lung disease. As such, proper treatment depends on the underlying cause. For cyanosis caused by exposure to cold, maintaining a warm environment can be effective, whereas supplemental oxygen administration may be required under conditions of chronic disease.

■ CARBON DIOXIDE TRANSPORT

MOLECULAR FATE OF CARBON DIOXIDE IN BLOOD

The solubility of CO_2 in blood is about 20 times that of O_2; therefore, considerably more CO_2 than O_2 is present in simple solution at equal partial pressures. The CO_2 that diffuses into RBCs is rapidly hydrated to H_2CO_3 because of the presence of carbonic anhydrase (**Figure 35–3**). H_2CO_3 dissociates to H^+ and HCO_3^-, and the H^+ is buffered, primarily by hemoglobin, while the HCO_3^- enters the plasma. Some of the CO_2 in the red cells reacts with the amino groups of hemoglobin and other proteins (R), forming **carbamino compounds.** Because deoxyhemoglobin binds more H^+ than oxyhemoglobin and forms carbamino compounds more readily, binding of O_2 to hemoglobin reduces its affinity for CO_2. The **Haldane effect** refers to the increased capacity of deoxygenated hemoglobin to bind and carry CO_2. Consequently, venous blood carries more CO_2 than arterial blood, CO_2 uptake is facilitated in the tissues, and CO_2 release is facilitated in the lungs. About 11% of the CO_2 added to the blood in the systemic capillaries is carried to the lungs as carbamino-CO_2.

CHLORIDE SHIFT

Because the rise in the HCO_3^- content of red cells is much greater than that in plasma as the blood passes through the capillaries, about 70% of the HCO_3^- formed in the red cells enters the plasma. The excess HCO_3^- leaves the red cells in exchange for Cl^- (Figure 35–3). This process is mediated by **anion exchanger 1,** a major membrane protein in the RBC. Because of this **chloride shift,** the Cl^- content of the red cells in venous blood is significantly greater than that in arterial blood. The chloride shift occurs rapidly and is essentially complete within 1 s. Note that for each CO_2 molecule added to a red cell, there is an increase of one osmotically active particle in the cell—either an HCO_3^- or a Cl^- (Figure 35–3). Consequently, the red cells take up water

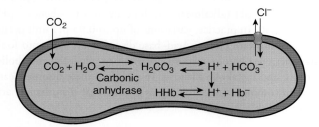

FIGURE 35–3 Fate of CO_2 in the red blood cell. Upon entering the red blood cell, CO_2 is rapidly hydrated to H_2CO_3 by carbonic anhydrase. H_2CO_3 is in equilibrium with H^+ and its conjugate base, HCO_3^-. H^+ can interact with deoxyhemoglobin, whereas HCO_3^- can be transported outside of the cell via anion exchanger 1 (AE1 or Band 3). In effect, for each CO_2 molecule that enters the red cell, there is an additional HCO_3^- or Cl^- in the cell.

TABLE 35–2 Fate of CO_2 in blood.

In plasma
1. Dissolved
2. Formation of carbamino compounds with plasma protein
3. Hydration, H^+ buffered, HCO_3^- in plasma
In red blood cells
1. Dissolved
2. Formation of carbamino-Hb
3. Hydration, H^+ buffered, 70% of HCO_3^- enters the plasma
4. Cl^- shifts into cells; mOsm in cells increases

and increase in size. In the lungs, the Cl^- moves back out of the cells and they shrink.

SPATIAL DISTRIBUTION OF CARBON DIOXIDE IN BLOOD

For convenience, the various fates of CO_2 in the plasma and red cells are summarized in Table 35–2. The extent to which they increase the capacity of the blood to carry CO_2 is indicated by the difference between the lines indicating the dissolved CO_2 and the total CO_2 in the dissociation curves for CO_2 shown in Figure 35–4. Of the approximately 49 mL of CO_2 in each deciliter of arterial blood (Table 35–1), 2.6 mL is dissolved, 2.6 mL is in carbamino compounds, and 43.8 mL is in HCO_3^-. In the tissues, 3.7 mL of CO_2 per dL of blood is added; 0.4 mL stays in solution, 0.8 mL forms carbamino compounds, and 2.5 mL forms HCO_3^-. Consequently, the pH of the blood drops from 7.40 to 7.36. In the lungs, the processes are reversed, and the 3.7 mL of

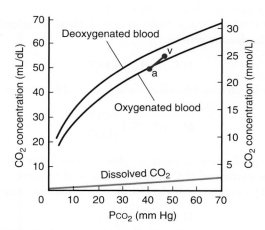

FIGURE 35–4 CO_2 dissociation curves. The arterial point (a) and the venous point (v) indicate the total CO_2 content found in arterial blood and venous blood of normal resting humans. Note the low amount of CO_2 that is dissolved (orange trace) compared to that which can be carried by other means (Table 35–2). (Modified with permission from Schmidt RF, Thews G: *Human Physiology.* New York: Springer; 1983.)

CO_2 is discharged into the alveoli. In this manner, 200 mL of CO_2 per minute at rest and much larger amounts during exercise are transported from the tissues to the lungs and excreted. It is worth noting that this amount of CO_2 is equivalent in 24 h to over 12,500 mEq of H^+.

ACID–BASE BALANCE & GAS TRANSPORT

The major source of acids in the blood under normal conditions is through cellular metabolism. The CO_2 formed by metabolism in the tissues is in large part hydrated to H_2CO_3, resulting in the large total H^+ load noted above. However, most of the CO_2 is excreted in the lungs, and the small quantities of the remaining H^+ are excreted by the kidneys.

BUFFERING IN THE BLOOD

Acid and base shifts in the blood are largely controlled by three main buffers in blood: (1) proteins, (2) hemoglobin, and (3) the carbonic acid–bicarbonate system. Plasma **proteins** are effective buffers because both their free carboxyl and their free amino groups dissociate.

The second buffer system is provided by the dissociation of the imidazole groups of the histidine residues in **hemoglobin.** In the pH 7.0–7.7 range, the free carboxyl and amino groups of hemoglobin contribute relatively little to its buffering capacity. However, the hemoglobin molecule contains 38 histidine residues, and on this basis—plus the fact that hemoglobin is present in large amounts—the hemoglobin in blood has six times the buffering capacity of the plasma proteins. In addition, the action of hemoglobin is unique because the imidazole groups of deoxyhemoglobin (Hb) dissociate less than those of oxyhemoglobin (HbO_2), making Hb a weaker acid and therefore a better buffer than HbO_2.

The third and major buffer system in blood is the **carbonic acid–bicarbonate system:**

$$H_2CO_3 \rightleftarrows H^+ + HCO_3^-$$

The Henderson–Hasselbalch equation for this system is

$$pH = pK + \log\frac{[HCO_3^-]}{[H_2CO_3]}$$

The pK for this system in an ideal solution is low (about 3), and the amount of H_2CO_3 is small and hard to measure accurately. However, in the body, H_2CO_3 is in equilibrium with CO_2:

$$H_2CO_3 \rightleftarrows CO_2 + H_2O$$

If the pK is changed to pK′ (apparent ionization constant due to less than ideal conditions for the solution) and $[CO_2]$ is substituted for $[H_2CO_3]$, the pK′ is 6.1:

$$pH = 6.10 + \log\frac{[HCO_3^-]}{[CO_2]}$$

The clinically relevant form of this equation is:

$$pH = 6.10 + \log\frac{[HCO_3^-]}{0.0301\ P_{CO_2}}$$

since the amount of dissolved CO_2 is proportional to the partial pressure of CO_2 and the solubility coefficient of CO_2 in mmol/L/mm Hg is 0.0301. $[HCO_3^-]$ cannot be measured directly, but pH and P_{CO_2} can be measured with suitable accuracy and $[HCO_3^-]$ can then be calculated.

The pK′ of this system is still low relative to the pH of the blood, but the system is one of the most effective buffer systems in the body because the amount of dissolved CO_2 is controlled by respiration (ie, it is an "open" system). Additional control of the plasma concentration of HCO_3^- is provided by the kidneys. When H^+ is added to the blood, HCO_3^- declines as more H_2CO_3 is formed. If the extra H_2CO_3 were not converted to CO_2 and H_2O and the CO_2 excreted in the lungs, the H_2CO_3 concentration would rise. Without CO_2 removal to reduce H_2CO_3, sufficient H^+ addition that would halve the plasma HCO_3^- would alter the pH 7.4 to 6.0. However, such an H^+ concentration increase is tolerated because: (1) extra H_2CO_3 that is formed is removed and (2) the H^+ rise stimulates respiration and therefore produces a drop in P_{CO_2}, so that some additional H_2CO_3 is removed. The net pH after such an increase in H^+ concentration is actually 7.2 or 7.3.

There are two additional factors that make the carbonic acid–bicarbonate system such a good biologic buffer. First, the reaction $CO_2 + H_2O \rightleftarrows H_2CO_3$ proceeds slowly in either direction unless the enzyme **carbonic anhydrase** is present. There is no carbonic anhydrase in plasma, but there is an abundant supply in RBCs, spatially confining and controlling the reaction. Second, the presence of hemoglobin in the blood increases the buffering of the system by binding free H^+ produced by the hydration of CO_2 and allowing for movement of the HCO_3^- into the plasma.

■ ACIDOSIS & ALKALOSIS

The pH of the arterial plasma is normally 7.40 and that of venous plasma slightly lower. A decrease in pH below the norm **(acidosis)** is technically present whenever the arterial pH is below 7.40 and an increase in pH **(alkalosis)** is technically present whenever pH is above 7.40. In practice, variations of up to 0.05 pH unit occur without untoward effects. Acid–base disorders are split into four categories: respiratory acidosis, respiratory alkalosis, metabolic acidosis, and metabolic alkalosis. In addition, these disorders can occur in combination. Some causes of acid–base disturbances are shown in Table 35–3.

RESPIRATORY ACIDOSIS

Any short-term rise in arterial P_{CO_2} results in **respiratory acidosis.** Recall that CO_2 that is retained is in equilibrium with H_2CO_3, which in turn is in equilibrium with HCO_3^-. The effective rise in plasma HCO_3^- means that a new equilibrium is reached

TABLE 35–3 Plasma pH, HCO₃⁻, and Pco₂ values in various typical disturbances of acid–base balance.ᵃ

Condition	pH	HCO₃⁻ (mEq/L)	Pco₂ (mm Hg)	Cause
Normal	7.40	24.1	40	
Metabolic acidosis	7.28	18.1	40	NH₄Cl ingestion
	6.96	5.0	23	Diabetic acidosis
Metabolic alkalosis	7.50	30.1	40	NaHCO₃ ingestion
	7.56	49.8	58	Prolonged vomiting
Respiratory acidosis	7.34	25.0	48	Breathing 7% CO₂
	7.34	33.5	64	Emphysema
Respiratory alkalosis	7.53	22.0	27	Voluntary hyperventilation
	7.48	18.7	26	Three-week residence at 4000-m altitude

ᵃIn the diabetic acidosis and prolonged vomiting examples, respiratory compensation for primary metabolic acidosis and alkalosis has occurred, and the Pco₂ has shifted from 40 mm Hg. In the emphysema and high-altitude examples, renal compensation for primary respiratory acidosis and alkalosis has occurred and has made the deviations from normal of the plasma HCO₃⁻ larger than they would otherwise be.

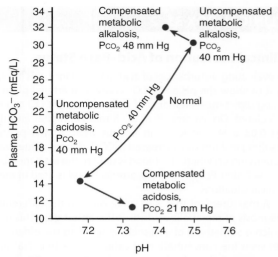

FIGURE 35–5 Acid–base paths during metabolic acidosis. Changes in true plasma pH, HCO₃⁻, and Pco₂ at rest, during metabolic acidosis and alkalosis, and following respiratory compensation are plotted. Metabolic acidosis or alkalosis causes changes in pH along the Pco₂ isobar line (middle line). Respiratory compensation moves pH toward normal by altering Pco₂ (top and bottom arrows).

at a lower pH. The pH change observed at any increase in Pco₂ during respiratory acidosis depends on the buffering capacity of the blood. Initial changes occur independently of any compensatory mechanism; that is, they are those of **uncompensated respiratory acidosis**.

RESPIRATORY ALKALOSIS

Any short-term lowering of Pco₂ below what is needed for proper CO₂ exchange results in **respiratory alkalosis.** The decreased CO₂ shifts the equilibrium of the carbonic acid–bicarbonate system to effectively lower [H⁺] and increase pH. As in respiratory acidosis, initial pH changes corresponding to respiratory alkalosis are those that occur independently of any compensatory mechanism and are thus **uncompensated respiratory alkalosis**.

METABOLIC ACIDOSIS & ALKALOSIS

Blood pH changes can also arise by nonrespiratory mechanism. **Metabolic acidosis** occurs when strong acids are added to blood. If, for example, a large amount of acid is ingested (eg, aspirin overdose), acids in the blood are quickly increased. The H₂CO₃ that is formed is converted to H₂O and CO₂, and the CO₂ is rapidly excreted via the lungs. This is the situation in **uncompensated metabolic acidosis.** Note that in contrast to respiratory acidosis, metabolic acidosis does not include a change in Pco₂; the shift toward metabolic

acidosis occurs along an isobar line (Figure 35–5). When the free [H⁺] level falls as a result of addition of alkali, or more commonly, the removal of large amounts of acid (eg, following vomiting), **metabolic alkalosis** results. In uncompensated metabolic alkalosis the pH rises along the isobar line (Figure35–5).

RESPIRATORY & RENAL COMPENSATION

Uncompensated acidosis and alkalosis as described above are seldom seen because of compensation systems. The two main compensatory systems are **respiratory compensation** and **renal compensation.**

The respiratory system compensates for metabolic acidosis or alkalosis by altering ventilation, and consequently, the Pco₂, which can directly change blood pH. Respiratory mechanisms are fast. In response to metabolic acidosis, ventilation is increased, resulting in a decrease of Pco₂ and a subsequent increase in pH toward normal (Figure 35–5). In response to metabolic alkalosis, ventilation is decreased, Pco₂ is increased, and a subsequent decrease in pH occurs. Because respiratory compensation is a quick response, the graphical representation in Figure 35–5 overstates the two-step adjustment in blood pH. In actuality, as soon as metabolic acidosis begins, respiratory compensation is invoked and the large shifts in pH depicted do not occur.

For complete compensation from respiratory or metabolic acidosis/alkalosis, renal compensatory mechanisms are invoked. The kidney responds to acidosis by actively secreting fixed acids

CLINICAL BOX 35-2

Clinical Evaluation of Acid–Base Status

In evaluating disturbances of acid–base balance, it is important to know the pH and HCO_3^- content of arterial plasma. Using direct measurements of pH and P_{CO_2}, $[HCO_3^-]$ can be calculated. On average, P_{CO_2} is ~8 mm Hg higher and the pH 0.03–0.04 unit lower in venous than arterial plasma resulting in 2 mmol/L increased $[HCO_3^-]$. Venous values vary depending on where the blood is drawn; the local metabolism will alter P_{CO_2}. Therefore, arterial blood is used in most clinical situations.

A measurement that is of some value in the differential diagnosis of metabolic acidosis is the **anion gap.** This gap, which is something of a misnomer, refers to the difference between the concentration of cations other than Na^+ and the concentration of anions other than Cl^- and HCO_3^- in the plasma. It consists for the most part of proteins in anionic form, HPO_4^{2-}, SO_4^{2-}, and organic acids; a normal value is about 12 mEq/L. It is increased when the plasma concentration of K^+, Ca^{2+}, or Mg^+ is decreased; when the concentration of (or the charge on) plasma proteins is increased; or when organic anions such as lactate or foreign anions accumulate in blood. It is decreased when cations are increased or when plasma albumin is decreased. The anion gap is increased in metabolic acidosis due to ketoacidosis, lactic acidosis, and other forms of acidosis in which organic anions are increased.

CLINICAL BOX 35-3

Effects of Hypoxia on Cells and Selected Tissues
Effects on Cells

Hypoxia causes the production of transcription factors (hypoxia-inducible factors; HIFs). These are made up of α and β subunits. In normally oxygenated tissues, the α subunits are rapidly ubiquitinated and destroyed. However, in hypoxic cells, the α subunits dimerize with β subunits, and the dimers activate genes that produce several proteins including angiogenic factors and erythropoietin, among others.

Effects on the Brain

In hypoxemia and the other generalized forms of hypoxia, the brain is affected first. A sudden drop in the inspired P_{O_2} to less than 20 mm Hg, which occurs, for example, when cabin pressure is suddenly lost in a plane flying above 16,000 m, can cause loss of consciousness in 10–20 s and death in 4–5 min. Less severe hypoxia causes a variety of mental aberrations not unlike those produced by alcohol: impaired judgment, drowsiness, dulled pain sensibility, excitement, disorientation, loss of time sense, and headache. Other symptoms include anorexia, nausea, vomiting, tachycardia, and, when the hypoxia is severe, hypertension. The rate of ventilation is increased in proportion to the severity of the hypoxia of the carotid chemoreceptor cells.

Respiratory Stimulation

Dyspnea is by definition difficult or labored breathing in which the person is conscious of shortness of breath; **hyperpnea** is the general term for an increase in the rate or depth of breathing regardless of the patient's subjective sensations. **Tachypnea** is rapid, shallow breathing. In general, a normal individual is not conscious of respiration until ventilation is doubled, and breathing is not uncomfortable until ventilation is tripled or quadrupled. Whether or not a given level of ventilation is uncomfortable also appears to depend on a variety of other factors. Hypercapnia and, to a lesser extent, hypoxia cause dyspnea. An additional factor is the effort involved in moving the air in and out of the lungs (the work of breathing).

while retaining filtered HCO_3^-. In contrast, the kidney responds to alkalosis by decreasing H^+ secretion and by decreasing the retention of filtered HCO_3^-. Clinical evaluations of acid–base status are discussed in **Clinical Box 35–2** and the role of the kidneys in acid–base homeostasis is discussed in more detail in Chapter 38.

■ HYPOXIA

Hypoxia is O_2 deficiency at the tissue level. Numerous classifications for hypoxia have been used, but the more traditional four-type system still has considerable utility if the definitions of the terms are kept clearly in mind. The four categories are (1) **hypoxemia** (sometimes termed **hypoxic hypoxia**), in which the P_{O_2} of the arterial blood is reduced; (2) **anemic hypoxia,** in which the arterial P_{O_2} is normal but the amount of hemoglobin available to carry O_2 is reduced; (3) **ischemic** or **stagnant hypoxia,** in which the blood flow to a tissue is so low that adequate O_2 is not delivered to it despite a normal P_{O_2} and hemoglobin concentration; and (4) **histotoxic hypoxia,** in which the amount of O_2 delivered to a tissue is adequate but, because of the action of a toxic agent, the tissue cells cannot make use of the O_2 supplied to them. Some specific effects of hypoxia on cells and tissues are discussed in **Clinical Box 35–3**.

■ HYPOXEMIA

By definition, hypoxemia is a condition of reduced arterial P_{O_2}. Hypoxemia is a problem in normal individuals at high altitudes and is a complication of pneumonia and a variety of other diseases of the respiratory system.

EFFECTS OF DECREASED BAROMETRIC PRESSURE

Despite a stable composition of air at increasing altitude, there is a drop in total barometric pressure **(Figure 35–6)**, resulting in a drop in P_{O_2}. At 3000 m above sea level, the alveolar P_{O_2} is

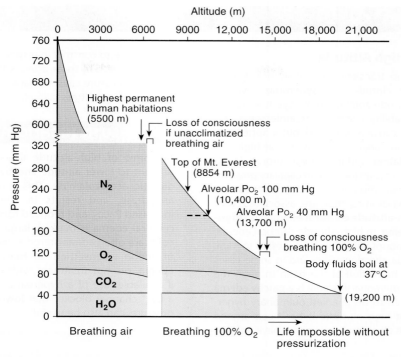

FIGURE 35–6 **Composition of alveolar air in individuals breathing air (0–6100 m) and 100% O₂ (6100–13,700 m).** The minimal alveolar P_{O_2} that an unacclimatized person can tolerate without loss of consciousness is about 35–40 mm Hg. Note that with increasing altitude, the alveolar P_{CO_2} drops because of the hyperventilation due to hypoxic stimulation of the carotid and aortic chemoreceptors. The fall in barometric pressure with increasing altitude is not linear because air is compressible.

about 60 mm Hg and there is enough hypoxic stimulation of the chemoreceptors under normal breathing to cause increased ventilation. As one ascends higher, the alveolar P_{O_2} falls less rapidly and the alveolar P_{CO_2} declines because of the hyperventilation. The resulting fall in arterial P_{CO_2} produces respiratory alkalosis. A number of compensatory mechanisms operate over a period of time to increase altitude tolerance (**acclimatization**), but in unacclimatized persons, mental symptoms such as irritability appear at about 3700 m. At 5500 m, the hypoxic symptoms are severe; and at altitudes above 6100 m (20,000 ft), consciousness is usually lost.

HYPOXIC SYMPTOMS & BREATHING OXYGEN

Some of the effects of high altitude can be offset by breathing 100% O₂. Under these conditions, the total atmospheric pressure becomes the limiting factor in altitude tolerance.

The partial pressure of water vapor in the alveolar air is constant at 47 mm Hg, and that of CO₂ is normally 40 mm Hg, so that the lowest barometric pressure at which a normal alveolar P_{O_2} of 100 mm Hg is possible is 187 mm Hg, the pressure at about 10,400 m (34,000 ft). At greater altitudes, the increased ventilation due to the decline in alveolar P_{O_2} lowers the alveolar P_{CO_2} somewhat, but the maximum alveolar P_{O_2} that can be attained when breathing 100% O₂ at the ambient barometric pressure of

100 mm Hg at 13,700 m is ~40 mm Hg. At ~14,000 m, consciousness is lost in spite of the administration of 100% O₂. At 19,200 m, the barometric pressure is 47 mm Hg, and at or below this pressure the body fluids boil at body temperature. Some delayed effects of high altitude are discussed in **Clinical Box 35–4.**

ACCLIMATIZATION

Acclimatization to altitude is due to the operation of a variety of compensatory mechanisms. The respiratory alkalosis produced by the hyperventilation shifts the oxygen–hemoglobin dissociation curve to the left, but a concomitant increase in RBC 2,3-DPG tends to decrease the O₂ affinity of hemoglobin. The net effect is a small increase in P_{50}. The decrease in O₂ affinity makes more O₂ available to the tissues.

The initial ventilatory response to increased altitude is relatively small, because the alkalosis tends to counteract the stimulating effect of hypoxia. However, ventilation steadily increases over the next 4 days because the active transport of H⁺ into cerebrospinal fluid (CSF), or possibly a developing lactic acidosis in the brain, causes a fall in CSF pH that increases the response to hypoxia. After 4 days, the ventilatory response begins to decline slowly, but it takes years of residence at higher altitudes for it to decline to the initial level, if it is reached at all.

Erythropoietin secretion increases promptly on ascent to high altitude and then falls somewhat over the following 4 days as the ventilatory response increases and the arterial P_{O_2} rises.

CLINICAL BOX 35–4

Delayed Effects of High Altitude

Many individuals develop transient "mountain sickness" in response to changes in altitude. This syndrome develops 8–24 h after arrival at altitude and lasts 4–8 days. It is characterized by headache, irritability, insomnia, breathlessness, and nausea and vomiting. Its cause is unsettled, but it appears to be associated with cerebral edema. The low Po_2 at high altitude causes arteriolar dilation, and if cerebral autoregulation does not compensate, there is an increase in capillary pressure that favors increased transudation of fluid into brain tissue.

Two more serious syndromes that are associated with high-altitude illness: **high-altitude cerebral edema** and **high-altitude pulmonary edema**. In high-altitude cerebral edema, the capillary leakage in mountain sickness progresses to frank brain swelling, with ataxia, disorientation, and in some cases coma and death due to herniation of the brain through the tentorium. High-altitude pulmonary edema is a patchy edema of the lungs that is related to the marked pulmonary hypertension that develops at high altitude. It has been argued that it occurs because not all pulmonary arteries have enough smooth muscle to constrict in response to hypoxia, and in the capillaries supplied by those arteries, the general rise in pulmonary arterial pressure causes a capillary pressure increase that disrupts their walls (stress failure).

THERAPEUTIC HIGHLIGHTS

All forms of high-altitude illness are benefited by descent to lower altitude and by treatment with the diuretic acetazolamide. This drug inhibits carbonic anhydrase, and results in stimulated respiration, increased $Paco_2$, and reduced formation of CSF. When cerebral edema is marked, large doses of glucocorticoids are often administered as well. Their mechanism of action is unsettled. In high-altitude pulmonary edema, prompt treatment with O_2 is essential—and, if available, use of a hyperbaric chamber. Nifedipine, a Ca^{2+} channel blocker that lowers pulmonary artery pressure, can also be useful.

The increase in circulating RBCs triggered by the erythropoietin begins in 2–3 days and is sustained as long as the individual remains at high altitude. Compensatory changes also occur in the tissues. The mitochondria, which are the site of oxidative reactions, increase in number, and myoglobin increases, which facilitates the movement of O_2 into the tissues. The tissue content of cytochrome oxidase also increases.

■ DISEASES CAUSING HYPOXEMIA

Hypoxemia is the most common form of hypoxia seen clinically. The diseases that cause it can be roughly divided into those in which the gas exchange apparatus fails, those such as congenital heart disease in which large amounts of blood are shunted from the venous to the arterial side of the circulation, and those in which the respiratory pump fails. Some specific causes of hypoxemia are discussed in the following text.

VENTILATION–PERFUSION IMBALANCE

Patchy ventilation–perfusion imbalance is by far the most common cause of hypoxemia in clinical situations. In disease processes that prevent ventilation of some of the alveoli, the ventilation–blood flow ratios in different parts of the lung determine the extent to which systemic arterial Po_2 declines. If nonventilated alveoli are perfused, the nonventilated but perfused portion of the lung is in effect a right-to-left shunt, dumping unoxygenated blood into the left side of the heart. Lesser degrees of ventilation–perfusion imbalance are more common. In the example illustrated in **Figure 35–7**, the balanced ventilation–perfusion example on the left illustrates a uniform distribution throughout gas exchange. However, when ventilation is not in balance with perfusion, O_2 exchange is compromised. Note that the underventilated alveoli (B) have a low alveolar Po_2, whereas the overventilated alveoli (A) have a high alveolar Po_2 while both have the same blood flow. The unsaturation of the hemoglobin of the blood coming from B is not completely compensated by the slightly greater saturation of the blood coming from A, because hemoglobin is normally nearly saturated in the lungs and the higher alveolar Po_2 adds only a little more O_2 to the hemoglobin than it normally carries. Consequently, the arterial blood is unsaturated. The CO_2 content of the arterial blood is generally normal in such situations, since extra loss of CO_2 in overventilated regions can balance diminished loss in underventilated areas.

VENOUS-TO-ARTERIAL SHUNTS

When a cardiovascular abnormality such as an interatrial septal defect permits large amounts of unoxygenated venous blood to bypass the pulmonary capillaries and dilute the oxygenated blood in the systemic arteries ("right-to-left shunt"), chronic hypoxemia and cyanosis (**cyanotic congenital heart disease**) result. Administration of 100% O_2 raises the O_2 content of alveolar air but has little effect on hypoxia due to venous-to-arterial shunts. This is because the deoxygenated venous blood does not have the opportunity to get to the lung to be oxygenated.

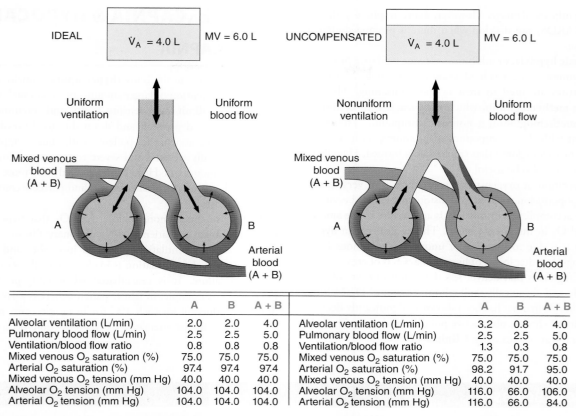

		A	B	A + B		A	B	A + B
Alveolar ventilation (L/min)		2.0	2.0	4.0	Alveolar ventilation (L/min)	3.2	0.8	4.0
Pulmonary blood flow (L/min)		2.5	2.5	5.0	Pulmonary blood flow (L/min)	2.5	2.5	5.0
Ventilation/blood flow ratio		0.8	0.8	0.8	Ventilation/blood flow ratio	1.3	0.3	0.8
Mixed venous O_2 saturation (%)		75.0	75.0	75.0	Mixed venous O_2 saturation (%)	75.0	75.0	75.0
Arterial O_2 saturation (%)		97.4	97.4	97.4	Arterial O_2 saturation (%)	98.2	91.7	95.0
Mixed venous O_2 tension (mm Hg)		40.0	40.0	40.0	Mixed venous O_2 tension (mm Hg)	40.0	40.0	40.0
Alveolar O_2 tension (mm Hg)		104.0	104.0	104.0	Alveolar O_2 tension (mm Hg)	116.0	66.0	106.0
Arterial O_2 tension (mm Hg)		104.0	104.0	104.0	Arterial O_2 tension (mm Hg)	116.0	66.0	84.0

FIGURE 35–7 Comparison of ventilation/blood flow relationships in health and disease. Left: "Ideal" ventilation/blood flow relationship. **Right:** Nonuniform ventilation and uniform blood flow, uncompensated. $\dot{V}_A$, alveolar ventilation; MV, respiratory minute volume. See the text for details. (Reproduced with permission from Comroe JH Jr, et al: *The Lung: Clinical Physiology and Pulmonary Function Tests*, 2nd ed. Year Book; 1962.)

■ OTHER FORMS OF HYPOXIA

Anemic hypoxia is not severe at rest unless the hemoglobin deficiency is marked, because 2,3-DPG increases in the RBCs. However, anemic patients may have considerable difficulty during exercise because of a limited ability to increase O_2 delivery to the active tissues.

Small amounts of carbon monoxide (CO) are formed in the body, and this gas may function as a chemical messenger. In larger amounts, CO is poisonous. Outside the body, it is formed by incomplete combustion of carbon. CO is toxic because it reacts with hemoglobin to form **carboxyhemoglobin (COHb)** which does not take up O_2. CO poisoning is often listed as a form of anemic hypoxia because the amount of hemoglobin that can carry O_2 is reduced, but the total hemoglobin content of the blood is unaffected by CO. The affinity of hemoglobin for CO is 210 times its affinity for O_2, and COHb liberates CO very slowly. An additional difficulty is that when COHb is present, the dissociation curve of the remaining HbO_2 shifts to the left, decreasing the amount of O_2 released. This is why an anemic individual who has 50% of the normal amount of HbO_2 may be able to perform moderate work, whereas an individual with HbO_2 reduced to the same level because of the formation of COHb is seriously incapacitated.

Because of the affinity of CO for hemoglobin, progressive COHb formation occurs when the alveolar P_{CO} is greater than 0.4 mm Hg. However, the amount of COHb formed depends on the duration of exposure to CO as well as the concentration of CO in the inspired air and the alveolar ventilation. The symptoms of CO poisoning are those of any type of hypoxia, especially headache and nausea, but there is little stimulation of respiration, since P_{O_2} remains normal in the arterial blood, keeping the carotid and aortic chemoreceptors from stimulation. The cherry-red color of COHb is visible in the skin, nail beds, and mucous membranes. The symptoms produced by chronic exposure to sublethal concentrations of CO are those of progressive brain damage, including mental changes and, sometimes, a parkinsonism-like state. Treatment of CO poisoning consists of immediate termination of the exposure and adequate ventilation, by artificial respiration if necessary. Ventilation with O_2 is preferable to ventilation with fresh air, since O_2 hastens the dissociation of COHb. Hyperbaric oxygenation (see below) is useful in this condition.

Ischemic hypoxia, or stagnant hypoxia, is due to slow circulation and is a problem in organs such as the kidneys and heart during shock. The liver and possibly the brain are damaged by ischemic hypoxia in heart failure. The blood flow to the lung is normally very large, and it takes prolonged hypotension to produce significant damage. However, acute respiratory distress syndrome (ARDS) can develop when there is prolonged circulatory collapse.

Histotoxic hypoxia, or inhibition of tissue oxidative processes, is most commonly the result of cyanide poisoning. Methylene blue or nitrites are used to treat cyanide poisoning. They act by forming **methemoglobin,** which then reacts with cyanide to form **cyanmethemoglobin,** a nontoxic compound. The extent of treatment with these compounds is, of course, limited by the amount of methemoglobin that can be safely formed. Hyperbaric oxygenation may also be useful.

Administration of oxygen-rich gas mixtures is of very limited value in hypoperfusion, anemic, and histotoxic hypoxia because all that can be accomplished in this way is an increase in the amount of dissolved O_2 in the arterial blood. This is also true in hypoxemia when it is due to shunting of unoxygenated venous blood past the lungs. In other forms of hypoxemia, O_2 is of great benefit. Treatment regimens that deliver less than 100% O_2 are of value both acutely and chronically, and administration of O_2 24 h/day for 2 years in this manner has been shown to significantly decrease the mortality of chronic obstructive pulmonary disease. O_2 toxicity and therapy are discussed in **Clinical Box 35–5.**

■ HYPERCAPNIA & HYPOCAPNIA

HYPERCAPNIA

Retention of CO_2 in the body (**hypercapnia**) initially stimulates respiration. Retention of larger amounts produces such symptoms as confusion, diminished sensory acuity and, eventually, coma with respiratory depression and death due to depression of the central nervous system. In patients with these symptoms, the P_{CO_2} is markedly elevated and severe respiratory acidosis is present. Large amounts of HCO_3^- are excreted, but more HCO_3^- is reabsorbed, raising the plasma HCO_3^- and partially compensating for the acidosis.

CO_2 is so much more soluble than O_2 that hypercapnia is rarely a problem in patients with pulmonary fibrosis. However, it does occur in ventilation–perfusion inequality and when for any reason alveolar ventilation is inadequate in the various forms of pump failure. It is exacerbated when CO_2 production is increased. For example, in febrile patients there is a 13% increase in CO_2 production for each 1°C rise in temperature, and a high carbohydrate intake increases CO_2 production because of the

---

CLINICAL BOX 35–5

Administration of Oxygen & Its Potential Toxicity

It is interesting that while O_2 is necessary for life in aerobic organisms, it is also toxic. Indeed, 100% O_2 has been demonstrated to exert toxic effects not only in animals but also in bacteria, fungi, cultured animal cells, and plants. The toxicity seems to be due to the production of reactive oxygen species including superoxide anion (O_2^-) and H_2O_2. When 80–100% O_2 is administered to humans for periods of 8 h or more, the respiratory passages become irritated, causing substernal distress, nasal congestion, sore throat, and coughing.

A chronic condition characterized by lung cysts and densities (**bronchopulmonary dysplasia**) develops in some infants treated with O_2 for respiratory distress syndrome. This syndrome may be a manifestation of O_2 toxicity. Another complication in these infants is **retinopathy of prematurity (retrolental fibroplasia),** the formation of opaque vascular tissue in the eyes, which can lead to serious visual defects. The retinal receptors mature from the center to the periphery of the retina, and they use considerable O_2. This causes the retina to become vascularized in an orderly manner. Oxygen treatment before maturation is complete provides the needed O_2 to the photoreceptors, and consequently the normal vascular pattern fails to develop. Evidence indicates that this condition can be prevented or ameliorated by treatment with vitamin E, which exerts an anti-oxidant effect and, in animals, by growth hormone inhibitors.

Administration of 100% O_2 at increased pressure accelerates the onset of O_2 toxicity, with the production not

only of tracheobronchial irritation but also of muscle twitching, ringing in the ears, dizziness, convulsions, and coma. The speed with which these symptoms develop is proportional to the pressure at which the O_2 is administered; for example, at 4 atm, symptoms develop in 30 min in half the patients, whereas at 6 atm, convulsions develop in a few minutes.

On the other hand, exposure to 100% O_2 at 2–3 atm can increase dissolved O_2 in arterial blood to the point that arterial O_2 tension is greater than 2000 mm Hg and tissue O_2 tension is 400 mm Hg. If exposure is limited to 5 h or less at these pressures, O_2 toxicity is not a problem. Therefore, **hyperbaric O_2 therapy** in closed tanks is used to treat diseases in which improved oxygenation of tissues cannot be achieved in other ways. It is of demonstrated value in carbon monoxide poisoning, radiation-induced tissue injury, gas gangrene, very severe blood loss anemia, diabetic leg ulcers, and other wounds that are slow to heal, and rescue of skin flaps and grafts in which the circulation is marginal. It is also the primary treatment for decompression sickness and air embolism.

In hypercapnic patients in severe pulmonary failure, the CO_2 level may be so high that it depresses rather than stimulates respiration. Some of these patients keep breathing only because the carotid and aortic chemoreceptors drive the respiratory center. If the hypoxic drive is withdrawn by administering O_2, breathing may stop. During the resultant apnea, the arterial P_{O_2} drops but breathing may not start again, as P_{CO_2} further depresses the respiratory center. Therefore, O_2 therapy in this situation must be started with care.

increase in the respiratory quotient. Normally, alveolar ventilation increases and the extra CO_2 is expired, but it accumulates when ventilation is compromised.

HYPOCAPNIA

Hypocapnia is the result of hyperventilation. During voluntary hyperventilation, the arterial P_{CO_2} falls from 40 mm Hg to as low as 15 mm Hg while the alveolar P_{O_2} rises to 120–140 mm Hg.

The more chronic effects of hypocapnia are seen in neurotic patients who chronically hyperventilate. Cerebral blood flow may be reduced 30% or more because of the direct constrictor effect of hypocapnia on the cerebral vessels. The cerebral ischemia causes light-headedness, dizziness, and paresthesias. Hypocapnia also increases cardiac output. It has a direct constrictor effect on many peripheral vessels, but it depresses the vasomotor center, so that the blood pressure is usually unchanged or only slightly elevated.

Other consequences of hypocapnia are due to the associated respiratory alkalosis, the blood pH being increased to 7.5 or 7.6. The plasma HCO_3^- level is low, but HCO_3^- reabsorption is decreased because of the inhibition of renal acid secretion by the low P_{CO_2}. The body total calcium level does not change, but the plasma Ca^{2+} level falls and hypocapnic individuals can develop carpopedal spasm, a positive Chvostek sign, and other signs of tetany.

CHAPTER SUMMARY

- Partial pressure differences between air and blood for O_2 and CO_2 dictate a net flow of O_2 into the blood and CO_2 out of the blood in the pulmonary system.
- The amount of O_2 in the blood is determined by the amount dissolved (minor) and the amount bound (major) to hemoglobin. Each hemoglobin molecule contains four subunits that each can bind O_2. Hemoglobin O_2 binding is cooperative and also affected by pH, temperature, and the concentration of 2,3-DPG.
- CO_2 in blood is rapidly converted into H_2CO_3 due to the activity of carbonic anhydrase. CO_2 also readily forms carbamino compounds with blood proteins (including hemoglobin). The rapid net loss of CO_2 allows more CO_2 to dissolve in blood.
- The pH of plasma is 7.4. A decrease in plasma pH is termed **acidosis** and an increase of plasma pH is termed **alkalosis.** A short-term change in arterial P_{CO_2} due to decreased ventilation results in respiratory acidosis. A short-term change in arterial P_{CO_2} due to increased ventilation results in respiratory alkalosis. Metabolic acidosis occurs when strong acids are added to the blood, and metabolic alkalosis occurs when strong bases are added to (or strong acids are removed from) the blood.
- Respiratory compensation to acidosis or alkalosis involves quick changes in ventilation. Such changes effectively change the P_{CO_2} in the blood plasma. Renal compensation mechanisms are much slower and involve H^+ secretion or HCO_3^- reabsorption.
- Hypoxia is a deficiency of O_2 at the tissue level. Hypoxia has powerful consequences at the cellular, tissue, and organ level.

MULTIPLE-CHOICE QUESTIONS

For all questions, select the single best answer unless otherwise directed.

1. Arterial and venous blood was drawn from an individual. When comparing the two draws using a sensitive pH meter, it was noticed that the pH of the arterial blood was 7.40 while the pH of the venous blood was 7.36. How do CO_2 differences in arterial versus venous blood account for these normal readings?
   A. CO_2 released from metabolism is acidic.
   B. Increased carbamino compounds are acidic and alter the pH.
   C. CO_2 bound to hemoglobin releases H^+ and increase acidity.
   D. Cl^- shift in RBCs increases acidity in the plasma.
   E. Increased CO_2 in venous blood results in increased HCO_3^- and H^+, which decreases pH.

2. In a laboratory experiment, a researcher was able to take whole blood, separate out various components, and compare the ability to hold onto O_2. Each of the modified blood samples was exposed to O_2 as a gas with a P_{O_2} of 100 mm Hg and allowed to reach equilibrium. Which of the following samples showed the poorest ability to hold onto O_2?
   A. Whole blood with a slightly raised pH
   B. Whole blood devoid of hemoglobin
   C. Whole blood with raised CO_2 content
   D. Whole blood at a raised temperature
   E. Whole blood devoid of 2,3-DPG

3. Blood is isolated in the laboratory and RBCs are carefully separated from the rest of the plasma. Each of these isolates is exposed to the same amount of CO_2 gas and, pH and HCO_3^- are measured. Assuming proteins and enzymes in the plasma and RBCs were working properly, which of the following would be an expected result?
   A. The blood plasma isolate had higher pH and decreased $[HCO_3^-]$ compared with the RBC isolate.
   B. The blood plasma isolate had lower pH and increased $[HCO_3^-]$ compared with the RBC isolate.
   C. The blood plasma isolate had lower pH and decreased $[HCO_3^-]$ compared with the RBC isolate.
   D. The blood plasma isolate had higher pH and increased $[HCO_3^-]$ compared with the RBC isolate.
   E. The blood plasma isolate had similar pH and similar $[HCO_3^-]$ compared with the RBC isolate.

4. A student is brought into the campus clinic after a bout of vomiting. He is breathing normally, but complains of dizziness and numbness in his extremities. As you suspected, a quick check of the blood plasma shows an increase in serum $[HCO_3^-]$ and elevated plasma pH. You deduce the following and treat accordingly.
   A. Metabolic acidosis
   B. Respiratory acidosis
   C. Respiratory alkalosis
   D. Metabolic alkalosis

5. Two friends are running up a familiar hill to finish out a jog. They increase their breathing rate and depth as they near to the top of the hill. They both reach the finish and stop for a minute to "catch their breath." Runner A turned to the other and says "we started to hyperventilate there at the top of the hill." Runner B responded by saying "I don't

think you used that term correctly." Why is Runner B correct here?

A. Hyperventilation refers to continual rapid breathing. Since both runners were able to catch their breaths, hyperventilation did not occur.

B. Hyperventilation refers to an increased breathing pattern that results in a ventilation/perfusion mismatch. The observed increase was a normal response to maintain ventilation/perfusion matching.

C. Hyperventilation refers to a slowing down in breathing rate and a reduced depth of breathing.

D. Hyperventilation cannot occur during exercise.

6. A young man is struck in the chest area during a game of pickup basketball. He shows immediate signs of chest soreness and difficulty breathing but is otherwise alert. He is taken to an urgent care center where he is diagnosed with atelectasis and is treated with an incentive spirometer, which is sufficient to reverse breathing difficulties and fully re-inflate his lungs. What would be the expected result from extended atelectasis?

A. A reduced arterial Po_2 due to ventilation/perfusion that approaches zero in the affected alveoli

B. An increased arterial Po_2 due to an increase in ventilation/perfusion in the affected alveoli

C. An increase in physiological dead space

D. A reduced arterial Pco_2 due to ventilation/perfusion that approaches zero in the affected alveoli

7. A young couple was spending their afternoon on a picnic. After their picnic, the young woman got down on her knee, pulled out a small box with a ring and proposed. The man was taken aback, said yes, and began to hyperventilate. The quick thinking bride-to-be grabbed a paper bag and instructed her fiancé to slow his breathing and use the bag to rebreathe his exhaled breath. What change in the lung was she worried about and why does a paper bag work to prevent this condition?

A. Metabolic acidosis; rebreathing exhaled air with a higher Pco_2 than environmental airs reestablishes a proper blood $[CO_2]$.

B. Metabolic alkalosis; rebreathing humidified the air to better allow for proper CO_2 exchange.

C. Respiratory alkalosis due to hyperventilation; rebreathing CO_2 reestablishes a proper blood $[CO_2]$.

D. Respiratory acidosis due to hyperventilation; rebreathing CO_2 reestablishes a proper blood $[CO_2]$.

E. The hyperventilation results in a drying of the air; rebreathing exhaled air humidifies the air and allows for proper O_2 exchange.

8. A couple in Colorado was keeping warm in the winter with their wood stove. They left the stove unattended throughout the night. In the morning, the couple arose and complained to each other about dizziness, nausea, fatigue, and headache. At that time they noticed small crack in the venting system of their stove, and called 911 to report possible CO poisoning. They removed themselves from the house and, after several hours of breathing normal air, their symptoms were gone. How did the CO affect O_2 transport in their blood?

A. CO directly interacts with carbonic anhydrase and prevents $CO + H_2O \leftrightarrow H_2CO_3$, lowering CO_2 and the ability to regulate breathing.

B. CO interacts with tissue cytochromes to cause cell death.

C. CO outcompetes O_2 for hemoglobin, resulting in anemic hypoxia.

D. CO interferes with blood flow, resulting in ischemic hypoxia.

9. Through various clinical trials between 1980 and 2005, it was observed that hypoxemic patients with chronic COPD (ie, FEV_1/FVC ~30%) could be treated with 100% O_2 to increase arterial Po_2 within 20 min. However, it was also shown that at least a subset of these individuals experienced increased arterial Pco_2, or hypercapnia, after 20 min of 100% O_2. While minute ventilation can drop rapidly within the first few minutes of 100% O_2 treatment, this usually recovered within 5 min, and thus hypoventilation could be ruled out as a cause of hypercapnia. Which of the following could account for the observed hypercapnia?

A. Decreased ventilation/perfusion due to increased anatomical dead space in response to increased O_2.

B. Increased ventilation/perfusion due to decreased total dead space in response to increased O_2.

C. Decreased ventilation/perfusion due to increased perfusion of conducting airway.

D. Increased ventilation/perfusion due to decreased anatomic dead space in response to increased O_2.

E. Decreased ventilation/perfusion ratio due to increased total dead space in response to increased O_2.

10. A 59-year-old woman comes to the emergency department with an acute onset of shortness of breath. She states to the attending physicians that she recently sustained a fractured fibula in her right leg and has had slightly elevated blood pressure for several years. A lung scan demonstrates a perfusion defect in the lower right lobe. Which of the following occurs if blood flow to the alveolar units in the region of the perfusion defect is totally obstructed by a pulmonary embolism?

A. There will be a reduced arterial Po_2 due to venous to arterial shunt.

B. The Po_2 of the alveoli affected by the embolism will be equal to Po_2 in the inspired air.

C. The anatomical dead space is decreased.

D. The ventilation/perfusion of the alveoli in the affected area goes to zero.

E. The Po_2 of the alveolus will be equal to the mixed venous Po_2.

ANSWERS

1. The correct answer is **E.** CO_2 is higher in venous blood (extra 3.7 mL/dL). The action of carbonic anhydrase quickly converts CO_2 and H_2O into H_2CO_3, which can dissociate into HCO_3^- and H^+. The net increase in CO_2 naturally results in more acidic blood. The process is reversed when the blood passes through the lung and the additional CO_2 is moved from the blood to the alveoli. While it is true that CO_2 is released from metabolism that occurs in the tissue (**A**) and that additional carbamino groups (**B**) including with hemoglobin (**C**), none of these are acidic (eg, H^+ generating) and thus can be ruled out. The Cl^- shift (**D**) refers to the electroneutral exchange of HCO_3^- with Cl^- across the RBC membrane; this does not alter H^+ concentration and can be ruled out.

2. The correct answer is **B.** Upon equilibrium with a Po_2 of 100 mm Hg, normal blood will have 0.3 mL of dissolved

oxygen and 20.1 mL of O_2 bound to hemoglobin. As one can see, in the absence of hemoglobin, this greater than 98% of the O_2 is lost from the blood. Changes in pH (**A**), caused by changes in CO_2 (**C**) content or by other means, changes in temperature (**D**), or changes in 2,3-DPG, all can alter the ability for hemoglobin to carry O_2. However, none of these changes prohibits hemoglobin binding, and thus their changes are minimal compared to a loss of hemoglobin.

3. The correct answer is **A**. Carbonic anhydrase is found in RBC and is the enzyme that catalyzes the reaction $CO_2 + H_2O \leftrightarrow H_2CO_3$; H_2CO_3 quickly reaches equilibrium with H^+ and its conjugate base, HCO_3^-. Thus, in the presence of carbonic anhydrase, there would be a decrease in pH (increase in H^+) and an increase in HCO_3^-. Because carbonic anhydrase is not typically found in the blood plasma, relative to RBC, blood plasma would show a higher pH (ruling out **B, C,** and **E**) and a decreased [HCO_3^-] (ruling out **B, D,** and **E**) when compared with RBC.

4. The correct answer is **D**. Metabolic alkalosis refers to nonrespiratory increases in plasma pH. Loss of body acids due to repeated vomiting is equivalent to increase in the body's bases, or alkalosis. Because there is a loss of acid from the body, both metabolic acidosis (**A**) and respiratory acidosis (**B**) can be eliminated. Since the patient is breathing normally, a hypoventilation that could lead to respiratory alkalosis (**C**) can be eliminated.

5. The correct answer is **B**. Increased in ventilation due to aerobic activity is a normal response to the need for increased oxygen due to increased muscle metabolism and blood flow and results in proper ventilation/perfusion matching. By definition, hyperventilation is an increased breathing pattern that results in a ventilation/perfusion mismatch, "blowing off of CO_2 and respiratory alkalosis." Thus, not every increase in breathing rate/depth is hyperventilation and **A** can be ruled out. Hypoventilation refers to a reduced breathing pattern that results in ventilation/perfusion mismatching, ruling out **C**. Although more commonly associated in nonexercise environment, hyperventilation can occur during exercise and **D** is ruled out.

6. The correct answer is **A**. A temporary and partial lung collapse can be caused by an impact injury. During the time of alveolar collapse, inspired air cannot enter the affected alveoli, and assuming perfusion of the area is still occurring, blood will not be reoxygenated and this shunt will effectively lower arterial P_{O_2} and increase arterial P_{CO_2} (ruling out **D**). Since it is ventilation that goes to zero and perfusion that is constant, there is no increase in ventilation/perfusion and **B** can be ruled out. Dead space refers to gas-filled areas in the lung where gas exchange does not occur; since a collapse alveolus does not fill with gas, it does not represent an increase in dead space and **C** can be ruled out.

7. The correct answer is **C**. Rapid breathing has the effect of "blowing off CO_2" and altering the blood gases. The fast exchange of gas in the alveoli tends to drop arterial P_{CO_2}, which results in an increase in blood pH or respiratory alkalosis. Because blood pH increases, both **A** and **D** can be eliminated. One beneficial effect of breathing into a paper bag

is that subsequent inhalations will have higher P_{CO_2}, and thus prevent rapid changes in blood pH. Cases of metabolic acidosis or alkalosis are, by definition, pathological changes in pH due to nonrespiratory changes, and thus **A** and **B** can be ruled out. While the rebreathing of inspired air would likely include more humidified air than normally inspired, this would not greatly change O_2 or CO_2 exchange, ruling out **B** and **E**.

8. The correct answer is **C**. CO binds to hemoglobin with a much greater affinity than O_2. This has two large effects on O_2 transfer: (1) there is less hemoglobin available for O_2 binding; and (2) CO stays on hemoglobin much longer, keeping hemoglobin unavailable for O_2 transport. Because effective hemoglobin is reduced, this is considered an anemic hypoxia. CO has no effect on carbonic anhydrase activity, ruling out **A**. CO can be toxic to tissue cytochromes to cause cellular dysfunction and death. However, this toxicity would only occur at concentrations that result in death from lack of O_2 transport, and thus **B** is ruled out. While ischemic hypoxia refers to low tissue O_2 in response to reduced blood flow; however, CO has no effect on blood flow, thus, **D** is not correct.

9. The correct answer is **E**. Hypercapnia refers to an increase in arterial P_{CO_2}. This can occur when alveoli are well perfused in the absence of proper ventilation, a decrease in ventilation/perfusion, and results in a shunt. The lung has inherent physiologic mechanisms to maintain proper ventilation/perfusion. Under conditions of poor ventilation of an alveolus, as occurs in COPD, is a local hypoxic pulmonary vasoconstriction, where the low oxygen in the alveolus provides feedback to the local vasculature and limits perfusion to the hypoxic alveoli, thus preventing a ventilation/perfusion mismatch. Upon introduction of 100% O_2, the hypoxic feedback may be relieved even without proper ventilation resulting in increased perfusion. In effect, there is an increase in total dead space and decrease in ventilation/perfusion. Because there is a net decrease in ventilation/perfusion, answers above that indicate an increased in ventilation/perfusion, **B** and **D** can be eliminated. Anatomical dead space refers to naturally occurring areas in the lung where gas exchange does not occur (eg, trachea and bronchi). Observed changes are in the respiratory region and refer to total dead space. Answers that refer to changes in anatomical dead space **A** and **D** or O_2 exchange in the conducting airway (**C**) are thus eliminated.

10. The answer is **B**. The pulmonary emboli will prevent perfusion of the functional alveoli in the area, eliminate the opportunity for gas exchange and leave the alveolar P_{O_2} unchanged (and **E** can be ruled out). Because the emboli prevent venous blood from moving and mixing with arterial blood, no shunt occurs and **A** can be ruled out. Anatomical dead space refers to the space in a healthy lung where no ventilation occurs. In the stated case, emboli would increase (not decrease) total or physiologic dead space. For these two reasons, **C** can be ruled out. Ventilation is unchanged by the emboli and perfusion goes to zero. Thus, the ventilation/perfusion ratio goes to infinity and **D** can be ruled out.

Regulation of Respiration

- Locate the pre-Bötzinger complex and describe its role in producing spontaneous respiration.
- Identify the location and probable functions of the dorsal and ventral groups of respiratory neurons, the pneumotaxic center, and the apneustic center in the brainstem.
- List the specific respiratory functions of the vagus nerves and the respiratory receptors in the carotid body, the aortic body, and the ventral surface of the medulla oblongata.
- Describe and explain the ventilatory responses to increased CO_2 concentrations and decreased O_2 concentrations in the inspired air.
- Describe the effects of each of the main nonchemical factors that influence respiration.
- Describe the effects of exercise on ventilation and O_2 exchange in the tissues.
- Define periodic breathing and explain its occurrence in various disease states.

INTRODUCTION

Spontaneous respiration is produced by rhythmic discharge of motor neurons that innervate the respiratory muscles. This discharge is dependent on nerve impulses from the brain; breathing stops if the spinal cord is transected above the origin of the phrenic nerves. The rhythmic discharges from the brain that produce spontaneous respiration are regulated by alterations in arterial Po_2, Pco_2, and H^+ concentration, and this chemical control of breathing is supplemented by a number of nonchemical influences. The physiologic bases for these phenomena are discussed in this chapter.

■ NEURAL CONTROL OF BREATHING

CONTROL SYSTEMS

Two separate neural mechanisms regulate respiration. One is responsible for voluntary control and the other for automatic control. The voluntary system is located in the cerebral cortex and sends impulses to the respiratory motor neurons via the corticospinal tracts. The automatic system is driven by a group of pacemaker cells in the medulla. Impulses from these cells activate motor neurons in the cervical and thoracic spinal cord that innervate inspiratory muscles. Those in the cervical cord activate the diaphragm via the phrenic nerves, and those in the thoracic spinal cord activate the external intercostal muscles.

The motor neurons to the expiratory muscles are inhibited when those supplying the inspiratory muscles are active, and vice versa. Although spinal reflexes contribute to this **reciprocal innervation,** it is due primarily to activity in descending pathways. Impulses in these descending pathways excite agonists and inhibit antagonists. The one exception to the reciprocal inhibition is a small amount of activity in phrenic axons for a short period after inspiration. The function of this postinspiratory output appears to break the lung's elastic recoil and make respiration smooth.

MEDULLARY SYSTEMS

The main components of the **respiratory control pattern generator** responsible for automatic respiration are located in the medulla. Rhythmic respiration is initiated by a small group of synaptically coupled pacemaker cells in the **pre-Bötzinger** (pre-BÖTC) **complex** on either side of the medulla between the nucleus ambiguus and the lateral reticular nucleus (**Figure 36–1**). These neurons discharge rhythmically, and they produce rhythmic discharges in phrenic motor neurons. They also contact the hypoglossal nuclei, and the tongue is involved in the regulation of airway resistance.

Neurons in the pre-BÖTC complex discharge rhythmically in brain slice preparations in vitro, and if the slices become hypoxic, discharge changes to one associated with gasping. Addition of cadmium to the slices causes occasional sigh-like discharge patterns. There are NK1 receptors and μ-opioid receptors on these neurons, and, in vivo, substance P stimulates and opioids inhibit respiration. Depression of respiration is a side effect that limits the use of opioids in the treatment of pain. In addition, dorsal and ventral groups of respiratory neurons are present in the medulla (**Figure 36–2**). However, lesions of these neurons do not abolish respiratory activity, and they apparently project to the pre-BÖTC pacemaker neurons.

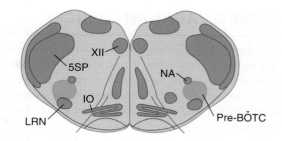

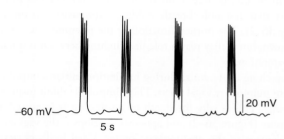

FIGURE 36–1 **Pacemaker cells in the pre-Bötzinger (pre-BÖTC) complex. Top:** Anatomic diagram of the pre-BÖTC from a neonatal rat. **Bottom:** Sample rhythmic discharge tracing of neurons in the pre-BÖTC complex from a brain slice of a neonatal rat. IO, inferior olive; LRN, lateral reticular nucleus; NA, nucleus ambiguus; XII, nucleus of 12th cranial nerve; 5SP, spinal nucleus of trigeminal nerve. (Modified with permission from Feldman JC, Gray PA: Sighs and gasps in a dish, *Nat Neurosci.* 2000 June;3(6):531–532.)

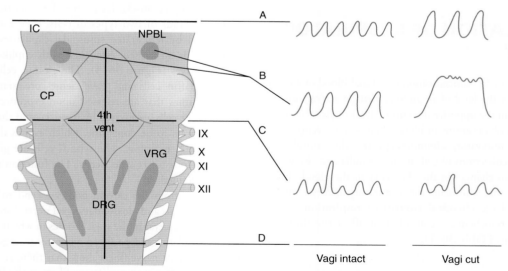

FIGURE 36–2 **Respiratory neurons in the brainstem.** Dorsal view of brainstem; cerebellum removed. The effects of various lesions and brainstem transections are shown; the spirometer tracings at the right indicate the depth and rate of breathing. If a lesion is introduced at D, breathing ceases. The effects of higher transections, with and without vagus nerves transection, are shown (see the text for details). CP, middle cerebellar peduncle; DRG, dorsal group of respiratory neurons; IC, inferior colliculus; NPBL, nucleus parabrachialis (pneumotaxic center); VRG, ventral group of respiratory neurons; 4th vent, fourth ventricle. The roman numerals identify cranial nerves. (Modified with permission from Mitchell RA, Berger A: State of the art: Review of neural regulation of respiration. *Am Rev Respir Dis.* 1975 Feb;111(2):206–224.)

PONTINE & VAGAL INFLUENCES

Although the rhythmic discharge of medullary neurons concerned with respiration is spontaneous, it is modified by neurons in the pons and afferents in the vagus from receptors in the airways and lungs. An area known as the **pneumotaxic center** in the medial parabrachial and Kölliker-Fuse nuclei of the dorsolateral pons contains neurons active during inspiration and neurons active during expiration. When this area is damaged, respiration becomes slower and tidal volume greater, and when the vagi are also cut in anesthetized animals, there are prolonged inspiratory spasms that resemble breath holding (**apneusis;** section B in Figure 36–2). The normal function of the pneumotaxic center is unknown, but it may play a role in switching between inspiration and expiration.

Stretching of the lungs during inspiration initiates impulses in afferent pulmonary vagal fibers. These impulses inhibit inspiratory discharge. This is why the depth of inspiration is increased after vagotomy (Figure 36–2) and apneusis develops if the vagi are cut after damage to the pneumotaxic center. Vagal feedback activity does not alter the rate of rise of the neural activity in respiratory motor neurons.

When the activity of the inspiratory neurons is increased in intact animals, the rate and the depth of breathing are increased. The depth of respiration is increased because the lungs are stretched to a greater degree before the amount of vagal and pneumotaxic center inhibitory activity is sufficient to overcome the more intense inspiratory neuron discharge. The respiratory rate is increased because the after-discharge in the vagal and possibly the pneumotaxic afferents to the medulla is rapidly overcome.

■ REGULATION OF RESPIRATORY ACTIVITY

A rise in the P_{CO_2} or H^+ concentration of arterial blood or a drop in its P_{O_2} increases the level of respiratory neuron activity in the medulla; changes in the opposite direction have a slight inhibitory effect. The effects of variations in blood chemistry on ventilation are mediated via respiratory **chemoreceptors**—the carotid and aortic bodies and collections of cells in the medulla and elsewhere that are sensitive to changes in the chemistry of the blood. They initiate impulses that stimulate the respiratory center. Superimposed on this basic **chemical control of respiration**, other afferents provide nonchemical controls that affect breathing in particular situations (Table 36–1).

■ CHEMICAL CONTROL OF BREATHING

The chemical regulatory mechanisms adjust ventilation in such a way that the alveolar P_{CO_2} is normally held constant, the effects of excess H^+ in the blood are combated, and the P_{O_2} is raised when

TABLE 36–1   Stimuli affecting the respiratory center.

Chemical control
CO_2 (via CSF and brain interstitial fluid H^+ concentration)
(via carotid and aortic bodies)
Nonchemical control
Vagal afferents from receptors in the airways and lungs
Afferents from the pons, hypothalamus, and limbic system
Afferents from proprioceptors
Afferents from baroreceptors: arterial, atrial, ventricular, pulmonary

it falls to a potentially dangerous level. The respiratory minute volume is proportional to the metabolic rate, but the link between metabolism and ventilation is CO_2, not O_2. The receptors in the carotid and aortic bodies are stimulated by a rise in the P_{CO_2} or H^+ concentration of arterial blood or a decline in its P_{O_2}. After denervation of the carotid chemoreceptors, the response to a drop in P_{O_2} is abolished; the predominant effect of hypoxia after denervation of the carotid bodies is a direct depression of the respiratory center. The response to changes in arterial blood H^+ concentration in the pH 7.3–7.5 range is also abolished, although larger changes exert some effect. The response to changes in arterial P_{CO_2}, on the other hand, is affected only slightly; it is reduced no more than 30–35%.

CAROTID & AORTIC BODIES

There is a carotid body near the carotid bifurcation on each side, and there are usually two or more aortic bodies near the arch of the aorta (Figure 36–3). Each carotid and aortic body (**glomus**) contains islands of two types of cells, type I and type II cells, surrounded by fenestrated sinusoidal capillaries. The type I or **glomus cells** are closely associated with cuplike endings of the afferent nerves (Figure 36–4). The glomus cells resemble adrenal chromaffin cells and have dense-core granules containing catecholamines that are released upon exposure to hypoxia and cyanide. The cells are excited by hypoxia, and the principal transmitter appears to be dopamine, which excites the nerve endings by way of D_2 receptors. The type II cells are glia-like, and each surrounds four to six type I cells. The function of type II cells is not fully defined.

Afferents from the carotid bodies ascend to the medulla via the carotid sinus and glossopharyngeal nerves, and fibers from the aortic bodies ascend in the vagi. Studies in which one carotid body has been isolated and perfused while recordings are being taken from its afferent nerve fibers show that there is a graded increase in impulse traffic in these afferent fibers as the P_{O_2} of the perfusing blood is lowered (Figure 36–5) or the P_{CO_2} is raised. Type I glomus cells have O_2-sensitive K^+ channels, whose conductance is reduced in proportion to the degree of hypoxia to which they are exposed. This reduces the K^+ efflux, depolarizing the cell and causing Ca^{2+} influx that leads to an excitation of the afferent nerve endings.

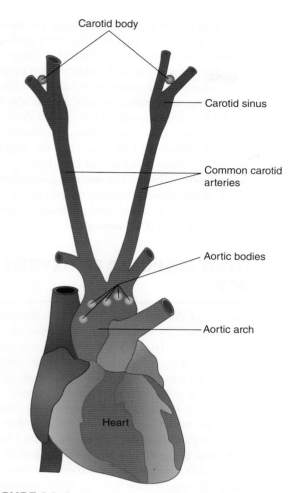

FIGURE 36–3 **Location of carotid and aortic bodies.** Carotid bodies are positioned near a major arterial baroreceptor, the carotid sinus. Aortic bodies are shown near the aortic arch.

The blood flow in each 2 mg carotid body is about 0.04 mL/min, or 2000 mL/100 g of tissue/min compared with a blood flow of 54 mL or 420 mL per 100 g/min in the brain and kidneys, respectively. Because the blood flow per unit of tissue is so enormous, the O_2 needs of the cells can be met largely by dissolved O_2 alone. Therefore, the receptors are not stimulated in conditions such as anemia or carbon monoxide poisoning, in which the amount of dissolved O_2 in the blood reaching the receptors is generally normal, even though the combined O_2 in the blood is markedly decreased. The receptors are stimulated when the arterial Po_2 is low or when the amount of O_2 delivered to the receptors per unit time is decreased.

Because of their anatomic location, the aortic bodies have not been studied in as great detail as the carotid bodies. Their responses are probably similar but of lesser magnitude. In humans in whom both carotid bodies have been removed but the aortic bodies left intact, the responses are essentially the same as those following denervation of both carotid and aortic bodies in animals: little change in ventilation at rest, but the ventilatory response to hypoxia is lost and the ventilatory response to CO_2 is reduced by 30%.

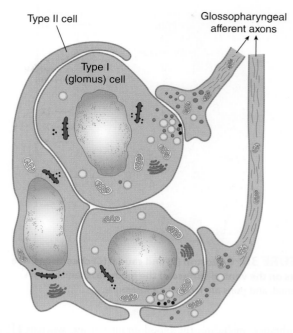

FIGURE 36–4 **Organization of the carotid body.** Type I (glomus) cells contain catecholamines. When exposed to hypoxia, they release their catecholamines, which stimulate the cuplike endings of the carotid sinus nerve fibers in the glossopharyngeal nerve. The glia-like type II cells surround the type I cells and probably have a sustentacular function.

CHEMORECEPTORS IN THE BRAINSTEM

The chemoreceptors that mediate the hyperventilation produced by increases in arterial Pco_2 after the carotid and aortic bodies are denervated are located in the medulla oblongata and consequently are called **medullary chemoreceptors.** They are separate from the dorsal and ventral respiratory neurons and are located on the ventral surface of the medulla (**Figure 36–6**). The chemoreceptors monitor the H^+ concentration of cerebrospinal fluid (CSF), including the brain interstitial fluid. CO_2 readily penetrates

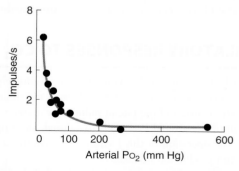

FIGURE 36–5 **Effect of Pco_2 on afferent nerve firing.** The rate of discharge of a single afferent fiber from the carotid body (circles) is plotted at several Po_2 values and fitted to a line. A sharp increase in firing rate is observed as Po_2 falls below normal resting levels (ie, near 100 mm Hg). (Used with permission of S. Sampson.)

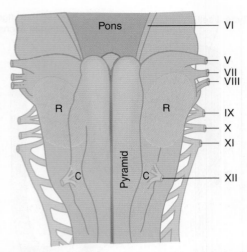

FIGURE 36–6 Rostral (R) and caudal (C) chemosensitive areas on the ventral surface of the medulla. Cranial nerves, pyramid, and pons are labeled for reference.

membranes, including the blood–brain barrier, whereas H^+ and HCO_3^- penetrate slowly. The CO_2 that enters the brain and CSF is promptly hydrated; H_2CO_3 dissociates, so that the local H^+ concentration rises. In this manner, the H^+ concentration in brain interstitial fluid parallels the arterial PCO_2. Increase in spinal fluid H^+ concentration proportionately stimulates respiration.

VENTILATORY RESPONSES TO CHANGES IN ACID–BASE BALANCE

In metabolic acidosis there is pronounced respiratory stimulation. The induced hyperventilation decreases alveolar PCO_2 ("blows off CO_2") and thus produces a compensatory fall in blood H^+ concentration. Conversely, in metabolic alkalosis ventilation is depressed and the arterial PCO_2 rises, raising the H^+ concentration toward normal. If there is an increase in ventilation that is not secondary to a rise in arterial H^+ concentration, the drop in PCO_2 lowers the H^+ concentration below normal (**respiratory alkalosis**); conversely, hypoventilation that is not secondary to a fall in plasma H^+ concentration causes **respiratory acidosis**.

VENTILATORY RESPONSES TO CO_2

The arterial PCO_2 is normally maintained at 40 mm Hg. When arterial PCO_2 rises as a result of increased tissue metabolism, ventilation is stimulated and the rate of pulmonary excretion of CO_2 increases until the arterial PCO_2 falls to normal, shutting off the stimulus. The operation of this feedback mechanism keeps CO_2 excretion and production in balance.

When a gas mixture containing CO_2 is inhaled, the alveolar PCO_2 rises, elevating the arterial PCO_2 and stimulating ventilation as soon as the blood that contains more CO_2 reaches the medulla. CO_2 elimination is increased, and the alveolar PCO_2 drops toward normal. This is why relatively large increments in the PCO_2 of

inspired air (eg, 15 mm Hg) produce relatively slight increments in alveolar PCO_2 (eg, 3 mm Hg). However, the PCO_2 does not drop to normal, and a new equilibrium is reached at which the alveolar PCO_2 is slightly elevated and the hyperventilation persists as long as CO_2 is inhaled. This results in an essentially linear relationship between respiratory minute volume and the alveolar PCO_2. Of course, this linearity has an upper limit. When the PCO_2 of the inspired gas is close to the alveolar PCO_2, elimination of CO_2 becomes difficult. When the CO_2 content of the inspired gas is more than 7%, the alveolar and arterial PCO_2 begin to rise abruptly in spite of hyperventilation. The resultant accumulation of CO_2 in the body (**hypercapnia**) depresses the central nervous system, including the respiratory center, and produces headache, confusion, and eventually coma (**CO_2 narcosis**).

VENTILATORY RESPONSE TO OXYGEN DEFICIENCY

When the O_2 content of the inspired air is decreased, respiratory minute volume is increased. The stimulation is slight when the PO_2 of the inspired air is more than 60 mm Hg, and marked stimulation of respiration occurs only at lower PO_2 values. However, any decline in arterial PO_2 below 100 mm Hg produces increased discharge in the nerves from the carotid and aortic chemoreceptors. There are two reasons why this increase in impulse traffic does not increase ventilation to any extent in normal individuals until the PO_2 is less than 60 mm Hg. First, because hemoglobin (Hb) is a weaker acid than HbO_2, there is a slight decrease in the H^+ concentration of arterial blood when the arterial PO_2 falls and hemoglobin becomes less saturated with O_2. The fall in H^+ concentration tends to inhibit respiration. In addition, any increase in ventilation that does occur lowers the alveolar PCO_2, and this also tends to inhibit respiration. Therefore, the stimulatory effects of hypoxia on ventilation are not clearly manifest until they become strong enough to override the counterbalancing inhibitory effects of a decline in arterial H^+ concentration and PCO_2.

The effects on ventilation of decreasing the alveolar PO_2 while holding the alveolar PCO_2 constant are shown in **Figure 36–7**. When the alveolar PCO_2 is stabilized at a level 2–3 mm Hg above normal, there is an inverse relationship between ventilation and the alveolar PO_2 even in the 90–110 mm Hg range; but when the alveolar PCO_2 is fixed at lower than normal values, there is no stimulation of ventilation by hypoxia until the alveolar PO_2 falls below 60 mm Hg.

EFFECTS OF HYPOXIA ON THE CO_2 RESPONSE CURVE

When the converse experiment is performed—that is, when the alveolar PO_2 is held constant while the response to varying amounts of inspired CO_2 is tested—a linear response is obtained (**Figure 36–8**). When the CO_2 response is tested at different fixed PO_2 values, the slope of the response curve changes, with the slope increased when alveolar PO_2 is decreased. In other words, hypoxia makes the individual more sensitive to an increase in arterial PCO_2. However, the

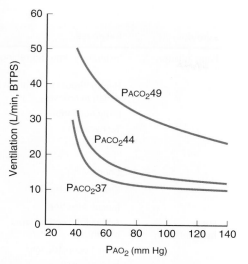

FIGURE 36–7 Ventilation at various alveolar Po₂ values when Pco₂ is held constant. Note the dramatic effect on the ventilatory response to Pao₂ when Paco₂ is increased. (Data from Loeschke HH and Gertz KH.)

alveolar Pco₂ level at which the curves in Figure 36-8 intersect is unaffected. In the normal individual, this threshold value is just below the normal alveolar Pco₂, indicating that normally there is a very slight but definite "CO₂ drive" of the respiratory area.

EFFECT OF H⁺ ON THE CO₂ RESPONSE

The stimulatory effects of H⁺ and CO₂ on respiration appear to be additive and not, like those of CO₂ and O₂, complexly interrelated. In metabolic acidosis, the CO₂ response curves are similar to those in Figure 36–8, except that they are shifted to the left. In other words,

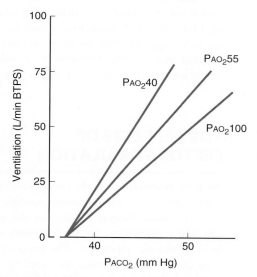

FIGURE 36–8 Fan of lines showing CO₂ response curves at various fixed values of alveolar Po₂. Decreased Pao₂ results in a more sensitive response to Paco₂.

the same amount of respiratory stimulation is produced by lower arterial Pco₂ levels. It has been calculated that the CO₂ response curve shifts 0.8 mm Hg to the left for each nanomole rise in arterial H⁺. About 40% of the ventilatory response to CO₂ is removed if the increase in arterial H⁺ produced by CO₂ is prevented. As noted above, the remaining 60% is probably due to the effect of CO₂ on spinal fluid or brain interstitial fluid H⁺ concentration.

■ NONCHEMICAL INFLUENCES ON RESPIRATION

RESPONSES MEDIATED BY RECEPTORS IN THE AIRWAYS & LUNGS

Receptors in the airways and lungs are innervated by myelinated and unmyelinated vagal fibers. The unmyelinated fibers are C fibers. The receptors innervated by myelinated fibers are commonly divided into **slowly adapting receptors** and **rapidly adapting receptors** on the basis of whether sustained stimulation leads to prolonged or transient discharge in their afferent nerve fibers (Table 36–2). The other group of receptors presumably consists of the endings of C fibers, and they are divided into pulmonary and bronchial subgroups on the basis of their location.

The shortening of inspiration produced by vagal afferent activity is mediated by slowly adapting receptors, as are the **Hering–Breuer reflexes**. The Hering–Breuer inflation reflex is an increase in the duration of expiration produced by steady lung inflation, and the Hering–Breuer deflation reflex is a decrease in the duration of expiration produced by marked deflation of the lung. Because the rapidly adapting receptors are stimulated by chemicals such as histamine, they have been called **irritant receptors**. Activation of rapidly adapting receptors in the trachea causes coughing, bronchoconstriction, and mucus secretion, and activation of rapidly adapting receptors in the lung may produce hyperpnea.

Because the C fiber endings are close to pulmonary vessels, they have been called J (juxtacapillary) receptors. They are stimulated by hyperinflation of the lung, but they respond as well to intravenous or intracardiac administration of chemicals such as capsaicin. The reflex response that is produced is apnea followed by rapid breathing, bradycardia, and hypotension (**pulmonary chemoreflex**). A similar response is produced by receptors in the heart (**Bezold–Jarisch reflex** or the **coronary chemoreflex**). The physiologic role of this reflex is uncertain, but it probably occurs in pathologic states such as pulmonary congestion or embolization, in which it is produced by endogenously released substances.

COUGHING & SNEEZING

Coughing begins with a deep inspiration followed by forced expiration against a closed glottis. This increases the intrapleural pressure to 100 mm Hg or more. The glottis is then suddenly opened, producing an explosive outflow of air at velocities up to 965 km (600 mi) per hour. Sneezing is a similar expiratory effort with a continuously open glottis. These reflexes help expel irritants and

TABLE 36–2 Airway and lung receptors.

Vagal Innervation	Type	Location in Interstitium	Stimulus	Response
Myelinated	Slowly adapting	Among airway smooth muscle cells (?)	Lung inflation	Inspiratory time shortening
				Hering–Breuer inflation and deflation reflexes
				Bronchodilation
				Tachycardia
	Rapidly adapting	Among airway epithelial cells	Lung hyperinflation	Hyperpnea
		Exogenous and endogenous substances (eg, histamine, prostaglandins)		Cough
				Bronchoconstriction
				Mucus secretion
Unmyelinated C fibers	Pulmonary C fibers	Close to blood vessels	Lung hyperinflation	Apnea followed by rapid breathing
	Bronchial C fibers	Exogenous and endogenous substances (eg, capsaicin, bradykinin, serotonin)		Bronchoconstriction
				Bradycardia
				Hypotension
				Mucus secretion

Modified with permission from Berger AJ, Hornbein TF: Control of respiration. In: Patton HD, et al: *Textbook of Physiology*, 21st ed, Vol 2. Saunders, 1989.

keep airways clear. Other aspects of innervation are considered in a special case (Clinical Box 36–1).

RESPIRATORY COMPONENTS OF VISCERAL REFLEXES

Inhibition of respiration and closure of the glottis during vomiting, swallowing, and sneezing not only prevent the aspiration of food

or vomitus into the trachea but, in the case of vomiting, fix the chest so that contraction of the abdominal muscles increases the intra-abdominal pressure. Similar glottic closure and inhibition of respiration occur during voluntary and involuntary straining.

Hiccup is a spasmodic contraction of the diaphragm and other inspiratory muscles that produces an inspiration during which the glottis suddenly closes. The glottic closure is responsible for the characteristic sensation and sound. Hiccups occur in the fetus in utero as well as throughout extrauterine life. Their function is unknown.

Yawning is a peculiar "infectious" respiratory act whose physiologic basis and significance are uncertain. Like hiccuping, it occurs in utero, and it occurs in fish and tortoises as well as mammals. The view that it is needed to increase O_2 intake has been discredited. Underventilated alveoli have a tendency to collapse, and it has been suggested that the deep inspiration and stretching them open prevents the development of atelectasis. Yawning increases venous return to the heart, which may benefit the circulation.

CLINICAL BOX 36–1

Lung Innervation & Patients with Heart–Lung Transplants

Transplantation of the heart and lungs is an established treatment for severe pulmonary disease and other conditions. In individuals with transplants, the recipient's right atrium is sutured to the donor heart, and the donor heart does not reinnervate, so the resting heart rate is elevated. The donor trachea is sutured to the recipient's just above the carina, and afferent fibers from the lungs do not regrow. Consequently, healthy patients with heart–lung transplants provide an opportunity to evaluate the role of lung innervation in normal physiology. Their cough responses to stimulation of the trachea are normal because the trachea remains innervated, but their cough responses to stimulation of the smaller airways are absent. Their bronchi tend to be dilated to a greater degree than normal. In addition, they have the normal number of yawns and sighs, indicating that these do not depend on innervation of the lungs. Finally, they lack Hering–Breuer reflexes, but their pattern of breathing at rest is normal, indicating that these reflexes do not play an important role in the regulation of resting respiration in humans.

RESPIRATORY EFFECTS OF BARORECEPTOR STIMULATION

Afferent fibers from the baroreceptors in the carotid sinuses, aortic arch, atria, and ventricles relay to the respiratory neurons, as well as the vasomotor and cardioinhibitory neurons in the medulla. Impulses in them inhibit respiration, but the inhibitory effect is slight and of little physiologic importance. The hyperventilation in shock is due to chemoreceptor stimulation caused by acidosis and hypoxia secondary to local stagnation of blood flow, and is not baroreceptor-mediated. The activity of inspiratory neurons affects blood pressure and heart rate, and activity in the vasomotor and cardiac areas in the medulla may have minor effects on respiration.

EFFECTS OF SLEEP

Respiration is less rigorously controlled during sleep than in the waking state, and brief periods of apnea occur in normal sleeping adults. Changes in the ventilatory response to hypoxia vary. If the P_{CO_2} falls during the waking state, various stimuli from proprioceptors and the environment maintain respiration, but during sleep, these stimuli are decreased and a decrease in P_{CO_2} can cause apnea. During rapid eye movement (REM) sleep, breathing is irregular and the CO_2 response is highly variable.

■ RESPIRATORY ABNORMALITIES

ASPHYXIA

In asphyxia produced by occlusion of the airway, acute hypercapnia and hypoxia develop together. Stimulation of respiration is pronounced, with violent respiratory efforts. Blood pressure and heart rate rise sharply, catecholamine secretion is increased, and blood pH drops. Eventually the respiratory efforts cease, the blood pressure falls, and the heart slows. Asphyxiated animals can still be revived at this point by artificial respiration, although they are prone to ventricular fibrillation. If artificial respiration is not started, cardiac arrest occurs in 4–5 min.

PERIODIC BREATHING

The acute effects of voluntary hyperventilation demonstrate the interaction of the chemical mechanisms regulating respiration. When a normal individual hyperventilates for 2–3 min, then stops and permits respiration to continue without exerting any voluntary control over it, a period of apnea occurs. This is followed by a few shallow breaths and then by another period of apnea, followed again by a few breaths (**periodic breathing**). The cycles may last for some time before normal breathing is resumed. The apnea apparently is due to a lack of CO_2 because it does not occur following hyperventilation with gas mixtures containing 5% CO_2. During the apnea, the alveolar P_{O_2} falls and the P_{CO_2} rises. Breathing resumes because of hypoxic stimulation of the carotid and aortic chemoreceptors before the CO_2 level has returned to normal. A few breaths eliminate the hypoxic stimulus, and breathing stops until the alveolar P_{O_2} falls again. Gradually, however, the P_{CO_2} returns to normal, and normal breathing resumes. Changes in breathing patterns can be symptomatic of disease (Clinical Box 36–2).

CLINICAL BOX 36–2

Periodic Breathing in Disease

Cheyne–Stokes Respiration
Periodic breathing occurs in various disease states and is often called Cheyne–Stokes respiration. It is seen most commonly in patients with heart failure and uremia, but it occurs also in patients with brain disease and during sleep in some normal individuals. Some of the patients with Cheyne–Stokes respiration have increased sensitivity to CO_2. The increased response is apparently due to disruption of neural pathways that normally inhibit respiration. In these individuals, CO_2 causes relative hyperventilation, lowering the arterial P_{CO_2}. During the resultant apnea, the arterial P_{CO_2} again rises to normal, but the respiratory mechanism again overresponds to CO_2. Breathing ceases, and the cycle repeats.

Another cause of periodic breathing in patients with cardiac disease is prolongation of the lung-to-brain circulation time, so that it takes longer for changes in arterial gas tensions to affect the respiratory area in the medulla. When individuals with a slower circulation hyperventilate, they lower the P_{CO_2} of the blood in their lungs, but it takes longer than normal for the blood with a low P_{CO_2} to reach the brain. During this time, the P_{CO_2} in the pulmonary capillary blood continues to be lowered, and when this blood reaches the brain, the low P_{CO_2} inhibits the respiratory area, producing apnea. In other words, the respiratory control system oscillates because the negative feedback loop from lungs to brain is abnormally long.

Sleep Apnea
Episodes of apnea during sleep can be central in origin (ie, due to failure of discharge in the nerves producing respiration) or they can be due to airway obstruction (**obstructive sleep apnea**). Apnea can occur at any age and can be produced when the pharyngeal muscles relax during sleep. In some cases, failure of the genioglossus muscles to contract during inspiration contributes to the blockage. The genioglossus muscles pull the tongue forward, and without (or with weak) contraction the tongue can obstruct the airway. After several increasingly strong respiratory efforts, the patient wakes up, takes a few normal breaths, and falls back to sleep. Apneic episodes are most common during REM sleep, when the muscles are most hypotonic. The symptoms are loud snoring, morning headaches, fatigue, and daytime sleepiness. When severe and prolonged, the condition can lead to hypertension and its complications. Frequent apneas can lead to numerous brief awakenings during sleep and to sleepiness during waking hours. With this in mind, it is not surprising to find that the incidence of motor vehicle accidents in sleep apnea patients is seven times greater than it is in the general driving population.

THERAPEUTIC HIGHLIGHTS

Treatment of sleep apnea depends on the patient and on the cause (if known). Treatments range from mild to moderate interventions to surgery. Interventions including positional therapy, dental appliances that rearrange the architecture of the airway, avoidance of muscle relaxants (eg, alcohol) or drugs that reduce respiratory drive, or continuous positive airway pressure. Because sleep apnea is increased in overweight or obese individuals, weight loss can also be effective.

■ EFFECTS OF EXERCISE

Exercise provides a physiologic example to explore many of the control systems discussed above. Of course, many cardiovascular and respiratory mechanisms must operate in an integrated fashion if the O_2 needs of the active tissue are to be met and the extra CO_2 and heat removed from the body during exercise. Circulatory changes increase muscle blood flow while maintaining adequate circulation in the rest of the body. In addition, there is an increase in the extraction of O_2 from the blood in exercising muscles and an increase in ventilation. This provides extra O_2, eliminates some of the heat, and excretes extra CO_2.

CHANGES IN VENTILATION

During exercise, the amount of O_2 entering the blood in the lungs is increased because the amount of O_2 added to each unit of blood and the pulmonary blood flow per minute are increased. The Po_2 of blood flowing into the pulmonary capillaries falls from 40 to 25 mm Hg or less, so that the alveolar-capillary Po_2 gradient is increased and more O_2 enters the blood. Blood flow per minute is increased from 5.5 L/min to as much as 20–35 L/min. The total amount of O_2 entering the blood therefore increases from 250 mL/min at rest to values as high as 4000 mL/min. The amount of CO_2 removed from each unit of blood is increased, and CO_2 excretion increases from 200 mL/min to as much as 8000 mL/min. The increase in O_2 uptake is proportional to work load, up to a maximum. Above this maximum, O_2 consumption levels off and the blood lactate level continues to rise (Figure 36–9). The lactate comes from muscles in which aerobic resynthesis of energy stores cannot keep pace with their utilization, and an **oxygen debt** is being incurred.

Ventilation increases abruptly with the onset of exercise, which is followed after a brief pause by a further, more gradual increase.

With moderate exercise, the increase is due mostly to an increase in the depth of respiration; this is accompanied by an increase in the respiratory rate when the exercise is more strenuous. Ventilation abruptly decreases when exercise ceases, which is followed after a brief pause by a more gradual decline to preexercise values. The abrupt increase at the start of exercise is presumably due to psychic stimuli and afferent impulses from proprioceptors in muscles, tendons, and joints. The more gradual increase is presumably humoral, even though arterial pH, Pco_2, and Po_2 remain constant during moderate exercise. The increase in ventilation is proportional to the increase in O_2 consumption, but several physiologic changes—body temperature, plasma K^+ levels, CO_2 concentrations, and more—contribute to this response in moderate exercise.

When exercise becomes more vigorous, buffering of the increased amounts of lactic acid that are produced liberates more CO_2, and this further increases ventilation. The response to graded exercise is shown in **Figure 36–10**. With increased production of acid, the increases in ventilation and CO_2 production remain proportional, so alveolar and arterial CO_2 change relatively little (**isocapnic buffering**). Because of the increased ventilation, alveolar Po_2 increases. With further accumulation of lactic acid, the increase in ventilation outstrips CO_2 production and alveolar Pco_2 falls, as does arterial Pco_2. The decline in arterial Pco_2

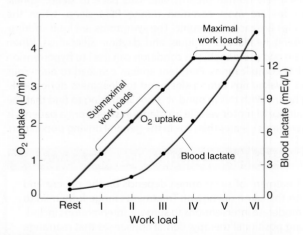

FIGURE 36–9 Relation between work load, blood lactate level, and O_2 uptake. I–VI, increasing workloads produced by increasing the speed and grade of a treadmill on which the subjects worked. (Reproduced with permission from Mitchell JH, Blomqvist G: Maximal oxygen uptake. *N Engl J Med.* 1971 May 6;284(18): 1018–1022.)

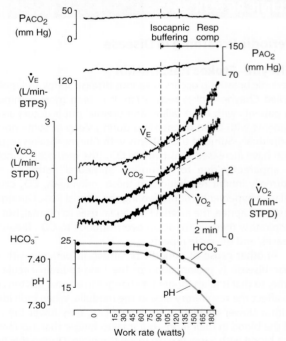

FIGURE 36–10 Physiologic responses to work rate during exercise. Changes in alveolar Pco_2, alveolar Po, ventilation ($\dot{V}_E$) consumption production ($\dot{V}co_2$) consumption ($\dot{V}o_2$) arterial HCO_3^-, and arterial pH with graded increases in work by an adult male on a bicycle ergometer. Resp comp, respiratory compensation; STPD, standard temperature (0°C) and pressure (760 mm Hg), dry. Dashed lines emphasize deviation from linear response. See the text for additional details. (Reproduced with permission from Wasserman K: Breathing during exercise. *N Engl J Med.* 1978 Apr 6;298(14):780–785.)

provides respiratory compensation for the metabolic acidosis produced by the additional lactic acid. The additional increase in ventilation produced by the acidosis depends on the carotid bodies and does not occur if they are removed.

The respiratory rate after exercise does not reach basal levels until the O_2 debt is repaid. This may take as long as 90 min. The stimulus to ventilation after exercise is not the arterial P_{CO_2}, which is normal or low, or the arterial P_{O_2}, which is normal or high, but the elevated arterial H^+ concentration due to the lactic acidemia. The magnitude of the O_2 debt is the amount by which O_2 consumption exceeds basal consumption from the end of exertion until the O_2 consumption has returned to preexercise basal levels.

CHANGES IN THE TISSUES

Maximum O_2 uptake during exercise is limited by the maximum rate at which O_2 is transported to the mitochondria in the exercising muscle. However, this limitation is not normally due to deficient O_2 uptake in the lungs, and hemoglobin in arterial blood is saturated even during the most severe exercise.

During exercise, the contracting muscles use more O_2, and the tissue P_{O_2} and the P_{O_2} in venous blood from exercising muscle fall nearly to zero. As more O_2 diffuses from the blood, the P_{O_2} of the blood in the muscles drops, and more O_2 is removed from hemoglobin. Because the capillary bed of contracting muscle is dilated and many previously closed capillaries are open, the mean distance from the blood to the tissue cells is greatly decreased; this facilitates the movement of O_2 from blood to cells. The oxygen–hemoglobin dissociation curve is steep in the P_{O_2} range below 60 mm Hg, and a relatively large amount of O_2 is supplied for each drop of 1 mm Hg in P_{O_2} (see Figure 35–2). Additional O_2 is supplied because, as a result of the accumulation of CO_2 and the rise in temperature in active tissues—and perhaps because of a rise in red blood cell 2,3-diphosphoglycerate (2,3-DPG)—the dissociation curve shifts to the right. The net effect is a threefold increase in O_2 extraction from each unit of blood. Because this increase is accompanied by a 30-fold or greater increase in blood flow, it permits the metabolic rate of muscle to rise as much as 100-fold during exercise.

EXERCISE TOLERANCE & FATIGUE

What determines the maximum amount of exercise that can be performed by an individual? Obviously, exercise tolerance has a time as well as an intensity dimension. For example, a fit young man can produce a power output on a bicycle of about 700 W for 1 min, 300 W for 5 min, and 200 W for 40 min. It used to be argued that the limiting factors in exercise performance were the rate at which O_2 could be delivered to the tissues or the rate at which O_2 could enter the body in the lungs. These factors play a role, but it is clear that other factors also contribute and that exercise stops when the sensation of **fatigue** progresses to the sensation of exhaustion. Fatigue is produced in part by bombardment of the brain by neural impulses from muscles, and the decline in

blood pH produced by lactic acidosis also makes one feel tired, as does the rise in body temperature, dyspnea, and, perhaps, the uncomfortable sensations produced by activation of the J receptors in the lungs.

CHAPTER SUMMARY

- Breathing is under both voluntary control (located in the cerebral cortex) and automatic control (driven by pacemaker cells in the medulla). There is a reciprocal innervation to expiratory and inspiratory muscles in that motor neurons supplying expiratory muscles are inactive when motor neurons supplying inspiratory muscles are active, and vice versa.
- The pre-BÖTC complex on either side of the medulla contains synaptically coupled pacemaker cells that allow for rhythmic generation of breathing. The spontaneous activity of these neurons can be altered by neurons in the pneumotaxic center, although the full regulatory function of these neurons on normal breathing is not understood.
- Breathing patterns are sensitive to chemicals in the blood through activation of respiratory chemoreceptors. There are chemoreceptors in the carotid and aortic bodies and in collections of cells in the medulla. These chemoreceptors respond to changes in P_{O_2} and P_{CO_2} as well as H^+ to regulate breathing.
- Receptors in the airway are additionally innervated by slowly adapting and rapidly adapting myelinated vagal fibers. Slowly adapting receptors can be activated by lung inflation. Rapidly adapting receptors, or irritant receptors, can be activated by irritants and result in cough or even hyperpnea.
- Receptors in the airway are also innervated by unmyelinated vagal fibers (C fibers) that are typically found next to pulmonary vessels. They are stimulated by hyperinflation (or exogenous substances including capsaicin) and lead to the pulmonary chemoreflex. The physiologic role for this response is not fully understood.

MULTIPLE-CHOICE QUESTIONS

For all questions, select the single best answer unless otherwise directed.

1. In an experimental system, the pre-BÖTC is eliminated and its main function is taken over by outside electrical stimulation. The investigator has full control of firing amplitude and rate, and can directly measure the downstream muscle response. While the investigator tried many different patterns and measurements, which of the following best substituted for normal pre-BÖTC activity during quiet respiration?
    A. Rhythmic bursts of ~2 s of impulses and 5 s of rest that resulted in contraction of expiratory muscles
    B. Large single neuron impulses every 10–12 s directed at dorsal respiratory group (DRG) and resulting in inspiratory muscle contraction
    C. Large single neuron impulses every 10–12 s directed at ventral respiratory group (VRG), and resulting in inspiratory muscle contraction
    D. Rhythmic bursts of ~2 s of impulses and 5 s of rest that resulted in contraction of inspiratory muscles
    E. Rhythmic bursts of ~2 s of impulses and 5 s of rest directed at the DRG, and resulting in expiratory muscle contraction

2. A professor and his student meet up in a gym and sit in adjoining stationary bikes and begin a light conversation. As time goes by, the chitchat is replaced by determination and the two find themselves pedaling their bikes at exceptional speeds. The extensive work of the leg muscles requires anaerobic respiration and results in raised levels of circulating lactic acid, which in turn increases ventilation. Eventually the student realizes that it is hopeless to keep up the pace and returns to a more normal cadence and more chitchat about current events. Which of the following is true concerning the transduction of the net increase in lactic acid to increased ventilation?

   A. Acid sensing in receptors responsible for the transduction are located in the medulla oblongata.
   B. Acid sensing in receptors responsible for the transduction are located in the carotid bodies.
   C. Acid sensing in receptors responsible for the transduction are located in the lung parenchyma.
   D. Acid sensing in receptors responsible for the transduction are located in the aortic baroreceptors.
   E. Acid sensing in receptors responsible for the transduction are located in the trachea and large bronchi.

3. In the nights leading up to a respiratory physiology exam, a student was suffering from a recurring nightmare. In this nightmare a knife-wielding horse was chasing the student through the streets and threatening to cut off his ability for spontaneous respiration. Assuming the horse was proficient in its threat, and that only breathing would be affected, which of the following answers would allow the knife-wielding horse to be successful?

   A. Transection of the brainstem above the pons
   B. Transection of the brainstem at the caudal end of the medulla
   C. Bilateral vagotomy
   D. Bilateral vagotomy combined with transection of the brainstem at the superior border of the pons
   E. Transection of the spinal cord at the level of the first thoracic segment

4. You are invited to a conference on pulmonary physiology in an airtight conference room at sea level. Prior to the meeting, the P_{CO_2} in the room is ~0.2 mm Hg. However, you arrive 1 h late and find that the room P_{CO_2} has increased to 20 mm Hg. When you enter the room, you rapidly respond to the increased P_{CO_2} with an increase in minute ventilation. Assuming that your central chemoreceptors are working correctly, what is the proper order for the following physiologic events: (1) decreased CSF pH; (2) increased arterial P_{CO_2}; (3) increased CSF P_{CO_2}; (4) stimulation of medullary chemoreceptors; (5) increased alveolar P_{CO_2}?

   A. 1, 2, 3, 4, 5
   B. 4, 1, 3, 2, 5
   C. 3, 4, 5, 1, 2
   D. 5, 2, 3, 1, 4
   E. 5, 3, 2, 4, 1

5. A carotid body was removed and studied in the laboratory. Within this sophisticated preparation, the following physiological responses could be recorded: (1) depolarization of type I glomus cells; (2) excitation of afferent nerve endings; (3) reduced conductance of hypoxia-sensitive K^+ channels in type I glomus cells; (4) Ca^{2+} entry into type I glomus cells; (5) decreased K^+ efflux. Assuming the isolated carotid body

could faithfully reproduce an in vivo response, what sequence would the above physiologic responses occur following an exposure to hypoxia?

   A. 1, 3, 4, 5, 2
   B. 1, 4, 2, 5, 3
   C. 3, 4, 5, 1, 2
   D. 3, 1, 4, 5, 2
   E. 3, 5, 1, 4, 2

6. After several years of experimentation, a researcher developed a drug that could directly stimulate the carotid bodies. After several more years of experimentation, the same researcher developed a way to deliver the drug intravenously and with limited side effects. While the researcher was confident that the drug worked in her preclinical mouse model, she wanted to develop a dose/response curve for the drug in a preclinical dog model. Following injection of the drug into the dog, which of the following would be a measure of a successful response?

   A. A decrease in the pH of arterial blood
   B. A decrease in the P_{CO_2} of arterial blood
   C. An increase in the HCO_3^- concentration of arterial blood
   D. An increase in urinary Na^+ excretion
   E. An increase in plasma Cl^-

7. In a laboratory that studies ventilation responses to blood and CSF components, several sophisticated setups are available to quickly change gas and ionic components of blood plasma. In a given day a newer member of the laboratory was able to successfully alter known blood and CSF parameters and record the expected ventilatory changes. As all experiments were successful, the laboratory member thought it would be prudent to run a control experiment and alter a blood or CSF component that did not change ventilation. Which of the following components of blood or CSF could be used as this control (ie, their alteration does *not* affect respiration)?

   A. Arterial HCO_3^- concentration
   B. Arterial H^+ concentration
   C. Arterial Na^+ concentration
   D. CSF CO_2 concentration
   E. CSF H^+ concentration

8. A 36-year-old man visits his physician at the request of his wife, who has noticed that in addition to his long history of snoring, she has recently observed episodes of apnea that extend for 1–2 min during his sleep. His physician recommends an overnight sleep study (polysomnography). In the study, records of respiratory activity, blood O_2 levels, heart rate, brain activity, and eye and leg movements are collected and analyzed. Following data analysis, the patient is informed that he has a central sleep apnea, or dysfunctional response of the central chemoreceptors that is present during sleep. Central chemoreceptors are stimulated by which one of the following?

   A. Loss of CSF
   B. Increase in CSF pH
   C. Rhythmic firing of pre-BÖTC neurons
   D. Increase in brain blood P_{CO_2}
   E. Decrease in brain blood P_{O_2}

9. A 30-year-old healthy woman visited the pulmonary clinic for a full respiratory test as part of a clinical study. During the study she was monitored for ventilatory response to

changes in P_{O_2} and P_{CO_2} as well as responses to voluntary changes in ventilation rate. During large inspirations and long expirations, the patient demonstrated normal slowing of respiratory frequency (Hering–Breuer reflex). The main lung receptors that sense changes in expiration and initiate the Hering–Breuer reflex are which of the following?

A. Peripheral chemoreceptors
B. Irritant receptors (rapidly adapting pulmonary stretch receptors)
C. Pulmonary C fibers (or J fibers)
D. Bronchial C fibers
E. Slowly adapting pulmonary stretch receptors

10. A 5-month-old infant was admitted to the hospital for evaluation because of repeated episodes of sleep apnea. During a ventilatory response test, his ventilation did not increase when arterial P_{CO_2} was increased, but decreased during hyperoxia. Which of the following could best explain this infant's apnea?

A. Bronchospasm
B. Decreased irritant receptor sensitivity
C. Diaphragm fatigue
D. Dysfunctional central chemoreceptors
E. Peripheral chemoreceptor hypersensitivity

ANSWERS

1. The correct answer is **C**. The pre-BÖTC is the rhythmic or pattern generator for the control of breathing. The rhythmic firing is largely communicated through the phrenic nerve for contraction of the diaphragm and control of inspiration. Expiration occurs as the diaphragm relaxes and is not a target for activation of the pre-BÖTC, ruling out **A** and **E**. The activation pattern generated by the pre-BÖTC includes many neurons and many firings, ruling out **B** and **C**. The DRG and VRG can provide upstream input to the pre-BÖTC to regulate the firing pattern but do not contribute downstream of the pre-BÖTC for muscle contraction, further ruling out **B** and **C**.

2. The correct answer is **B**. The accumulation of lactic acid, as occurs in the switch from aerobic to anaerobic metabolism during exercise, leads to an increase in alveolar ventilation primarily through the stimulation of the peripheral chemoreceptors. Central chemoreception (**A**) can respond to changes in pH via changes in [H^+] by sensing P_{CO_2} changes across the blood–brain barrier. However, the blood–brain barrier is not permeant to lactic acid, and thus it would not stimulate this region. Peripheral chemoreceptors include carotid bodies found in the carotid sinus, ruling out both **C** and **E**. The aortic baroreceptors (**D**) are found adjacent to the carotid bodies; however, these receptors are responsible for detecting changes in blood pressure, not changes in acids, and can be ruled out.

3. The correct answer is **B**. The horse would be aiming to cut off the work of the pre-BÖTC in directing phrenic nerve activity that stimulates inspiratory muscles. The pre-BÖTC is located in the medulla, so a transection at the caudal end would cut off this activity, where transection above the pons (**A**) would leave communication between the pre-BÖTC and phrenic nerve connection intact. Since the phrenic nerve exits the spinal column at C3, any transection of a thoracic segment would leave the breathing circuit intact, and (**E**) can be eliminated. Pulmonary vagal fibers contribute feedback to the breathing center that can alter breathing patterns. However,

bilateral vagotomy does not in itself eliminate breathing, eliminating **C** and **D**.

4. The correct answer is **D**. Upon entering the room you breathe in the CO_2-enriched air that subsequently raises alveolar P_{CO_2} (5). This limits the ability for CO_2 exchange at the alveoli and results in an increase in arterial P_{CO_2} (2). Because CO_2 can cross the blood–brain barrier, it then raises the CSF P_{CO_2} (3). An increased CSF P_{CO_2} will result in an increased [H^+], or lowered pH (1), and stimulate central chemoreceptors in the medulla (4).

5. The correct answer is **E**. In vivo, the carotid body is thought to sense decreases in P_{O_2} in the type I glomus cell through the actions of hypoxia-sensitive K^+ channels (5). This type of K^+ channel gating reduces K^+ efflux from the type I glomus cell (3) and leads to a depolarization (1). The depolarization gates Ca^{2+} channels, leading to Ca^{2+} entry (4) and neurotransmitter release to activate afferent nerve endings (2) that provide the low P_{O_2} information to the brain.

6. The correct answer is **B**. The carotid bodies are normally stimulated upon an increase in arterial P_{CO_2} and function to return P_{CO_2} to normal levels. Drug stimulation would mirror this drop in P_{CO_2}, which is accompanied by decreases in both H^+ and HCO_3^-, eliminating **A** and **C**. A change in blood pH does not have any effect on Na^+ excretion, thereby eliminating **D**. Lowering of P_{CO_2} could affect HCO_3^- movement from the plasma to RBCs in exchange for plasma Cl^-; however, the net change would be a decrease in plasma Cl^- and so **E** can be eliminated.

7. The correct answer is **C**. Changes in blood Na^+ concentrations do not affect breathing patterns. Changes in arterial HCO_3^- (**A**) also alter P_{CO_2} and pH, both of which can be sensed by chemoreceptors to alter respiration. Arterial [H^+] (**B**) can be monitored by peripheral chemoreceptors and indirectly, via P_{CO_2} changes, by central chemoreceptors. While chemoreceptors in the CSF lead to altered respiration by sensing increased [H^+] concentration, it is P_{CO_2} that passes through the blood–brain barrier and indirectly raises [H^+] through the action of carbonic anhydrase. Thus, both **D** and **E** can be ruled out.

8. The correct answer is **D**. The central chemoreceptors ultimately sense increased [H^+] in the CSF and then provide feedback to the respiratory pattern generators to alter ventilation. The change in [H^+] concentration in the CSF occurs following an increase in P_{CO_2} that can pass the blood–brain barrier into the CSF, where carbonic anhydrase catalyzes the conversion of $CO_2 + H_2O$ to H_2CO_3, which quickly dissociates into $H^+ + HCO_3^-$. CSF (**A**) is kept constant under normal conditions and can be ruled out as part of central chemoreceptor signaling. An increase in CSF pH (**B**) would correspond to a decrease in [H^+], and thus would not stimulate chemoreceptors. The central chemoreceptors do not receive signaling from the pre-BÖTC (**C**), rather they initiate signaling that ultimately regulates the respiratory control centers. Central chemoreceptors are insensitive to the brain blood P_{O_2}, and thus (**E**) can be ruled out.

9. The correct answer is **E**. Slowly adapting pulmonary stretch receptors are found in the airway smooth muscle and are stimulated after a large inspiration or extended expiration. As the name implies, their activation is relatively long acting. Peripheral chemoreceptors (**A**) monitor blood gases and pH, but neither of these would be expected to be changed in a healthy individual following large inspiration/extended

expiration. Irritant receptors (**B**) are found in the airway and responds rapidly to noxious chemicals to produce cough or sneeze, and can be ruled out. Pulmonary C fibers (**C**), also known as juxtacapillary or "J" fibers, are located close to the blood vessels in the alveoli. Their activation results in rapid, shallow breathing, or even apnea, and thus can be ruled out. Bronchial C fibers (**D**) are found next the blood vessels in the bronchial circulation and also respond to noxious chemicals. Their stimulation can result in rapid breathing and apnea as well as increased mucus secretion, and can be ruled out.

10. The correct answer is **D**. Changes in blood gases are communicated to the respiratory control center in the brain by chemoreceptors. While peripheral chemoreceptors, the aortic and carotid bodies are sensitive to Po_2, Pco_2, and pH, the central chemoreceptors are solely responsive to changes in pH, and more specifically [H^+]. While the lack of response to Pco_2 could be through central (via changes in pH) or peripheral receptors, the proper response to Po_2 suggests that the peripheral receptors are intact and working properly, ruling out (**E**). Bronchospasms refer to sudden contraction of bronchial muscles and are not associated with sleep apnea, ruling out (**A**). Irritant receptor activation (**B**) can result in sneeze and cough that would disrupt the airway; however, any decrease in their activity would not provide feedback to the respiratory control center. Isolated diaphragm fatigue (**C**) can be ruled out in that it is highly unlikely in an infant and would result in difficulty breathing in wakeful hours.

SECTION VII RENAL PHYSIOLOGY

Renal Function & Micturition

OBJECTIVES

After reading this chapter, you should be able to:

- Describe the morphology of a typical nephron and its blood supply.
- Define autoregulation and list the major theories advanced to explain autoregulation in the kidneys.
- Define glomerular filtration rate, describe how it can be measured, and list the major factors affecting it.
- Outline tubular handling of Na$^+$ and water.
- Discuss tubular reabsorption and secretion of glucose and K$^+$.
- Describe how the countercurrent mechanism in the kidney operates to produce hypertonic or hypotonic urine.
- List the major classes of diuretics; understand how each operates to increase urine flow.
- Describe the voiding reflex.

■ FUNCTIONAL ANATOMY

THE NEPHRON

The basic unit of the kidney is the **nephron**, made up of the renal tubule and its glomerulus. The size of the kidneys varies between species, as does the number of nephrons they contain. Each human kidney has approximately 1 million nephrons. The specific structures of the nephron are shown in diagrammatic manner in **Figure 37–1**.

The glomerulus is formed by the invagination of a tuft of capillaries into the dilated, blind end of the nephron (**Bowman's capsule**). The capillaries are supplied by an **afferent arteriole** and drained by the **efferent arteriole,** and it is from the glomerulus that the filtrate is formed. The diameter of the afferent arteriole is larger than the efferent arteriole. Two cellular layers separate the blood from the glomerular filtrate in Bowman's capsule: the capillary endothelium and the specialized epithelium of the capsule. The endothelium of the glomerular capillaries is fenestrated with pores. The endothelium of the glomerular capillaries is completely surrounded by the glomerular basement membrane along with specialized cells called podocytes. **Podocytes** have numerous pseudopodia that interdigitate to form **filtration slits** along the

capillary wall. The glomerular basement membrane, the basal lamina, does not contain visible gaps or pores. Stellate cells called **mesangial cells** are located between the basal lamina and the endothelium. Mesangial cells are contractile, play a role in the regulation of glomerular filtration, secrete the extracellular matrix, take up immune complexes, and are a target in glomerular disease.

Functionally, the glomerular membrane permits the free passage of neutral substances up to 4 nm in diameter and almost totally excludes those with diameters greater than 8 nm. However, the charge on molecules as well as their diameters affects their passage into Bowman's capsule.

The **proximal convoluted tubule** is made up of a single layer of cells that interdigitate with one another and are united by apical tight junctions. The luminal edges of the cells have a striated **brush border** made up of many microvilli.

The proximal convoluted tubule straightens and the next portion of the nephron is the **loop of Henle.** The descending portion of the loop and the proximal portion of the ascending limb are made up of thin, permeable cells. Farther on, the thick portion of the ascending limb (**TALH**) (Figure 37–1) is made up of thick cells containing many mitochondria. Nephrons with glomeruli in the outer portions of the renal cortex have short loops of Henle (**cortical nephrons**), whereas those with glomeruli in the

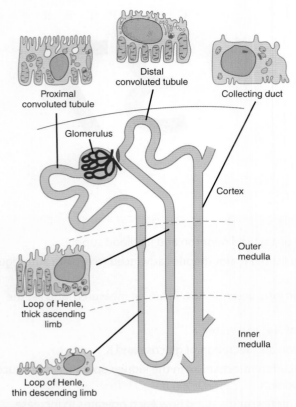

FIGURE 37–1 Diagram of a nephron. The main histologic features of the cells that make up each portion of the tubule are also shown.

juxtamedullary region of the cortex (**juxtamedullary nephrons**) have long loops extending down into the medullary pyramids. Typically, only 15% of the nephrons have long loops.

The thick end of the TALH reaches the glomerulus of the nephron from which the tubule arose and nestles between its afferent and efferent arterioles. Specialized cells at the end form the **macula densa,** which is particularly close to the afferent arteriole. The macula densa and the renin-secreting **granular cells** in the afferent arteriole form the **juxtaglomerular apparatus.**

The **distal convoluted tubule** starts at the macula densa, with no distinct brush border. The distal tubules coalesce to form **collecting ducts** that pass through the renal cortex and medulla to empty into the pelvis of the kidney at the apexes of the medullary pyramids. The epithelium of the collecting ducts is made up of **principal cells (P cells)** and **intercalated cells (I cells).** The P cells, which predominate, are relatively tall and have few organelles. They are involved in Na^+ reabsorption and vasopressin-stimulated water reabsorption. The I cells, which are present in smaller numbers, have more microvilli, cytoplasmic vesicles, and mitochondria. They are involved with acid secretion and HCO_3^- transport.

BLOOD VESSELS

The **afferent arterioles** are short, straight branches of the interlobular arteries. Each divides into multiple capillary branches to form the tuft of vessels in the glomerulus. The capillaries coalesce

to form the **efferent arteriole,** which in turn breaks up into capillaries that supply the tubules (**peritubular capillaries**) before draining into the interlobular veins. The glomerular capillaries are the only capillaries in the body that drain into arterioles. However, there is relatively little smooth muscle in the efferent arterioles. The efferent arteriole from each glomerulus breaks up into capillaries that supply a number of different nephrons.

The capillaries draining the tubules of the cortical nephrons form a peritubular network, whereas the efferent arterioles from the juxtamedullary glomeruli drain not only into a peritubular network, but also into vessels that form hairpin loops (the **vasa recta**). These loops dip into the medullary pyramids alongside the loops of Henle. The descending vasa recta have a nonfenestrated endothelium that contains a facilitated transporter for urea, and the ascending vasa recta have a fenestrated endothelium, consistent with their function in conserving solutes.

LYMPHATICS

The kidneys have an abundant lymphatic supply that drains via the thoracic duct into the venous circulation in the thorax.

INNERVATION OF THE RENAL VESSELS

The renal nerves travel along the renal blood vessels as they enter the kidney. They contain many postganglionic sympathetic efferent fibers and a few afferent fibers. The sympathetic fibers are distributed primarily to the afferent and efferent arterioles, the proximal and distal tubules, and the juxtaglomerular apparatus. In addition, there is a dense noradrenergic innervation of the TAHL.

Nociceptive afferents that mediate pain with kidney disease parallel the sympathetic efferents and enter the spinal cord in the thoracic and upper lumbar dorsal roots. Other renal afferents presumably mediate a **renorenal reflex** by which an increase in ureteral pressure in one kidney leads to a decrease in efferent nerve activity to the contralateral kidney. This decrease permits an increase in its excretion of Na^+ and water.

■ RENAL CIRCULATION

BLOOD FLOW

In a resting adult, the kidneys receive approximately 25% of the cardiac output. Renal blood flow can be measured with electromagnetic or other types of flow meters, or it can be determined by applying the Fick principle (see Chapter 30) to the kidney; that is, by measuring the amount of a given substance taken up per unit of time and dividing this value by the arteriovenous difference for the substance across the kidney. Because the kidney filters plasma, the **renal plasma flow** (RPF) equals the amount of a substance excreted per unit of time divided by the renal arteriovenous difference as long as the amount in the red cells is unaltered during passage through the kidney.

RPF can be measured by infusing p-aminohippuric acid (PAH) and determining its urine and plasma concentrations. PAH is filtered by the glomeruli and secreted by the tubular cells, so that its **extraction ratio** (arterial concentration minus renal venous concentration divided by arterial concentration) is high. For example, when PAH is infused at low doses, 90% of the PAH in arterial blood is removed in a single circulation through the kidney. It has therefore become commonplace to calculate the "RPF" by dividing the amount of PAH in the urine by the plasma PAH level, ignoring the level in renal venous blood. The value obtained should be called the **effective renal plasma flow (ERPF)** to indicate that the level in renal venous plasma was not measured.

$$ERPF = \frac{U_{PAH}\dot{V}}{P_{PAH}} = \text{Clearance of PAH}\,(C_{PAH})$$

Example:
Concentration of PAH in urine (U_{PAH}): 14 mg/mL
Urine flow (UV): 0.9 mL/min
Concentration of PAH in plasma (P_{PAH}): 0.02 mg/mL

$$ERPF = \frac{14 \times 0.9}{0.02}$$
$$= 630\,\text{mL/min}$$

It should be noted that the ERPF determined in this way is the **clearance** of PAH. The concept of clearance is discussed in detail below.

ERPF can be converted to actual RPF:
Average PAH extraction ratio: 0.9

$$\frac{ERP}{\text{Extraction ratio}} = \frac{630}{0.9} = \text{Actural RPF} = 700\,\text{mL/min}$$

From the RPF, the renal blood flow can be calculated by dividing by 1 minus the hematocrit:
Hematocrit (Hct): 45%

$$\text{Renal blood flow} = RPF \times \frac{1}{1-Hct}$$
$$= 700 \times \frac{1}{0.55}$$
$$= 1273\,\text{mL/min}$$

REGULATION OF THE RENAL BLOOD FLOW

Both vasodilators and vasoconstrictors can affect renal blood flow.

FUNCTIONS OF THE RENAL NERVES

Stimulation of the renal nerves increases renin secretion by a direct action of released norepinephrine on β_1-adrenergic receptors on the juxtaglomerular cells (see Chapter 38), and it increases Na^+ reabsorption, probably by a direct action of norepinephrine on

renal tubular cells or by angiotensin II effects. The proximal and distal tubules and the TALH are richly innervated.

Strong stimulation of the sympathetic noradrenergic nerves to the kidneys causes a marked decrease in renal blood flow. This effect is mediated by α_1-adrenergic receptors and to a lesser extent by postsynaptic α_2-adrenergic receptors. When systemic blood pressure falls, the vasoconstrictor response produced by decreased discharge in the baroreceptor nerves includes renal vasoconstriction.

AUTOREGULATION OF RENAL BLOOD FLOW

Autoregulation is defined as when renal vascular resistance varies with the pressure so that renal blood flow is relatively constant.

REGIONAL BLOOD FLOW & OXYGEN CONSUMPTION

The main function of the renal cortex is filtration of large volumes of blood through the glomeruli, so it is not surprising that the renal cortical blood flow is relatively great and little oxygen is extracted from the blood. The Po_2 of the cortex is about 50 mm Hg. On the other hand, maintenance of the osmotic gradient in the medulla requires a relatively low blood flow. However, metabolic work is being done, particularly to reabsorb Na^+ in the TAHL, so relatively large amounts of O_2 are extracted from the blood in the medulla. The Po_2 of the medulla is about 15 mm Hg. This makes the medulla vulnerable to hypoxia if flow is reduced further.

■ GLOMERULAR FILTRATION

MEASURING GFR

Glomerular filtration rate (GFR) is the amount of plasma ultrafiltrate formed each minute. A substance used to measure GFR must be freely filtered through the glomeruli and must be neither secreted nor reabsorbed by the tubules, should be nontoxic and not metabolized by the body.

Renal plasma clearance is the *volume of plasma* from which a substance is completely removed by the kidney in a given amount of time (usually minutes). The amount of that substance that appears in the urine per unit of time is the result of the renal filtering of a certain number of milliliters of plasma that contained this amount. GFR and clearance are measured in mL/min.

Therefore, if the substance is designated by the letter X, the GFR is equal to the concentration of X in urine (U_X) times the **urine flow** per unit of time (**V**) divided by the **arterial plasma level** of X (P_X), or $/P_X$. **This value is called the clearance of X (C_X).**

When using inulin, a loading dose is administered intravenously, followed by a sustaining infusion to keep the arterial plasma level constant. After the inulin has equilibrated with body fluids, an accurately timed urine specimen is collected and a plasma sample obtained halfway through the collection. Plasma and urinary inulin concentrations are determined and the clearance is calculated:

$$U_{IN} = 35\,mg/mL$$
$$\dot{V} = 0.9\,mL/min$$
$$P_{IN} = 0.25\,mg/mL$$
$$C_{IN} = \frac{U_{IN}\,\dot{V}}{P_{IN}} = \frac{35 \times 0.9}{0.25}$$
$$C_{IN} = 126\,mL/min$$

Clearance of creatinine (C_{Cr}) can also be used to determine GFR. However, some creatinine is secreted by the tubules; thus the clearance of creatinine will be slightly higher than inulin. In spite of this, the clearance of endogenous creatinine is a reasonable estimate of GFR as the values agree quite well with the GFR values measured with inulin.

CONTROL OF GFR

The factors governing filtration across the glomerular capillaries are the same as those governing filtration across all other capillaries (see Chapter 31), that is, the size of the capillary bed, the permeability of the capillaries, and the hydrostatic and osmotic pressure gradients across the capillary wall. For each nephron:

$$GFR = K_f[(P_{GC} - P_T) - (\pi_{GC} - \pi_T)]$$

where K_f, the glomerular ultrafiltration coefficient, is the product of the glomerular capillary wall hydraulic conductivity (ie, its permeability) and the effective filtration surface area. P_{GC} is the mean hydrostatic pressure in the glomerular capillaries, P_T the mean hydrostatic pressure in the tubule (Bowman's space), π_{GC} the oncotic pressure of the plasma in the glomerular capillaries, and π_T the oncotic pressure of the filtrate in the tubule (Bowman's space).

PERMEABILITY

The permeability of the glomerular capillaries is about 50 times that of the capillaries in skeletal muscle. Neutral substances with effective molecular diameters of less than 4 nm are freely filtered, and the filtration of neutral substances with diameters of more than 8 nm approaches zero. Between these values, filtration is inversely proportional to diameter. However, sialoproteins in the glomerular capillary wall are negatively charged, and negative charges repel negatively charged substances in blood, with the result that filtration of anionic substances 4 nm in diameter is less than half that of neutral substances of the same size. This probably explains why albumin, with an effective molecular diameter of approximately 7 nm, normally has a glomerular concentration only 0.2% of its plasma concentration rather than the higher concentration that would be expected on the basis of diameter alone; circulating albumin is negatively charged. Conversely, filtration of cationic substances is greater than that of neutral substances.

The amount of protein in the urine is normally less than 100 mg/day, and most of this is not filtered but comes from shed tubular cells. The presence of significant amounts of albumin in the urine is called **albuminuria**. In nephritis, the negative charges in the glomerular wall are dissipated, and albuminuria can occur for this reason without an increase in the size of the "pores" in the membrane.

SIZE OF THE CAPILLARY BED

K_f can be altered by the mesangial cells, with contraction of these cells producing a decrease in K_f that is largely due to a reduction in the surface area available for filtration.

HYDROSTATIC & OSMOTIC PRESSURE

The pressure in the glomerular capillaries is higher than that in other capillary beds. Furthermore, the vessels "downstream" from the glomeruli, the efferent arterioles, have a relatively high resistance. The capillary hydrostatic pressure is opposed by the hydrostatic pressure in Bowman's capsule. It is also opposed by the oncotic pressure gradient across the glomerular capillaries ($\pi_{GC} - \pi_T$). π_T is normally negligible, and the gradient is essentially equal to the oncotic pressure of the plasma proteins.

CHANGES IN GFR

Variations in the factors discussed in the preceding paragraphs and listed in Table 37–1 have predictable effects on the GFR. Changes in renal vascular resistance as a result of autoregulation tend to stabilize filtration pressure, but when the mean systemic arterial pressure drops below the autoregulatory range (Figure 37–2), GFR drops sharply. The GFR tends to be maintained when efferent arteriolar constriction is greater than afferent constriction, but either type of constriction decreases blood flow to the tubules.

TABLE 37–1　Factors affecting the glomerular filtration rate.

Changes in renal blood flow
Changes in glomerular capillary hydrostatic pressure
Changes in systemic blood pressure
Afferent or efferent arteriolar constriction
Changes in hydrostatic pressure in Bowman's capsule
Ureteral obstruction
Edema of kidney inside tight renal capsule
Changes in concentration of plasma proteins: dehydration, hypoproteinemia, etc (minor factors)
Changes in K_f
Changes in glomerular capillary permeability
Changes in effective filtration surface area

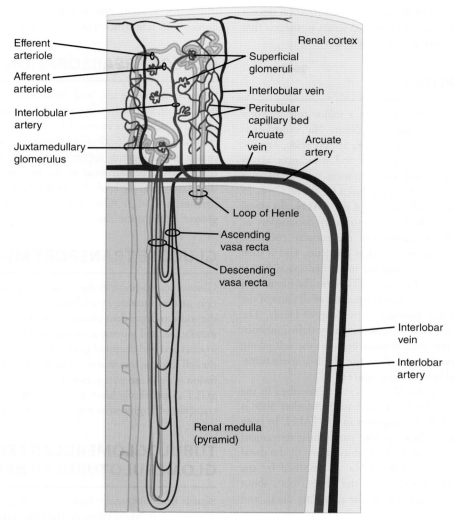

FIGURE 37–2 **Renal circulation.** Interlobar arteries divide into arcuate arteries, which give off interlobular arteries in the cortex. The interlobular arteries provide an afferent arteriole to each glomerulus. The efferent arteriole from each glomerulus breaks up into capillaries that supply blood to the renal tubules. Venous blood enters interlobular veins, which in turn flow via arcuate veins to the interlobar veins. (Modified with permission from Boron WF, Boulpaep EL: *Medical Physiology.* Saunders, 2009.)

FILTRATION FRACTION

The ratio of the GFR to the RPF, the **filtration fraction**, is normally 0.16–0.20. The GFR varies less than the RPF. When there is a fall in systemic blood pressure, the GFR falls less than the RPF because of efferent arteriolar constriction, and consequently the filtration fraction rises.

■ MECHANISMS OF TUBULAR REABSORPTION & SECRETION

Small proteins and some peptide hormones are reabsorbed in the proximal tubules by endocytosis. Other substances are secreted or reabsorbed in the tubules by passive diffusion between cells and through cells by facilitated diffusion down chemical or electrical gradients or active transport against such gradients. Movement is by way of ion channels, exchangers, cotransporters, and pumps.

The pumps and other transporters in the luminal membrane are different from those in the basolateral membrane. Like transport systems elsewhere, renal active transport systems have a maximal rate, or **transport maximum (Tm)**, at which they can transport a particular solute. Thus, the amount of a particular solute transported is proportional to the amount present up to the Tm for the solute, but at higher concentrations, the transport mechanism is **saturated** and there is no appreciable increment in the amount transported. However, the Tms for some systems are high, and it is difficult to saturate them.

The tubular epithelium, like that of the small intestine, is a **leaky epithelium** in that the tight junctions between cells permit the passage of some water and electrolytes. The degree to which leakage by this **paracellular pathway** contributes to the net flux of fluid and solute into and out of the tubules is controversial since it is difficult to measure, but current evidence seems to suggest that it is a significant factor in the proximal tubule.

Na⁺ REABSORPTION

The reabsorption of Na^+ and Cl^- plays a major role in body electrolyte and water homeostasis. In addition, Na^+ transport is coupled to the movement of H^+, glucose, amino acids, organic acids, phosphate, and other electrolytes and substances across the tubule walls. The principal cotransporters and exchangers in the various parts of the nephron are listed in Table 37–2. In the proximal tubules, the thick portion of the TALH, the distal tubules, and the collecting ducts, Na^+ moves by cotransport or exchange from the tubular lumen into the tubular epithelial cells down its concentration and electrical gradients, and is then actively pumped from these cells into the interstitial space. Na^+ is pumped into the interstitium by Na, K-ATPase in the basolateral membrane. Thus, Na^+ is actively transported out of all parts of the renal tubule except the thin portions of the loop of Henle. The tubular cells along the nephron are connected by tight junctions at their luminal edges, but there is space between the cells along the rest of their lateral borders. Much of the Na^+ is actively transported into these **lateral intercellular spaces**.

Normally about 60% of the filtered Na^+ is reabsorbed in the proximal tubule, primarily by Na–H exchange. Another 30% is absorbed via the Na–2Cl–K cotransporter in the TALH. In both of these segments of the nephron, passive paracellular movement of Na^+ also contributes to overall Na^+ reabsorption. In the distal convoluted tubule 7% of the filtered Na^+ is absorbed by the Na–Cl cotransporter. The remainder of the filtered Na^+, about 3%, is absorbed via ENaC channels in the collecting ducts, and

TABLE 37–2 Transport proteins involved in the movement of Na^+ and Cl^- across the apical membranes of renal tubular cells.[a]

Site	Apical Transporter	Function
Proximal tubule	Na/glucose CT	Na⁺ uptake, glucose uptake
	Na⁺/Pᵢ CT	Na⁺ uptake, Pᵢ uptake
	Na⁺ amino acid CT	Na⁺ uptake, amino acid uptake
	Na/lactate CT	Na⁺ uptake, lactate uptake
	Na/H exchanger	Na⁺ uptake, H⁺ extrusion
	Cl/base exchanger	Cl⁻ uptake
Thick ascending limb	Na–K–2Cl CT	Na⁺ uptake, Cl⁻ uptake, K⁺ uptake
	Na/H exchanger	Na⁺ uptake, H⁺ extrusion
	K⁺ channels	K⁺ extrusion (recycling)
Distal convoluted tubule	NaCl CT	Na⁺ uptake, Cl⁻ uptake
Collecting duct	Na⁺ channel (ENaC)	Na⁺ uptake

[a]Uptake indicates movement from tubular lumen to cell interior, extrusion is movement from cell interior to tubular lumen. CT, cotransporter; Pᵢ, inorganic phosphate.

Data from Schnermann JB, Sayegh EI: *Kidney Physiology*. Lippincott-Raven, 1998.

this is the portion that is regulated by aldosterone to permit homeostatic adjustments in Na^+ balance.

GLUCOSE REABSORPTION

Glucose, amino acids, and bicarbonate are reabsorbed along with Na^+ in the early portion of the proximal tubule. Glucose is typical of substances removed from the urine by secondary active transport. Essentially all of the glucose is reabsorbed, and no more than a few milligrams appear in the urine per 24 h. The amount reabsorbed is proportional to the amount filtered and hence to the plasma glucose level (P_G) times the GFR up to the transport maximum (Tm_G). When the Tm_G is exceeded, the amount of glucose in the urine rises.

GLUCOSE TRANSPORT MECHANISM

Glucose reabsorption in the kidneys is similar to glucose reabsorption in the intestine (see Chapter 26). Glucose and Na^+ bind to the sodium-dependent glucose transporter (SGLT)-2 in the apical membrane, and glucose is carried into the cell as Na^+ moves down its electrical and chemical gradient. The Na^+ is then pumped out of the cell into the interstitium, and the glucose exits by facilitated diffusion via glucose transporter (GLUT)-2 into the interstitial fluid. SGLT-2 specifically binds the D isomer of glucose, and the rate of transport of D-glucose is many times greater than that of L-glucose.

TUBULOGLOMERULAR FEEDBACK & GLOMERULOTUBULAR BALANCE

Signals from the renal tubule in each nephron feed back to affect filtration in its glomerulus. As the rate of flow through the TALH and first part of the distal tubule increases, GFR in the same nephron decreases, and, conversely, a decrease in flow increases the GFR. This process, known as **tubuloglomerular (TG) feedback**, maintains the constancy of the load delivered to the distal tubule.

The sensor for this response is the **macula densa**. The amount of fluid entering the distal tubule at the end of the TALH depends on the amount of Na^+ and Cl^- in it. The Na^+ and Cl^- enter the macula densa cells via the Na–K–2Cl cotransporter in their apical membranes. The increased Na^+ causes an increase in Na, K-ATPase activity and the resultant increase in ATP hydrolysis causes more adenosine to be formed. Adenosine is secreted from the basal membrane of the cells, and acts via adenosine A_1 receptors on macula densa cells to increase their release of Ca^{2+} to the vascular smooth muscle in the afferent arterioles. This causes afferent vasoconstriction and a resultant decrease in GFR.

Conversely, an increase in GFR causes an increase in the reabsorption of solutes, and consequently of water, primarily in the proximal tubule, so that in general the percentage of the solute reabsorbed is held constant. This process is called **glomerulotubular balance**, and it is particularly prominent for Na^+. The change in Na^+ reabsorption occurs within seconds after a change in filtration, so it seems unlikely that an extrarenal humoral factor is involved. Alternatively, one mediating factor is the oncotic pressure in the peritubular capillaries. When the GFR is high, there is a relatively large increase in the oncotic pressure of the plasma leaving the glomeruli via the efferent arterioles and hence in their capillary branches. This increases the reabsorption of Na^+ from the tubule.

WATER TRANSPORT

Normally, 180 L of fluid is filtered through the glomeruli each day, while the average daily urine volume is about 1 L. The same load of solute can be excreted per 24 h in a urine volume of 500 mL with a concentration of 1400 mOsm/kg or in a volume of 23.3 L with a concentration of 30 mOsm/kg. At least 87% of filtered water is reabsorbed, even when the urine volume is 23 L; and the reabsorption of the remainder of the filtered water can be varied without affecting total solute excretion. Therefore, when the urine is concentrated, water is retained in excess of solute; and when it is dilute, water is lost from the body in excess of solute. Both facts have great importance in the regulation of the osmolality of the body fluids. A key regulator of water output is vasopressin acting on the collecting ducts.

PROXIMAL TUBULE

Rapid diffusion of water across cell membranes depends on the presence of water channels, integral membrane proteins called **aquaporins**. **Aquaporin-1** is localized to both the basolateral and apical membrane of the proximal tubules and its presence allows water to move rapidly out of the tubule along the osmotic gradients set up by active transport of solutes, and isotonicity is maintained. Because the ratio of the concentration in tubular fluid to the concentration in plasma (TF/P) of the nonreabsorbable substance inulin is 2.5–3.3 at the end of the proximal tubule, it follows that 60–70% of the filtered solute and 60–70% of the filtered water have been removed by the time the filtrate reaches this point.

LOOP OF HENLE

As noted above, the loops of Henle of the juxtamedullary nephrons dip deeply into the medullary pyramids before draining into the distal convoluted tubules in the cortex, and all the collecting ducts descend back through the medullary pyramids to drain at the tips of the pyramids into the renal pelvis. There is a graded increase in the osmolality of the interstitium of the pyramids in humans: The osmolality at the tips of the papillae can reach about 1200 mOsm/kg of H_2O, approximately four times that of plasma. The descending limb of the loop of Henle is permeable to water, due to the presence of **aquaporin-1** in both the apical and basolateral membranes, but the ascending limb is impermeable to water. Na^+, K^+, and Cl^- are cotransported out of the TALH. Therefore, the fluid in the descending limb of the loop of Henle becomes **hypertonic** as water moves out of the tubule into the

hypertonic interstitium. In the ascending limb it becomes more dilute because of the movement of Na^+ and Cl^- out of the tubular lumen, and when fluid reaches the top of the ascending limb (called the **diluting segment**), it is now **hypotonic** to plasma. In passing through the descending loop of Henle, another 15% of the filtered water is removed, so approximately 20% of the filtered water enters the distal tubule, and the TF/P of inulin at this point is about 5.

In the TALH, a carrier cotransports one Na^+, one K^+, and $2Cl^-$ from the tubular lumen into the tubular cells. This is another example of secondary active transport; the Na^+ is actively transported from the cells into the interstitium by Na, K-ATPase in the basolateral membranes of the cells, keeping the intracellular Na^+ low. The Na–K–2Cl cotransporter has 12 transmembrane domains with intracellular amino and carboxyl terminals. K^+ diffuses back into the tubular lumen and back into the interstitium via ROMK and other K^+ channels. The Cl^- moves into the interstitium via ClC–Kb channels.

DISTAL TUBULE

The distal tubule, particularly its first part, is in effect an extension of the TALH. It is relatively impermeable to water, and continued removal of the solute in excess of solvent further dilutes the tubular fluid.

COLLECTING DUCTS

The collecting ducts have two portions: a cortical portion and a medullary portion. The changes in osmolality and volume in the collecting ducts depend on the amount of **vasopressin** acting on the ducts. This antidiuretic hormone from the posterior pituitary gland increases the permeability of the collecting ducts to water. The key to the action of vasopressin on the collecting ducts is **aquaporin-2** stored in vesicles in the cytoplasm of principal cells. Vasopressin causes rapid insertion of these vesicles into the apical membrane of cells mediated via the vasopressin V_2 receptor, cyclic adenosine 5-monophosphate (cAMP), and protein kinase A.

In the presence of enough vasopressin to produce maximal antidiuresis, water moves out of the hypotonic fluid entering the cortical collecting ducts into the interstitium of the cortex, and the tubular fluid becomes isotonic, thus as much as 10% of the filtered water is removed. The isotonic fluid then enters the medullary collecting ducts with a TF/P inulin of about 20. An additional 5% or more of the filtrate is reabsorbed into the hypertonic interstitium of the medulla, producing a concentrated urine with a TF/P inulin of over 300. In humans, the osmolality of urine may reach 1400 mOsm/kg H_2O, almost five times the osmolality of plasma, with a total of 99.7% of the filtered water being reabsorbed.

When vasopressin is absent, the collecting duct epithelium is relatively impermeable to water. The fluid therefore remains hypotonic, and large amounts flow into the renal pelvis. In humans, the urine osmolality may be as low as 30 mOsm/kg of H_2O.

The impermeability of the distal portions of the nephron is not absolute; along with the salt that is pumped out of the collecting duct fluid, about 2% of the filtered water is reabsorbed in the absence of vasopressin. However, as much as 13% of the filtered water may be excreted, and urine flow may reach 15 mL/min or more.

THE COUNTERCURRENT MECHANISM

The concentrating mechanism depends on the maintenance of a gradient of **increasing osmolality** along the medullary pyramids. This gradient is produced by the operation of the loops of Henle as **countercurrent multipliers** and maintained by the operation of the vasa recta as **countercurrent exchangers**. A countercurrent system is a system in which the inflow runs parallel to, counter to, and in close proximity to the outflow for some distance. This occurs for both the loops of Henle and the vasa recta in the renal medulla (**Figure 37–3**).

The operation of each loop of Henle as a countercurrent multiplier depends on the high permeability of the thin descending limb to water (via aquaporin-1), the active transport of Na^+ and Cl^- out of the thick ascending limb, and the inflow of tubular fluid from the proximal tubule, with outflow into the distal tubule. The process can be explained using hypothetical steps leading to the normal equilibrium condition, although the steps do not occur in vivo. It is also important to remember that the equilibrium is maintained unless the osmotic gradient is washed out. Assume first a condition in which osmolality is 300 mOsm/kg of H_2O throughout the descending and ascending limbs and the medullary interstitium. Assume in addition that the pumps in

the thick ascending limb can pump 100 mOsm/kg of Na^+ and Cl^- from the tubular fluid to the interstitium, increasing interstitial osmolality to 400 mOsm/kg of H_2O. Water then moves out of the thin descending limb, and its contents equilibrate with the interstitium. However, fluid containing 300 mOsm/kg of H_2O is continuously entering this limb from the proximal tubule, so the gradient against which the Na^+ and Cl^- are pumped is reduced and more enters the interstitium. Meanwhile, hypotonic fluid flows into the distal tubule, and isotonic and subsequently hypertonic fluid flows into the ascending thick limb. The process keeps repeating, and the final result is a gradient of osmolality from the top to the bottom of the loop.

In juxtamedullary nephrons with longer loops and thin ascending limbs, the osmotic gradient is spread over a greater distance and the osmolality at the tip of the loop is greater. This is because the thin ascending limb is relatively impermeable to water but permeable to Na^+ and Cl^-. Therefore, Na^+ and Cl^- move down their concentration gradients into the interstitium, and there is additional passive countercurrent multiplication. The greater the length of the loop of Henle, the greater the osmolality that can be reached at the tip of the medulla.

The osmotic gradient in the medullary pyramids would not last long if the Na^+ and urea in the interstitial spaces were removed by the circulation. These solutes remain in the pyramids primarily because the vasa recta operate as countercurrent exchangers. The solutes diffuse out of the vessels conducting blood toward the cortex and into the vessels descending into the pyramid. Conversely, water diffuses out of the descending vessels and into the fenestrated ascending vessels. Therefore, the solutes tend to recirculate in the medulla and water tends to bypass it, so that hypertonicity is maintained. The water removed from the collecting ducts in the pyramids is also removed by the vasa recta and enters the general circulation. Countercurrent exchange is a passive process; it depends on movement of water and could not maintain the osmotic gradient along the pyramids if the process of countercurrent multiplication in the loops of Henle were to cease.

ROLE OF UREA

Urea contributes to the establishment of the osmotic gradient in the medullary pyramids and to the ability to form a concentrated urine in the collecting ducts. Urea transport is mediated by urea transporters, presumably by facilitated diffusion. There are at least four isoforms of the transport protein UT-A in the kidneys (UT-A1 to UT-A4); UT-B is found in the descending limbs of the vasa recta. Urea transport in the collecting duct is mediated by UT-A1 and UT-A3, and both are regulated by vasopressin. During antidiuresis, when vasopressin is high, the amount of urea deposited in the medullary interstitium increases, thus increasing the concentrating capacity of the kidney. In addition, the amount of urea in the medullary interstitium and, consequently, in the urine varies with the amount of urea filtered, and this in turn varies with the dietary intake of protein. Therefore, a high-protein diet increases the ability of the kidneys to concentrate the urine and a low-protein diet reduces the kidneys' ability to concentrate the urine.

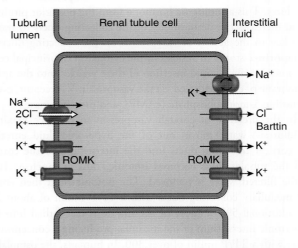

FIGURE 37–3 **NaCl transport in the thick ascending limb of the loop of Henle.** The Na–K–2Cl cotransporter moves these ions into the tubular cell by secondary active transport. Na^+ is transported out of the cell into the interstitium by Na, K-ATPase in the basolateral membrane of the cell. Cl^- exits in basolateral ClC–Kb Cl^- channels. Barttin, a protein in the cell membrane, is essential for normal ClC–Kb function. K^+ moves from the cell to the interstitium and the tubular lumen by ROMK and other K^+ channels.

OSMOTIC DIURESIS

The presence of large quantities of unreabsorbed solutes in the renal tubules causes an increase in urine volume called **osmotic diuresis**. Solutes that are not reabsorbed in the proximal tubules exert an appreciable osmotic effect as the volume of tubular fluid decreases and their concentration rises. Therefore, they "hold water in the tubules." In addition, the concentration gradient against which Na$^+$ can be pumped out of the proximal tubules is limited. Normally, the movement of water out of the proximal tubule prevents any appreciable gradient from developing, but Na$^+$ concentration in the fluid falls when water reabsorption is decreased because of the presence in the tubular fluid of increased amounts of unreabsorbable solutes. The limiting concentration gradient is reached, and further proximal reabsorption of Na$^+$ is prevented; more Na$^+$ remains in the tubule, and water stays with it. The result is that the loop of Henle is presented with a greatly increased volume of isotonic fluid. This fluid has a decreased Na$^+$ concentration, but the total amount of Na$^+$ reaching the loop per unit time is increased. In the loop, reabsorption of water and Na$^+$ is decreased because the medullary hypertonicity is decreased. The decrease is due primarily to decreased reabsorption of Na$^+$, K$^+$, and Cl$^-$ in the ascending limb of the loop because the limiting concentration gradient for Na$^+$ reabsorption is reached. More fluid passes through the distal tubule, and because of the decrease in the osmotic gradient along the medullary pyramids, less water is reabsorbed in the collecting ducts. The result is a marked increase in urine volume and excretion of Na$^+$ and other electrolytes.

Osmotic diuresis is produced by the administration of compounds such as mannitol and related polysaccharides that are filtered but not reabsorbed. It is also produced by naturally occurring substances when they are present in amounts exceeding the capacity of the tubules to reabsorb them. For example, in **diabetes mellitus**, if blood glucose is high, glucose in the glomerular filtrate is high, thus the filtered load will exceed the Tm$_G$ and glucose will remain in the tubules causing polyuria. Osmotic diuresis can also be produced by the infusion of large amounts of sodium chloride or urea.

It is important to recognize the difference between osmotic diuresis and water diuresis. In water diuresis, the amount of water reabsorbed in the proximal portions of the nephron is normal, and the maximal urine flow that can be produced is about 16 mL/min. In osmotic diuresis, increased urine flow is due to decreased water reabsorption in the proximal tubules and loops and very large urine flows can be produced. As the load of excreted solute is increased, the concentration of the urine approaches that of plasma in spite of maximal vasopressin secretion, because an increasingly large fraction of the excreted urine is isotonic proximal tubular fluid. If osmotic diuresis is produced in someone with diabetes insipidus, the urine concentration rises for the same reason.

"FREE WATER CLEARANCE"

In order to quantitate the gain or loss of water by excretion of a concentrated or dilute urine, the "free water clearance" (C$_{H_2O}$) is sometimes calculated. This is the difference between the urine volume and the clearance of osmoles (C$_{Osm}$):

$$C_{H_2O} = \dot{V} - \frac{U_{Osm} \dot{V}}{P_{Osm}}$$

where V the urine flow rate and U$_{Osm}$ and P$_{Osm}$ the urine and plasma osmolality, respectively. C$_{Osm}$ is the amount of water necessary to excrete the osmotic load in a urine that is isotonic with plasma. Therefore, C$_{H_2O}$ is negative when the urine is hypertonic and positive when the urine is hypotonic.

■ REGULATION OF Na$^+$ EXCRETION

Multiple regulatory mechanisms have evolved to control the excretion of Na$^+$. Through the operation of these regulatory mechanisms, the amount of Na$^+$ excreted is adjusted to equal the amount ingested over a wide range of dietary intakes, and the individual stays in Na$^+$ balance. When Na intake is high, or saline is infused, natriuresis occurs, whereas when ECF is reduced (for example, fluid loss following vomiting or diarrhea) a decrease in Na$^+$ excretion occurs.

Variations in Na$^+$ excretion are brought about by changes in GFR and changes in tubular reabsorption, primarily in the 3% of filtered Na$^+$ that reaches the collecting ducts. Factors affecting Na$^+$ reabsorption include the renin–angiotensin aldosterone system and other adrenocortical hormones, the circulating level of ANP and other natriuretic hormones, and the rate of tubular secretion of H$^+$ and K$^+$.

Na$^+$ retention in kidney disease has at least three causes: a reduction in the amount of Na$^+$ filtered; an increase in aldosterone secretion caused by a decline in plasma volume and activation of the renin–angiotensin system; and heart failure where there is a reduction in cardiac output.

EFFECTS OF ADRENOCORTICAL STEROIDS

Adrenal mineralocorticoids such as aldosterone increase tubular reabsorption of Na$^+$ in association with secretion of K$^+$ and H$^+$ and also Na$^+$ reabsorption with Cl$^-$. Mineralocorticoids act primarily in collecting ducts to increase the number of active epithelial sodium channels (ENaCs) in this part of the nephron. In Liddle syndrome, mutations in the genes that code for the β subunit and less commonly the γ subunit of ENaC cause the channels to become constitutively active in the kidney. This leads to Na$^+$ retention and hypertension.

Prolonged exposure to high levels of circulating mineralocorticoids does not cause edema in otherwise normal individuals because eventually the kidneys escape from the effects of the steroids. This **escape phenomenon**, which may be due to increased secretion of ANP, is discussed in Chapter 20. It appears to be reduced or absent in nephrosis, cirrhosis, and heart failure, and patients with these diseases continue to retain Na^+ and become edematous when exposed to high levels of mineralocorticoids

OTHER HUMORAL EFFECTS

Reduction of dietary intake of salt increases aldosterone secretion, producing marked but slowly developing decreases in Na^+ excretion. A variety of other humoral factors affect Na^+ reabsorption. PGE_2 causes a natriuresis, possibly by inhibiting Na, K-ATPase and increasing intracellular Ca^{2+}, which in turn inhibits Na^+ transport via ENaCs. Endothelin and IL-1 cause natriuresis, probably by increasing the formation of PGE_2. ANP and related molecules increase intracellular cyclic 3′,5′-guanosine monophosphate (cGMP), and this inhibits transport via ENaC. Inhibition of Na, K-ATPase by ouabain also increases Na^+ excretion. Angiotensin II increases reabsorption of Na^+ and HCO_3^- by an action on the proximal tubules. There is an appreciable amount of angiotensin-converting enzyme in the kidneys, and the kidneys convert 20% of the circulating angiotensin I to angiotensin II. In addition, angiotensin I is generated in the kidneys.

■ REGULATION OF K⁺ EXCRETION

Much of the filtered K^+ is removed from the tubular fluid by active reabsorption in the proximal tubules, and K^+ is then secreted into the fluid by the distal tubular cells. The rate of K^+ secretion is proportional to the rate of flow of the tubular fluid through the distal portions of the nephron, because with rapid flow there is less opportunity for the tubular K^+ concentration to rise to a value that stops further secretion. In the absence of complicating factors, the amount secreted is approximately equal to the K^+ intake, and K^+ balance is maintained. In the collecting ducts, Na^+ is generally reabsorbed and K^+ is secreted. There is no rigid one-for-one exchange, and much of the movement of K^+ is passive. However, there is electrical coupling in the sense that intracellular migration of Na^+ from the lumen tends to lower the potential difference across the tubular cell, and this favors movement of K^+ into the tubular lumen. K^+ excretion is decreased when the amount of Na^+ reaching the distal tubule is small. In addition, if H^+ secretion is increased, K^+ excretion will decrease as K^+ is reabsorbed in collecting duct cells in exchange for H^+, via the action of the H, K-ATPase.

■ DIURETICS

Furosemide and the other loop diuretics inhibit the Na–K–2Cl cotransporter in the TALH (Table 37-3). They cause a marked natriuresis and kaliuresis. Thiazides act by inhibiting Na–Cl cotransport in the distal tubule causing less marked diuresis, but both loop diuretics and thiazides cause increased delivery of Na^+ (and fluid) to the collecting ducts, facilitating K^+ excretion.

TABLE 37-3 Mechanism of action of various diuretics.

Agent	Mechanism of Action
Water	Inhibits vasopressin secretion
Ethanol	Inhibits vasopressin secretion
Antagonists of V_2 vasopressin receptors such as tolvaptan	Inhibit action of vasopressin on collecting duct
Large quantities of osmotically active substances such as mannitol and glucose	Produce osmotic diuresis
Xanthines such as caffeine and theophylline	Decrease tubular reabsorption of Na^+ and increase GFR
Acidifying salts such as $CaCl_2$ and NH_4Cl	Supply acid load; H^+ is buffered, but an anion is excreted with Na^+ when the ability of the kidneys to replace Na^+ with H^+ is exceeded
Carbonic anhydrase inhibitors such as acetazolamide (Diamox)	Decrease H^+ secretion, with resultant increase in Na^+ and K^+ excretion
Metolazone (Zaroxolyn), thiazides such as chlorothiazide (Diuril)	Inhibit the Na–Cl cotransporter in the early portion of the distal tubule
Loop diuretics such as furosemide (Lasix), ethacrynic acid (Edecrin), and bumetanide	Inhibit the Na–K–2Cl cotransporter in the medullary thick ascending limb of the loop of Henle
K^+-retaining natriuretics such as spironolactone (Aldactone), triamterene (Dyrenium), and amiloride (Midamor)	Inhibit Na^+–K^+ "exchange" in the collecting ducts by inhibiting the action of aldosterone (spironolactone) or by inhibiting the ENaCs (amiloride)

Thus, K^+ depletion and hypokalemia are common complications. On the other hand, the so-called K^+-sparing diuretics act in the collecting duct by inhibiting the action of aldosterone or blocking ENaCs.

■ EFFECTS OF DISORDERED KIDNEY FUNCTION

LOSS OF CONCENTRATING & DILUTING ABILITY

In kidney disease, the urine becomes less concentrated and urine volume is often increased, producing the symptoms of **polyuria** and **nocturia** (waking up at night to void). The ability to form a dilute urine is often retained, but in advanced kidney disease, the osmolality of the urine becomes fixed at about that of plasma, indicating that the diluting and concentrating functions of the kidney have both been lost. The loss is due in part to disruption of the countercurrent mechanism, but a more important cause is a loss of functioning nephrons requiring the remaining nephrons to filter and excrete all of the osmotically active substances typically removed by both kidneys. This essentially is an osmotic diuresis. The increased filtration in the remaining nephrons eventually damages them, and thus more nephrons are lost. The eventual result of this positive feedback is complete kidney failure with **oliguria**, or even **anuria**.

UREMIA

When the breakdown products of protein metabolism accumulate in the blood, the syndrome known as **uremia** develops. The symptoms of uremia include lethargy, anorexia, nausea and vomiting, mental deterioration and confusion, muscle twitching, convulsions, and coma. The blood urea nitrogen (BUN) and creatinine levels are high, and the blood levels of these substances are used as an index of the severity of the uremia. The toxic substances that cause the symptoms of uremia can be removed by **hemodialysis**.

ACIDOSIS

Acidosis is common in chronic kidney disease because of failure to excrete the acid products of digestion and metabolism. In the rare syndrome of **renal tubular acidosis**, there is specific impairment of the ability to make the urine acidic, and other renal functions are usually normal. However, in most cases of chronic kidney disease the urine is maximally acidified, and acidosis develops because the total amount of H^+ that can be secreted is reduced because of impaired renal tubular production of NH_4^+.

■ THE BLADDER

FILLING AND EMPTYING

The walls of the ureters contain smooth muscle arranged in spiral, longitudinal, and circular bundles, but not distinct layers. Peristaltic contractions occurring one to five times per minute move the urine from the renal pelvis to the bladder. The ureters pass obliquely through the bladder wall and, although there are no ureteral sphincters, the ureters closed except during peristaltic waves, preventing reflux of urine.

The smooth muscle of the bladder are also is arranged in spiral, longitudinal, and circular bundles. Contraction of the circular muscle, which is called the **detrusor muscle**, is mainly responsible for emptying the bladder during urination (**micturition**). Muscle bundles pass on either side of the urethra, and these fibers are sometimes called the **internal urethral sphincter**, although they do not encircle the urethra. Farther along the urethra is a sphincter of skeletal muscle, the sphincter of the membranous urethra (**external urethral sphincter**). The bladder epithelium is made up of a superficial layer of flat cells and a deep layer of cuboidal cells. The bladder is also innervated.

The physiology of bladder emptying has not been completely elucidated. Micturition is fundamentally a spinal reflex facilitated and inhibited by higher brain centers subject to voluntary facilitation and inhibition. Urine enters the bladder without producing much increase in intravesical pressure until the viscus is well filled. In addition, like other types of smooth muscle, the bladder muscle has the property of plasticity; when it is stretched, the tension initially produced is not maintained. The relation between intravesical pressure and volume can be measured by inserting a catheter and emptying the bladder, then recording the pressure while the bladder is filled with 50-mL increments of water or air (**cystometry**). A plot of intravesical pressure against the volume of fluid in the bladder is called a **cystometrogram**. At first there is an initial rise in pressure when the first increments in volume are produced (Ia); then a long, nearly flat segment as further increments are produced (Ib); and finally, a sudden, sharp rise in pressure as the micturition reflex is triggered (II). The first urge to void is felt at a bladder volume of about 150 mL, and a marked sense of fullness at about 400 mL. The flatness of segment Ib is a manifestation of the law of Laplace. This law states that the pressure in a spherical viscus is equal to twice the wall tension divided by the radius. In the case of the bladder, the tension increases as the organ fills, but so does the radius. Therefore, the pressure increase is slight until the organ is relatively full.

During micturition, the perineal muscles and external urethral sphincter are relaxed, the detrusor muscle contracts, and urine passes out through the urethra.

REFLEX CONTROL

The bladder smooth muscle has some inherent contractile activity; however, when its nerve supply is intact, stretch receptors in the bladder wall initiate a reflex contraction. Fibers in the pelvic nerves are the afferent limb of the voiding reflex, and the parasympathetic fibers to the bladder that constitute the efferent limb also travel in these nerves. The reflex is integrated in the sacral portion of the spinal cord. In the adult, the volume of urine in the bladder that normally initiates a reflex contraction is about 300–400 mL.

Threshold for the voiding reflex, like the stretch reflexes, is adjusted by the activity of facilitatory and inhibitory centers in the brainstem. There is a facilitatory area in the pontine region and an inhibitory area in the midbrain. After transection of the brainstem just above the pons, the threshold is lowered and less bladder filling is required to trigger it, whereas after transection at the top of the midbrain, the threshold for the reflex is essentially normal. There is another facilitatory area in the posterior hypothalamus. The bladder can be made to contract by voluntary facilitation of the spinal voiding reflex when it contains only a few milliliters of urine. Voluntary contraction of the abdominal muscles aids the expulsion of urine by increasing the intra-abdominal pressure, but voiding can be initiated without straining even when the bladder is nearly empty.

EFFECTS OF DEAFFERENTATION

When the sacral dorsal roots are cut, such as **tabes dorsalis** in humans, all reflex contractions of the bladder are abolished. The bladder becomes distended, thin-walled, and hypotonic, although some contractions still occur because of the intrinsic response of the smooth muscle to stretch.

EFFECTS OF DENERVATION

When the afferent and efferent nerves are both destroyed, as they may be by tumors of the cauda equina or filum terminale, the bladder is flaccid and distended for a while. Gradually, however, the muscle of the "decentralized bladder" becomes active, with many contraction waves that expel dribbles of urine out of the urethra. The bladder becomes shrunken and the bladder wall hypertrophied. The reason for the difference between the small, hypertrophic bladder seen in this condition and the distended, hypotonic bladder seen when only the afferent nerves are interrupted is not known.

EFFECTS OF SPINAL CORD TRANSECTION

After spinal cord transection, the bladder is flaccid and unresponsive. It becomes overfilled, and urine dribbles through the sphincters (**overflow incontinence**). After spinal shock has passed, the voiding reflex returns, although there is no voluntary control and no inhibition or facilitation from higher. Some paraplegic patients train themselves to initiate voiding by pinching or stroking their thighs, provoking a mild mass reflex. In some instances, the voiding reflex becomes hyperactive, bladder capacity is reduced, and the wall becomes hypertrophied. This type of bladder is sometimes called the **spastic neurogenic bladder**.

CHAPTER SUMMARY

- Plasma enters the kidneys and is filtered in the glomerulus. As the filtrate passes down the nephron and through the tubules its volume is reduced and water and solutes are removed (tubular reabsorption) and waste products are secreted (tubular secretion).

- A nephron consists of an individual renal tubule and its glomerulus. Each tubule has several segments, beginning with the proximal tubule, followed by the loop of Henle (descending and ascending limbs), the distal convoluted tubule, the connecting tubule, and the collecting duct.

- The kidneys receive just under 25% of the cardiac output and RPF can be measured by infusing PAH and determining its urine and plasma concentrations.

- Renal blood flow enters the glomerulus via the afferent arteriole and leaves via the efferent arteriole (whose diameter is smaller). Renal blood flow is regulated by norepinephrine (constriction, reduction of flow), dopamine (vasodilation, increases flow), angiotensin II (constricts), prostaglandins (dilation in the renal cortex and constriction in the renal medulla), and acetylcholine (vasodilation).

- GFR can be measured by a substance that is freely filtered and neither reabsorbed nor secreted in the tubules, is nontoxic, and is not metabolized by the body. Inulin meets these criteria and is extensively used to measure GFR.

- Urine is stored in the bladder before voiding (micturition). The micturition response involves reflex pathways but is under voluntary control.

MULTIPLE-CHOICE QUESTIONS

For all questions, select the single best answer unless otherwise directed.

1. The greatest fraction of filtered sodium is reabsorbed in what portion of the nephron?
   A. Proximal tubule
   B. Loop of Henle
   C. Distal tubule
   D. Cortical collecting duct
   E. Medullary collecting duct

2. In the absence of vasopressin, the greatest fraction of filtered water is absorbed in the
   A. proximal tubule.
   B. loop of Henle.
   C. distal tubule.
   D. cortical collecting duct.
   E. medullary collecting duct.

3. If the clearance of a substance that is freely filtered is less than that of inulin,
   A. there is net reabsorption of the substance in the tubules.
   B. there is net secretion of the substance in the tubules.
   C. the substance is neither secreted nor reabsorbed in the tubules.
   D. the substance becomes bound to protein in the tubules.
   E. the substance is secreted in the proximal tubule to a greater degree than in the distal tubule.

4. Glucose reabsorption occurs in the
   A. proximal tubule.
   B. loop of Henle.
   C. distal tubule.
   D. cortical collecting duct.
   E. medullary collecting duct.

5. On which of the following does aldosterone exert its greatest effect?
   A. Glomerulus
   B. Proximal tubule
   C. Thin portion of the loop of Henle
   D. Thick portion of the loop of Henle
   E. Cortical collecting duct

6. What is the clearance of a substance when its concentration in the plasma is 10 mg/dL, its concentration in the urine is 100 mg/dL, and urine flow is 2 mL/min?
   A. 2 mL/min
   B. 10 mL/min
   C. 20 mL/min
   D. 200 mL/min
   E. Clearance cannot be determined from the information given

7. As urine flow increases during osmotic diuresis,
   A. the osmolality of urine falls below that of plasma.
   B. the osmolality of urine increases because of the increased amounts of nonreabsorbable solute in the urine.
   C. the osmolality of urine approaches that of plasma because plasma leaks into the tubules.
   D. the osmolality of urine approaches that of plasma because an increasingly large fraction of the excreted urine is isotonic proximal tubular fluid.
   E. the action of vasopressin on the renal tubules is inhibited.

8. A physiologist is studying the effect of food additives on GFR in order to determine what additives should be avoided in individuals with CKD. A caffeine was found to affect urine output through an effect on GFR. What is the effect and the mechanism involved?

    A.   Increase urine output; afferent arteriole vasodilation
    B.   Increase urine output; efferent arteriole vasodilation
    C.   Increase urine output; afferent arteriole vasoconstriction
    D.   Increase urine output; efferent arteriole vasoconstriction
    E.   Decrease urine output; afferent arteriole vasodilation
    F.   Decrease urine output; efferent arteriole vasodilation
    G.   Decrease urine output; afferent arteriole vasoconstriction
    H.   Decrease urine output; efferent arteriole vasoconstriction

9. A 20-year-old woman comes to the clinic for a routine physical that she needs as part of her application for work as a summer camp counselor. The physical exam was WNL. Her urinalysis shows a trace of protein. A defect in what cells could be causing the leakage of protein?

    A.   Mesangial cells
    B.   Bowman's capsule cells
    C.   Pericytes
    D.   Podocytes

10. A 53-year-old man comes to the clinic to participate in a clinical trial to evaluate a new epilepsy drug. Prior to the study laboratory work is done and a 24-h urine collection is made. The man's serum creatinine is 2.3 mg/dL, urine creatinine is 89.2 mg/dL, and his urine output volume per day is 2250 mL/day. What is his approximate GFR?

    A.   6 mL/min
    B.   60 mL/min
    C.   87 mL/min
    D.   120 mL/min
    E.   600 mL/min

ANSWERS

1. The correct answer is **A.** The majority of filtered sodium is reabsorbed in the proximal tubule. The final determination of sodium reabsorption is completed in the medullary collecting duct.

2. The correct answer is **A.** The proximal tubule the major site of filtered water reabsorption.

3. The correct answer is **A.** Clearance is the amount of a substance that is filtered and is present in the urine. If the amount of the substance in the urine is less than that of inulin which is filtered but not reabsorbed or secreted, that substance must be reabsorbed in the tubules.

4. The correct answer is **A.** The transport maximum of glucose is in the proximal tubule, not any other tubular segment.

5. The correct answer is **E.** Cortical collecting duct where aldosterone is responsible for sodium reabsorption via ENaC transporters.

6. The correct answer is **C.** ([urine]/[plasma]) × urine flow = (100 mg/dL/10 mg/dL) × 2 mL/min = 20 mL/min

7. The correct answer is **D.** As urine output increases, the amount of the solutes in the urine increase and the osmolality of urine approaches that of plasma. The majority of solute in the urine makes it isotonic since the majority is isotonic proximal tubular fluid.

8. The correct answer is **A.** Caffeine causes vasodilation of the afferent arteriole which would increase GFR and urine output. A decrease in efferent arteriole resistance would decrease GFR leading to a decrease in urine output. An increase in afferent resistance would also decrease GFR.

9. The correct answer is **D.** Podocytes form the filtration slits along the glomerular capillary wall, and a defect in them would cause leakage of protein into the urine.

10. The correct answer is **B.** U/P × UV: ((89.2 mg/dL/2.3 mg/dL) × (2250 mL/day))/1440 min/day

Regulation of Extracellular Fluid Composition & Volume

- Describe how the tonicity (osmolality) of the extracellular fluid is maintained by alterations in water intake and vasopressin secretion.

- Discuss the effects of vasopressin, the receptors on which it acts, and how its secretion is regulated.

- Describe how the volume of the extracellular fluid is maintained by alterations in renin and aldosterone secretion.

- Outline the cascade of reactions that lead to the formation of angiotensin II and its metabolites in the circulation.

- List the functions of angiotensin II and the receptors on which it acts to carry out these functions.

- Describe the structure and functions of atrial natriuretic peptide (ANP), B-type natriuretic peptide (BNP), and C-type natriuretic peptide (CNP) and the receptors on which they act.

- Describe the site and mechanism of action of erythropoietin, and the feedback regulation of its secretion.

■ VASOPRESSIN AND DEFENSE OF TONICITY

The defense of the tonicity of the extracellular fluid (ECF) is primarily the function of the vasopressin-secreting and thirst mechanisms. The total body osmolality is directly proportional to the total body sodium plus the total body potassium divided by the total body water, so that changes in the osmolality of the body fluids occur when a mismatch exists between the amount of these electrolytes and the amount of water ingested or lost from the body. When the effective osmotic pressure of the plasma rises, vasopressin secretion is increased and the thirst mechanism is stimulated; water is retained in the body, diluting the hypertonic plasma; and water intake is increased. Conversely, when the plasma becomes hypotonic, vasopressin secretion is decreased and "solute-free water" (water in excess of solute) is excreted. In this way, the tonicity of the body fluids is maintained within a narrow normal range. In health, plasma osmolality ranges from 280 mOsm/kg of H_2O to 295 mOsm/kg

of H_2O, with vasopressin secretion maximally inhibited at 285 mOsm/kg and stimulated at higher values.

There are at least three kinds of vasopressin receptors: V_{1A}, V_{1B}, and V_2. All are G-protein–coupled. The V_{1A} and V_{1B} receptors act through phosphatidylinositol hydrolysis to increase the intracellular Ca^{2+} concentration. The V_2 receptors act through G_s to increase cyclic adenosine 3′,5′-monophosphate (cAMP) levels. The half-life of vasopressin is 18 min.

Vasopressin is often called the **antidiuretic hormone (ADH)** since it acts on the kidney to reduce water excretion by increasing collecting duct permeability. The urine becomes concentrated, and volume decreases, and body fluid osmolality decreases. In the absence of vasopressin, urine is hypotonic to plasma, excreted volume is increased, and there is a net water loss. Consequently, the osmolality of the body fluid rises.

The mechanism by which vasopressin exerts its antidiuretic effect is activated by **V_2 receptors** and involves aquaporin-2 in the apical (luminal) membranes of the principal cells of the collecting ducts. Movement of water across membranes by simple diffusion is augmented by movement through the aquaporin-2 channels. These channels are stored in endosomes inside the cells, and vasopressin causes their rapid translocation to the luminal membranes.

Although V_{1A} receptors mediate its vasoconstrictor actions, vasopressin plays little role in blood pressure control since it also acts on the area postrema of the brain to reduce cardiac output.

V_{1B} receptors (also called V_3 receptors) are unique to the anterior pituitary, where they mediate increased secretion of adrenocorticotropic hormone (ACTH).

Vasopressin is stored in the posterior pituitary and released into the bloodstream in response to nerve fiber impulses. When plasma osmotic pressure is above 285 mOsm/kg, vasopressin secretion occurs. Vasopressin secretion is regulated by osmoreceptors in the anterior hypothalamus that are outside the blood–brain barrier and appear to be located in the circumventricular organs, primarily the organum vasculosum of the lamina terminalis (OVLT). Changes in vasopressin secretion occur when osmolality is changed as little as 1%. In this way, the osmolality of the plasma in normal individuals is tightly maintained close to 285 mOsm/L.

Vasopressin secretion is increased when ECF volume is low, and decreased when ECF volume is high. There is an inverse relationship between the rate of vasopressin secretion and the rate of discharge in afferents from stretch receptors in the low- and high-pressure portions of the vascular system. The low-pressure receptors are those in the great veins, right and left atria, and pulmonary vessels; the high-pressure receptors are those in the carotid sinuses and aortic arch. Exponential increases in plasma vasopressin occur when blood pressure decreases. However, the low-pressure receptors monitor the fullness of the vascular system, and moderate decreases in blood volume that reduce central venous pressure without lowering arterial pressure can also increase plasma vasopressin.

Thus, the low-pressure receptors are the primary mediators of volume effects on vasopressin secretion. Impulses pass from them via the vagi to the nucleus of the tractus solitarius (NTS). An inhibitory pathway projects from the NTS to the caudal ventrolateral medulla (CVLM), and there is a direct excitatory pathway from the CVLM to the hypothalamus. Angiotensin II (Ang II) reinforces the response to hypovolemia and hypotension by acting on the circumventricular organs to increase vasopressin secretion, in the renal tubules to increase sodium reabsorption, and in the vascular system to cause vasoconstriction.

Hypovolemia and hypotension produced by conditions such as hemorrhage release large amounts of vasopressin, and in the presence of hypovolemia, the osmotic response curve is shifted to the left. Its slope is also increased. The result is water retention and reduced plasma osmolality. This includes hyponatremia, since Na^+ is the most abundant osmotically active component of the plasma.

CLINICAL IMPLICATIONS

Volume and other nonosmotic stimuli can interfere with the osmotic control of vasopressin secretion. For example, patients who have had surgery may have elevated levels of plasma vasopressin because of pain and hypovolemia, and this may cause low plasma osmolality and dilutional hyponatremia.

Diabetes insipidus is the syndrome that results when there is a vasopressin deficiency (**central diabetes insipidus**) or when the kidneys fail to respond to the hormone (**nephrogenic diabetes insipidus**). The symptoms of diabetes insipidus are passage of large amounts of dilute urine (**polyuria**) and the drinking of large amounts of fluid (**polydipsia**), provided the thirst mechanism is intact. Polydipsia keeps these patients healthy, and if their sense of thirst is depressed for any reason, dehydration that can be fatal develops.

Another cause of diabetes insipidus is inability of the kidneys to respond to vasopressin (**nephrogenic diabetes insipidus**). There are two types: in one, the gene for the V_2 receptor gene on the X chromosome is mutated (a recessive trait), making the receptor unresponsive; the other type is due to mutations in the autosomal gene for aquaporin-2 preventing the water channel from locating to the apical membrane of the collecting duct.

Vasopressin deficiency is caused by disease processes in the supraoptic and paraventricular nuclei, the hypothalamohypophysial tract, or the posterior pituitary gland, 30% of clinical cases are due to neoplastic lesions of the hypothalamus, either primary or metastatic; 30% are posttraumatic; 30% are idiopathic; and the remainder are due to vascular lesions, infections, systemic diseases such as sarcoidosis that affect the hypothalamus, or mutations in the gene for prepropressophysin. Symptoms that develop after surgical removal of the posterior lobe of the pituitary may be temporary if the distal ends of the supraoptic and paraventricular fibers are only damaged, because the fibers recover, make new vascular connections, and begin to secrete vasopressin again.

Synthetic peptides, such as 1-deamino-8-D-arginine vasopressin (desmopressin; dDAVP), have high antidiuretic activity with little pressor activity, making them valuable in the treatment of vasopressin deficiency.

■ DEFENSE OF VOLUME

The volume of the ECF is determined primarily by the total amount of osmotically active solute in the ECF. Because Na^+ and Cl^- are by far the most abundant osmotically active solutes in ECF, and because changes in Cl^- are to a great extent secondary to changes in Na^+, the amount of Na^+ in the ECF is the most important determinant of ECF volume. Therefore, the mechanisms that control Na^+ balance are the major mechanisms defending ECF volume. Ang II stimulates aldosterone and vasopressin secretion, and causes thirst. Ang II is one of the most potent vasoconstrictors in the body which can help maintain blood pressure in physiological conditions and cause hypertension in pathological conditions.

Expansion of the ECF volume increases the secretion of atrial natriuretic peptide (ANP) and B-type natriuretic peptide (BNP) by the heart causing natriuresis and diuresis.

In disease states, loss of water from the body (**dehydration**) causes a moderate decrease in ECF volume, due to loss from both intracellular and ECF compartments. Excessive loss of Na^+ in the stools (diarrhea), urine (severe acidosis, adrenal insufficiency), or sweat (heat prostration) decreases ECF volume markedly and eventually leads to shock.

When ECF volume is decreased, blood pressure falls, glomerular capillary pressure declines, and glomerular filtration rate (GFR) falls, reducing the amount of Na^+ filtered. Tubular reabsorption of Na^+ is increased, in part because the secretion of aldosterone is increased and due to the release in Ang II in response to the drop in blood pressure. Other changes in Na^+ excretion occur too rapidly to be solely due to changes in aldosterone secretion. For example, rising from the supine to the standing position increases aldosterone secretion.

■ THE RENIN–ANGIOTENSIN SYSTEM

RENIN

Renin is an aspartyl protease enzyme that converts angiotensinogen to angiotensin I (Ang I). The synthesis of Ang I is the rate-limiting step in the synthesis of Ang II. Ang I is converted to Ang II via the action of the angiotensin-converting enzyme (**ACE**), a dipeptidyl peptidase. Renin is synthesized as a prepro-hormone (prorenin) and is mainly released from the granular cells of the juxtamedullary apparatus in the kidney. However, prorenin can also be secreted by other organs, including the ovaries. Active renin has a half-life in the circulation of 80 min or less.

Renin in kidney and bloodstream is produced by the **juxtaglomerular cells (JG cells)** (Figure 38–1). These epithelioid cells are located in the media of afferent arterioles as they enter the glomeruli. The membrane-lined secretory granules in JG cells contain renin. Renin secretion is regulated by s factors including the intrarenal baroreceptor mechanism that causes renin secretion to decrease when arteriolar pressure at the level of the JG cells increases and to increase when arteriolar pressure falls. Another renin-regulating sensor is in the macula densa. Renin secretion is inversely proportional to the amount of Na^+ and Cl^- entering the distal tubules from the loop of Henle. Na^+ and Cl^- enter macula densa cells via the $Na–K–2Cl^-$ transporters in their apical membranes, and this increase triggers a reduction in renin secretion in JG cells in adjacent afferent arterioles. Renin secretion also varies inversely with the plasma K^+ level, but the effect of K^+ appears to be mediated by the changes in Na^+ and Cl^- delivery to the macula densa. Ang II also feeds back to inhibit renin secretion by a direct action on JG cells. Vasopressin inhibits renin secretion but the mechanism is not clear. Finally, increased activity of the sympathetic nervous system increases renin secretion. The increase is mediated both by increased circulating catecholamines and by norepinephrine secreted by postganglionic renal sympathetic nerves. Catecholamines act mainly on β_1-adrenergic receptors on JG cells and renin release is mediated by an increase in intracellular cAMP.

Circulating angiotensinogen is found in the α_2-globulin fraction of the plasma, is synthesized in the liver and its circulating level is increased by glucocorticoids, thyroid hormones, estrogens, several cytokines, and Ang II.

ACE hydrolyses histidyl-leucine from the inactive Ang I, forming the octapeptide **Ang II**. It also inactivates bradykinin. Increased tissue bradykinin that occurs when ACE is inhibited acts on B_2 receptors to produce the cough that is an annoying side of treatment with ACE inhibitors. Most of the converting enzyme that forms Ang II in the circulation is located in endothelial cells. Much of the conversion occurs as the blood passes through the lungs, but conversion also occurs in many other parts of the body.

Ang II is metabolized rapidly; its half-life in the circulation in humans is 1–2 min. An aminopeptidase (**ACE2**) removes the aspartic acid (Asp) residue from the amino terminal of the peptide. The resulting heptapeptide has physiologic activity and is called **angiotensin III or more commonly, Ang (1–7)**. Removal of a second amino terminal residue from angiotensin III produces the hexapeptide sometimes called angiotensin IV.

Plasma renin activity (PRA) is an indication of renin levels, and is measured by determining the amount of Ang I produced by a sample to which endogenous angiotensinogen is added using radioimmunoassay. **Plasma renin concentration (PRC)** can also be measured if angiotensinogen is not added to the sample. Normal PRA in supine subjects eating a normal amount of sodium is approximately 1 ng of Ang I generated per milliliter per hour. The plasma Ang II concentration in such subjects is about 25 pg/mL (approximately 25 pmol/L).

Ang I functions solely as the precursor of Ang II. Ang II produces arteriolar constriction and a rise in systolic and diastolic blood pressure. Ang II also acts directly on the adrenal cortex to increase the secretion of aldosterone, and the **renin–angiotensin system (RAS)** is a major regulator of aldosterone secretion, often called the **renin–angiotensin–aldosterone system (RAAS)**. Additional actions of Ang II include facilitation of the release of norepinephrine by a direct action on postganglionic sympathetic neurons, contraction of mesangial cells with a resultant decrease in GFR, and a direct effect on the renal tubules to increase Na^+ reabsorption.

Ang II also acts on the brain to decrease the sensitivity of the baroreflex, and this potentiates the pressor effect of Ang II. In addition, Ang II acts on the brain to increase water intake and increase the secretion of vasopressin and ACTH. It does not penetrate the blood–brain barrier, but triggers these responses by acting on the circumventricular organs, four small structures in the brain that are outside the blood–brain barrier.

Ang III or **Ang (1–7)** causes vasodilation and is increased in the presence of hormones such as estrogens.

The biological activity of the RAS is mediated by two classes of Ang II receptors. AT_1 receptors are G-protein–coupled (G_q) to phospholipase C, and Ang II increases the cytosolic free Ca^{2+} level, and numerous tyrosine kinases. In vascular smooth muscle, AT_1 receptors are associated with caveolae, and Ang II increases production of caveolin-1. The AT_1 receptor gene is located on chromosome 3.

There are also AT_2 receptors encoded by a gene on the X chromosome. Like the AT_1 receptors, they have seven transmembrane domains and are G-protein–coupled to activate various phosphatases that in turn antagonize growth effects and open K^+ channels. In addition, Ang II binds to AT_2 receptors to increase NO in certain tissues, therefore increasing intracellular cyclic 3,5-guanosine monophosphate (cGMP). Ang (1–7) is also thought to have its vasodilator activity via AT_2 receptors. AT_1 receptors in arterioles

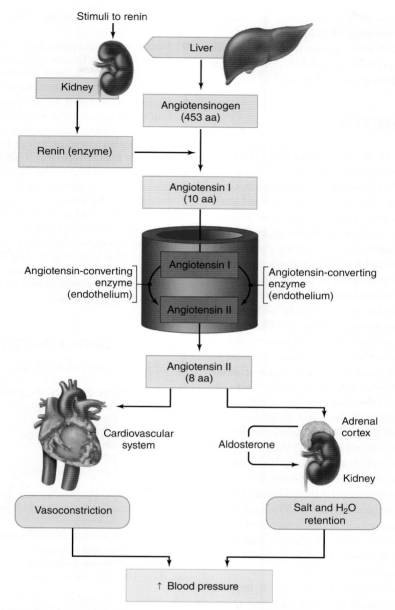

FIGURE 38–1 **Summary of the renin–angiotensin system and the stimulation of aldosterone secretion by angiotensin II.** The plasma concentration of renin is the rate-limiting step in the renin–angiotensin system; therefore, it is the major determinant of plasma angiotensin II concentration.

and in the adrenal cortex are regulated in opposite ways: an excess of Ang II downregulates the vascular receptors, but up-regulates the adrenocortical receptors.

■ HORMONES OF THE HEART & OTHER NATRIURETIC FACTORS

Two **natriuretic hormones** are secreted by the heart. The muscle cells in the atria and, to a much lesser extent in the ventricles, contain secretory granules that increase in number when NaCl intake is increased and ECF expanded.

The first natriuretic hormone isolated from the heart was **ANP**. ANP was subsequently isolated from other tissues, including the brain. A second natriuretic polypeptide **BNP** (also known as **brain natriuretic peptide**) is also present in the brain, but more is present in the human heart, including the ventricles. A third member of this family has been named **CNP**, but very little is present in the heart and the circulation, and it appears to be primarily a paracrine mediator.

ANP and BNP act on the kidneys to increase Na$^+$ excretion. They appear to produce this effect by dilating afferent arterioles and relaxing mesangial cells. Both of these actions increase GFR. In addition, they act on the renal tubules to inhibit

Na⁺ reabsorption. Other actions include an increase in capillary permeability, leading to extravasation of fluid and a decline in blood pressure. In addition, they relax vascular smooth muscle in arterioles and venules. These peptides also inhibit renin secretion and counteract the pressor effects of catecholamines and Ang II.

■ ERYTHROPOIETIN

When an individual bleeds or becomes hypoxic, hemoglobin synthesis is enhanced, and production and release of red blood cells from the bone marrow (**erythropoiesis**) are increased. Conversely, when the red cell volume is increased above normal levels by transfusion, the erythropoietic activity of the bone marrow decreases. These adjustments are brought about by changes in the circulating level of **erythropoietin,** a circulating glycoprotein produced in the kidney (85%) and liver (15%). Erythropoietin is produced in the peritubular capillary bed of the kidney. Erythropoietin increases the number of erythropoietin-sensitive committed stem cells in bone marrow that are converted to red blood cell precursors and subsequently to mature erythrocytes. The receptor for erythropoietin is a linear protein with a single transmembrane domain that is a member of the cytokine receptor superfamily that has tyrosine kinase activity, and activates a cascade of serine and threonine kinases resulting in inhibited apoptosis of red cells and their increased growth and development. The principal site of inactivation of erythropoietin is the liver, and the hormone has a half-life in the circulation of about 5 h. However, the increase in circulating red cells that it triggers takes 2–3 days to appear, since red cell maturation is a relatively slow process. Recombinant erythropoietin is available for clinical use as epoetin alfa, and is used in the treatment of the anemia associated with kidney failure; 90% of the patients with end-stage renal disease undergoing dialysis are anemic as a result of erythropoietin deficiency. Erythropoietin is also used to stimulate red cell production in individuals who are banking a supply of their own blood in preparation for autologous transfusions during elective surgery.

The usual stimulus for erythropoietin secretion is hypoxia, but secretion can also be stimulated by cobalt salts and androgens. Recent evidence suggests that the O₂ sensor regulating erythropoietin secretion in the kidneys and the liver is a heme protein that in the deoxy form stimulates and in the oxy form inhibits transcription of the erythropoietin gene to form erythropoietin mRNA. Secretion of the hormone is also facilitated by the alkalosis that develops at high altitudes. Like renin secretion, erythropoietin secretion is facilitated by catecholamines via a β-adrenergic mechanism, although the RAS is totally separate from the erythropoietin system.

CHAPTER SUMMARY

- Total body osmolality is directly proportional to the total body sodium plus the total body potassium divided by the total body water. Changes in the osmolality of the body fluids occur when a disproportion exists between the amount of

these electrolytes and the amount of water ingested or lost from the body.

- Vasopressin's main physiologic effect is the retention of water by the kidney by increasing the water permeability of the renal collecting ducts. Water is absorbed from the urine, the urine becomes concentrated, and its volume decreases.

- Vasopressin is stored in the posterior pituitary and released into the bloodstream in response to the stimulation of osmoreceptors or baroreceptors. Increases in secretion occur when osmolality is changed as little as 1%, thus keeping the osmolality of the plasma very close to 285 mOsm/L.

- The amount of Na⁺ in the ECF is the most important determinant of ECF volume, and mechanisms that control Na⁺ balance are the major mechanisms defending ECF volume. The main mechanism regulating sodium balance is the RAS, a hormone system that regulates blood pressure.

- The kidneys secrete the enzyme renin and renin acts in concert with ACE to form Ang II. Ang II acts directly on the adrenal cortex to increase the secretion of aldosterone. Aldosterone increases the retention of sodium from the urine via action on the renal collecting duct.

MULTIPLE-CHOICE QUESTIONS

For all questions, select the single best answer unless otherwise directed.

1. Dehydration increases the plasma concentration of all the following hormones *except*
   A. vasopressin.
   B. angiotensin II.
   C. aldosterone.
   D. norepinephrine.
   E. atrial natriuretic peptide.

2. In a patient who has become dehydrated, body water should be replaced by intravenous infusion of
   A. distilled water.
   B. 0.9% sodium chloride solution.
   C. 5% glucose solution.
   D. hyperoncotic albumin.
   E. 10% glucose solution.

3. Renin is secreted by
   A. cells in the macula densa.
   B. cells in the proximal tubules.
   C. cells in the distal tubules.
   D. granular cells in the juxtaglomerular apparatus.
   E. cells in the peritubular capillary bed.

4. Erythropoietin is secreted by
   A. cells in the macula densa.
   B. cells in the proximal tubules.
   C. cells in the distal tubules.
   D. granular cells in the juxtaglomerular apparatus.
   E. cells in the peritubular capillary bed.

5. When a woman who has been on a low-sodium diet for 8 days is given an intravenous injection of captopril, a drug that inhibits ACE, which of the following would be expected?
   A. Blood pressure to rise because cardiac output would fall
   B. Blood pressure to rise because peripheral resistance would fall
   C. Blood pressure to fall because cardiac output would fall

D. Blood pressure to fall because peripheral resistance would fall

E. PRA to fall because circulating Ang I level would rise

6. Which of the following would *not* be expected to increase renin secretion?
   A. Administration of a drug that blocks ACE
   B. Administration of a drug that blocks AT_1 receptors
   C. Administration of a drug that blocks β-adrenergic receptors
   D. Constriction of the aorta between the celiac artery and the renal arteries
   E. Administration of a drug that reduces ECF volume

7. Which of the following is *least* likely to contribute to the beneficial effects of ACE inhibitors in the treatment of heart failure?
   A. Vasodilation
   B. Decreased cardiac growth
   C. Decreased cardiac afterload
   D. Increased PRA
   E. Decreased plasma aldosterone

8. A 50-year-old woman comes into the emergency department with complaints of "hearing her heart beat." She is concerned that she may be having a heart attack. When her blood pressure is measured, it is elevated. The physician gives her a diuretic, and although the blood pressure drops, he decides to perform some additional tests to determine the cause of the hypertension. The woman's PRA level is elevated and CT scans show that her left kidney is smaller than her right. What is the physician's diagnosis likely to be?
   A. Myocardial infarction
   B. Stroke attack
   C. Renal artery stenosis
   D. Renal denervation

9. A scientist is performing studies on runners after a 10,000-m race. She finds that the urine of runners after the race is more concentrated and has reduced volume than before the race. What mechanism contributes to the change in urine concentration and output?
   A. Decrease in thirst response
   B. Increase in water permeability in the collecting duct
   C. Decrease in ADH secretion
   D. Increase in thirst during the race

10. A 56-year-old man is admitted to the ED with an acute myocardial infarction. The man was transferred to the CCU and was placed on 24 h intake and output. A few days later his 24 h urinary output was decreased lower than normal. An increase in which of the following contributes to the reduced urine flow in a patient with congestive heart failure and reduced effective circulating volume?
    A. ANP
    B. Urodilatin (renal natriuretic peptide)
    C. Renal perfusion pressure
    D. Renal sympathetic nerve activity
    E. Sodium delivery to the macula densa

ANSWERS

1. Answer is **E.** ANP is released by the atria in the presence of atrial pressure increase due to central volume increase.

2. Answer is **B.** Albumin will cause an increase in central volume expansion but will not affect extra-vascular volume. Dextrose 5% in water is often given for individuals with normovolemia, but not glucose that may cause insulin release and will be excreted once transport maximum is surpassed rather than affecting volume expansion. Distilled water will cause edema of brain tissue and extravascular tissue.

3. Answer is **D.** The JG cells are located close to the macula densa between afferent and efferent arterioles.

4. Answer is **E.** Erythropoietin is secreted by cells in the peritubular capillary bed of the kidney.

5. Answer is **D.** Captopril is an ACE inhibitor. A reduction in ACE would cause a reduction in Ang II. A low-sodium diet would cause RAS activation, renin release and elevated levels of Ang II. Blocking Ang II synthesis with captopril would reduce BP, cause a reduction in peripheral resistance, and cause an increase in cardiac output.

6. Answer is **B.** Blocking AT_1 receptors would affect bioactivity of Ang II, but not affect renin release.

7. Answer is **E.** Aldosterone causes volume loss that would be beneficial for heart failure.

8. Answer is **C.** The stenosis of the renal artery leads to the consequent increase in PRA to compensate for the reduction in the perfusion pressure in the stenotic kidney.

9. Answer is **B.** Fluid loss (dehydration) during the race leads to increase in ADH secretion leading to an increase in water permeability in the collecting duct allowing water retention but increase in urine concentration.

10. Answer is **D.** An increase in renal sympathetic nerve activity promotes a decrease in sodium and water excretion by decreasing GFR, increasing renin secretin, and increasing tubular sodium reabsorption. All the other factors would cause an increase in sodium and water excretion.

Acidification of the Urine & Bicarbonate Excretion

OBJECTIVES

After reading this chapter, you should be able to:

- Outline the processes involved in the secretion of H⁺ into the tubules and discuss the significance of these processes in the regulation of acid-base balance.
- Define acidosis and alkalosis, and give (in mEq/L and pH) the normal mean and the range of H⁺ concentrations in blood that are compatible with health.
- Describe the changes in blood chemistry that occur during the development of metabolic acidosis and metabolic alkalosis, and the respiratory and renal compensations for these conditions.
- Describe the changes in blood chemistry that occur during the development of respiratory acidosis and respiratory alkalosis, and the renal compensation for these conditions.

INTRODUCTION

The kidneys play a key role in the maintenance of acid–base balance and to do this they must excrete acid in the amount equivalent to the production of nonvolatile acids in the body. The production of nonvolatile acids will vary with diet, metabolism, and disease. The kidneys must also filter and reabsorb plasma bicarbonate, and thus prevent the loss of bicarbonate in the urine. Both processes are linked physiologically, due to the nephron's ability to secrete H⁺ ions into the filtrate.

■ RENAL H⁺ SECRETION

The cells of the proximal and distal tubules and the collecting ducts secrete hydrogen ions. The transporter that is responsible for H⁺ secretion in the proximal tubules is the Na–H exchanger (primarily NHE3) (**Figure 39–1**). This is an example of secondary active transport; Na^+ is moved from the inside of the cell to the interstitium by Na, K-ATPase on the basolateral membrane, which keeps intracellular Na^+ low, thus establishing the drive for Na^+ to enter the cell from the tubular lumen via the Na–H exchanger. The Na–H exchanger secretes H⁺ into the lumen in exchange for Na^+. The secreted H⁺ combines with filtered HCO_3^- to form H_2CO_3; the presence of **carbonic anhydrase** on the apical membrane of the proximal tubule catalyzes the formation of H_2O and CO_2 from H_2CO_3. The apical membrane of epithelial cells lining the proximal tubule is permeable to CO_2 and H_2O, and they enter the tubule rapidly. **Eighty percent of the filtered load of HCO_3^- is reabsorbed in the proximal tubule**.

Inside the cell, carbonic anhydrase is also present and can catalyze the formation of H_2CO_3 from CO_2 and H_2O. H_2CO_3 dissociates into H⁺ ions and HCO_3^-; the H⁺ is secreted into the tubular lumen, and the HCO_3^- that is formed diffuses into the interstitial fluid. Thus, for each H⁺ secreted, one Na^+ and one HCO_3^- enter the interstitial fluid. Because carbonic anhydrase catalyzes the formation of H_2CO_3, drugs that inhibit carbonic anhydrase depress both secretion of acid by the proximal tubules and the reactions that depend on it.

In the distal tubules and collecting ducts, H⁺ secretion is independent of Na^+ in the tubular lumen, and most H⁺ is secreted by an ATP-driven proton pump. Aldosterone acts on this pump to increase distal H⁺ secretion. Interstitial cells in this part of the renal tubule secrete acid and contain abundant carbonic anhydrase. The H⁺-translocating ATPase that produces H⁺ secretion is located in vesicles and in the apical cell membrane. In acidosis, the number of H⁺ pumps is increased by insertion of the vesicles into the apical cell membrane. Some of the H⁺ is also secreted

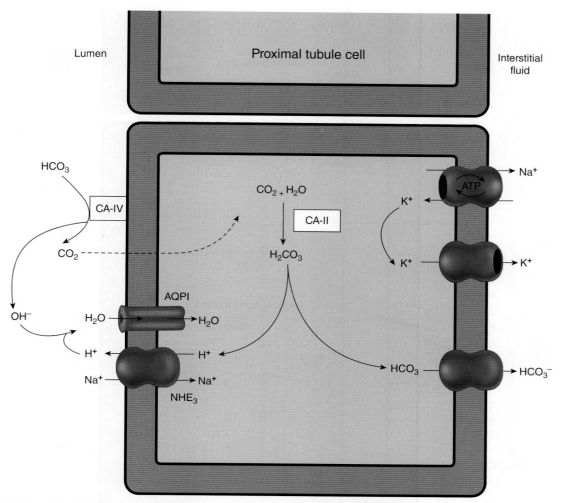

FIGURE 39–1 **Secretion of acid and reabsorption of filtered bicarbonate by proximal tubular cells in the kidney.** H⁺ is transported into the tubular lumen by NHE3 in exchange for Na⁺. Active transport by Na, K-ATPase is indicated by arrows. Dashed arrows indicate diffusion.

by H–K-ATPase. In addition, interstitial cells contain **anion exchanger 1** (AE1) in basolateral cell membranes. AE1 can function as a Cl/HCO_3 exchanger for the transport of HCO_3^- to the interstitial fluid.

REACTION WITH BUFFERS

The maximal H⁺ gradient against which the transport mechanisms can secrete corresponds with a urine pH of about 4.5; a H⁺ concentration 1000 times greater than the plasma H⁺ concentration. This is normally reached in the collecting ducts. Three important reactions in the tubular fluid remove free H⁺, permitting more acid to be excreted **(Figure 39–2)**. These are the reactions of H⁺ with HCO_3^- (bicarbonate) to form CO_2 and H_2O; H⁺ with HPO_4^{2-} (dibasic phosphate) to form $H_2PO_4^-$ (titratable acids), and H⁺ with NH_3 (ammonia) to form NH_4^+.

In an average diet, approximately 40% of acid (about 30 mEq/day) produced by the body during metabolic reactions is excreted as **titratable acid** (ie, phosphate system) and 60%

of acid (about 50 mEq/day) is excreted as NH_4^+. The pK′ of the bicarbonate system is 6.1, that of the dibasic phosphate system is 6.8, and that of the ammonia system is 9.0. The concentration of HCO_3^- in the plasma, and consequently in the glomerular filtrate, is normally about 24 mEq/L, whereas that of phosphate is only 1.5 mEq/L. Therefore, in the proximal tubule most of the secreted H⁺ reacts with HCO_3^- to form H_2CO_3, and this enters the cell as CO_2 and H_2O following the action of carbonic anhydrase in the brush border of the proximal tubule cells. The CO_2 entering the tubular cells adds to the pool of CO_2 available to form H_2CO_3. Because most of the H⁺ is removed from the tubule, the pH of the fluid is changed very little. This is the mechanism by which HCO_3^- is reabsorbed; for each mol of HCO_3^- removed from the tubular fluid, 1 mol of HCO_3^- diffuses from the tubular cells into the blood.

Secreted H⁺ also reacts with dibasic phosphate (HPO_4^{2-}) to form monobasic phosphate ($H_2PO_4^-$). This happens mainly in the distal tubules and collecting ducts where the phosphate that escapes proximal reabsorption is concentrated by the reabsorption of water.

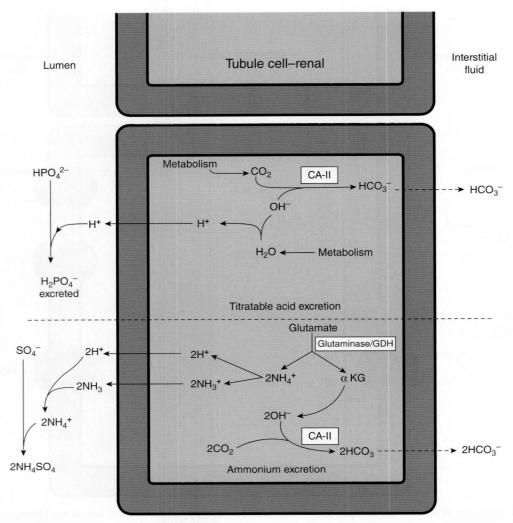

FIGURE 39–2 Titratable acid and ammonium formation. Top: Formation of monobasic phosphate. **Bottom:** Ammonium formation. Note that in each instance one Na^+ and one HCO_3^- enter the bloodstream for each H^+ secreted.

In the proximal tubule (where NH_3 is made) and in the distal tubules, the ammonia buffering system allows secreted H^+ to combine with NH_3. NH_4^+ is in equilibrium with NH_3 and H^+ in the cells. The pK′ of the ammonia system is 9.0, and the ammonia system is titrated only from the pH of the urine to pH 7.4, so it contributes very little to the titratable acidity. Because the pK′ of this reaction is 9.0, the ratio of NH_3 to NH_4^+ at pH 7.0 is 1:100 (Figure 39–3). NH_3 is lipid-soluble and diffuses across the cell membranes down its concentration gradient into the interstitial fluid and tubular urine. In the urine it reacts with H^+ to form NH_4^+, and the NH_4^+ remains "trapped" in the urine. Each H^+ ion that reacts with the buffers contributes to the urinary **titratable acidity,** which is measured by determining the amount of alkali that must be added to the urine to return its pH to 7.4, the pH of the glomerular filtrate. However, the titratable acidity obviously measures only a fraction of the acid secreted, since it does not account for the H_2CO_3 that has been converted to H_2O and CO_2.

The principal reaction producing NH_4^+ in cells is conversion of glutamine to glutamate that is catalyzed by **glutaminase** in tubular cells. **Glutamic dehydrogenase** catalyzes the conversion of glutamate to α-ketoglutarate, with the production of more NH_4^+. Subsequent metabolism of α-ketoglutarate utilizes $2H^+$, freeing $2HCO_3^-$.

The reabsorption of HCO_3^- is crucial to the maintenance of acid–base balance, as a loss of a single HCO_3^- ion in the urine would be the equivalent of adding a H^+ ion to the blood. The kidneys have the ability to replenish the body with new HCO_3^-. This occurs when H^+ are removed from the body as NH_4^+ or titratable acid, as there is formation of new bicarbonate within the cells, and this enters the blood.

AMMONIA SECRETION

In chronic acidosis, the amount of NH_4^+ excreted at any given urine pH increases, because more NH_3 enters the tubular urine. NH_3 secretion leads to removal of H^+ from the tubular fluid and further increases H^+ secretion by the renal tubules and excretion in

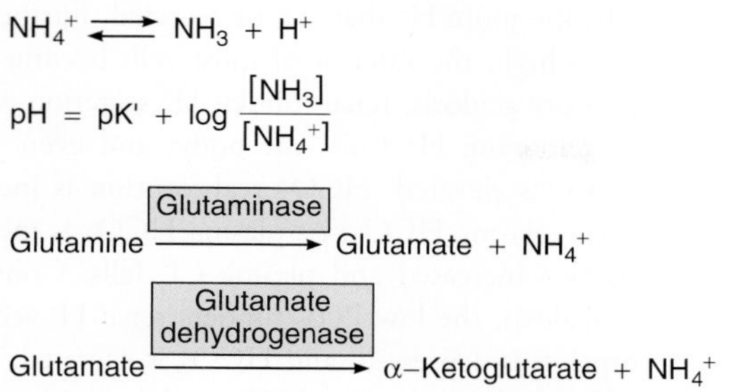

$$NH_4^+ \rightleftharpoons NH_3 + H^+$$

$$pH = pK' + \log \frac{[NH_3]}{[NH_4^+]}$$

Glutamine $\xrightarrow{\boxed{\text{Glutaminase}}}$ Glutamate + NH_4^+

Glutamate $\xrightarrow{\boxed{\begin{array}{c}\text{Glutamate}\\\text{dehydrogenase}\end{array}}}$ α–Ketoglutarate + NH_4^+

FIGURE 39–3 **Major reactions involved in ammonia production in the kidneys.**

the urine. Because the amount of phosphate buffer filtered at the glomerulus cannot be increased, urinary excretion of acid via the phosphate buffer system is limited. The production of NH_4^+ by the renal tubules is the only way the kidneys can remove even the normal amount, much less an increased amount, of nonvolatile acid produced in the body.

In the inner medullary cells of the collecting duct, the main process by which NH_3 is secreted into the urine and then changed to NH_4^+ is called **nonionic diffusion,** thereby maintaining the concentration gradient for diffusion of NH_3. In the proximal tubule, nonionic diffusion of NH_4^+ is less important because NH_4^+ can be secreted into the lumen, often by replacing H^+ via the Na–H exchanger.

FACTORS AFFECTING ACID SECRETION

Renal acid secretion is altered by changes in the intracellular P_{CO_2}, K^+ concentration, carbonic anhydrase level, and adrenocortical hormone concentration. When the P_{CO_2} is high (**respiratory acidosis**), more intracellular H_2CO_3 is available to buffer the hydroxyl ions and acid secretion is enhanced, whereas the reverse is true when the P_{CO_2} is low (**respiratory alkalosis**). K^+ depletion enhances acid secretion whereas K^+ excess in the cells inhibits acid secretion. When carbonic anhydrase is inhibited, acid secretion is inhibited because the formation of H_2CO_3 is decreased. Aldosterone and the other adrenocortical steroids that enhance tubular reabsorption of Na^+ also increase the secretion of H^+ and K^+.

BICARBONATE EXCRETION

Although the process of HCO_3^- reabsorption does not involve actual transport of this ion into the tubular cells, HCO_3^- reabsorption is proportional to the amount filtered over a relatively wide range. There is no demonstrable transport maximum, but HCO_3^- reabsorption is decreased when the extracellular fluid (ECF) volume is expanded (**Figure 39–4**). When the plasma HCO_3^- concentration is low, all the filtered HCO_3^- is reabsorbed; but when the plasma HCO_3^- concentration is high (ie, >26–28 mEq/L; the renal threshold for HCO_3^-), HCO_3^- appears in the urine and the urine becomes alkaline. Conversely, when the plasma HCO_3^- falls below about 26 mEq/L, the value at which

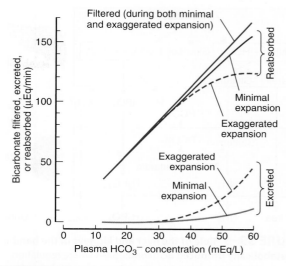

FIGURE 39–4 **Effect of ECF volume on HCO_3^- filtration, reabsorption, and excretion in rats.** The pattern of HCO_3^- excretion is similar in humans. The plasma HCO_3^- concentration is normally about 24 mEq/L. (Reproduced with permission from Purkerson ML, Lubowitz H, White RW, et al: On the influence of extracellular fluid volume expansion on bicarbonate reabsorption in the rat, *J Clin Invest.* 1969 Sep;48(9):1754-1760.)

all the secreted H^+ is being used to reabsorb HCO_3^-, more H^+ becomes available to combine with other buffer anions. Therefore, the lower the plasma HCO_3^- concentration drops, the more acidic the urine becomes and the greater its NH_4^+ content.

H⁺ BALANCE

H^+ concentrations in the body are expressed as pH, the negative logarithm of the H^+ concentration. A decrease in pH of 1 unit, for example from 7.0 to 6.0, represents a 10-fold increase in H^+ concentration. The pH notation is a useful because the H^+ concentrations are very low relative to those of other cations. For example, Na^+ concentration of arterial plasma that has been equilibrated with red blood cells is about 140 mEq/L, whereas the H^+ concentration is 0.00004 mEq/L, a pH of 7.40.

Since the pH of the arterial plasma is normally 7.40 and that of venous plasma slightly lower, technically, **acidosis** is present whenever the arterial pH is below 7.40, and **alkalosis** is present whenever pH is above 7.40, although variations of up to 0.05 pH unit occur without untoward effects. The H^+ concentrations in the ECF that are compatible with life cover an approximately fivefold range, from 0.00002 mEq/L (pH 7.70) to 0.0001 mEq/L (pH 7.00).

Amino acids are utilized in the liver for gluconeogenesis, leaving NH_4^+ and HCO_3^- as products from their amino and carboxyl groups (**Figure 39–5**). The NH_4^+ is incorporated into urea and the protons that are formed are buffered intracellularly by HCO_3^-, so little NH_4^+ and HCO_3^- escape into the circulation. However, metabolism of sulfur-containing amino acids produces H_2SO_4, and metabolism of phosphorylated amino acids such as phosphoserine produces H_3PO_4. These strong acids enter the circulation and present a major H^+ load to the buffers in the ECF. The H^+

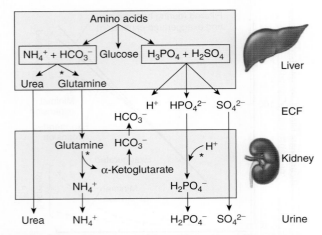

FIGURE 39–5   Role of the liver and kidneys in the handling of metabolically produced acid loads. Sites where regulation occurs are indicated by asterisks. (Modified with permission from Knepper MA, Burg MB, Orloff J, et al: Ammonium, urea, and systemic pH regulation. *Am J Physiol* 1987; July; 253(1 Pt 2):F199–F202.)

load from amino acid metabolism is normally about 50 mEq/day. The CO_2 formed by metabolism in the tissues is in large part hydrated to H_2CO_3, and the total H^+ load from this source is over 12,500 mEq/day. Most of the CO_2 is removed from the body by the lungs, and only small quantities of the H^+ remain to be excreted by the kidneys. Common sources of extra acid loads are strenuous exercise (lactic acid), diabetic ketosis (acetoacetic acid and β-hydroxybutyric acid), and ingestion of acidifying salts, such as NH_4Cl and $CaCl_2$, that in effect add HCl to the body. The failure of diseased kidneys to excrete normal amounts of acid is also a cause of acidosis. Fruits are the main dietary source of alkali. They contain Na^+ and K^+ salts of weak organic acids, and the anions of these salts are metabolized to CO_2, leaving $NaHCO_3$ and $KHCO_3$ in the body. $NaHCO_3$ and other alkalinizing salts are sometimes ingested in large amounts, but a more common cause of alkalosis is loss of acid from the body as a result of vomiting of gastric juice rich in HCl, which is equivalent to adding alkali to the body.

RENAL COMPENSATION TO RESPIRATORY ACIDOSIS & ALKALOSIS

A rise in arterial P_{CO_2} due to decreased ventilation causes **respiratory acidosis,** and conversely, a decline in P_{CO_2} causes **respiratory alkalosis.** Either respiratory acidosis or alkalosis cause changes in the kidneys that tend to **compensate** for the acidosis or alkalosis and adjust plasma pH toward normal.

HCO_3^- reabsorption in the renal tubules depends not only on the filtered load of HCO_3^-, which is the product of the glomerular filtration rate and the plasma HCO_3^- level, but also on the rate of H^+ secretion by renal tubular cells, since HCO_3^- is reabsorbed by exchange for H^+. The rate of H^+ secretion—and hence the rate of HCO_3^- reabsorption—is proportional to the arterial P_{CO_2}, probably because the more CO_2 that is available to form H_2CO_3 in

the tubular cells, the more H^+ that can be secreted. Furthermore, when the P_{CO_2} is high, the interior of most cells becomes more acidic. In respiratory acidosis, renal tubular H^+ secretion is therefore increased, removing H^+ from the body; and even though the plasma HCO_3^- is elevated, HCO_3^- reabsorption is increased, further raising the plasma HCO_3^-. As plasma HCO_3^- is increased, Cl^- excretion is also increased and plasma Cl^- falls. Conversely, in respiratory alkalosis, the low P_{CO_2} hinders renal H^+ secretion, HCO_3^- reabsorption is depressed, and HCO_3^- is excreted, further reducing the already low plasma HCO_3^- and lowering the pH toward normal.

METABOLIC ACIDOSIS AND RENAL COMPENSATION

When acids stronger than hemoglobin (Hb) and the other buffer acids are added to blood, **metabolic acidosis** is produced; and when the free H^+ level falls as a result of addition of alkali or removal of acid, **metabolic alkalosis** results. If H_2SO_4 is added, the H^+ is buffered and the Hb^-, negatively charged proteins ($Prot^-$), and HCO_3^- levels in plasma drop. The H_2CO_3 formed is converted to H_2O and CO_2, and the CO_2 is rapidly excreted via the lungs. This is the situation in **uncompensated** metabolic acidosis. However, acidosis is rarely uncompensated and in actuality, the rise in plasma H^+ stimulates respiration, so that the P_{CO_2} is reduced instead of rising or remaining constant. This **respiratory compensation** raises the pH even further. The **renal** compensatory mechanisms then bring about the excretion of the extra H^+ and return the buffer systems to normal.

The anions that replace HCO_3^- in the plasma in metabolic acidosis are filtered, each with a cation (principally Na^+), thus maintaining electrical neutrality. Renal tubular cells secrete H^+ into the tubular fluid in exchange for Na^+; for each H^+ secreted, one Na^+ and one HCO_3^- are added to the blood. Secreted H^+ reacts with HCO_3^- to form CO_2 and H_2O (bicarbonate reabsorption); with HPO_4^{2-} to form $H_2PO_4^-$; and with NH_3 to form NH_4^+. In this way, large amounts of H^+ can be secreted, permitting correspondingly large amounts of HCO_3^- to be returned to (in the case of bicarbonate reabsorption) or added to the depleted body stores and large numbers of cations to be reabsorbed. It is only when the acid load is very large that cations are lost with the anions, producing diuresis and depletion of body cation stores. In chronic acidosis, glutamine synthesis in the liver is increased, using some of the NH_4^+ that usually is converted to urea (Figure 39-5), and the glutamine provides the kidneys with an additional source of NH_4^+. NH_3 secretion increases over a period of days (adaptation of NH_3 secretion), further improving the renal compensation for acidosis. In addition, the metabolism of glutamine in the kidneys produces α-ketoglutarate, and this in turn is decarboxylated, producing HCO_3^-, which enters the bloodstream and helps buffer the acid load.

The overall reaction in blood when a strong acid such as H_2SO_4 is added is:

$$2NaHCO_3 + H_2SO_4 \rightarrow Na_2SO_4 + 2H_2CO_3$$

For each mol of H$^+$ added, 1 mol of NaHCO$_3$ is lost. The kidney, in effect, reverses the reaction:

$$Na_2SO_4 + 2H_2CO_3 \rightarrow 2NaHCO_3 + 2H^+ + SO_4^{2-}$$

and the H$^+$ and SO$_4^{2-}$ are excreted. Of course, H$_2$SO$_4$ is not excreted as such, the H$^+$ appears in the urine as titratable acidity and NH$_4^+$.

In metabolic acidosis, respiratory compensation tends to inhibit the renal response in the sense that the induced drop in Pco$_2$ hinders acid secretion, but it also decreases the filtered load of HCO$_3^-$ and so its net inhibitory effect is not great.

METABOLIC ALKALOSIS

In metabolic alkalosis, the plasma HCO$_3^-$ level and pH rise. The respiratory compensation is a decrease in ventilation produced by the decline in H$^+$ concentration, elevating the Pco$_2$. This brings the pH back toward normal while elevating the plasma HCO$_3^-$ level still further. The magnitude of this compensation is limited by the carotid and aortic chemoreceptor mechanisms, which drive the respiratory center if any appreciable fall occurs in the arterial Po$_2$. In metabolic alkalosis, more renal H$^+$ secretion is expended in reabsorbing the increased filtered load of HCO$_3^-$; and if the HCO$_3^-$ level in plasma exceeds 26–28 mEq/L, HCO$_3^-$ appears in the urine. The rise in Pco$_2$ inhibits the renal compensation by facilitating acid secretion, but its effect is relatively slight.

IMPLICATIONS OF URINARY pH CHANGES

Depending on the rates of the interrelated processes of acid secretion, NH$_4^+$ production, and HCO$_3^-$ excretion, the pH of the urine in humans varies from 4.5 to 8.0. Excretion of urine that is at a pH different from that of the body fluids has important implications for the body's electrolyte and acid–base economy. Acids are buffered in the plasma and cells, with the overall reaction being HA + NaHCO$_3$ → NaA + H$_2$CO$_3$. The H$_2$CO$_3$ forms CO$_2$ and H$_2$O, and the CO$_2$ is expired, while the NaA appears in the glomerular filtrate. To the extent that the Na$^+$ is replaced by H$^+$ in the urine, Na$^+$ is conserved in the body. Furthermore, for each H$^+$ excreted with phosphate or as NH$_4^+$, there is a net gain of one HCO$_3^-$ in the blood, replenishing the supply of this important buffer anion. Conversely, when base is added to the body fluids, the OH$^-$ are buffered, raising the plasma HCO$_3^-$. When the plasma level exceeds 28 mEq/L, the urine becomes alkaline and the extra HCO$_3^-$ is excreted in the urine. Because the rate of maximal H$^+$ secretion by the tubules varies directly with the arterial Pco$_2$, HCO$_3^-$ reabsorption is also affected by the Pco$_2$.

MULTIPLE-CHOICE QUESTIONS

For all questions, select the single best answer unless otherwise directed.

1. A 50-year-old man comes to see his primary care physician complaining of back pain and fatigue. His physician diagnoses him with multiple myeloma. He also has secondary light chain nephropathy that causes him to have chronic metabolic acidosis due to a reduction in proximal tubular reabsorption of bicarbonate. Assuming the man has no other renal disease and that his lung function is normal, which of the following responses is most likely seen in the patient?
   A. Increase in NH$_4^+$ in urine.
   B. Decreased synthesis of glutamine in the liver.
   C. Decrease in H$_2$PO$_4^-$ in the urine.
   D. Increase in arterial Pco$_2$.

2. A 25-year-old woman comes to the urgent care clinic complaining of burning on urination and needing to void frequently. She states she had a urinary tract infection (UTI) 2 years previously. On physical examination, the physician finds no suprapubic tenderness, and she is taking no medications. He orders a urinalysis to determine if a UTI is present. What is the lowest urinary pH that the physician would expect to see in the results of the urinalysis of this woman?
   A. 2.5
   B. 4.5
   C. 6.5
   D. 8.5

3. A 22-year-old woman arrives at the urgent care clinic complaining of lethargy and weakness. Upon examination, her blood pressure was 100/55 mm Hg, and her body mass index was 17 kg/m^2. She was taking no medications, had no significant medical history and denied any recent illness. She mentioned to the physician that she was afraid of gaining weight and had been taking diuretics to limit weight gain. The physician diagnosed diuretic abuse. What lab finding would be consistent with loop or thiazide diuretic abuse?
   A. Metabolic alkalosis.
   B. Hyperkalemia.
   C. Hypernatremia.
   D. Hyperchloridemia.

4. A 35-year-old woman had a sudden onset of hypertension. Previously her blood pressure was 110/70 mm Hg, but upon visiting the physician's office with complaints of headache, her blood pressure was increased to 150/90 mm Hg. Her laboratory workup came back showing elevated levels of aldosterone and reductions in renin. What serum electrolyte or acid–base abnormality would you expect to find?
   A. Metabolic acidosis
   B. Hyperchloridemia
   C. Hypokalemia
   D. Hyponatremia

5. An 18-year-old woman passed out at a party and was taken to the emergency room by her friends. They stated that she had been drinking alcoholic beverages heavily. Upon admission to the emergency room, she was only responsive to painful stimuli. Her laboratory tests showed that she had metabolic acidosis and had an increase in urinary ketone excretion. She was started on a glucose/saline drip intravenously and transferred to the intensive care unit. Over the next few days, urinary excretion of what compound would be expected to increase as her body restores normal acid–base balance?
   A. Urea
   B. Dibasic phosphate (HPO$_4^{2-}$)
   C. Protein
   D. Ammonium (NH$_4^+$)
   E. Monobasic phosphate (H$_2$PO$_4^-$)

6. A medical student is required to present a case study as part of his matriculation. While the student has excellent bedside manner and performs admirably in small groups, the idea of speaking to an audience is frightening to him. Just prior to the presentation, the student begins to hyperventilate, causing an immediate increase in blood pH. Why did the increase in blood pH occur?
   A. Hyperventilation activates neural mechanisms that remove acid from the blood.
   B. Hyperventilation makes Hb a stronger acid.
   C. Hyperventilation increases the P_{O_2} of the blood.
   D. Hyperventilation decreases the P_{CO_2} in the alveoli.
   E. The increased muscle work of increased breathing generates more CO_2.

7. A 56-year-old African American man has had consistent hemodialysis treatment for 2 years due to renal disease associated with sickle cell anemia. He has not had a sickle cell crisis in the past 3 years since he was compliant with his therapy; however, he recently missed his scheduled treatment. What would you expect his laboratory results to show when he came in for dialysis days later?
   A. Negative base excess
   B. A reduction in plasma creatinine concentration
   C. A reduction in blood urea nitrogen (BUN)
   D. No base excess

8. A new PhD student in a diabetes laboratory is working on a novel animal model for diabetes. The student is required to collect urine from control and diabetic mice and perform pH measurements on the urine. As expected, urine pH for the diabetic mice is quite low compared with controls. Prior to developing a project in the laboratory, the student presents the results at laboratory meeting and is required to discuss normal filtration in the kidney. How should she correctly describe the fate of filtered bicarbonate ions in an individual with normal renal function under normal acid–base conditions?
   A. All filtered bicarbonate is excreted into the urine.
   B. Excreted bicarbonate mostly derives from the proximal tubule.
   C. Filtered bicarbonate is mostly reabsorbed in the proximal tubule.
   D. Excreted bicarbonate mostly derives from secretion in the distal nephron.
   E. Very few bicarbonate ions are filtered.

9. A 1-month-old boy is brought to the pediatric emergency department with persistent vomiting. The mother said the baby started vomiting after feeding and the emesis is whitish-yellow with no blood. The baby is otherwise healthy and had an uncomplicated vaginal birth. The physician palpates an olive-sized mass in the epigastric area and suspects pyloric stenosis. What would the physician expect the baby's acid–base balance to be?
   A. Respiratory alkalosis.
   B. Metabolic acidosis.
   C. No acid–base disturbance
   D. Metabolic alkalosis

10. A 48-year-old woman visited her physician complaining of constant thirst and frequent urination. She was admitted to the hospital to determine the cause of her polydipsia and polyuria. She was not given fluids for 6 h, and no change in her urine osmolarity was measured during this time. When given an infusion of a nonpressor dose of an antidiuretic hormone (ADH) agonist, she experienced a rapid increase in urine osmolarity. What diagnosis is most likely to account for the woman's polydipsia and polyuria?
   A. Central diabetes insipidus
   B. Compulsive overconsumption of water
   C. Nephrogenic diabetes insipidus
   D. Type 1 diabetes mellitus
   E. Type 2 diabetes mellitus

ANSWERS

1. The correct answer is **A.** Metabolic acidosis stimulates renal ammoniagenesis and allows a net increase in H^+ excretion when NH_4^+ is lost in the urine. In chronic acidosis, the liver synthesis of glutamine is increased so that more NH_4^+ is produced, ruling out **B.** Increases rather than decreases in $H_2PO_4^-$ (**C**) and arterial P_{CO_2} (**D**) would be associated with chronic metabolic acidosis.

2. The correct answer is **B.** Typical urinary pH can vary widely between 4.5 and 8.0, but is usually around 6. Certain bacteria associated with UTIs (eg, *Proteus* sp.) produce urease, an enzyme that produces NH_4^+ from uric acid resulting in an increased urine pH upon infection. In contrast, *Escherichia coli*, a common cause of UTI, has no effect on urine pH.

3. The correct answer is **A.** Loop and thiazide diuretics can cause metabolic alkalosis due to their ability to increase Na^+ delivery to the collecting ducts and the resulting increase cellular uptake of Na^+ from the lumen by apical epithelial Na^+ channels (ENaCs). Increased intracellular Na^+ causes the basolateral Na/K exchanger to more actively exchange Na^+ for K^+, which is then passively secreted into the lumen through apical channels, resulting in K^+ loss. The increased delivery of K^+ to the collecting ducts facilitates the exchange of K^+ for H^+ by the H/K exchanger on the intercalated alpha cells, resulting in loss of H^+ in urine and metabolic alkalosis. Hyperkalemia (**B**) does not occur because K^+ is typically lost in the urine with diuretics. Hypernatremia (**C**) does not occur since Na^+ is reabsorbed in the distal nephron. Hyperchloridemia (**D**) is associated with metabolic acidosis and can also be ruled out.

4. The correct answer is **C.** Hypertension caused by Na^+ retention is a direct result of primary hyperaldosteronism. If she had hyponatremia (**D**), she would not be hypertensive. Aldosterone causes K^+ loss in the urine, resulting in the observed hypokalemia and drives renal H^+ secretion, causing metabolic alkalosis and eliminating **A**.

5. The correct answer is **D.** Renal ammoniagenesis is the major response to an increase in net acid excretion (as evidenced in this case by ketone excretion), and at the same time causes new bicarbonate to be produced to combat metabolic acidosis. Because there is no evidence of excessive dietary protein or of damage at the glomerular barrier, urea (**A**) and protein (**C**) increases can be ruled out. Phosphates (**B** and **E**) cannot be increased by filtration, and thus they would not be expected to change much and can be ruled out as answers.

6. The correct answer is **D.** Hyperventilation (ie, increased ventilation without complementary increase in perfusion) leads to a reduction in alveolar P_{CO_2} and subsequent arterial P_{CO_2}. Because of the action of carbonic anhydrase, the loss of blood

Pco$_2$ increases blood pH. Rebreathing expired air (eg, breathing into a paper bag) is a way of limiting CO$_2$ loss and changes in blood pH. Hyperventilation does not work through neural control of blood acids (**A**) and has no effect on the buffering capacity of Hb (**B**). The gradient for O$_2$ exchange between the alveolar space and blood remains very high and does not affect O$_2$ exchange, eliminating **C**. While increased muscle work of the diaphragm can consume more O$_2$ this will not appreciably change blood CO$_2$ or pH, eliminating **E**.

7. The correct answer is **A**. Because the patient has renal insufficiency, he will be in metabolic acidosis. Base excess is negative in metabolic acidosis, ruling out **D** and is positive in metabolic alkalosis. Since the man has renal insufficiency, both plasma creatinine (**B**) and BUN (**C**) would be elevated and not reduced.

8. The correct answer is **C**. Greater than 90% of filtered bicarbonate is reabsorbed by the proximal tubule, preventing loss of bicarbonate to the urine. Bicarbonate reabsorption is dependent on HCO$_3^-$ concentration. When the plasma HCO$_3^-$ concentration is low, all the filtered HCO$_3^-$ is reabsorbed; but when the plasma HCO$_3^-$ concentration is high, HCO$_3^-$ appears in the urine and the urine becomes alkaline.

9. The correct answer is **D**. Persistent emesis results in loss of stomach acids and net loss of H$^+$, resulting in increased pH and metabolic alkalosis, ruling out both **B** and **C**. Respiratory alkalosis refers to increases of blood pH in response to ventilation/perfusion mismatch; the act of emesis is not respiratory in nature and **A** can be ruled.

10. The correct answer is **A**. Restoration of urine concentrating ability with exogenous ADH infusion is consistent with a failure of endogenous ADH secretion and thus the diagnosis of central diabetes insipidus. The lack of response to ADH in the kidney is the hallmark of nephrogenic diabetes insipidus; thus addition of ADH would not be expected to change urine osmolarity had that been her diagnosis (rules out **C**). Lack of water consumption for 6 h should increase urine osmolarity in cases of compulsive water drinking (rules out **B**) or in individuals with diabetes mellitus (**D** and **E**).

Index

Page references accompanied by *b* signify a box; *f* a figure, photo, or illustration; *t* a table.